Teaching Atlas
of Thoracic Radiology

Teaching Atlas of Thoracic Radiology

Sebastian Lange, M.D.
Professor and Chairman
Department of Radiology
Knappschafts-Krankenhaus
Recklinghausen, Germany

Paul Stark, M.D.
Associate Professor
Department of Radiology
Brigham and Women's Hospital
Harvard University Medical School
Boston, Massachusetts, USA;
Professor of Radiology
Loma Linda University
School of Medicine
Loma Linda, California, USA

1042 illustrations

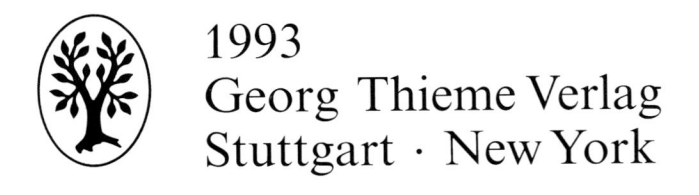

1993
Georg Thieme Verlag
Stuttgart · New York

Thieme Medical Publishers, Inc.
New York

Sebastian Lange, M.D.
Professor and Chairman,
Dept. of Radiology
Knappschafts-Krankenhaus
Dorstener Straße 151
4350 Recklinghausen
Germany

Paul Stark, M.D.
Associate Professor, Dept. of Radiology
Brigham and Women's Hospital
Harvard University School of Medicine
Boston, MA 02115
USA

Cover design: Renate Stockinger

Library of Congress Cataloging-in-Publication Data
Lange, Sebastian.
[Lehratlanten der radiologischen Diagnostik.
Lunge und Mediastinum. English]
Teaching atlas of thoracic radiology / Sebastian Lange, Paul Stark.
p. cm.
Includes bibliographical references and index.
1. Chest–Radiography–Atlases. I. Stark, Paul, 1944 – II. Title.
[DNLM: 1. Thoracic Radiography-atlases. WF 17 L274L]
RC 941. L3613 1993
617.5'407572 – dc 20
DNLM/DLC
for Library of Congress   92–49323 – CIP

This book is an authorized and revised translation of the German edition published and copyrighted 1991 by Georg Thieme Verlag, Stuttgart, Germany. Title of the German edition: Lehratlanten der radiologischen Diagnostik: Lunge und Mediastinum.

Some of the product names, patents and registered designs referred to in this book are in fact registered trademarks or proprietary names even though specific reference to this fact is not always made in the text. Therefore, the appearance of a name without designation as proprietary is not to be construed as a representation by the publisher that it is in the public domain.

This book, including all parts thereof, is legally protected by copyright. Any use, exploitation or commercialization outside the narrow limits set by copyright legislation, without the publisher's consent, is illegal and liable to prosecution. This applies in particular to photostat reproduction, copying, mimeographing or duplication of any kind, translating, preparation of microfilms, and electronic data processing and storage.

© 1993 Georg Thieme Verlag, Rüdigerstraße 14, 7000 Stuttgart 30, Germany
Thieme Medical Publishers, Inc., 381 Park Avenue South, New York, NY 10016

Typesetting by Fotosatz-Service Köhler, D-8700 Würzburg, typeset on Mono/Lasercomp 3000

Printed in Germany by K. Grammlich, D-7401 Pliezhausen

ISBN 3-13-791701-8   (GTV, Stuttgart)
ISBN 0-86577-467-6   (TMP, New York)   1 2 3 4 5 6

Important Note:

Medicine is an ever-changing science undergoing continual development. Research and clinical experience are continually expanding our knowledge, in particular our knowledge of proper treatment and drug therapy. Insofar as this book mentions any dosage or application, readers may rest assured that the authors, editors and publishers have made every effort to ensure that such references are in accordance with the state of knowledge at the time of production of the book.

Nevertheless this does not involve, imply, or express any guarantee or responsibility on the part of the publishers in respect of any dosage instructions and forms of application stated in the book. Every user is requested to examine carefully the manufacturers' leaflets accompanying each drug and to check, if necessary in consultation with a physician or specialist, whether the dosage schedules mentioned therein or the contraindications stated by the manufacturers differ from the statements made in the present book. Such examination is particularly important with drugs that are either rarely used or have been newly released on the market. Every dosage schedule or every form of application used is entirely at the user's own risk and responsibility. The authors and publishers request every user to report to the publishers any discrepancies or inaccuracies noticed.

Preface

The chest radiograph plays a crucial role in the diagnosis of intrathoracic disease. It is the backbone of thoracic radiology and is supplemented by cross-sectional imaging techniques. Radiologic findings have to be integrated with the clinical, laboratory, and histologic findings.

A teaching atlas can successfully demonstrate how imaging modalities combined with history and clinical picture can facilitate the quest for a correct diagnosis and expedite the subsequent therapy. This book contains twelve chapters and illustrates the most important normal variants and disease entities that affect the lungs and the mediastinum. The examples are related to the daily practice of a large hospital. Common diseases are described in more detail, although infrequent entities are also illustrated. Follow-up examinations which illustrate the longitudinal course of diseases are also included.

The reader is encouraged to analyze the individual illustrations and to try to reach a conclusion before reading the legends. This interactive approach to the atlas will improve learning and facilitate the retention of information.

We hope that this book will prove to be interesting, educational, useful, and that it will ultimately benefit the patients.

November, 1992 *Sebastian Lange*
Paul Stark

Contents

1. Normal Anatomy and Normal Variants ... 1

Normal Chest Radiographs	2	Pleura	10
Rib Cage Configurations	4	Interlobar Fissures	14
Chest Wall	6	Pulmonary Vessels	17
Soft Tissues	6	Bronchi	21
Bones	8	Mediastinum	23

2. Infections ... 27

Pneumonia	28	Granulomatous Form-Tuberculomas	56
Lobar Pneumonia	28	Cavitary Tuberculosis	58
Bronchopneumonia	36	Fibrous, Postprimary Tuberculosis	60
Interstitial Pneumonias	40	Intrapulmonary Calcifications	62
Chickenpox Pneumonia	42	Sarcoidosis	64
Chronic organizing Pneumonia	44	Fungal Diseases	71
Lung Abscess and Necrotizing Pneumonia	45	Echinococcal Disease	81
Tuberculosis	49	Collagen Vascular Diseases	83
Primary Tuberculous Complex	49	Wegener Granulomatosis	85
Tuberculous Pleurisy	49	Radiation Pneumonitis	86
Miliary Tuberculosis	51	Histiocytosis of Langerhans	89
Tuberculous Pneumonia	54		

3. Chronic Obstructive Lung Diseases ... 91

Emphysema	92	Bronchiectases	104
Emphysematous Bullae	94	Chronic Bronchitis	108
Vanishing Lung	100	Bronchiolitis Obliterans	108
Pericicatriceal Emphysema	102	Cystic Fibrosis	108
Swyer-James-Syndrome	103		

4. Pneumoconiosis ... 111

Types of Pneumoconiosis	112	Silicosis	120
Round Opacities	114	Asbestosis	122
Small, Irregular Opacities	116		
Large Opacities (Conglomerate Shadow, Progressive Massive Fibrosis)	118		

5. Neoplasms … 125

Bronchogenic Carcinoma … 126
   Peripheral Lung Cancer … 126
   Bronchoalveolar Cell Carcinoma … 131
   Atelectasis and Lung Cancer … 132
   Central Bronchogenic Carcinoma,
   Hilar Mass … 141
   Superior Sulcus Tumor;
   Pancoast Syndrome … 145
   Superior Vena Cava Obstruction:
   Esophageal Invasion … 147
Malignant Lymphoma … 149
Metastatic Disease … 156
   Nodular Metastasis … 156
   Lymphangitic Carcinomatosis … 160
Unusual Intrathoracic Tumors
and Related Conditions … 163

6. Vascular Disease … 167

Pulmonary Vascular Congestion … 168
   Pulmonary Edema … 173
   Chronic Pulmonary Venous Hypertension
   – Mitral Stenosis … 177
Pulmonary Embolism … 180
Discoid Atelectasis … 186

7. Trauma … 187

Traumatic Pneumothorax … 188
Pneumomediastinum … 191
Adult Respiratory Distress Syndrome (ARDS) … 192
Pulmonary Contusion, Traumatic Pneumatocele … 196
Lines, Tubes and Their Complications … 198
Postoperative Chest … 200

8. Congenital Malformations … 205

Bronchogenic Cysts … 206
Cystic-Adenomatoid Malformation … 208
Pulmonary Sequestration … 210
Vascular Malformations of the Lung … 214

9. Pleural Diseases … 217

Pleural Effusions … 218
   Subpulmonic Effusions, Intrafissural
   Collections of Fluid, Loculated Effusions … 220
Rounded Atelectasis … 225
Spontaneous Pneumothorax … 226
Pleural Thickening … 229
Plombage, Oleothorax … 231
Malignant Pleural Mesothelioma … 233

10. Mediastinum … 237

Goiters … 238
Thymic Hyperplasia and Thymoma … 240
Mediastinal Cysts and Lymphangiomas … 242
Thoracic Aorta … 246
Cardiac Diseases … 252
   Aortic Valvular Disease, Ventricular
   Aneurysms … 252
Mitral Valve Disease … 254
Septal Defects … 256
Tetralogy of Fallot, Patent Ductus Arteriosus,
Coarctation of the Aorta … 258
Pericardial Disease … 263

11. Diaphragm ... 267

Diaphragm Anomalies ... 268

12. Diseases of the Chest Wall ... 273

Thoracic Skeleton ... 274   Chest Wall Soft-Tissue Abnormalities ... 279

References ... 281

Index ... 285

1. Normal Anatomy and Normal Variants

1. Normal Anatomy and Normal Variants

Normal Chest Radiographs

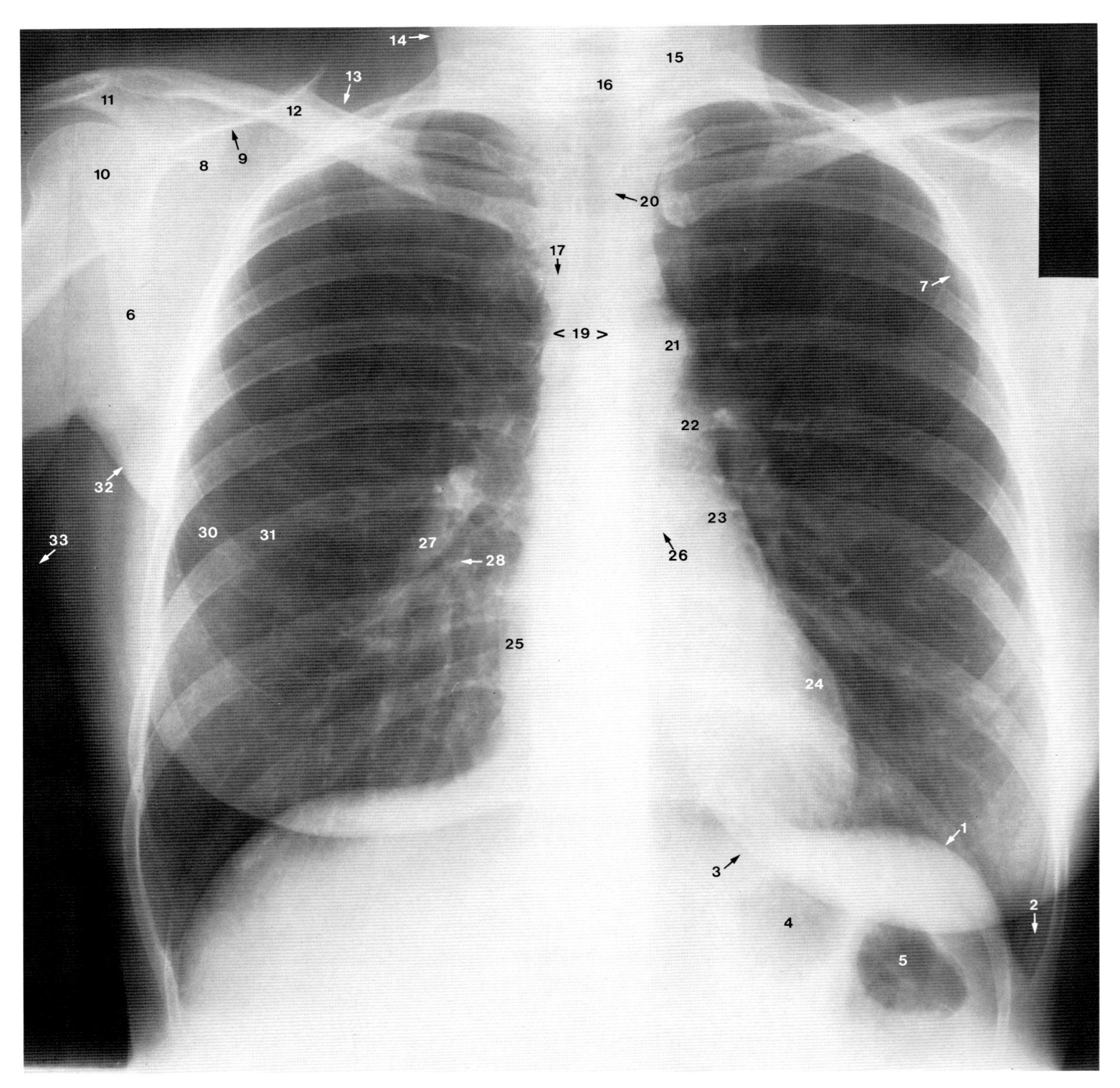

Fig. 1.1 **Frontal chest radiograph.**
Diaphragm (1), costophrenic sulcus (2), breast shadow (3), stomach bubble (4), colonic gas in splenic flexure (5), scapula, lateral border (6), scapula, medial border (7), coracoid process (8), spine of scapula (9), humeral head (10), acromioclavicular joint (11), clavicular shaft (12), companion shadow of clavicle (13), sternocleidomastoid muscle (14), transverse process, cervical spine (15), spinous process, cervical spine (16), pedicle (17), head of rib (18), trachea (19), posterior-superior junction line (20), aortic arch (21), main pulmonary artery segment (22), left atrial appendage (23), left ventricular border (24), right atrial border (25), descending thoracic aorta (26), interlobar pulmonary artery (27), bronchus intermedius (28), anterior segmental bronchus of left upper lobe seen on end (29), anterior rib (30), posterior rib (31), anterior axillary fold (32), posterior axillary fold (33).

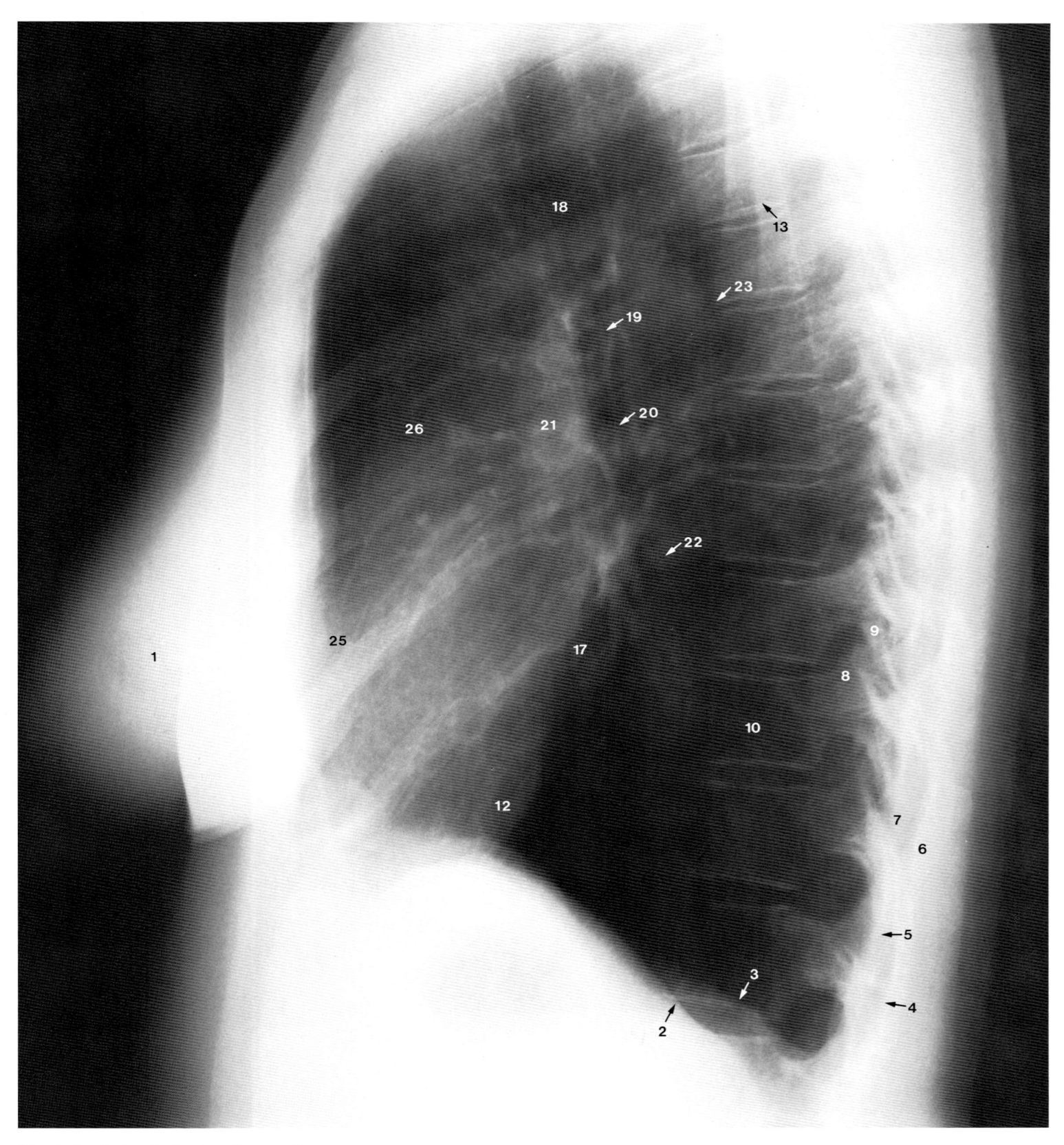

Fig. 1.2 **Lateral chest radiograph.**
Breast shadow (1), left hemidiaphragm, obscured anteriorly by cardiac silhouette (2), right hemidiaphragm, uninterrupted contour to sternum (3), left posterior costophrenic sulcus (4), right posterior costophrenic sulcus (5), right-sided ribs (6), left-sided ribs (7), superior facet (8), inferior facet (9), vertebral body (10), scapula, lateral border (13), left ventricle (12), left atrium (17), trachea (18), right upper lobe bronchus (19), left main bronchus (20), right pulmonary artery and right pulmonary veins (21), left lower lobe pulmonary arteries (22), aortic arch (23), right ventricle (25), ascending aorta (26).

References: 22, 42, 113, 149.

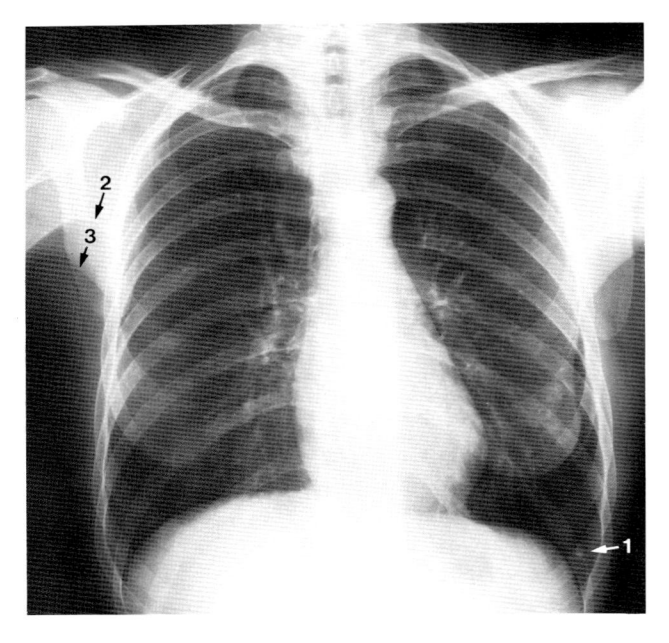

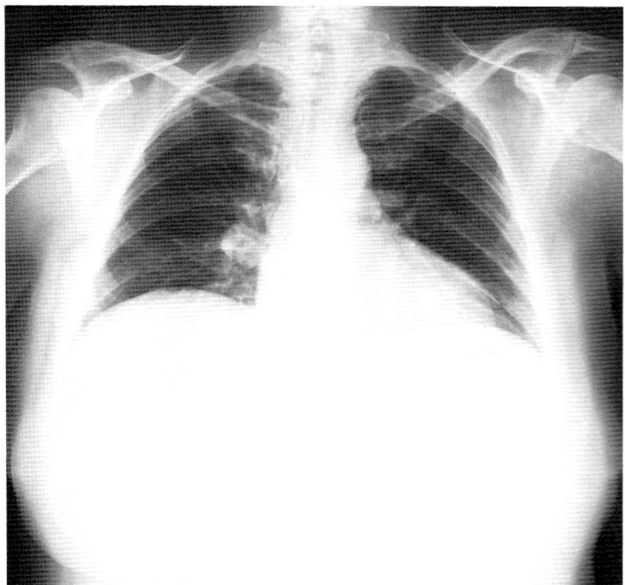

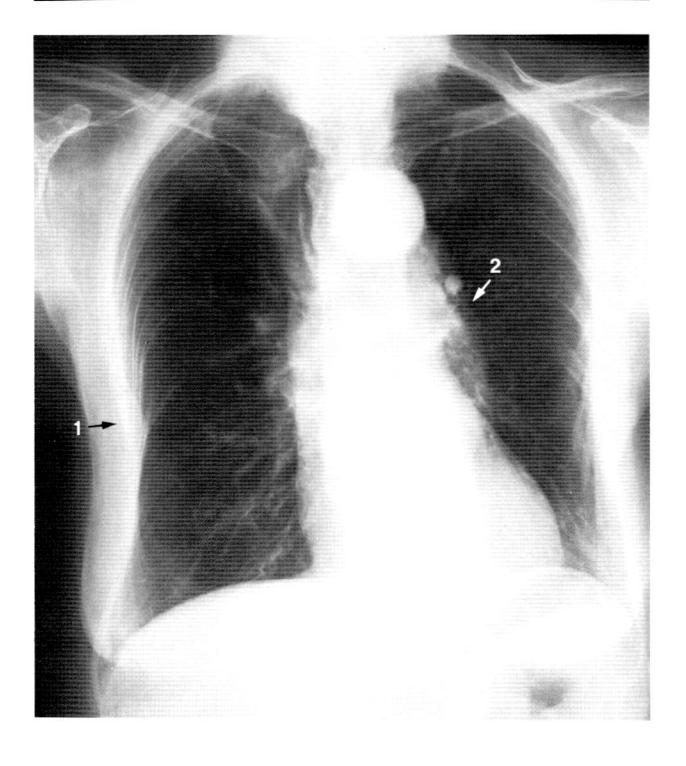

Rib Cage Configurations

Fig. 1.3 **Athletic individual.**
Ratio of vertical and horizontal maximal dimensions approaches 1. Calcified granuloma (1), axilla (2), anterior axillary fold (3), clavicular companion shadow and contour of sternocleidomastoid muscle (4).

Fig. 1.4 **Overweight individual.**
Ratio of vertical and horizontal maximal dimensions exceeds 1. High diaphragm, horizontal cardiac silhouette.

Fig. 1.5 **Bell-shaped chest in 89-year-old osteoporotic patient.**
Waist at the transition between middle and lower third of rib cage (1), tortuous aorta (2).

Fig. 1.6 **Scoliosis of thoracic spine.**
Asymmetric narrowing of left-sided intercostal spaces, when compared with right side.

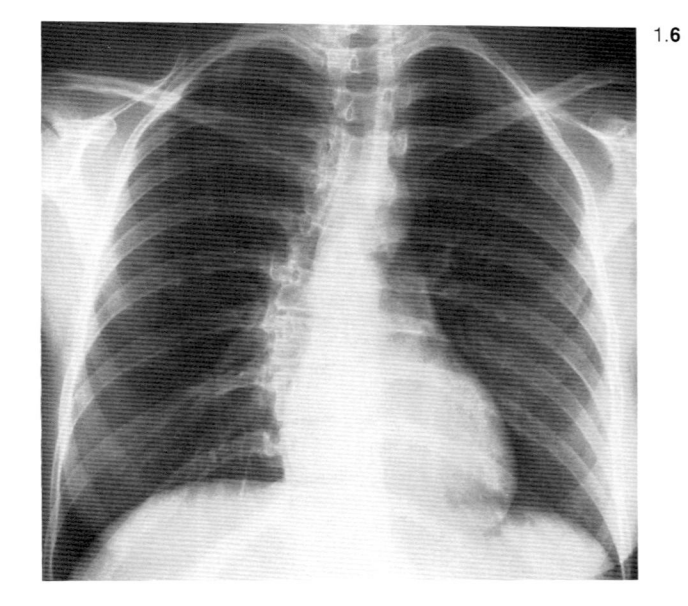

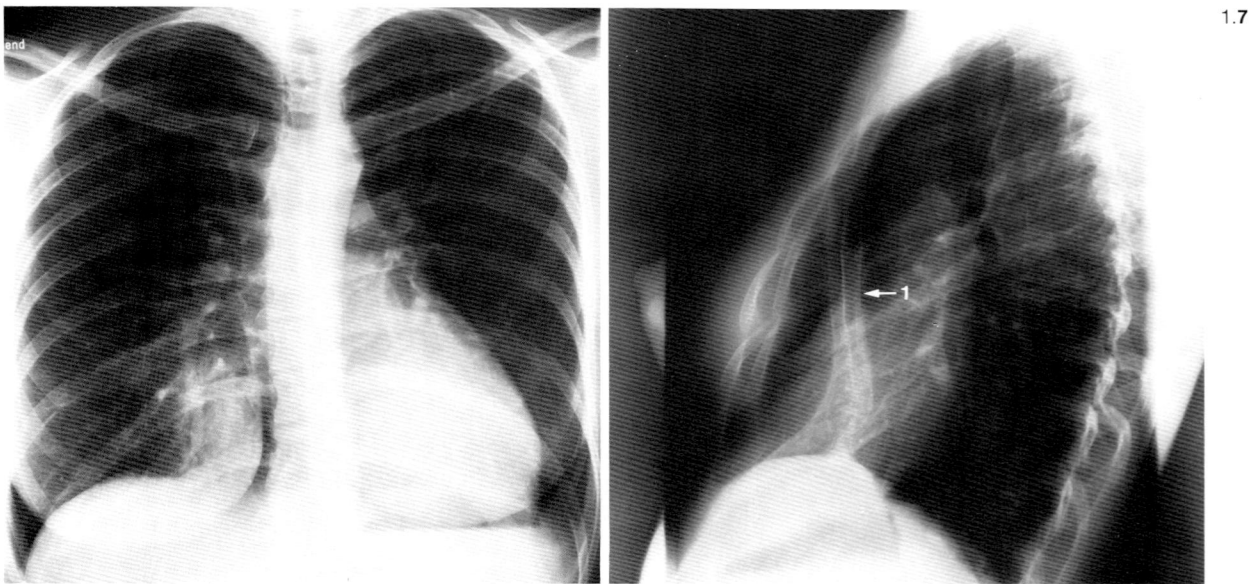

Fig. 1.7 **Pectus excavatum deformity.**
Sternal body (1) compresses and displaces the heart to the left. Prominent main pulmonary artery segment results from leftward rotation of cardiac silhouette.

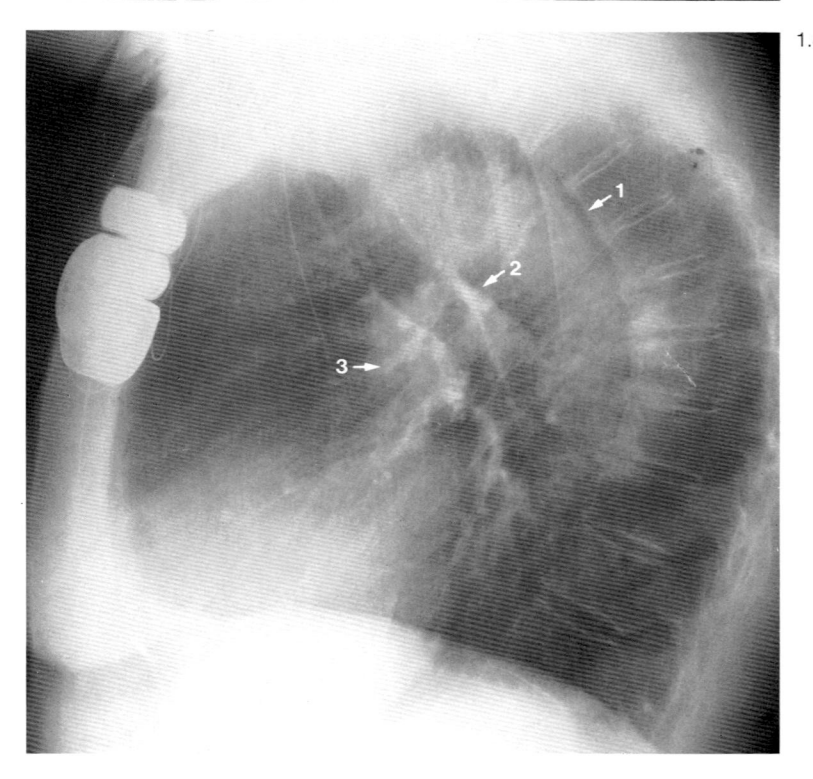

Fig. 1.8 **Hyperkyphosis.**
Increased sagittal diameter of the chest. Mild spondylosis deformans of thoracic spine. Pacemaker lead. Dilated aorta (1), enlarged left (2) and right (3) pulmonary arteries.

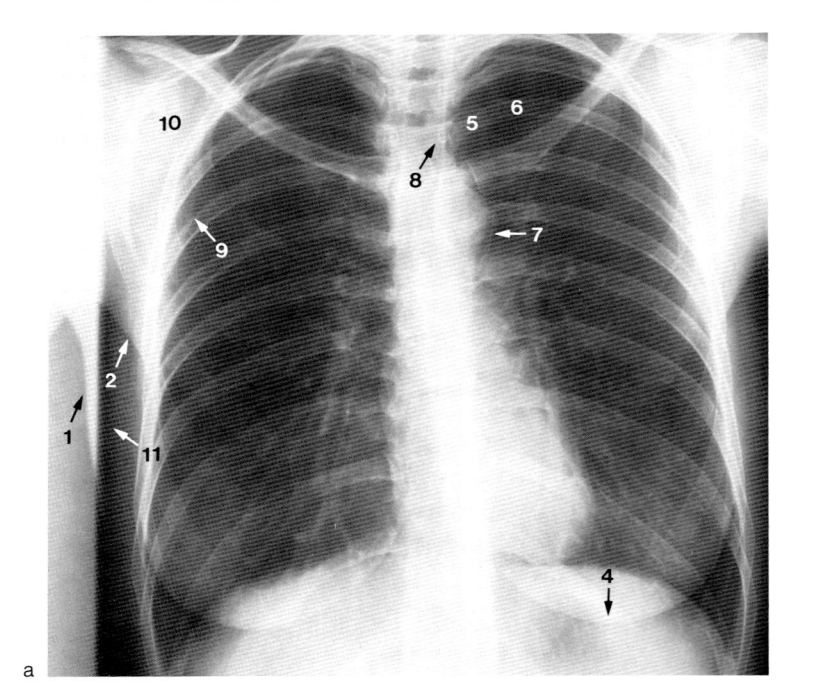

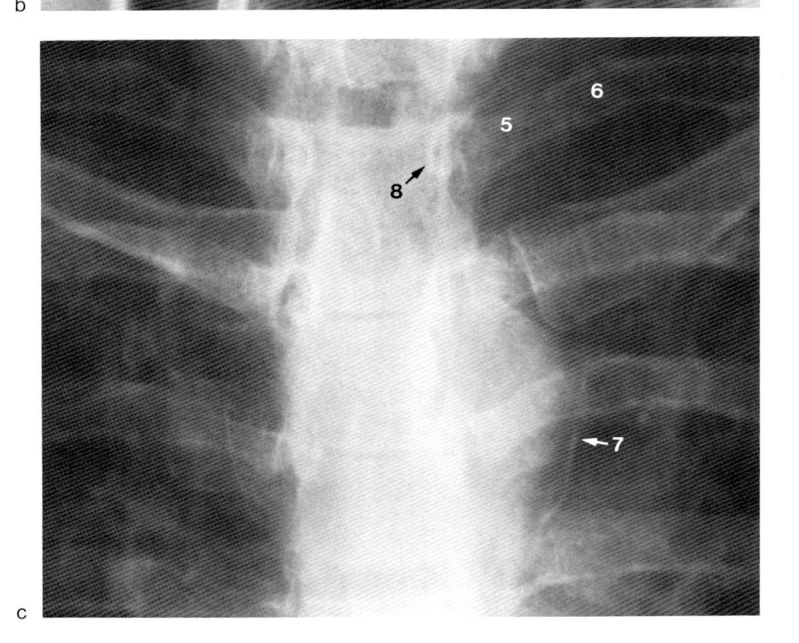

Chest Wall

Soft Tissues

Fig. 1.**9a–c** Posterior axillary fold (1), anterior axillary fold (2), axilla (3), breast shadow (4), transverse process (5), head of rib (6), manubrium sterni (7), pedicle (8), medial border of scapula (9), coracoid process (10), negative Mach-band outlines chest wall as a dark stripe. It results form lateral inhibition of retinal receptors at site of abrupt transition from dark to white surfaces.

Fig. 1.10 Lateral contour, sternocleidomastoid muscle (1), crossing between first anterior rib and third posterior rib (2), clavicle, companion shadow (3).

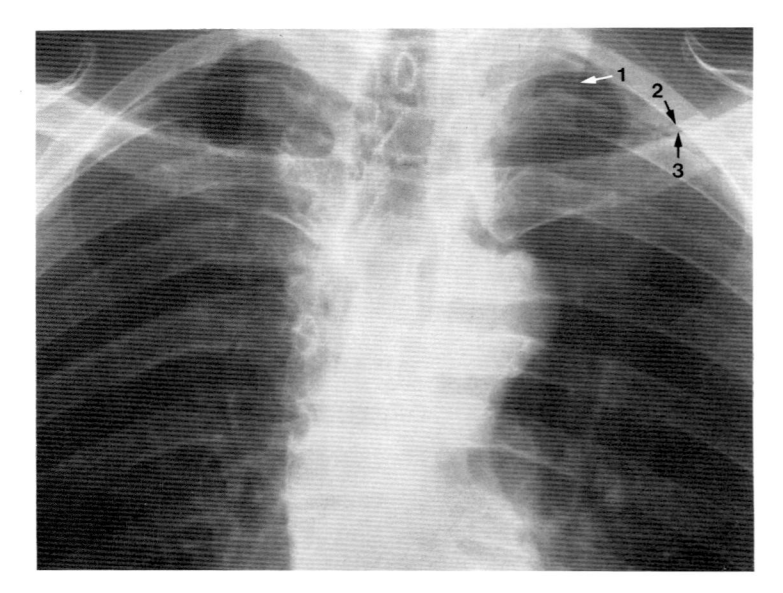

Fig. 1.11 Skinfold on supine radiograph (1).

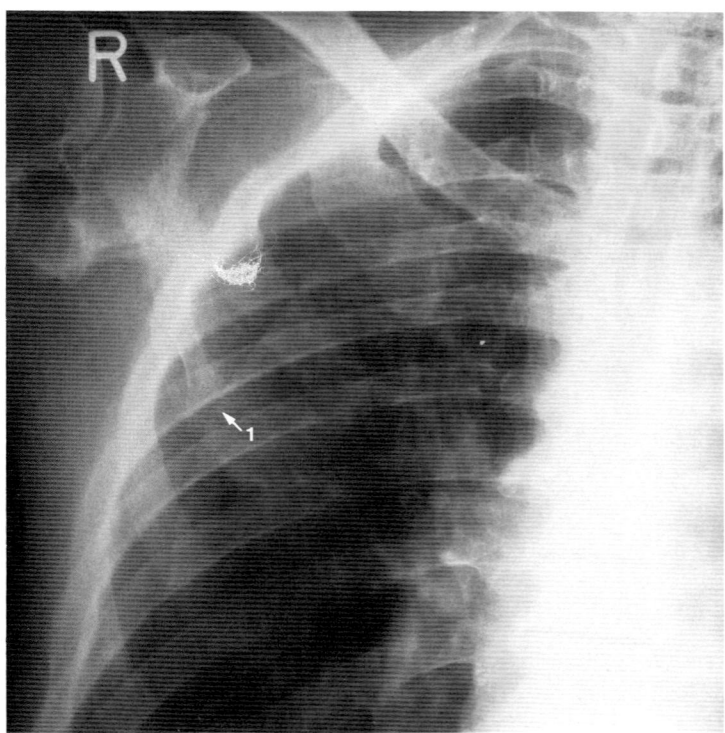

Fig. 1.12 Soft tissues, left arm (1), humeral head (2), humeral shaft (3), soft tissues, right arm (4), aortic arch (5), left pulmonary artery in epibronchial position (6), lateral border of scapula (7).

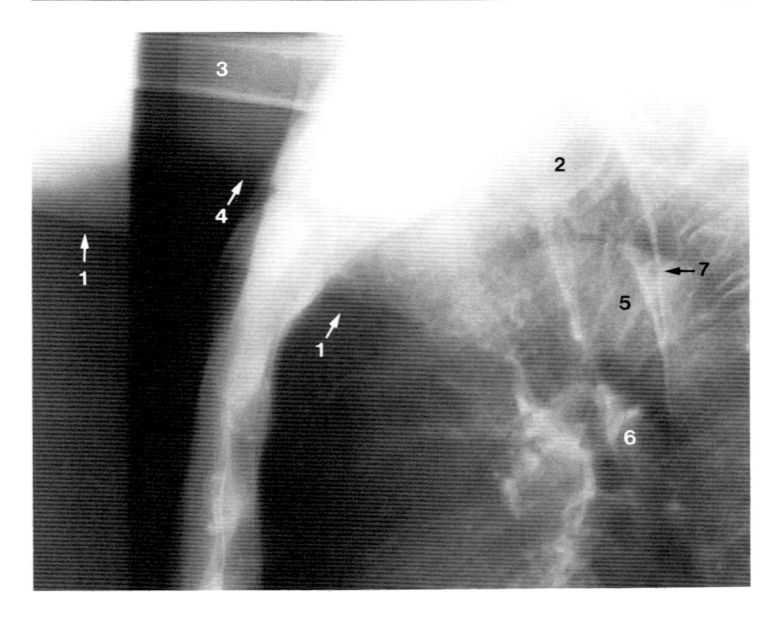

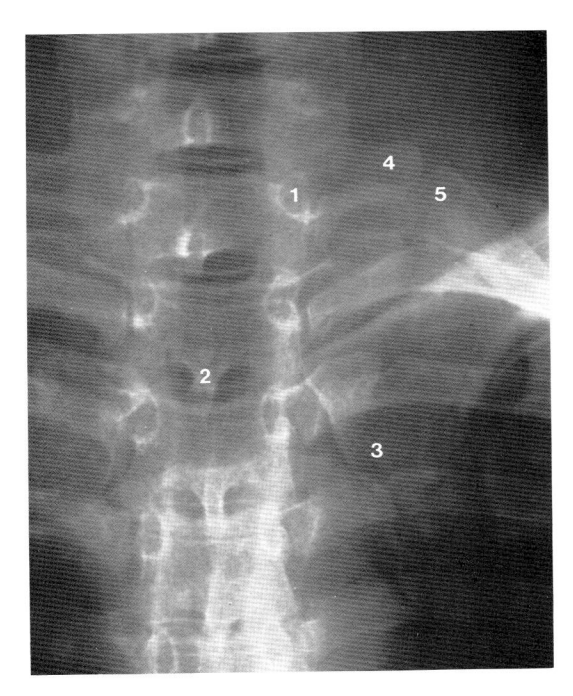

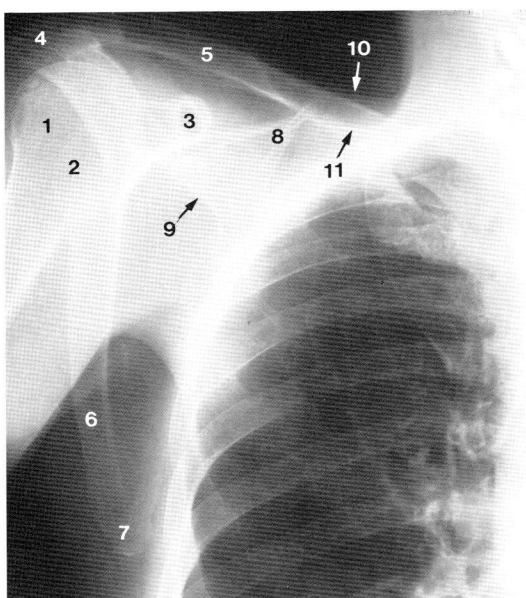

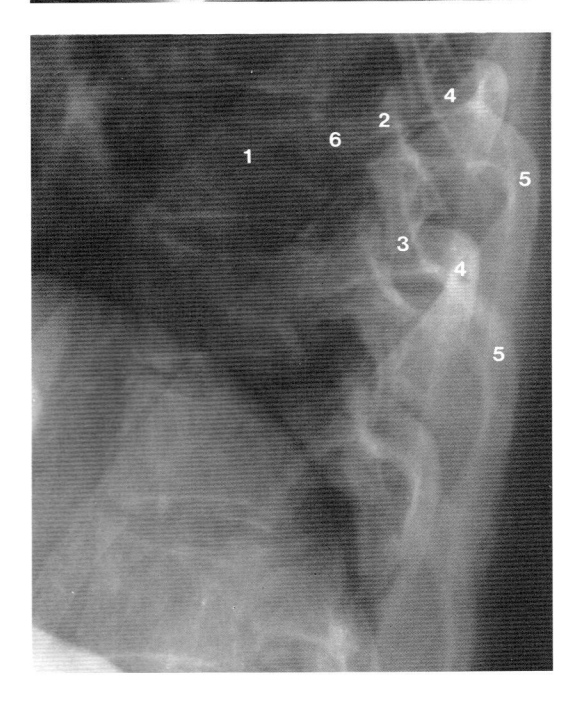

Bones

Fig. 1.13 Upper thoracic supine.
Pedicle (1), spinous process (2), clavicle and sternoclavicular joint (3), transverse process (4), costotransversal articulation with costal head (5). Vertebral end-plate seen as double contour due to inclination of central X-ray beam.

Fig. 1.14 Shoulder region.
Humeral head (1), glenoid fossa (2), coracoid process (3), acromion (4), clavicle (5), lateral border of scapula (6), inferior angle of scapula (7), superior angle of scapula (8), spine of scapula (9), companion shadow, clavicle (10), supraclavicular fossa seen in tangent (11).

Fig. 1.15 Lower thoracic spine.
Vertebral body (1), superior facet (2), inferior facet (3), rib (4), contralateral rib (5), pedicle (6).

Chest Wall

Fig. 1.**16a, b** Manubrium sterni (1), body of sternum (2), angle of Louis (between 1 and 2), breast soft tissue (3), nipple shadow (4), right hemidiaphragm seen completely (5), left hemidiaphragm subtending stomach bubble (6), left posterior costophrenic sulcus (8), right posterior costophrenic sulcus (9), calcified nucleus pulposus (10).

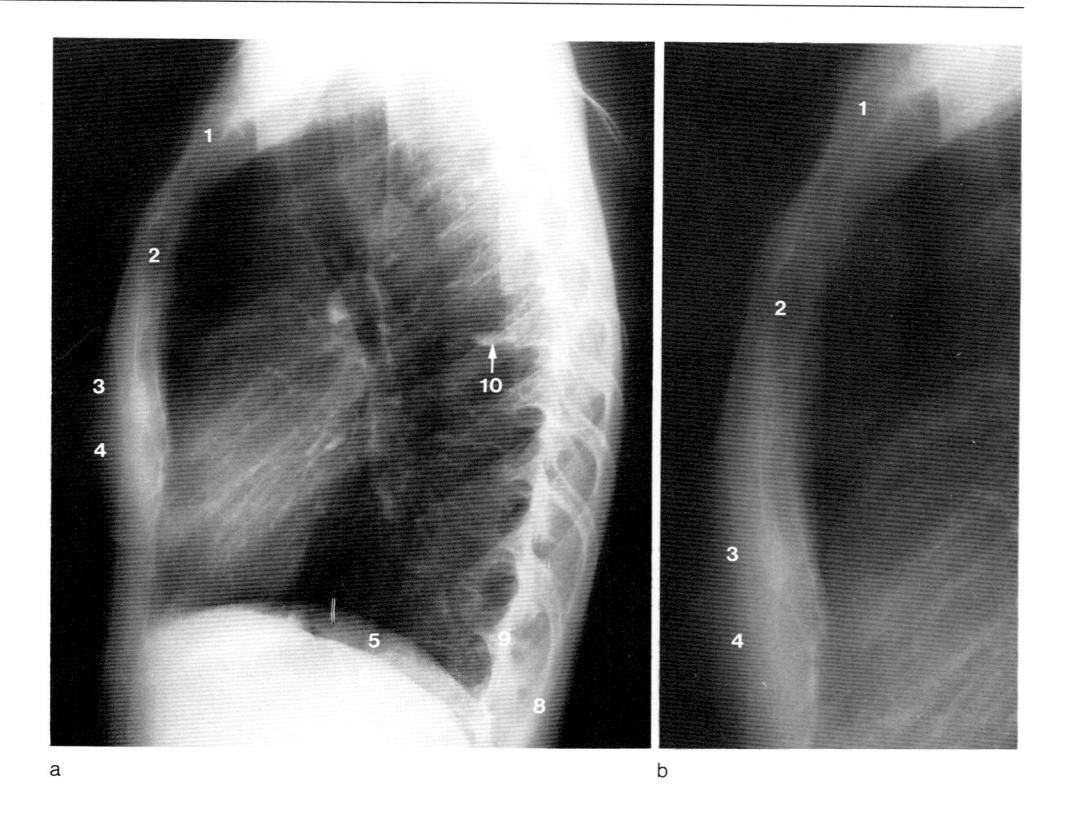

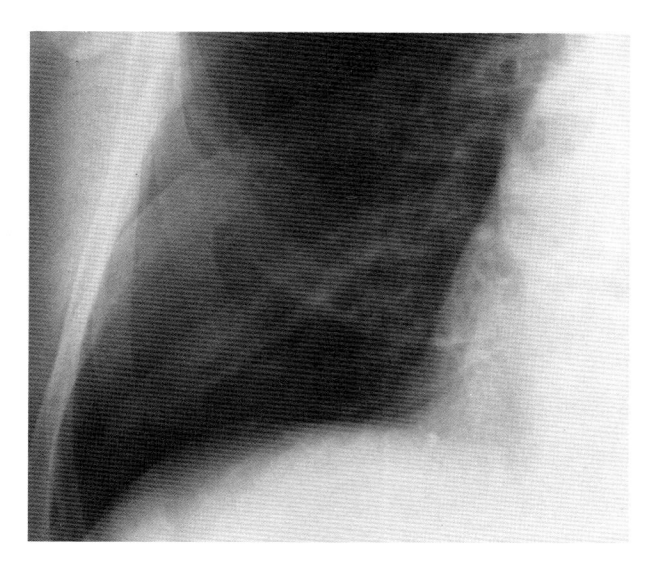

Fig. 1.**17** Bifid rib.

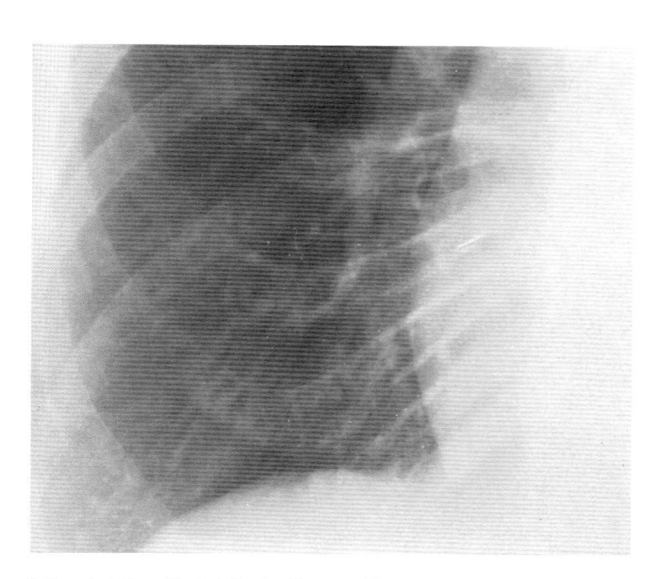

Fig. 1.**18** Calcified rib cartilages.

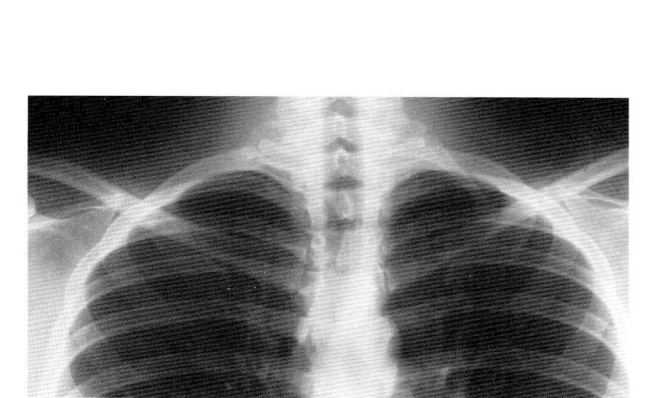

Fig. 1.**19a** Left-sided cervical rib.

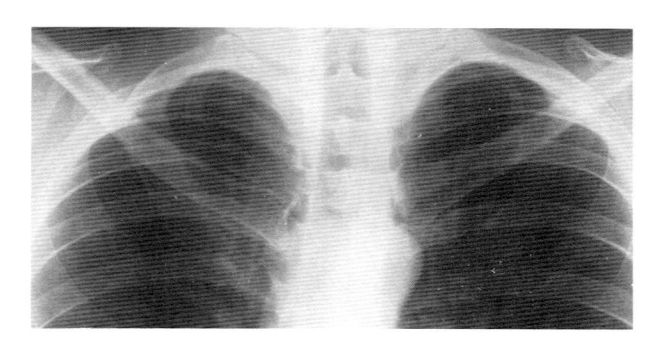

Fig. 1.**19b** Bilateral cervical ribs.

1. Normal Anatomy and Normal Variants

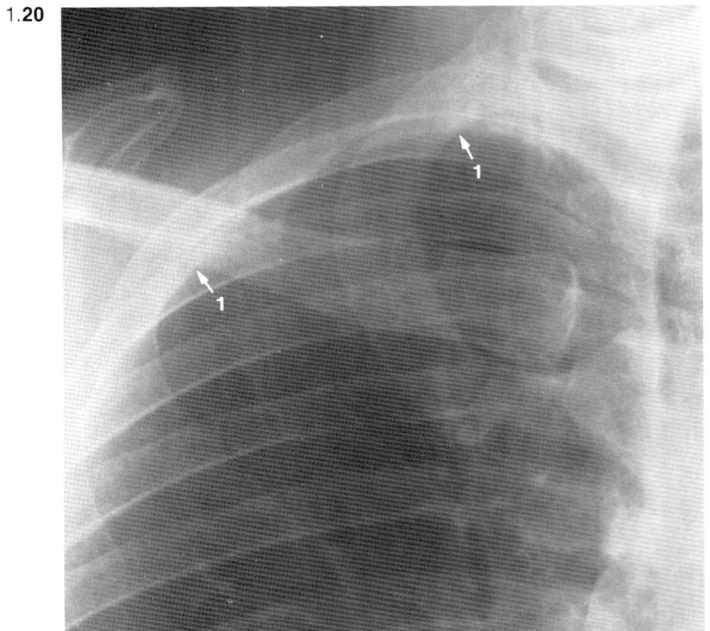

Pleura

The pleural space is lined by visceral and parietal pleura which glide over each other during respiratory motion. The visceral pleura has a thickness of less than 500 µm and is barely visible, particularly when a pneumothorax is present. Otherwise, the interface between the pleura and the adjacent organs is visible as a Mach band (retinal edge enhancement).

◁ Fig. 1.**20** Apical pleura (1). Note overlapping ribs 1 through 3.

◁ Fig. 1.**21** **Anterior inferior pleural reflection.**
Stomach bubble (1), anterior, retrosternal, and costal pleural margin, forming three interfaces (2), cardiac incisura (3), left posterior costophrenic sulcus (4), right posterior costophrenic sulcus (5).

Fig. 1.**22 a–c** **Anterior and posterior pleura.**
Pleural contour paralleling the chest wall. Anterior margin of lung in retrosternal (1) and retrocostal, parasternal location (2) (note three interfaces). Anterior left lung abuts on pericardial fat pad (3). It outlines the cardiac incisura. Left posterior costophrenic sulcus (4), right posterior costophrenic sulcus (5). Right posterior pleural edge (6). Left posterior pleura (7). Note white edge-enhancing Mach band.
▽

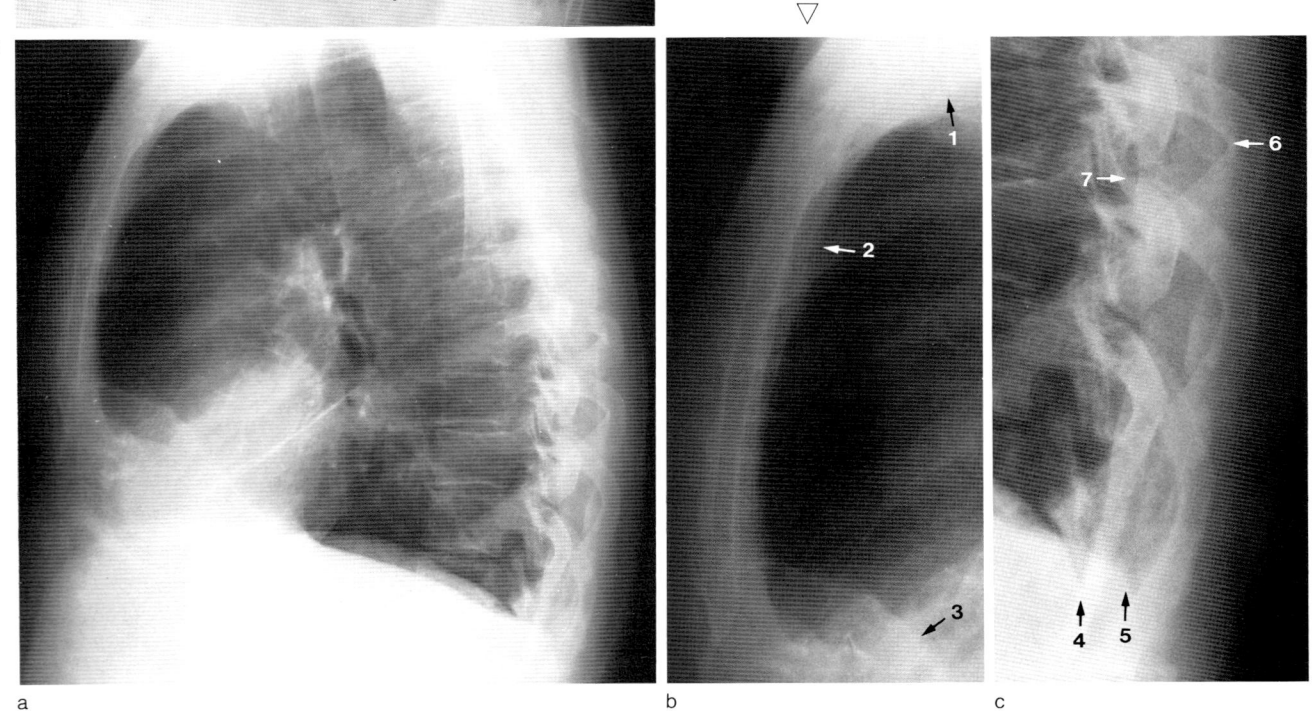

Fig. 1.**23 a, b** **Pericardial fat pad.**
Lung separates cardiac silhouette from anterior chest wall on superior CT sections and is replaced by pericardial fat on lower sections.

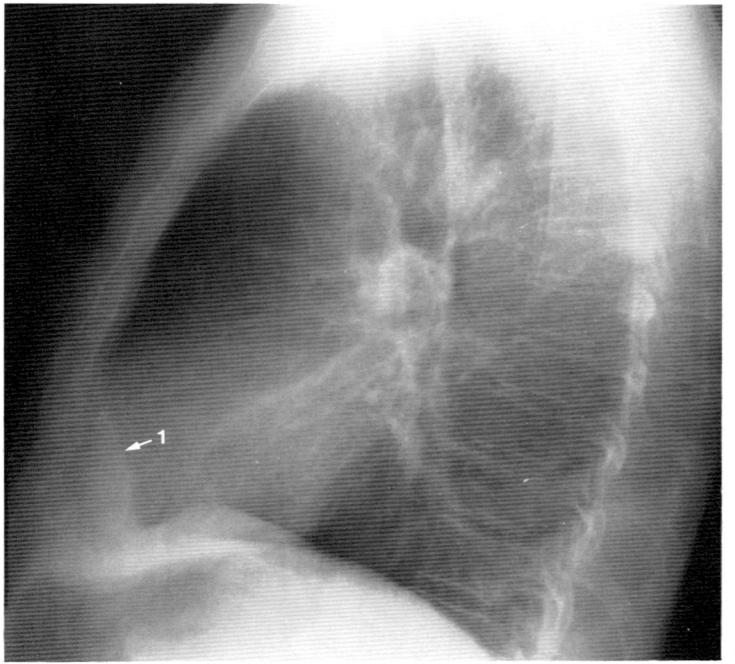

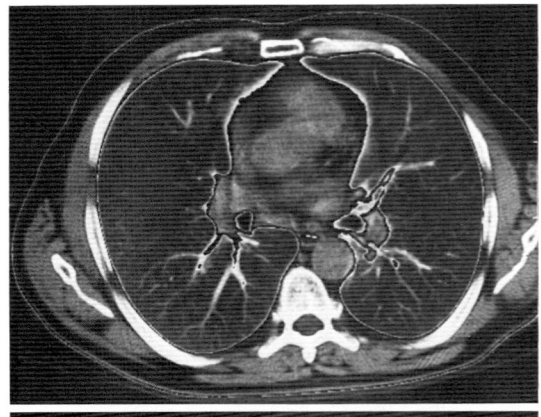

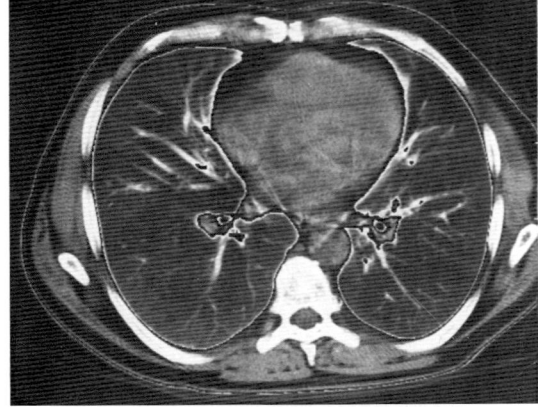

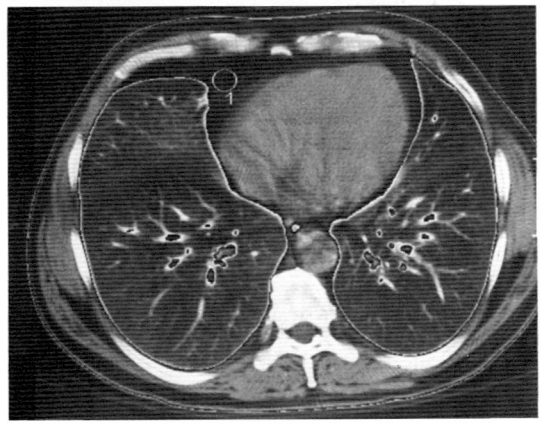

1. Normal Anatomy and Normal Variants

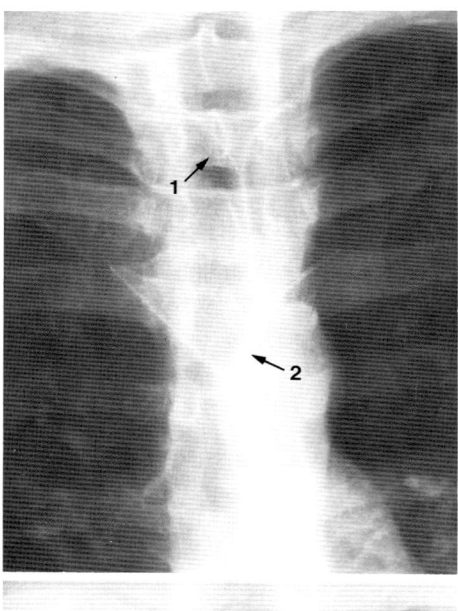

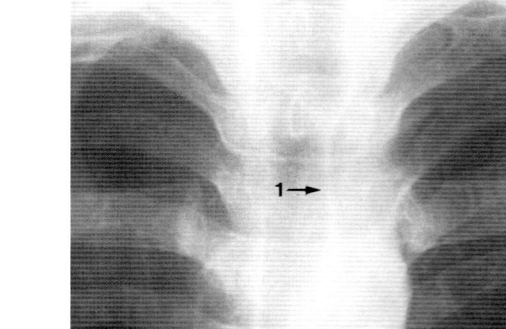

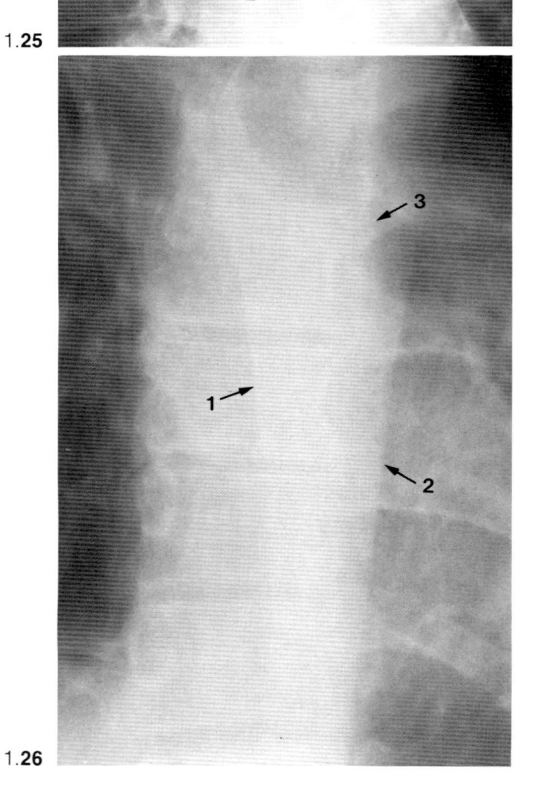

Fig. 1.24 Posterior superior junction line (1). Anterior junction line (2).

Fig. 1.25 Posterior superior junction line (1). Azygoesophageal stripe (2).

Fig. 1.26 Azygoesophageal stripe (1), paraspinal line (3), para-aortic line (2).

Fig. 1.27 Wide paraspinal stripe (1), paraspinal line (2), costotransversal articulations (3).

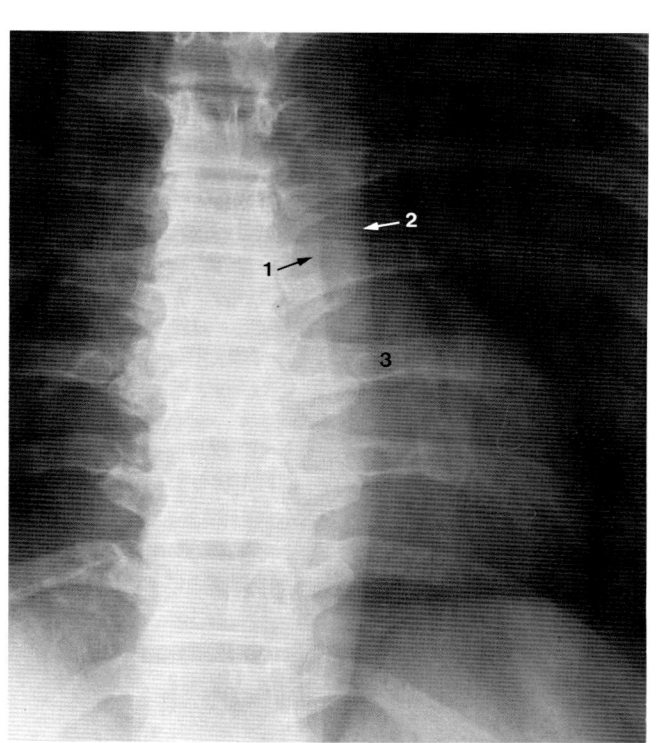

Fig. 1.**28 a, b** Posterior, superior junction line (1), azygoesophageal stripe (2), preaortic line, corresponding to left esophageal wall (3). Air in the esophagus can be seen occasionally in the interaorticobronchial segment, below the aortic arch.

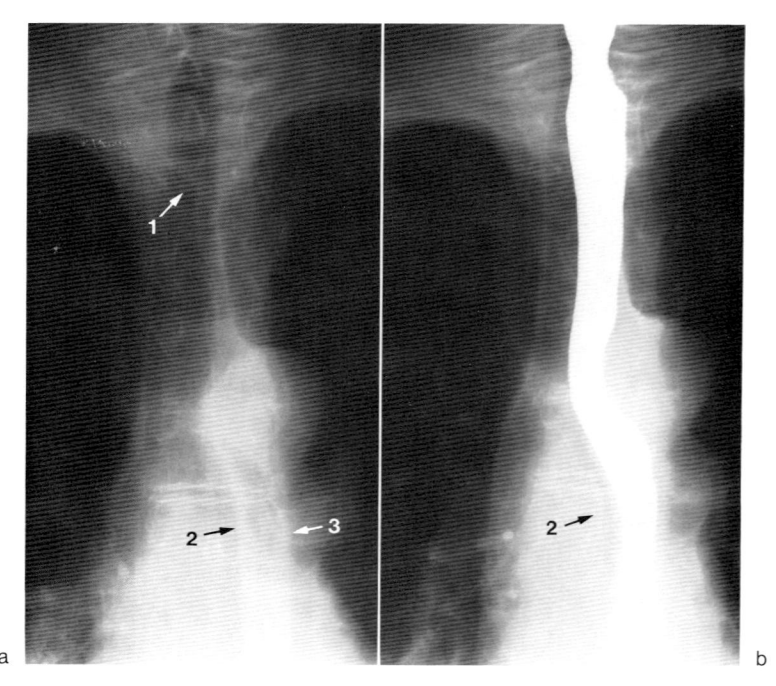

Fig. 1.**29** Aortic arch (1), aortic-pulmonic window (2), descending aorta (3).

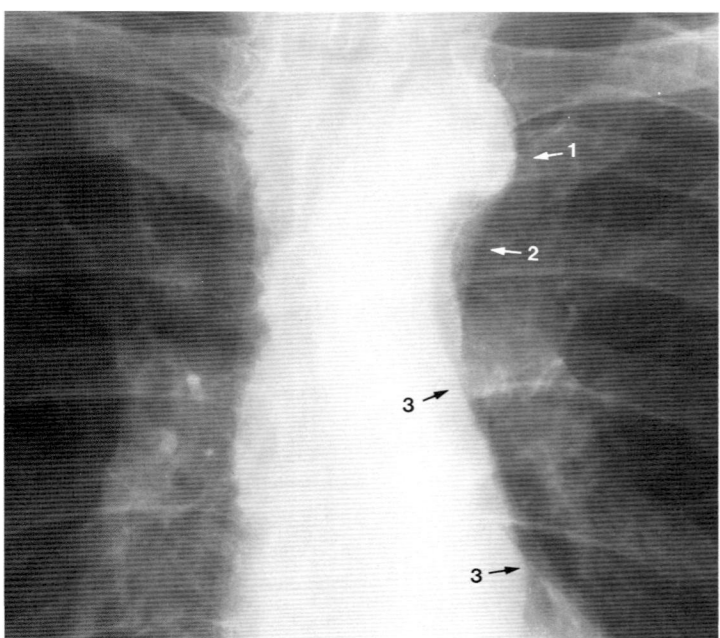

Fig. 1.**30 a–c** Aortic nipple (1) in patient with tuberculous cavity in left upper lobe. The left superior intercostal vein parallels the aortic arch and can be seen on end in 5–10% of normals. It can dilate significantly as a collateral pathway in superior vena caval obstruction.

References: 9, 88, 101, 167.

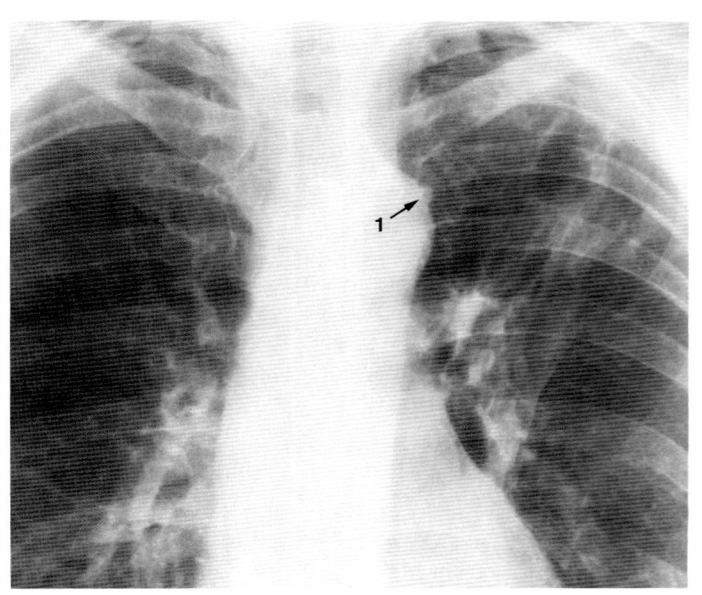

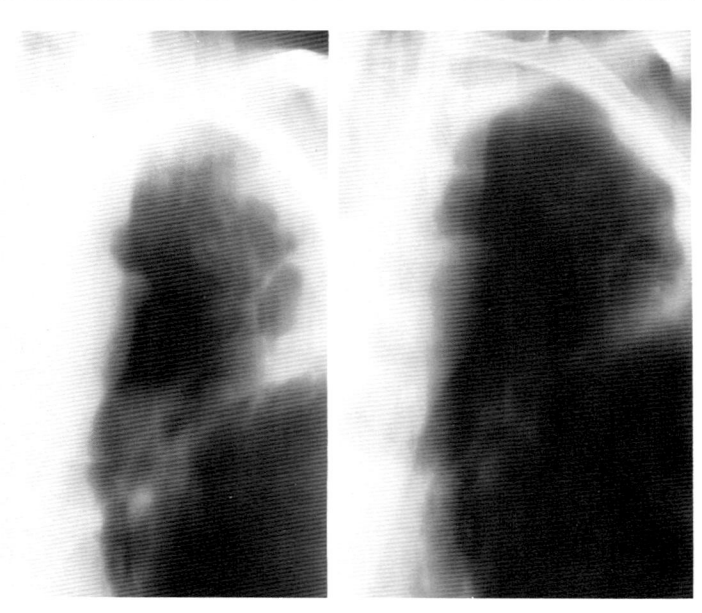

Interlobar Fissures

The interlobar fissures contain two layers of visceral pleura. They can be regularly seen on chest radiographs. In 50–70% they are incomplete, thus allowing for collateral ventilation between the lobes. In the lateral view, the minor and major fissures are frequently seen. On frontal radiographs, the minor fissure is seen in over 50% of cases. The inferior accessory fissure separates the mediobasal segment from the rest of the lower lobe and is present in 10% of the population. The superior accessory fissure separates the superior segment of the lower lobe from the basilar segments and is present in 6%. The azygos fissure contains four layers of pleura and separates part of the apical segment from the rest of the upper lobe. It is seen in 0.5% of normal people and is inconstant since it disappears with a pneumothorax.

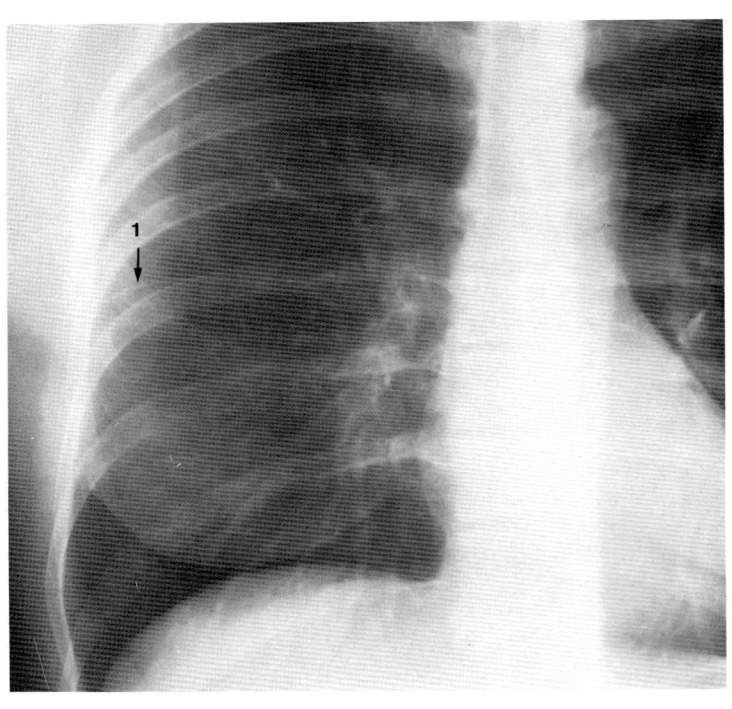

Fig. 1.31 **Minor fissure.**
Double contour (1) formed by tangential view of anterior and posterior aspect of fissure, which curves slightly.

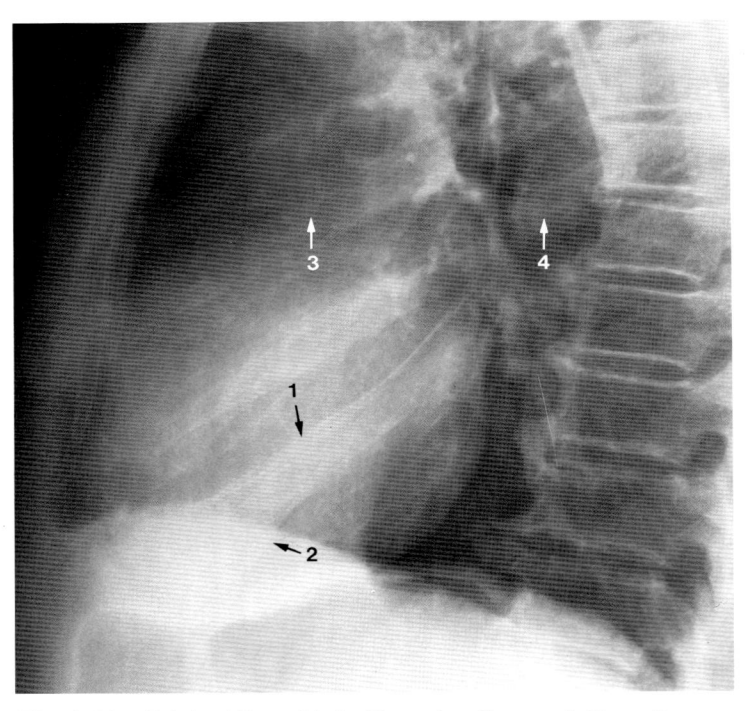

Fig. 1.32   Right (1) and left (2) major fissure. Minor fissure (3), superior accessory fissure (4).

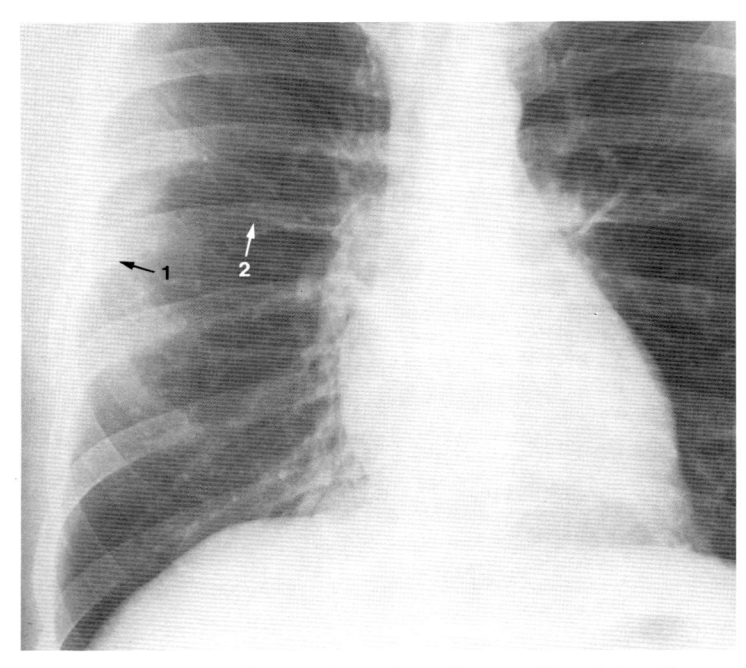

Fig. 1.33   Major fissure (1), minor fissure (2). Major fissure delineates lateral border of lower lobe. It is only rarely visible on frontal films as a discrete line or increased band of opacity, particularly when fat enters the fissure laterally. Lordotic projections increase the likelihood of seeing the major fissure on frontal films.

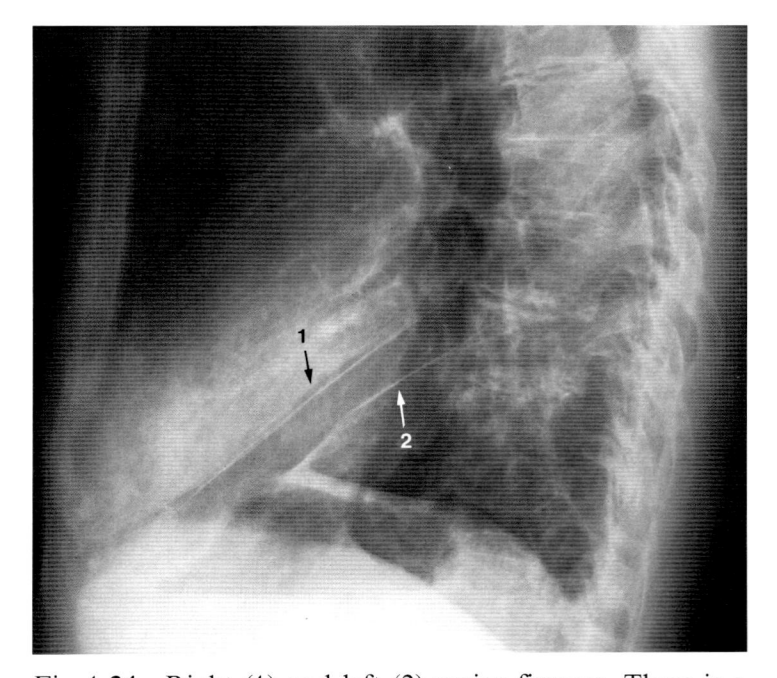

Fig. 1.34   Right (1) and left (2) major fissures. There is a slight loss of volume in the lower lobes, accounting for the elevation of the diaphragm.

Interlobar Fissures 15

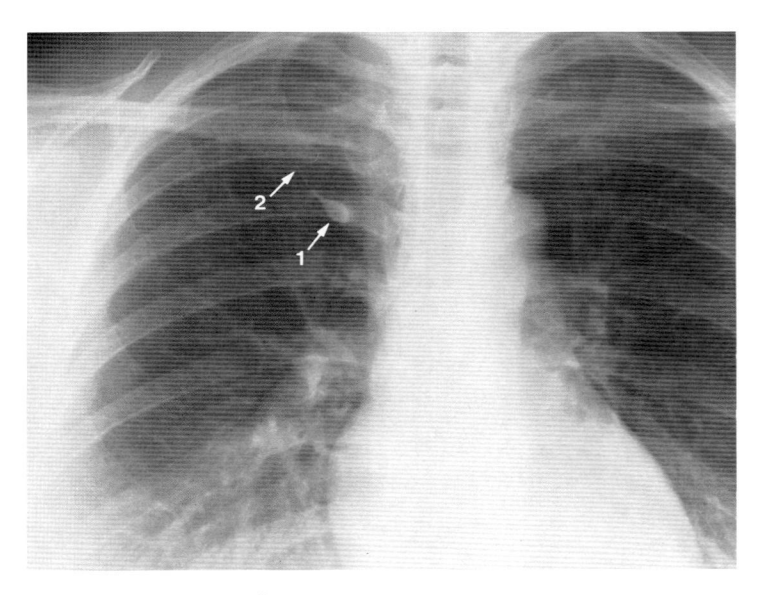

Fig. 1.35 **Azygos fissure.**
Azygos vein seen on end (1). Fissure (2) consists of two layers of visceral and two layers of parietal pleura.

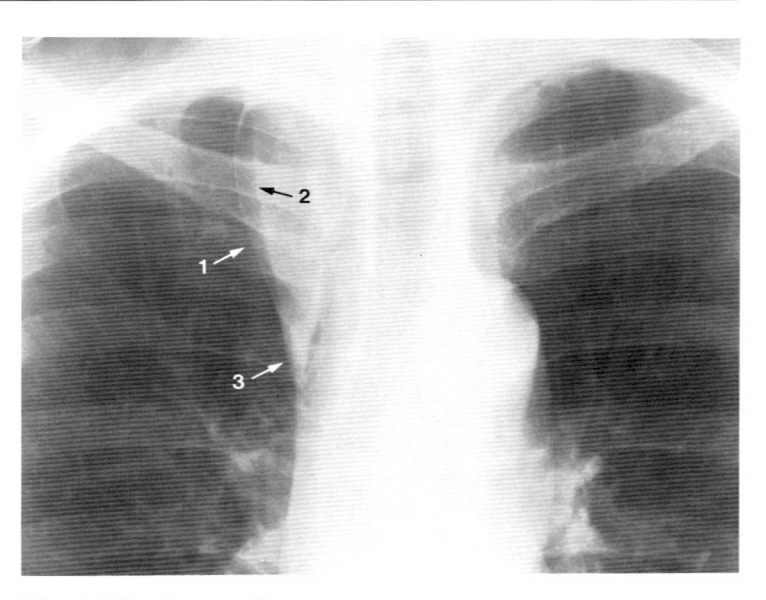

Fig. 1.36 **Azygos fissure.**
Pleura (1), superior vascular pedicle (2), azygos fissure (3).

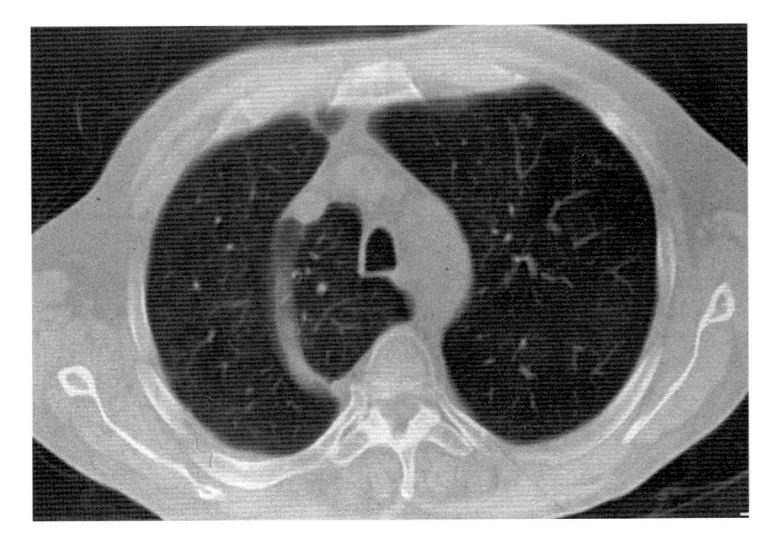

Fig. 1.37 CT scan of azygos fissure. Azygos vein courses through apical segment of right upper lobe.

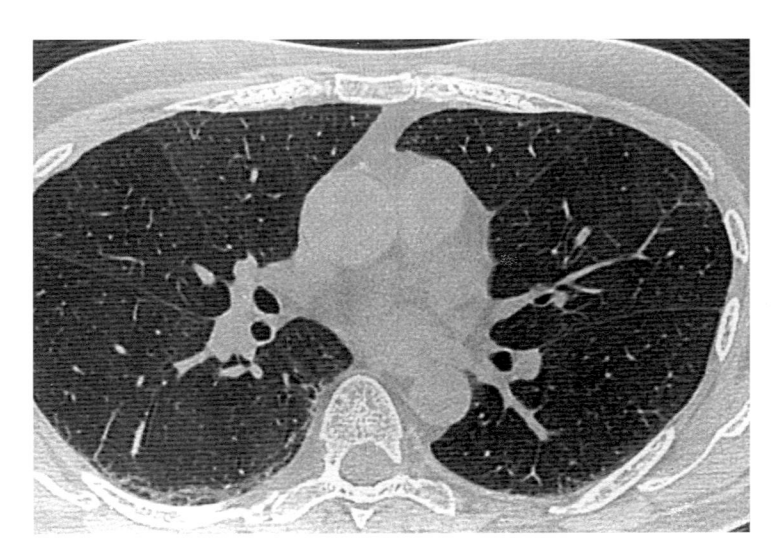

Fig. 1.38 CT scan demonstrates bilateral minor fissures.

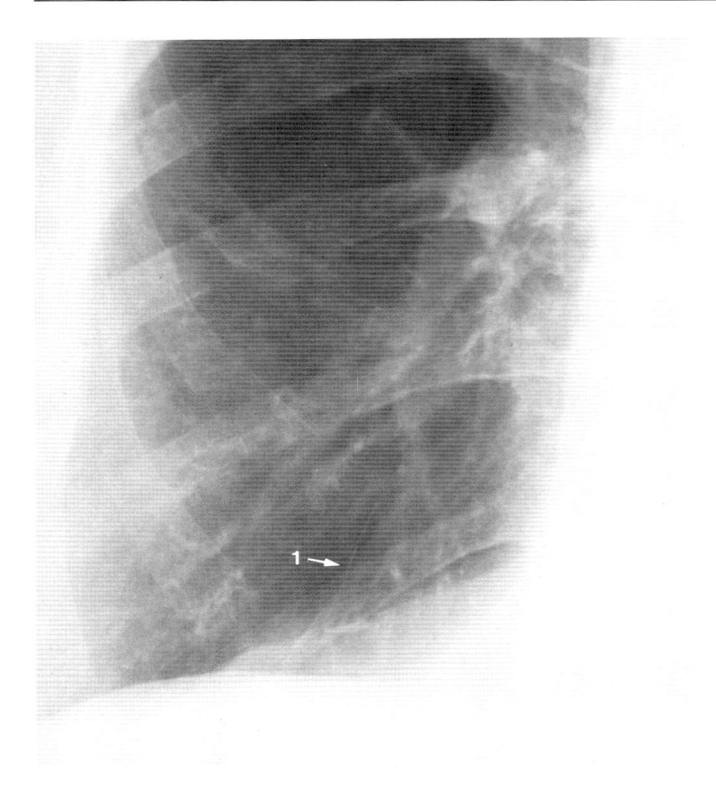

Fig. 1.39 Inferior accessory fissure (1).

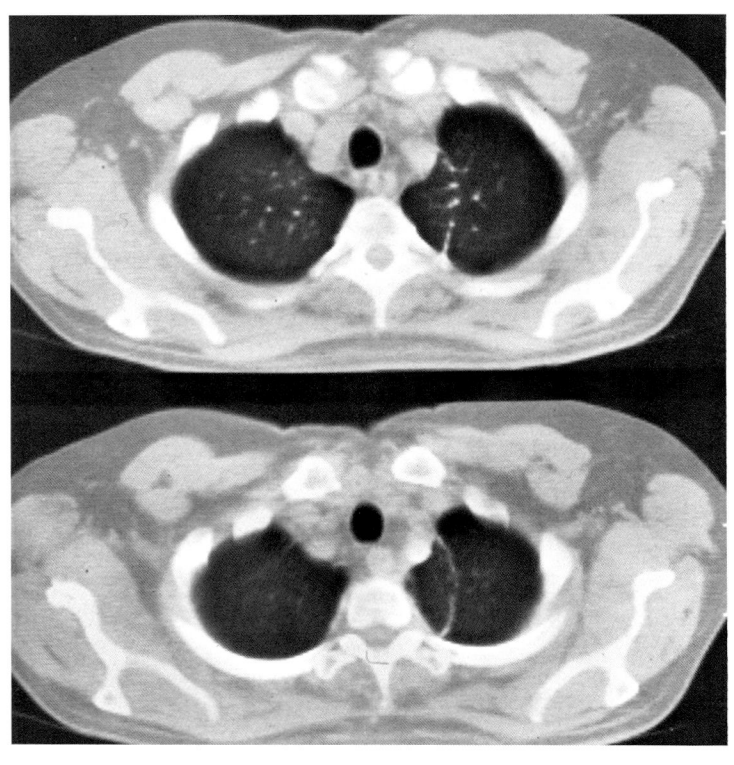

Fig. 1.40 Left-sided azygos fissure equivalent, likely containing a high hemiazygos vein.

References: 38, 45, 62, 136.

Pulmonary Vessels

Fig. 1.41 **Normal hilar vascular structures.**
Lower lobe pulmonary artery (1), lower lobe segmental pulmonary artery (2), upper lobe vessels (4).

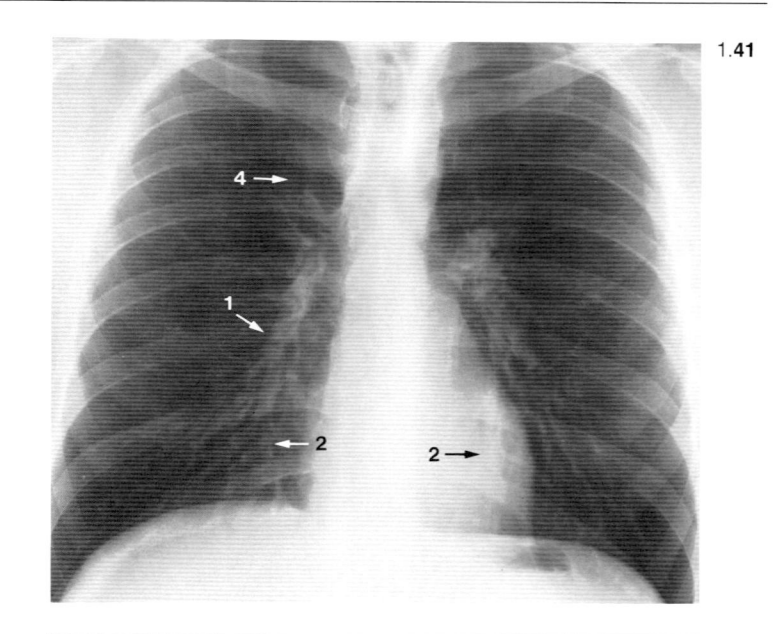

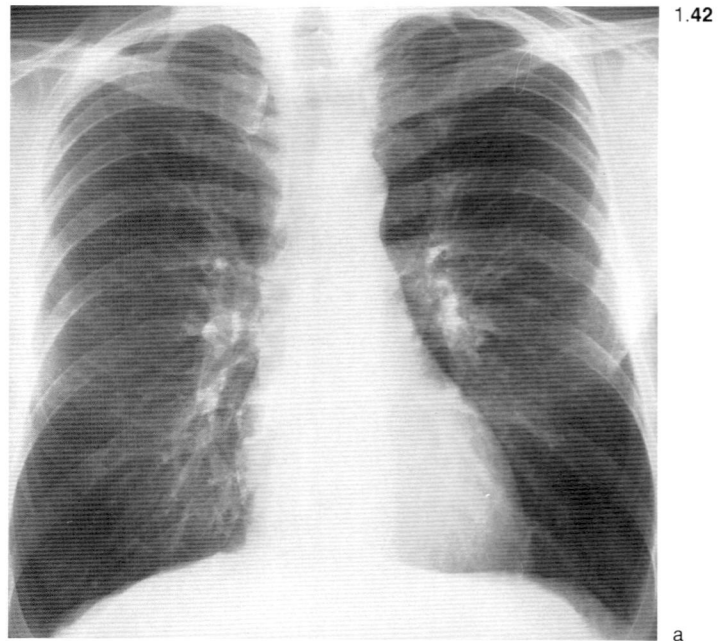

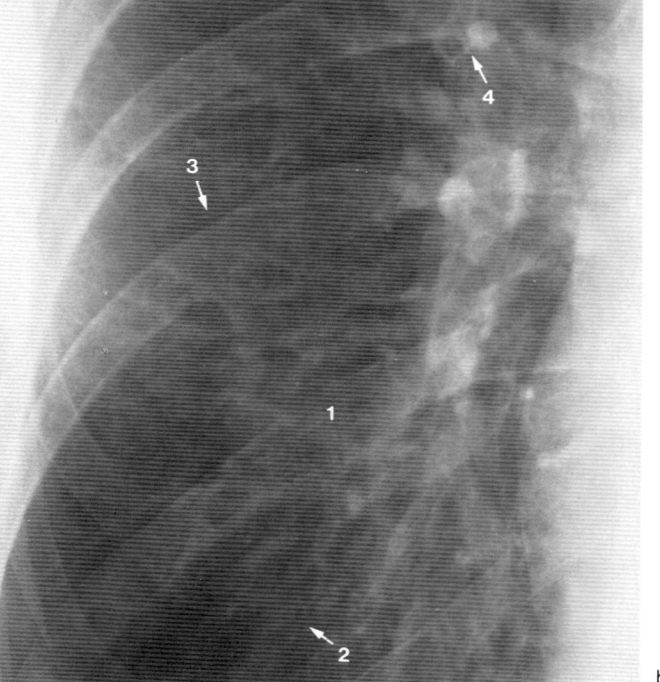

Fig. 1.42 a, b **Dilated hilar vascular structures.**
Horizontal lower lobe vessels represent pulmonary veins (1). Vertical basilar vascular structures represent pulmonary arteries (2). Minor fissure (3). Anterior segmental artery and bronchus seen on end, the so-called monocle sign (4).

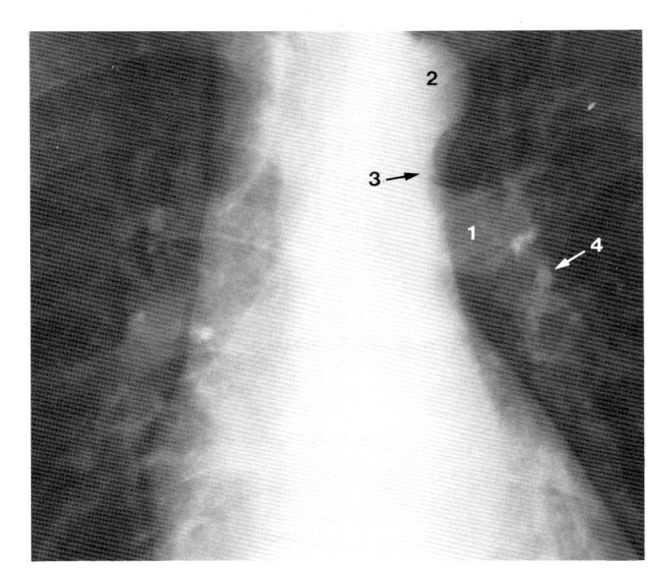

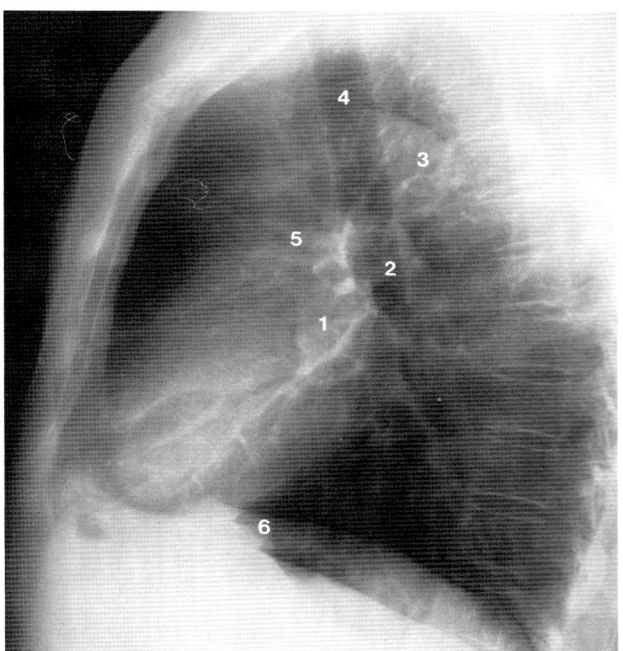

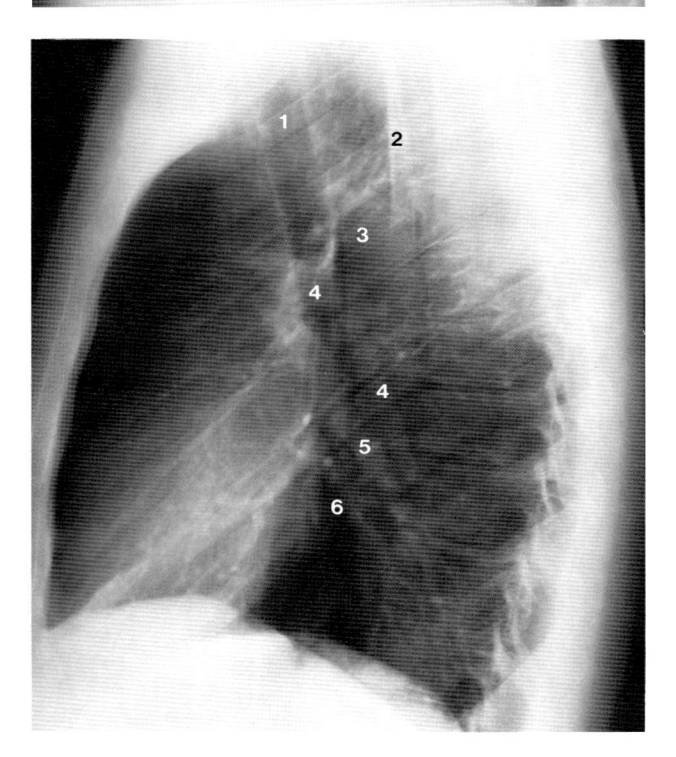

Fig. 1.43 **Hilar vessels.**
Left pulmonary artery (1), aortic arch (2), anterior closure of aortic-pulmonic window (3), segmental bronchus and artery of superior segment, left lower lobe, seen on end (4).

Fig. 1.44 Right hilar vascular structures in pretracheal location (1). The oval opacity is formed by the right pulmonary artery seen on end in its proximal horizontal course and the right superior pulmonary vein. Left pulmonary artery (2) is seen coursing above the left main bronchus. Aortic arch (3), trachea (4), superior pulmonary vein (5), inferior vena cava (6).

Fig. 1.45 Trachea (1), scapula (2), aortic arch (3), left pulmonary artery (4), lower lobe veins (5), located anterior to pulmonary artery branches.

Pulmonary Vessels

Fig. 1.46 a–e **Chest tomograms**
a AP tomogram at 10 cm from table top
b AP tomogram at 12 cm from table top
c AP tomogram at 14 cm from table top
d Lateral tomogram, 5 cm to the left of midline
e Lateral tomogram, 7 cm to the left of midline
1 Trachea
2 Aortic arch
3 Main bronchus
4 Interlobar artery
5 Superior segmental bronchus, lower lobe
6 Lower lobe bronchus
7 Laterobasal segmental veins
8 Upper lobe vein
9 Azygos vein
10 Pulmonary artery
11 Upper lobe bronchus
12 Lingula bronchus
13 Confluence of pulmonary vein into left atrium
14 Middle lobe bronchus
15 Upper lobe artery
16 Aorta
17 Anterior segmental artery, upper lobe
18 Anterior segmental bronchus, upper lobe

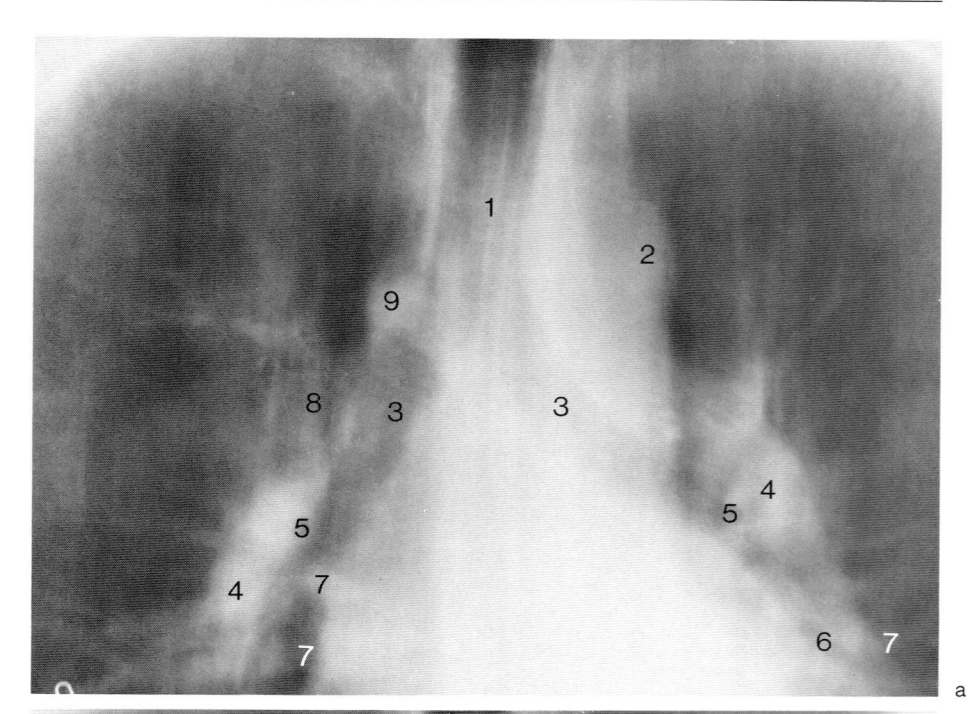

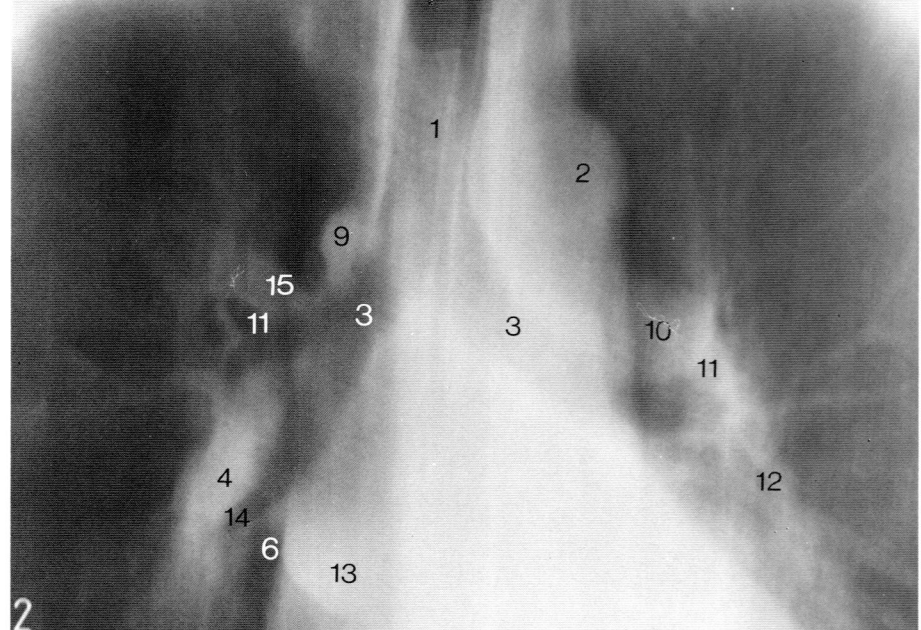

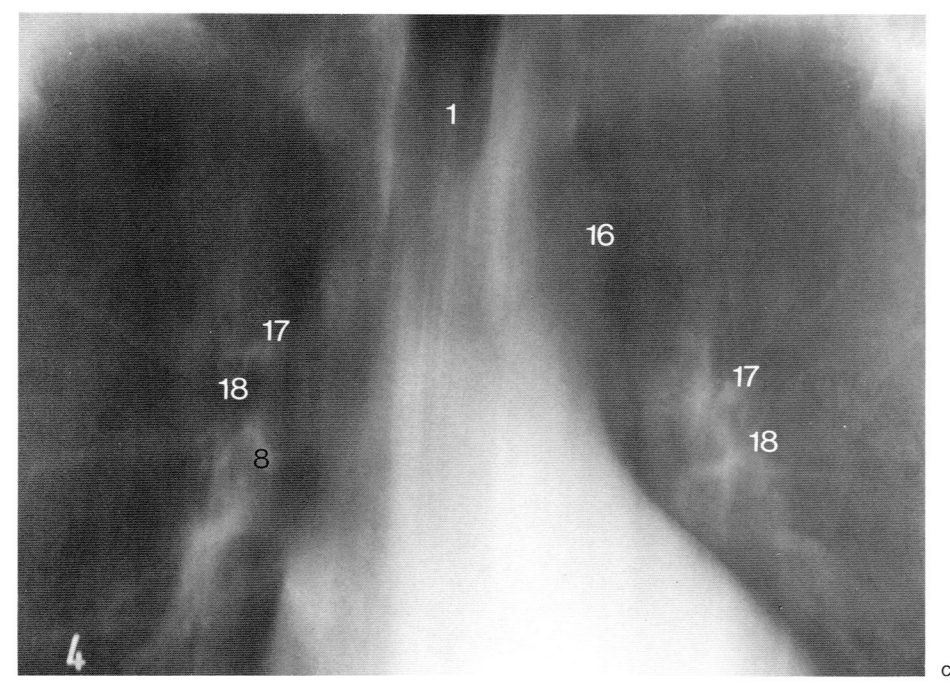

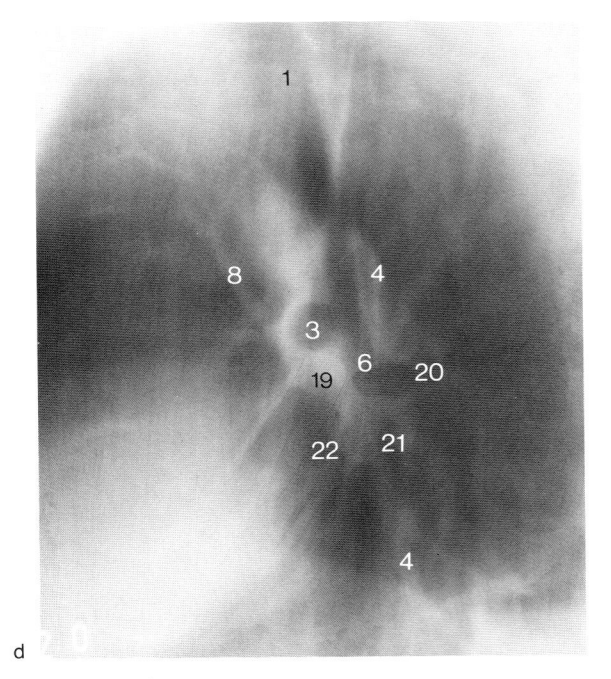

1 Trachea
3 Main bronchus
4 Interlobar artery
6 Lower lobe bronchus
8 Upper lobe vein
19 Venous confluence
20 Superior segment lower lobe, bronchus and artery

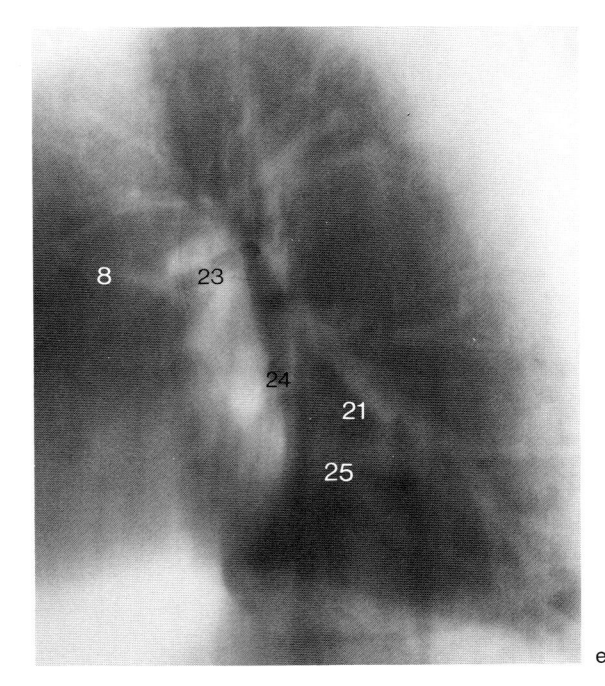

21 Posterobasal segment lower lobe, bronchus and artery
22 Anterobasal segment lower lobe, bronchus and artery
23 Anterior segment upper lobe, bronchus and artery
24 Lower lobe vein

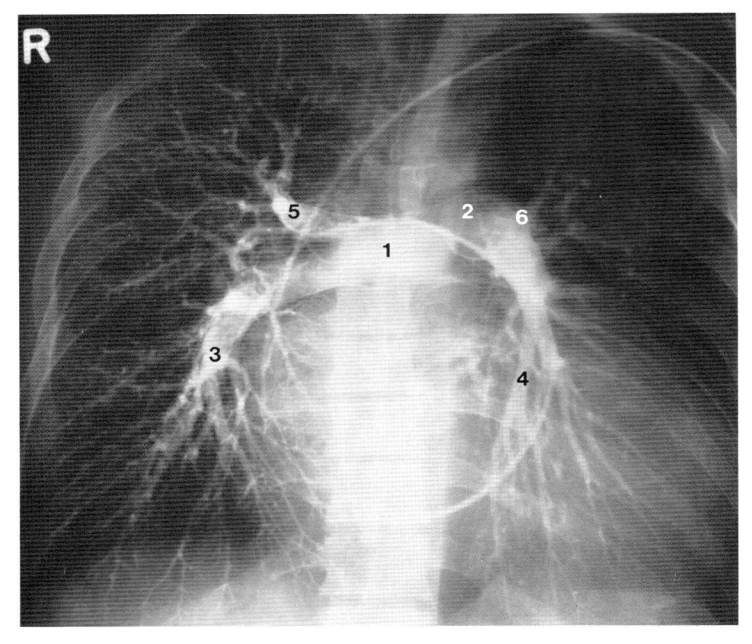

Fig. 1.47a **Pulmonary angiogram, arterial phase**
1 Right pulmonary artery
2 Main and left pulmonary arteries
3 Right lower lobe pulmonary artery
4 Left lower lobe pulmonary artery
5 Right upper lobe pulmonary artery
6 Left upper lobe pulmonary artery

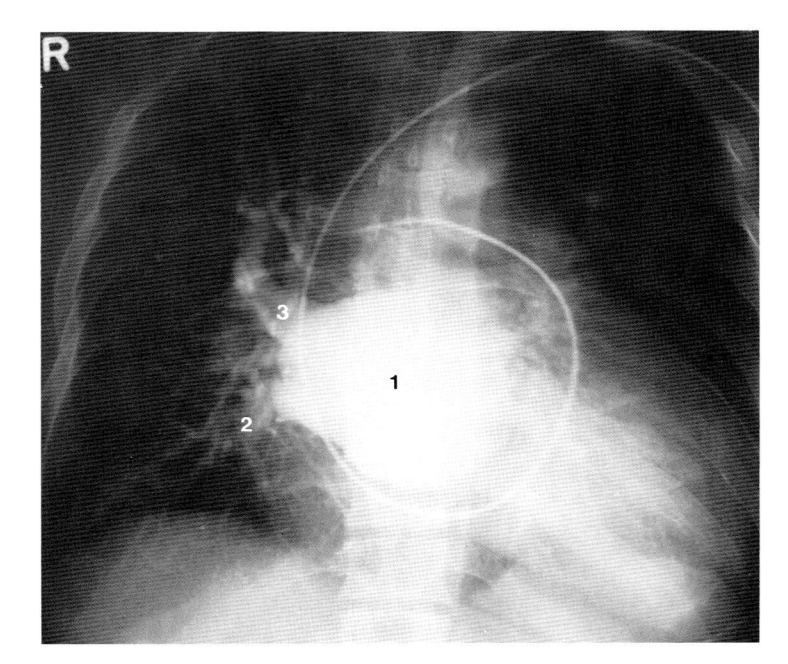

Fig. 1.47b **Venous phase**
1 Right atrium
2 Confluence of lower lobe veins
3 Confluence of upper lobe veins

Bronchi

Bronchography has largely been replaced as an investigative method by flexible bronchoscopy and computed tomography (CT). A normal bronchogram is used here only as a teaching tool for the optimal display of the bronchial anatomy.

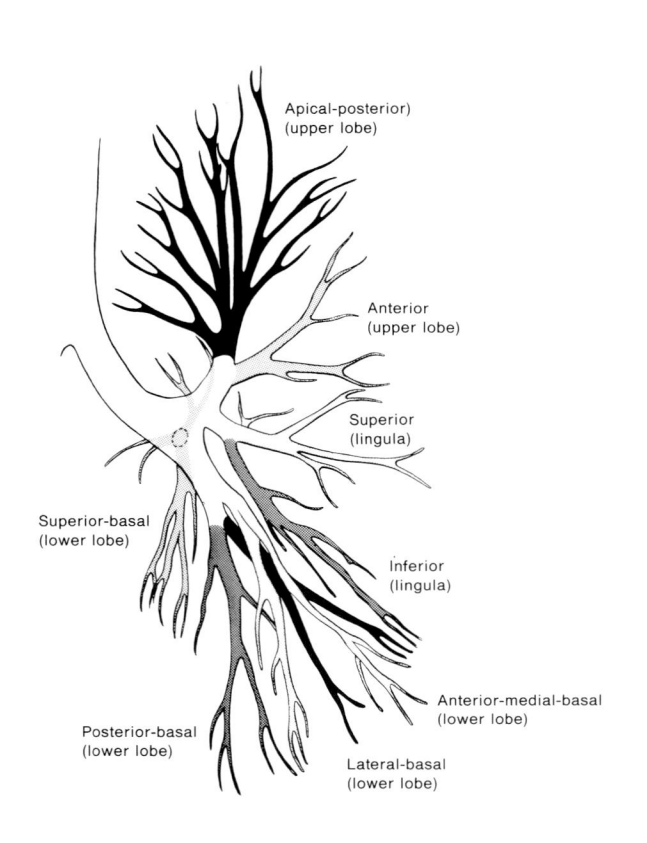

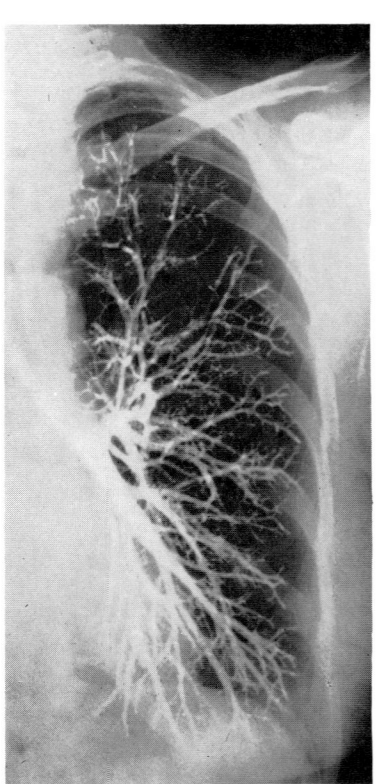

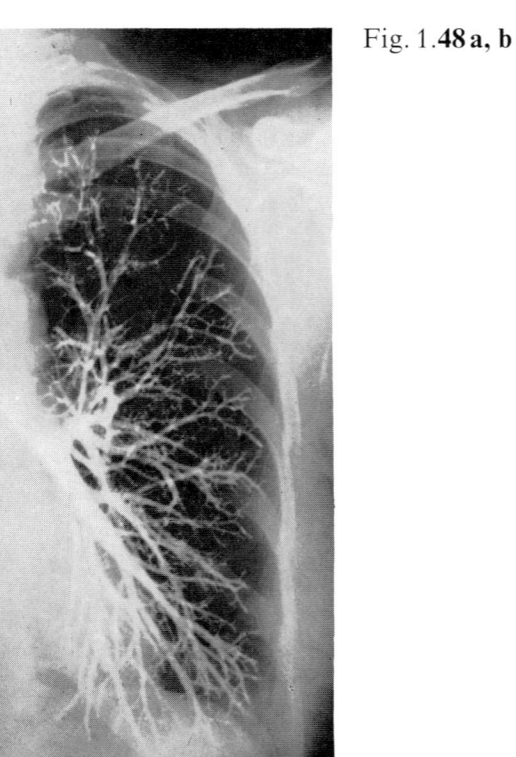

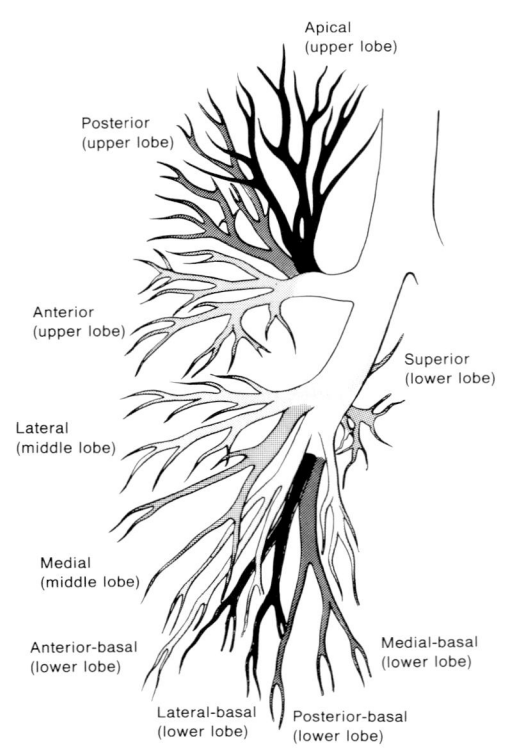

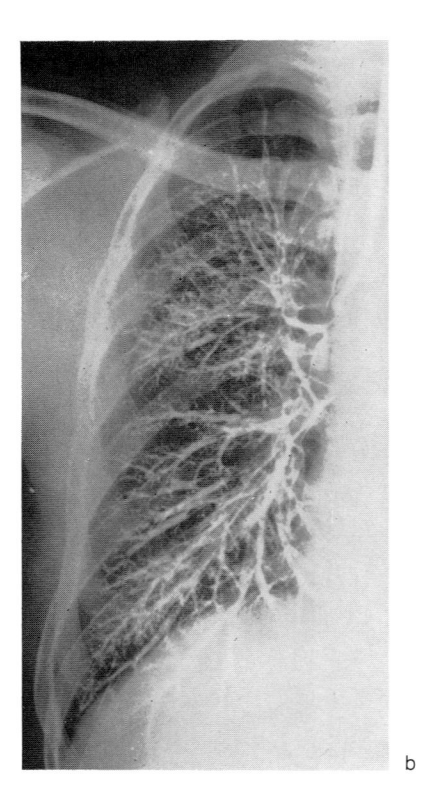

Fig. 1.**48 a, b**

22   1. Normal Anatomy and Normal Variants

Fig. 1.**49 a, b**

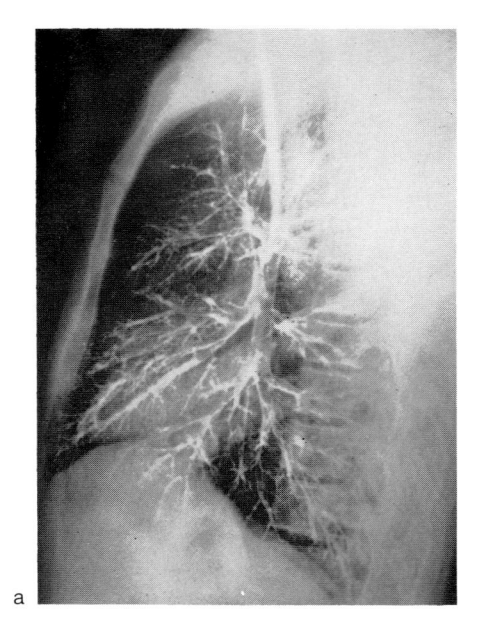

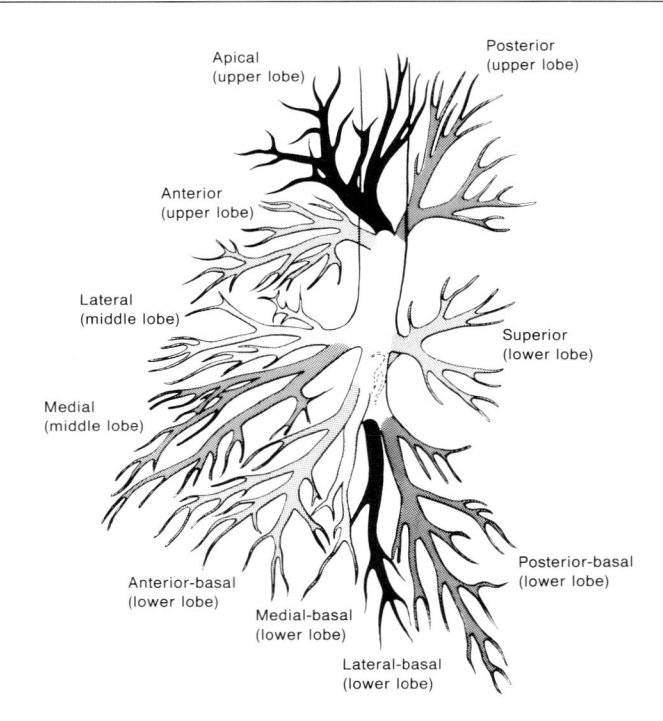

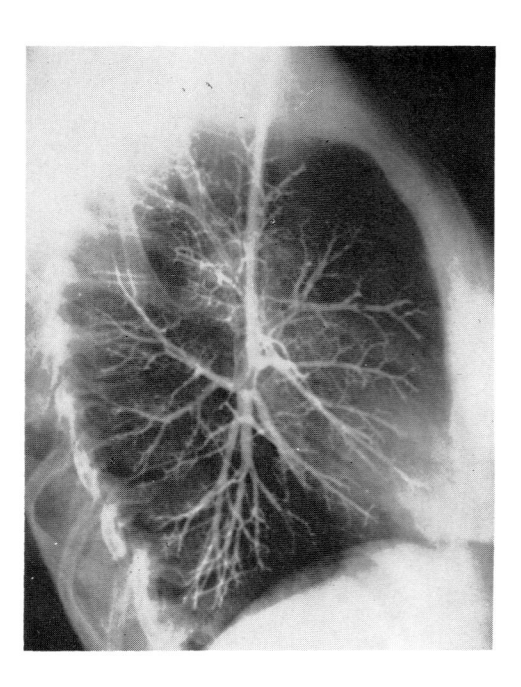

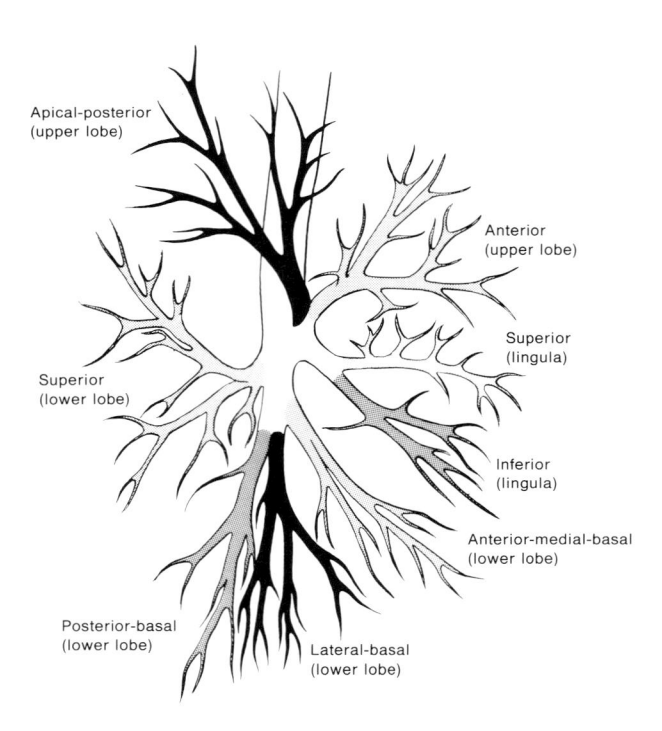

Mediastinum

The methods of choice for imaging mediastinal structures are CT and magnetic resonance imaging (MRI) with their high contrast resolution and cross-sectional image display devoid of the superimposition of structures. MRI can display the chest in coronal, sagittal, axial, and paraxial planes.

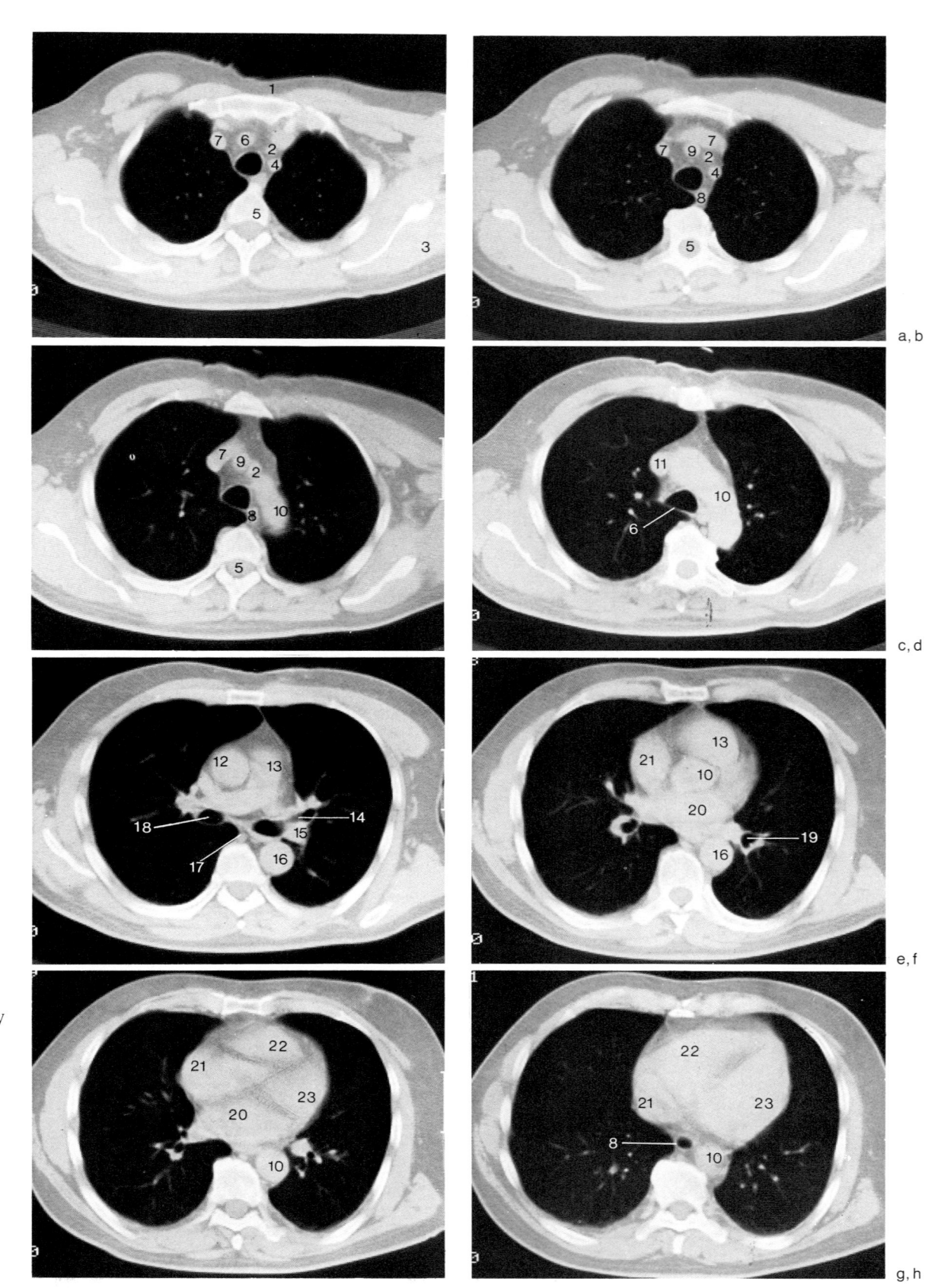

Fig. 1.**50 a–h**
Normal CT-anatomy
1 Sternum
2 Carotid artery
3 Scapula
4 Subclavian artery
5 Vertebra
6 Trachea
7 Subclavian vein
8 Esophagus
9 Brachiocephalic artery
10 Aorta
11 Vena cava
12 Ascending aorta
13 Main pulmonary artery
14 Upper lobe bronchus
15 Lower lobe artery
16 Ascending aorta
17 Azygos vein
18 Main bronchus
19 Lower lobe artery and vein
20 Left atrium
21 Right atrium
22 Right ventricle
23 Left ventricle

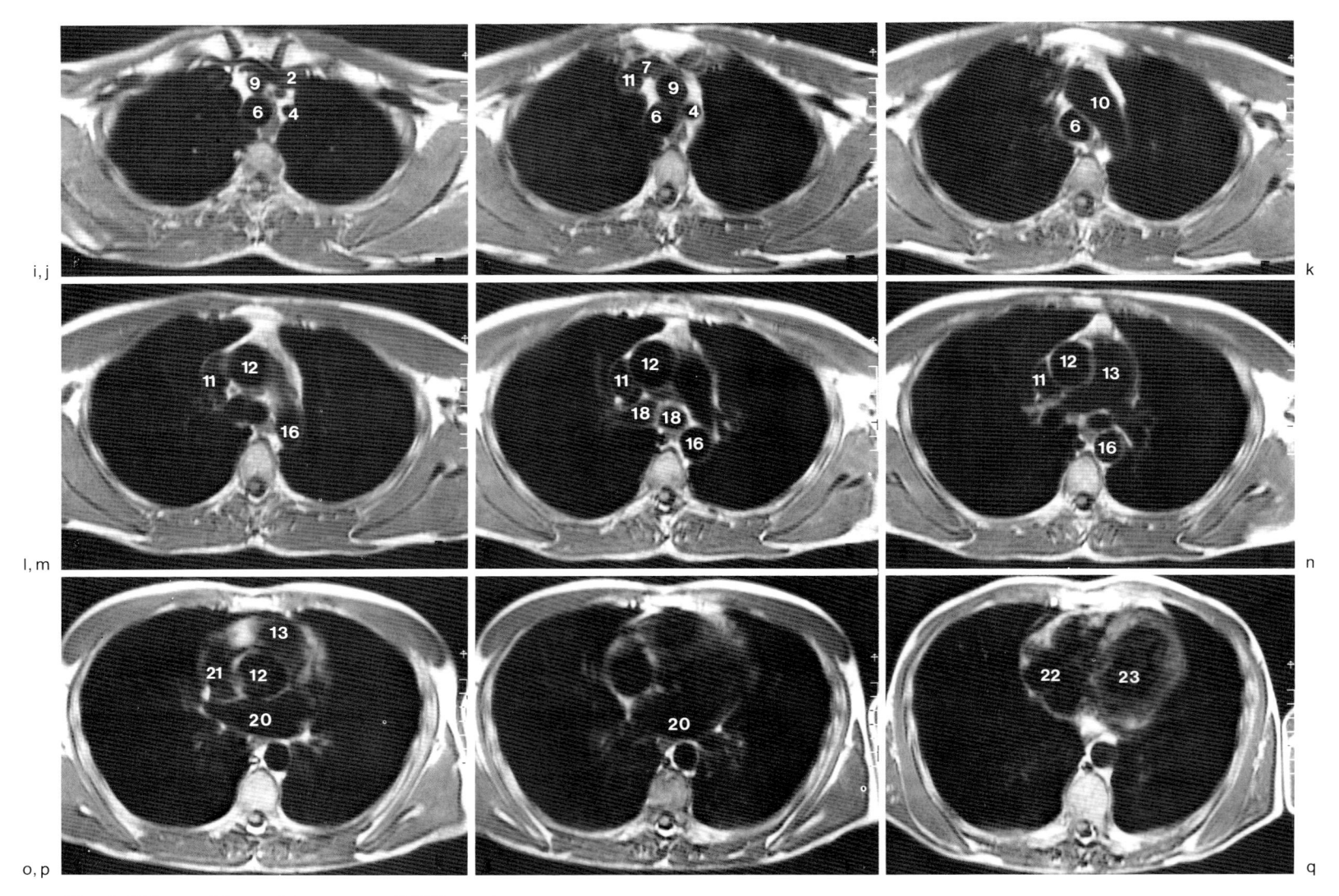

Fig. 1.50i–q **Normal transverse MRI anatomy**

- 2 Carotid artery
- 4 Subclavian artery
- 6 Trachea
- 7 Subclavian vein
- 9 Brachiocephalic artery
- 11 Vena cava
- 12 Ascending aorta
- 13 Main pulmonary artery
- 16 Ascending aorta
- 18 Main bronchus
- 20 Left atrium
- 21 Right atrium
- 22 Right ventricle
- 23 Left ventricle

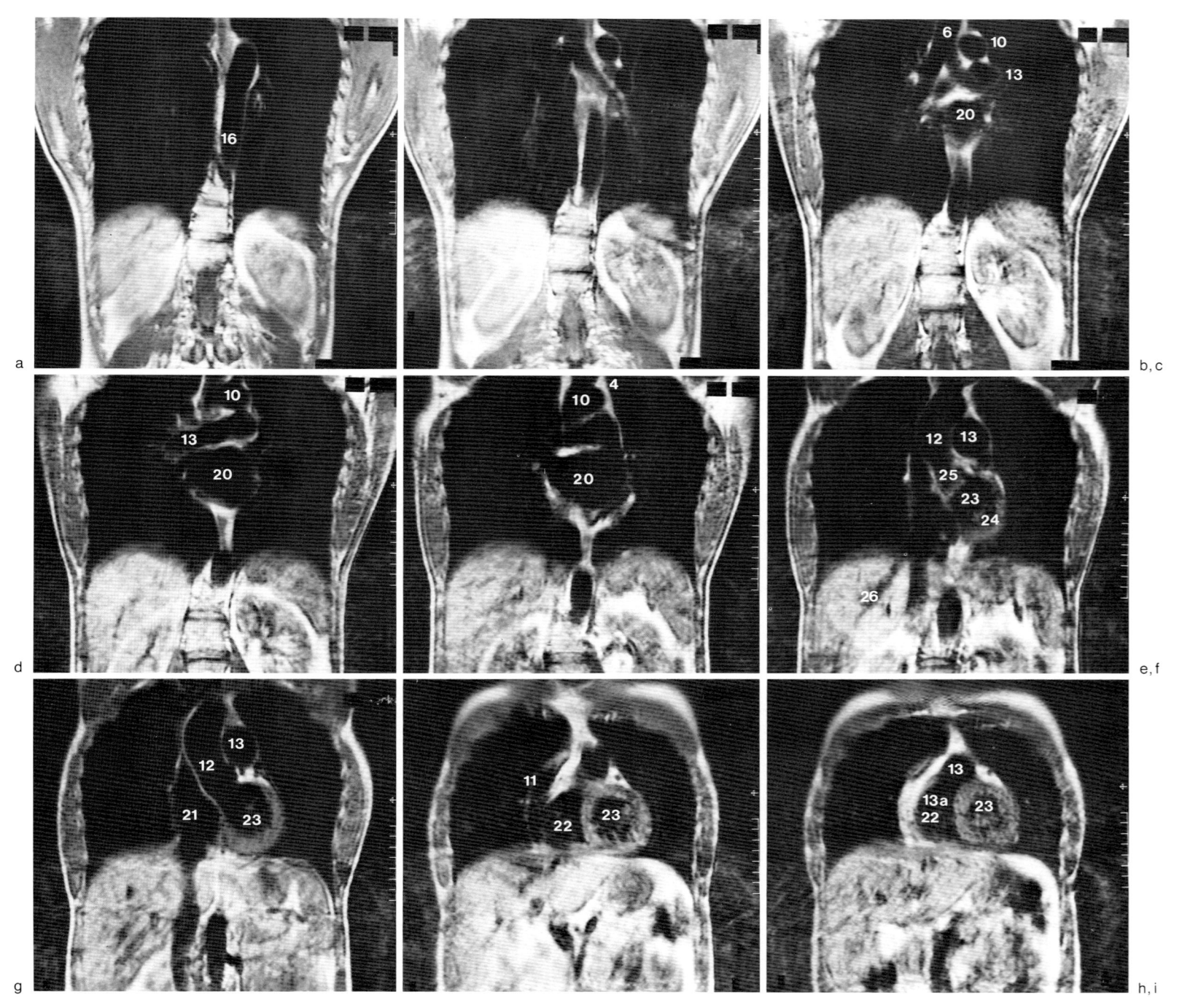

Fig. 1.51 a–i **Normal coronal MRI anatomy**

1 Sternum	11 Vena cava	19 Lower lobe bronchus and artery
2 Carotid artery	12 Ascending aorta	20 Left atrium
3 Scapula	12a Aortic valve	21 Right atrium
4 Subclavian artery	13 Main pulmonary artery	22 Right ventricle
5 Vertebra	13a Pulmonic valve	23 Left ventricle
6 Trachea	14 Upper lobe bronchus	24 Papillary muscle
7 Subclavian vein	15 Lower lobe artery	25 Aortic valve
8 Esophagus	16 Descending aorta	26 Hepatic vein
9 Brachiocephalic artery	17 Azygos vein	27 Mitral valve
10 Aorta	18 Main bronchus	28 Pulmonary veins

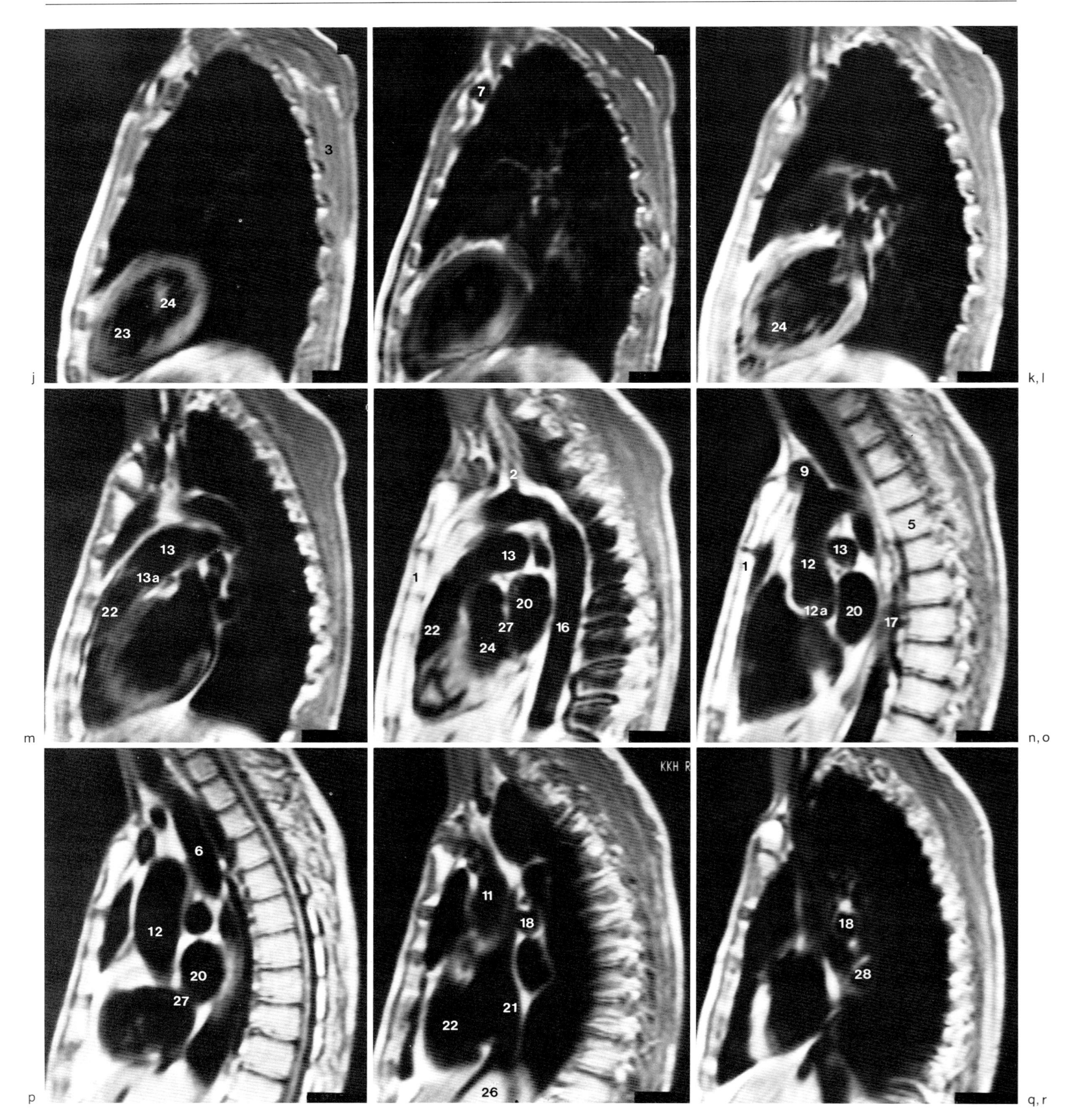

Fig. 1.51 j–r **Normal sagittal MRI anatomy**

2. Infections

Pneumonia

Pneumonia represents an infection of the lung parenchyma. It can be elicited by bacteria, mycoplasma, viruses, or fungi; it is characterized by a serofibrinous, cellular exudate in the interstitium and alveolar space. The prognosis of these infections has improved with the advent of antibiotics, yet pneumonia is still a major cause of morbidity and mortality and is the fifth most common cause of death in the USA. Histopathologically, pneumonia can be classified as lobar pneumonia, bronchopneumonia, and interstitial pneumonia. This classification correlates with the radiographic picture. It does not specify the causative organism. The radiologist's role is to diagnose the pneumonia, monitor its course, detect complications, and exclude other diseases that simulate pneumonia.

Lobar Pneumonia

This so-called airspace pneumonia is caused by bacteria, viruses, mycoplasma, and fungi. The consolidation starts in the peripheral lung and extends into surrounding alveoli via the pores of Cohn. It is confined to a lobe or segment, particularly if abutting a complete interlobar fissure. Radiologically, a homogeneous consolidation of the lung results. Air bronchograms are a conspicuous feature. The particular segment of lung involved can usually be identified on radiographs. Due to timely therapy with antibiotics, the classic lobar consolidation is now seen infrequently. The differential diagnosis shoud include tuberculous pneumonia, fungal pneumonias, bronchoalveolar cell carcinoma, lymphoma, pseudolymphoma alveolar sarcoidosis, and on rare occasions, BOOP (broncholitis obliterans with organizing pneumonia).

The diagnosis is facilitated by the presence of clinical symptoms including fever, sputum production, leukocytosis, hypoxemia, radiologic findings, as well as clearing after the institution of antibiotic therapy. Recurrent segmental or lobar consolidations are suspicious for bronchial obstruction with postobstructive pneumonia. Early cavitation and abscess formation are seen best on conventional tomographic or CT images.

Fig. 2.1 a–c **Extensive air space consolidation.**
50-year-old alcoholic with shaking chills and cough. Marked improvement after antibiotic therapy for 14 days.

Homogeneous opacification of middle and lower lung zones with patchy opacities at the extreme lung base and in the upper lobe. Note obscuration of part of the right heart border, indicating right middle lobe pneumonia, and obliteration of the right lower lobe pulmonary artery branches, indicative of a right lower lobe process. Clearly visible air bronchogram (1), pedicle (2), azygoesophageal stripe (3), inferior accessory fissure (4), spine of scapula (5), residual consolidation (6).

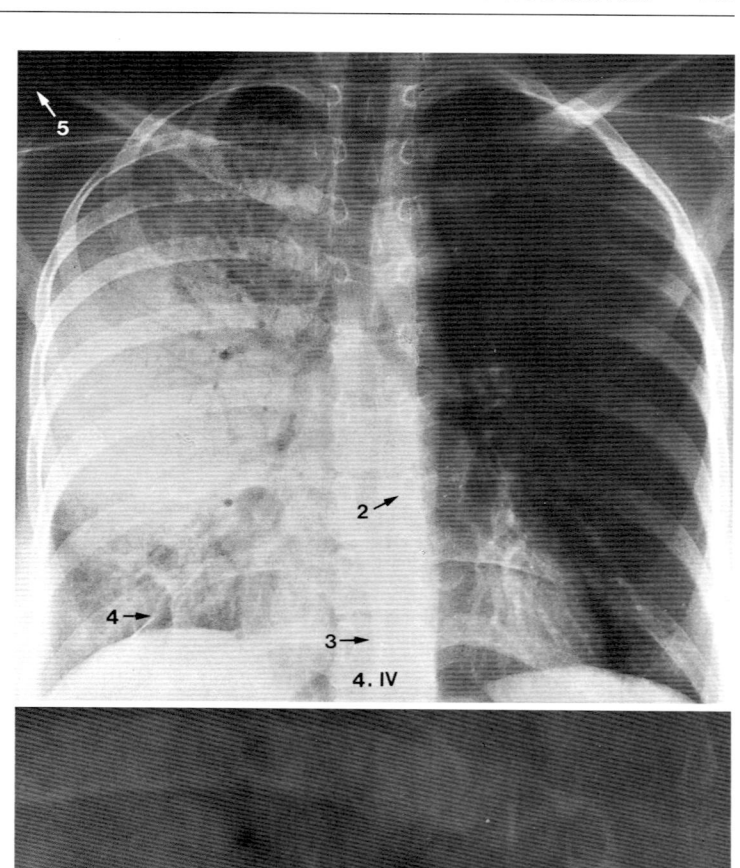

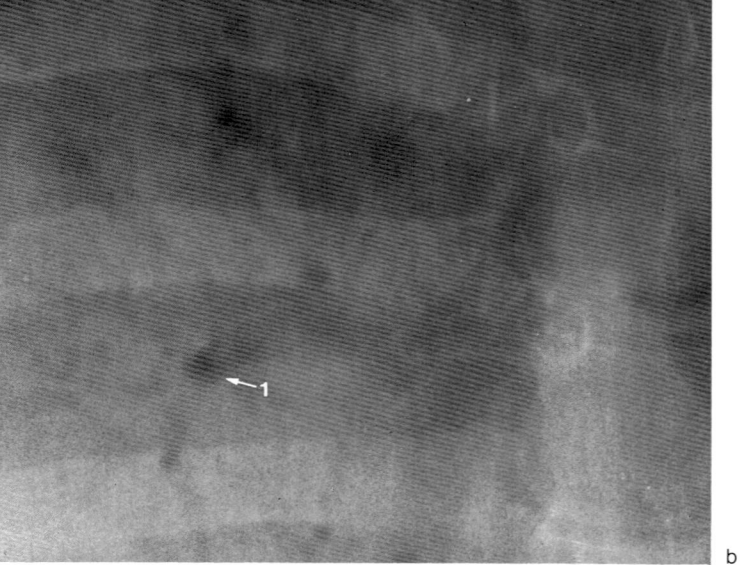

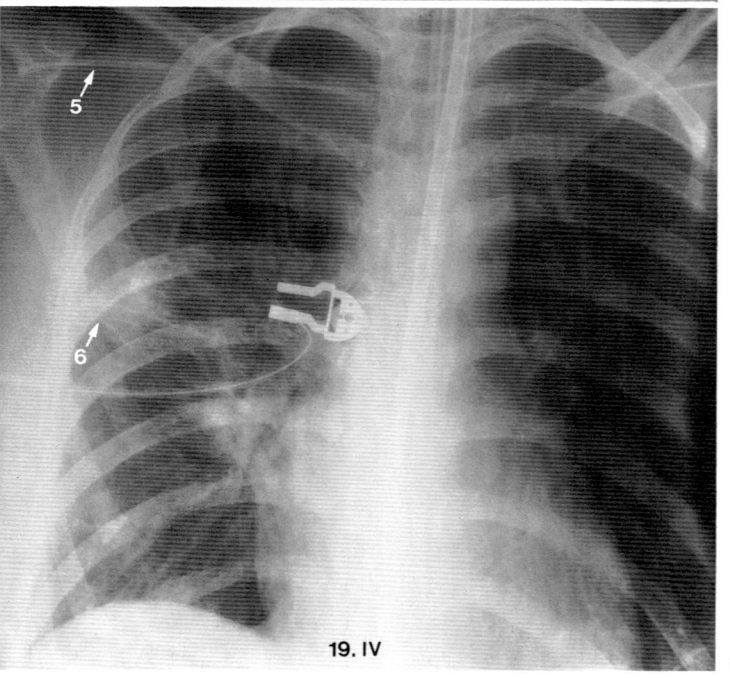

30 2. Infections

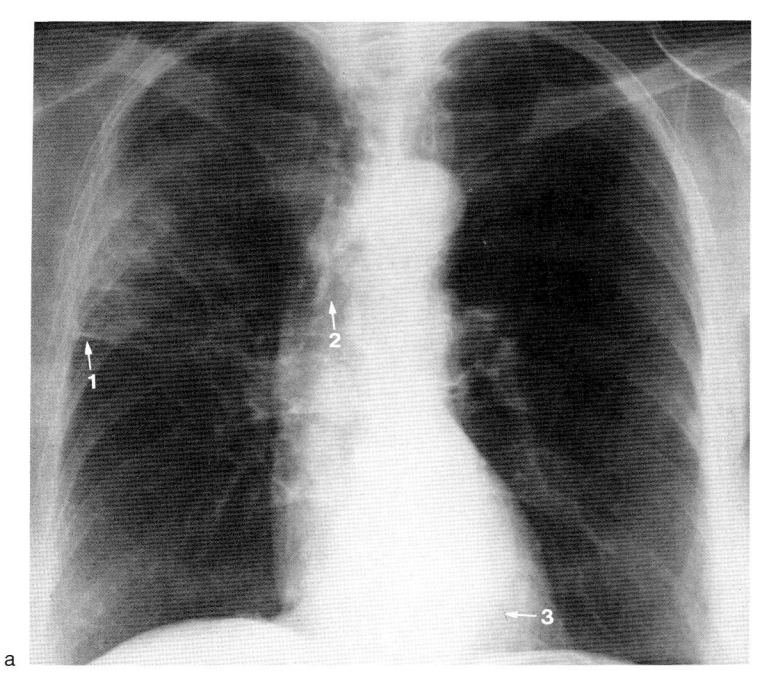

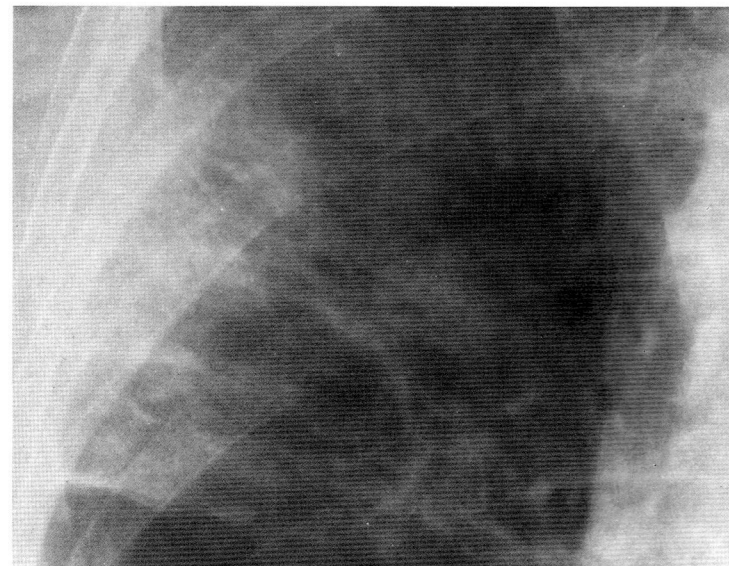

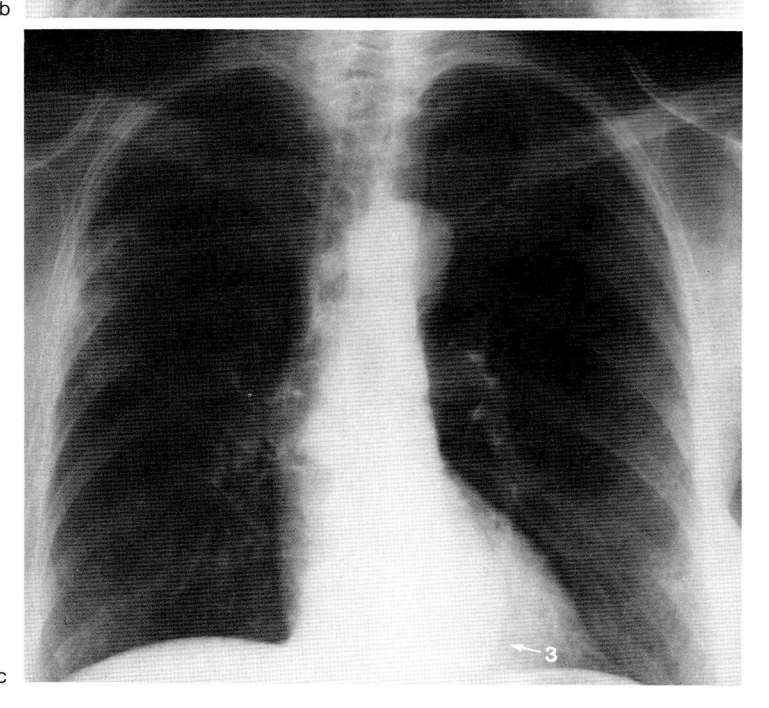

Fig. 2.2 a–c **Segmental pneumonia.**
72-year-old patient admitted with cough and 38.8 °C (102 °F) fever. Sputum culture yielded *Pseudomonas aeruginosa*. Near complete clearing after 10 days of antibiotic therapy (**c**).

Streaky opacification of anterior segment, right upper lobe, minor fissure (1), azygos vein (2), tortuous descending aorta (3).

Fig. 2.3 a–c **Pneumonia with parapneumonic effusion.**
40-year-old woman with abrupt onset of shaking chills, fever, cough, purulent expectoration containing *Aerobacter*. After 10 days of antibiotic therapy, nearly complete clearing of consolidation.

Homogeneous opacification of right upper lobe with relative sparing of apical segment. Right costophrenic sulcus blunted by small pleural effusion (1). The consolidation straddles the minor (2) and major (3) fissures, likely involving the so-called axillary subsegment of the right upper lobe. Air bronchogram (4), interlobar artery (5), lower lobe pulmonary veins (6), azygoesophageal recess (7), bronchus intermedius (8). Lateral view (**c**): contour of right hemidiaphragm is uninterrupted and has contact with right major fissure; contour of left hemidiaphragm is obliterated in its anterior third by contact with cardiac silhouette.

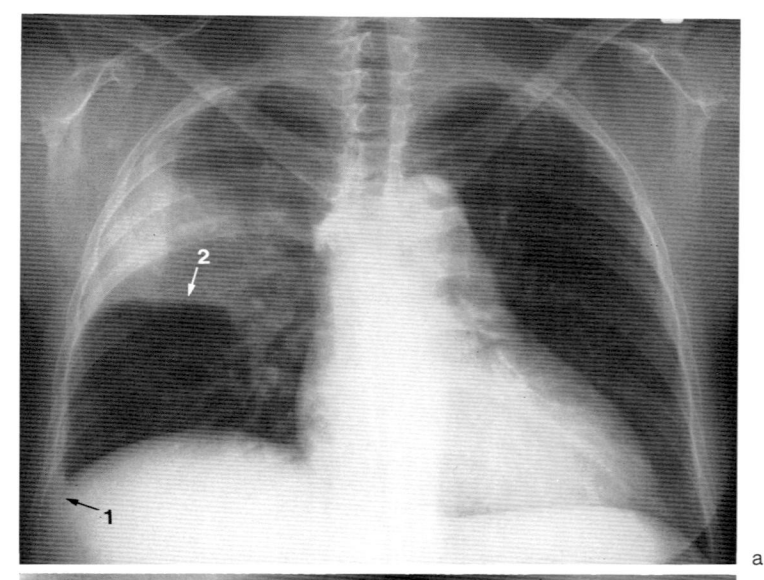

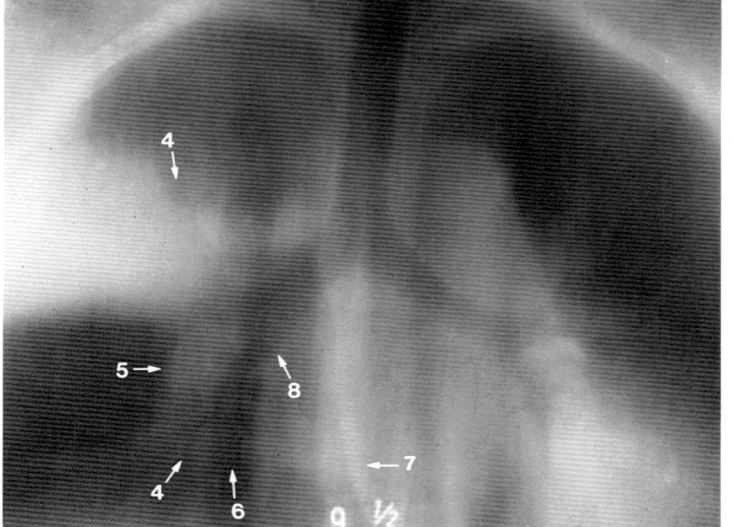

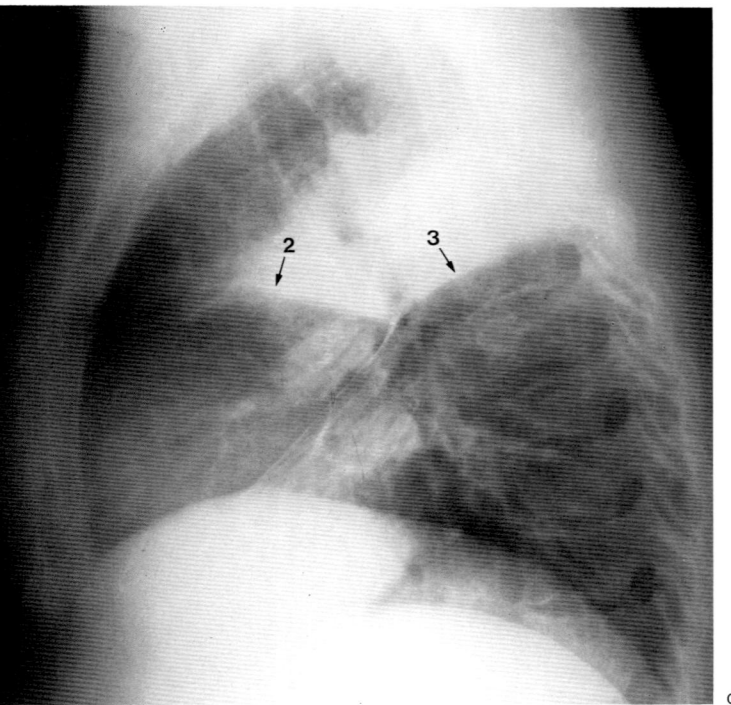

32   2. Infections

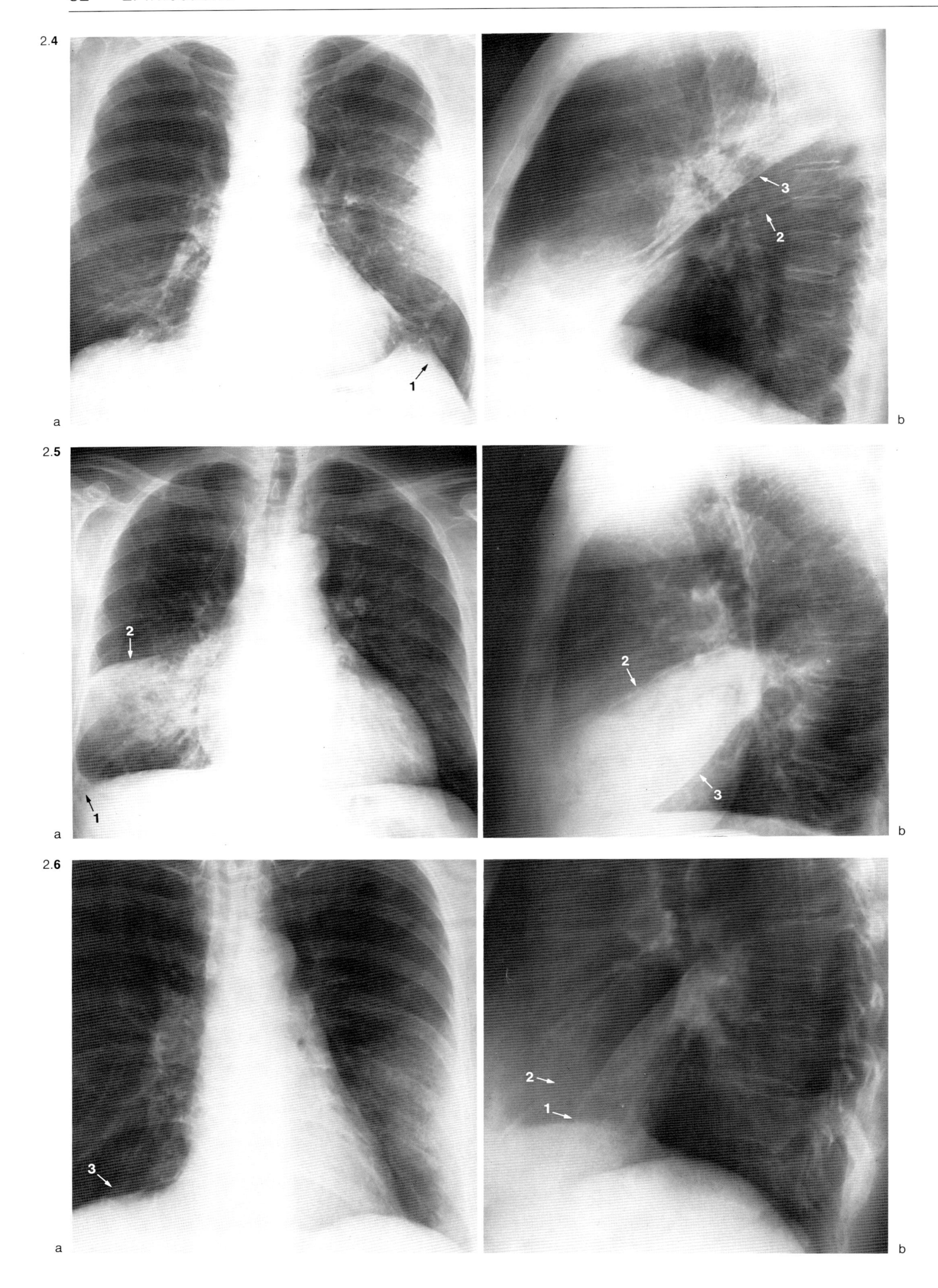

◁ **Fig. 2.4 a, b Pneumonia in apicoposterior segment of left upper lobe.**
56-year-old man.

Inhomogeneous opacification. Lateral view shows inferior demarcation of consolidation by left major fissure. Tenting of left diaphragmatic pleura forms juxtaphrenic peak (1) indicative of slight volume loss in left upper lobe. Right major fissure (2), left major fissure (3).

◁ **Fig. 2.5 a, b Right middle lobe pneumonia.**
79-year-old patient with coronary artery disease.

Homogeneous consolidation of right middle lobe. Small right pleural effusion (1), minor fissure (2) slightly displaced inferiorly due to loss of volume, major fissure (3), cardiac silhouette enlarged.

◁ **Fig. 2.6 a, b Pneumonia in anterobasal segment of left lower lobe.**
55-year-old patient.

Confluent opacification of left lower lobe abutting major fissure (1), right major fissure (2), inferior accessory fissure (3).

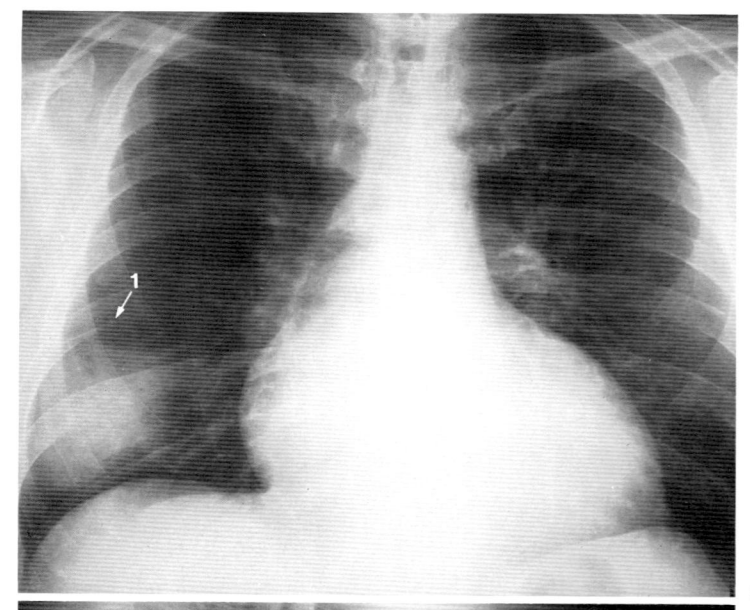

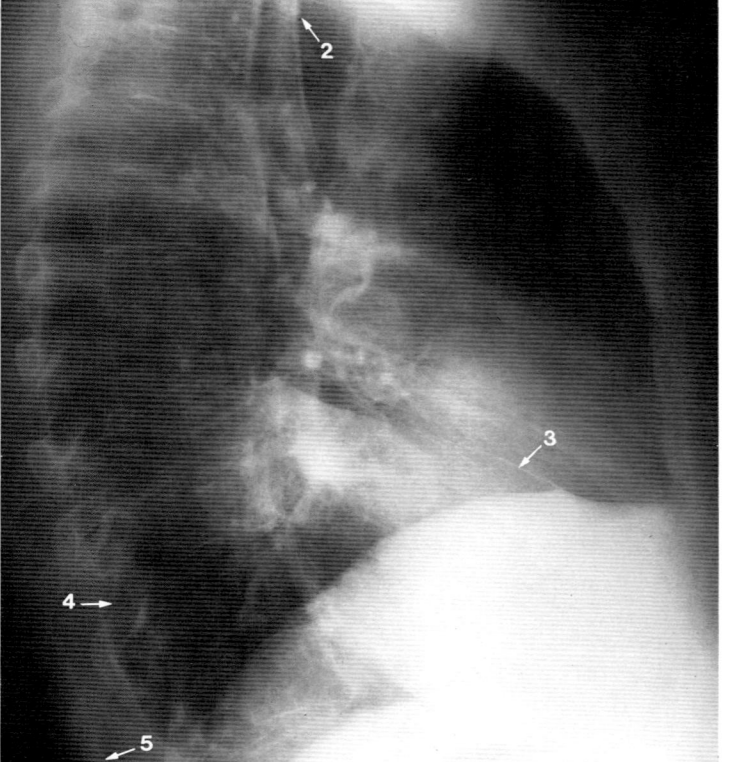

Fig. 2.7 a, b Pneumonia in anterobasal segment of right lower lobe.
48-year-old patient with alcoholic cardiomyopathy.

Homogeneous opacification of part of the right lower lobe. Cardiac silhouette enlarged. Minor fissure (1) has no contact with consolidation, scapula (2), right major fissure (3), right pleural effusion (4), left posterior pleura (5).

34   2. Infections

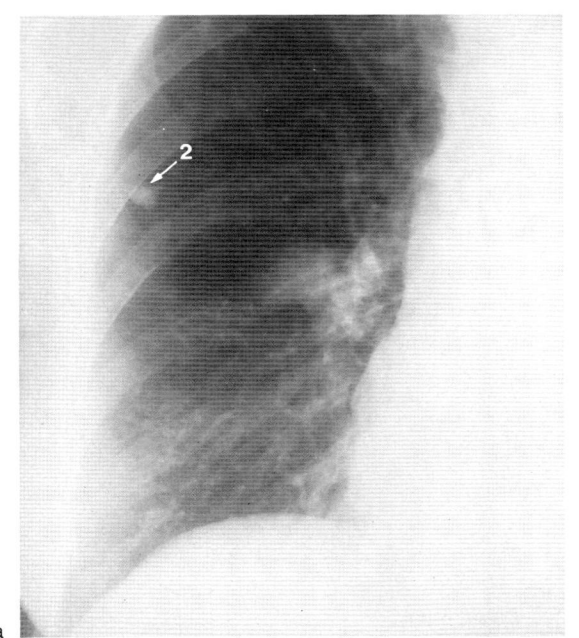

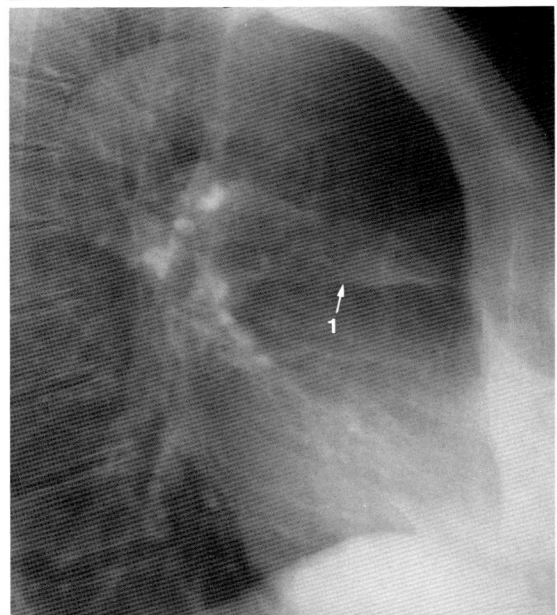

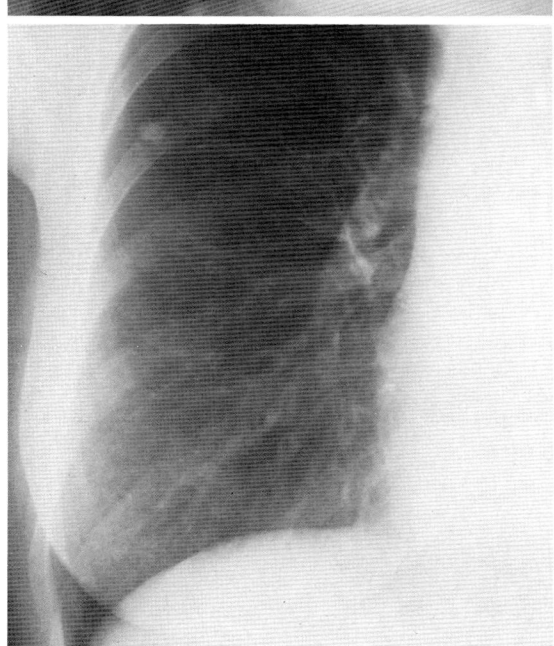

Fig. 2.8 a–c **Pneumonia in anterior segment of right upper lobe.**
61-year-old woman.

Rounded ill-defined opacity lateral to the hilus on the frontal view. It abuts on the minor fissure in the lateral view (1), calcified granuloma (2). Opacity cleared within a week without therapy.

Fig. 2.9 a–c   **Pneumonia in anterior segment of right upper lobe.**
Febrile patient.

Homogeneous opacity inferiorly marginated by the minor fissure (1), right major fissure (2), left major fissure (3), posterior tracheal wall (4). Pneumonia cleared within a week after antibiotic therapy.

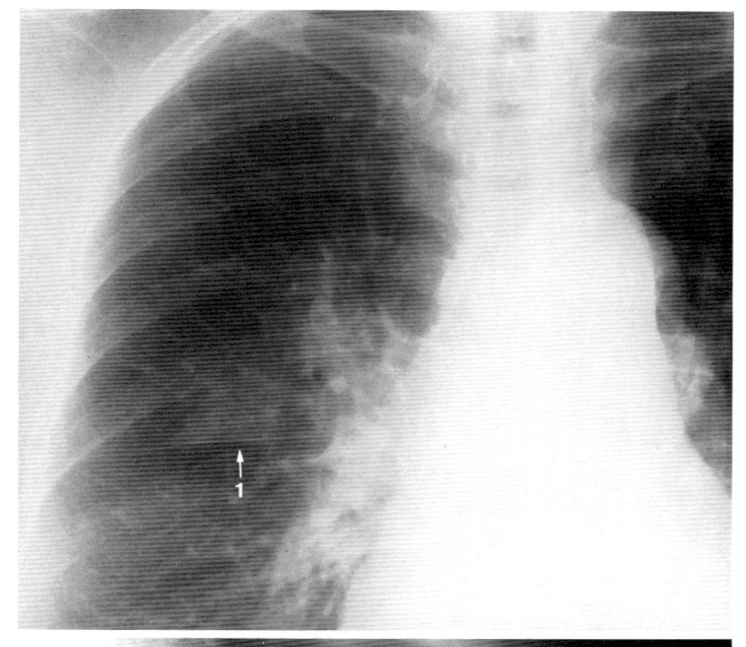

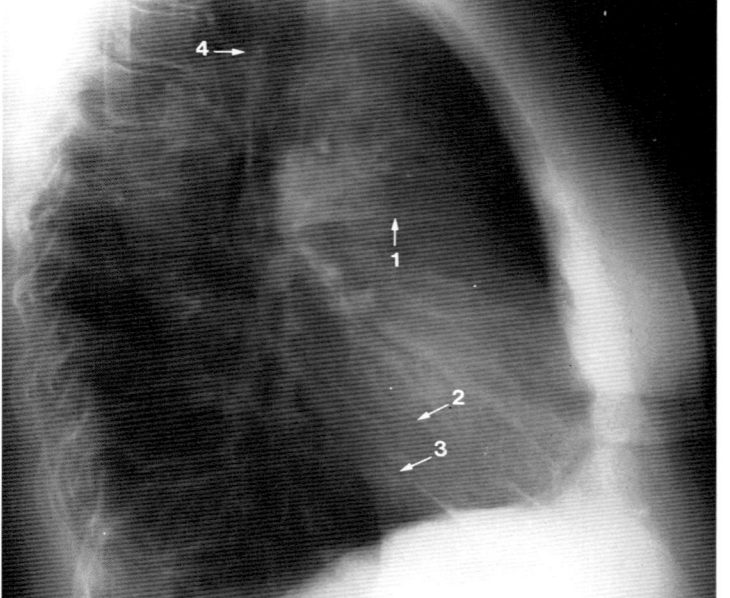

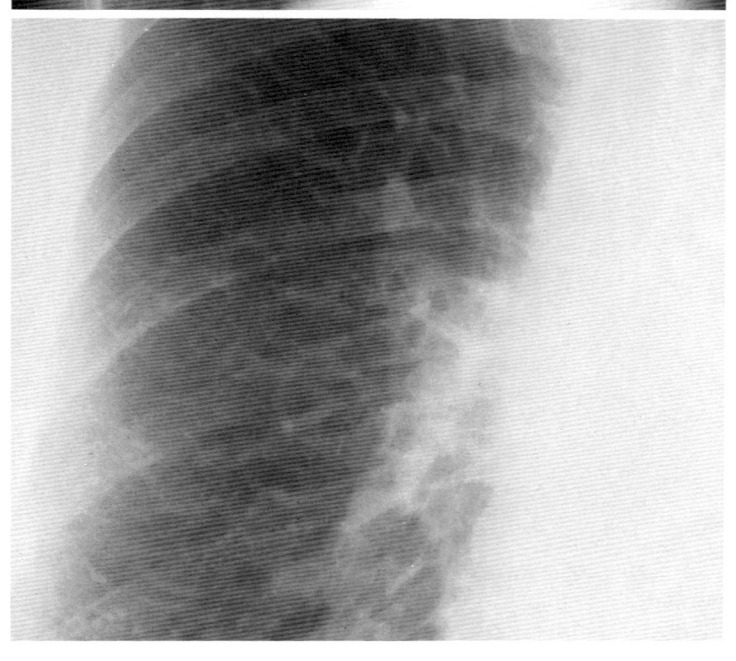

Bronchopneumonia

This is the most common form of pneumonia encountered in the hospital. The inflammation begins in the terminal and respiratory bronchioles rather than in the alveoli. It leads to necrotizing broncholitis and subsequent inflammation in the adjacent lung parenchyma. The process reaches the alveoli via the canals of Lambert, which connect the terminal bronchioles with the alveoli. Peribronchiolar foci of inflammation can encompass secondary lobules. The interlobular septa contain the spread of the inflammatory process even when microabscesses are formed. Bronchopneumonia is frequently multifocal, with well-aerated lung portions separating consolidated lung regions. On radiographs, the initial picture is that of a multifocal, patchy, even nodular process with a tendency for confluence in later stages.

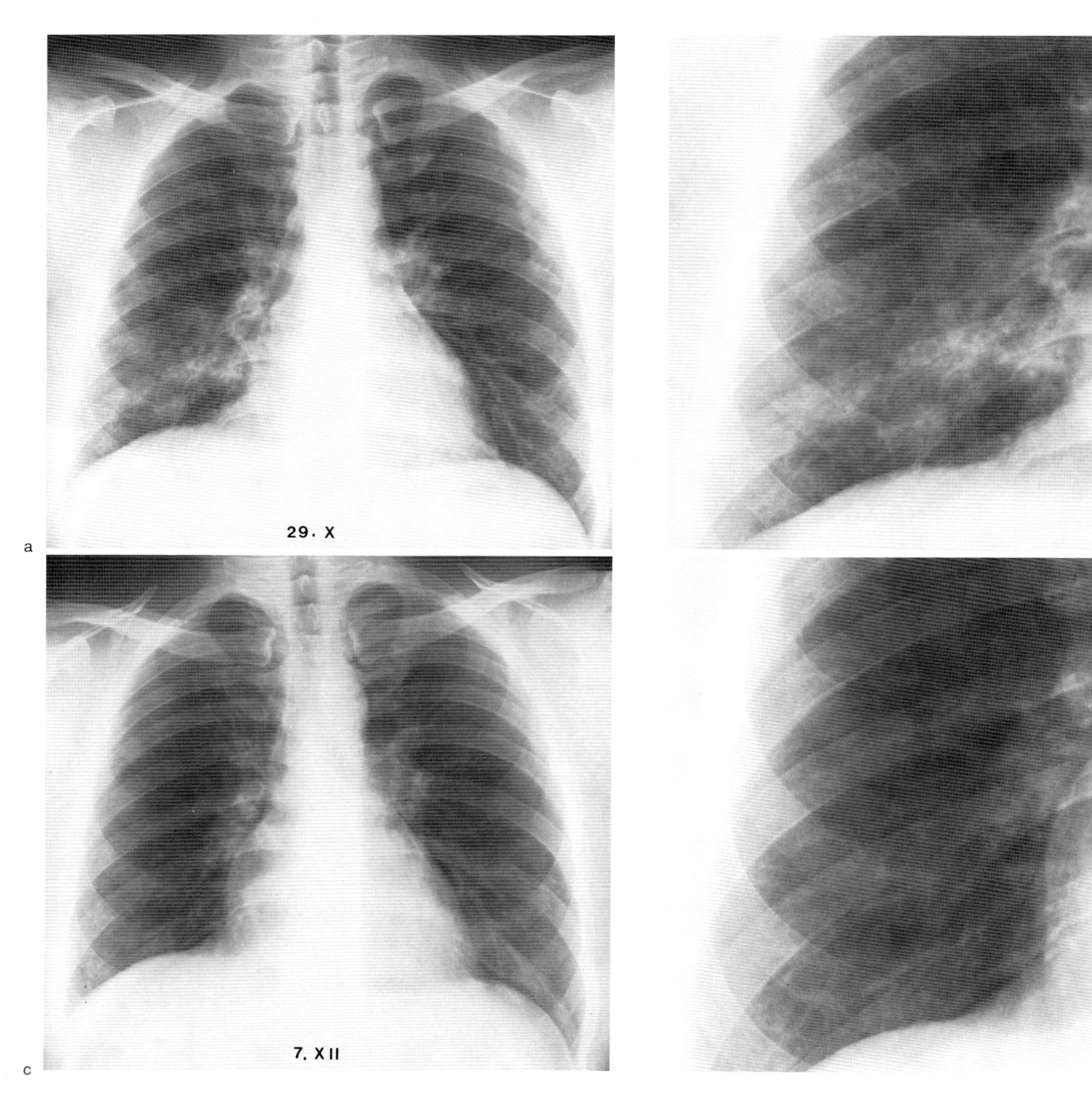

Fig. 2.10 a–d **Bronchopneumonia.**
29-year-old man with acute onset of fever and rapid response to antibiotic therapy. Patchy consolidation in right lower lung (a, b); obliteration of right heart border and right lower lobe pulmonary artery localize the pneumonia to the medial segment of the middle and lower lobes. Clearing on follow-up films (c, d).

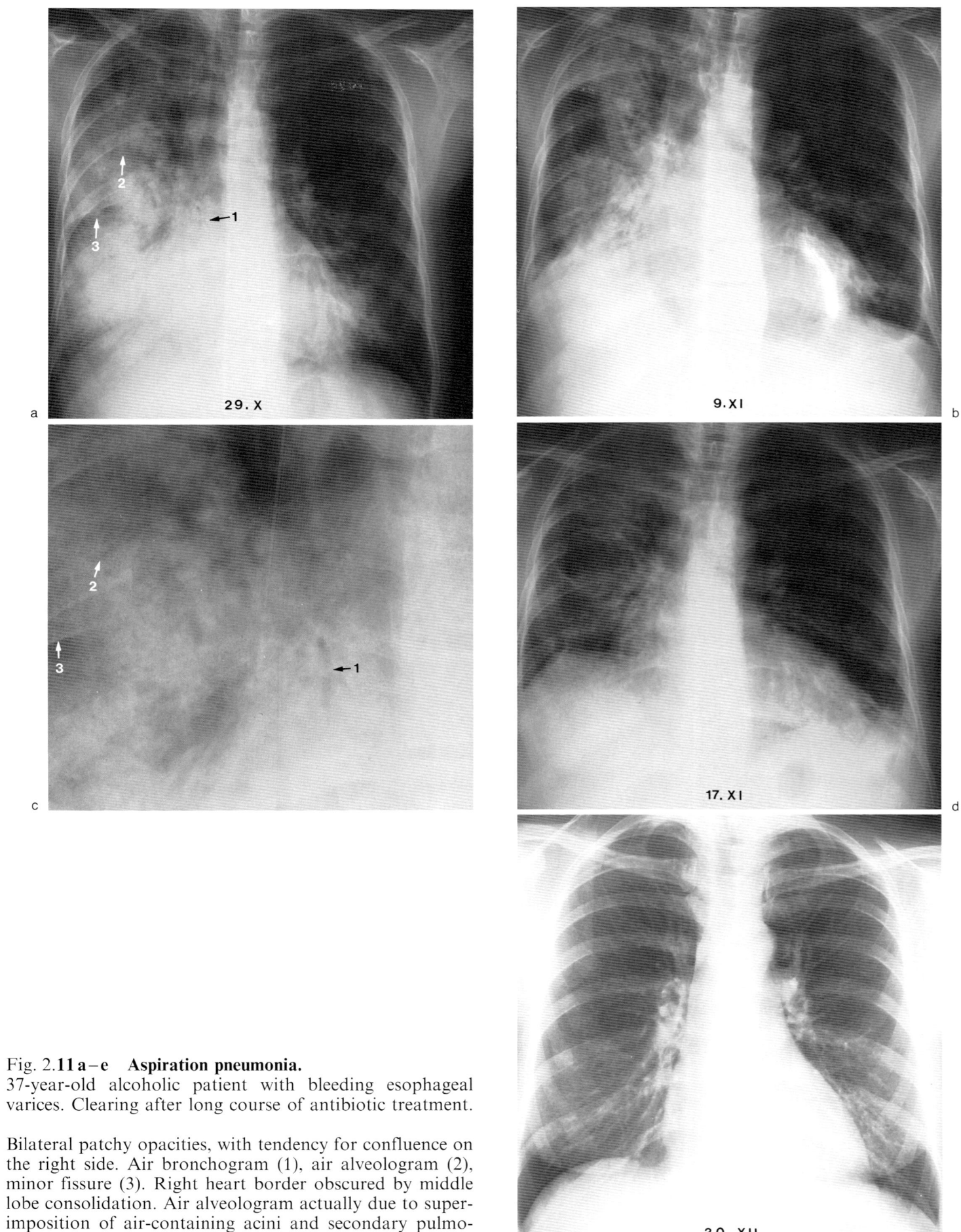

Pneumonia

Fig. 2.11 a–e Aspiration pneumonia.
37-year-old alcoholic patient with bleeding esophageal varices. Clearing after long course of antibiotic treatment.

Bilateral patchy opacities, with tendency for confluence on the right side. Air bronchogram (1), air alveologram (2), minor fissure (3). Right heart border obscured by middle lobe consolidation. Air alveologram actually due to superimposition of air-containing acini and secondary pulmonary lobules rather than alveoli.

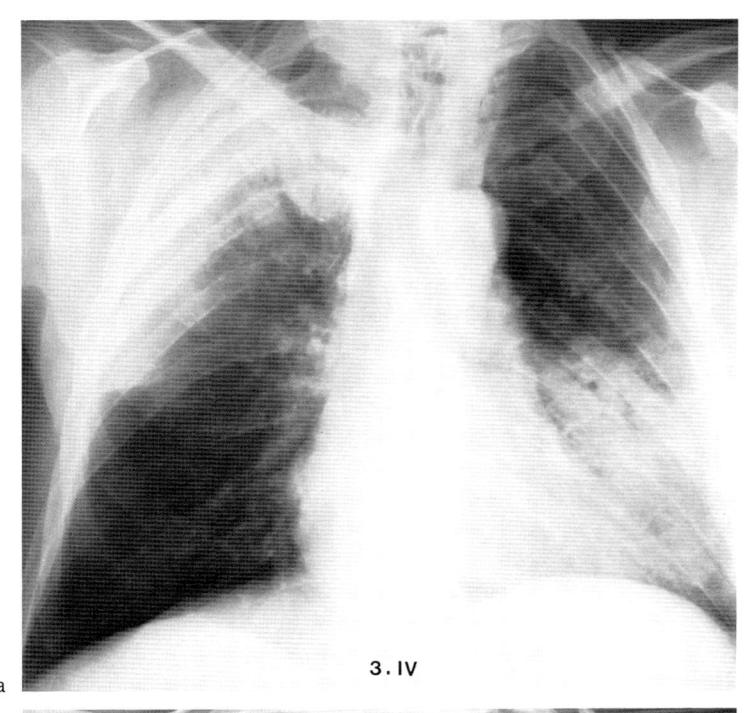

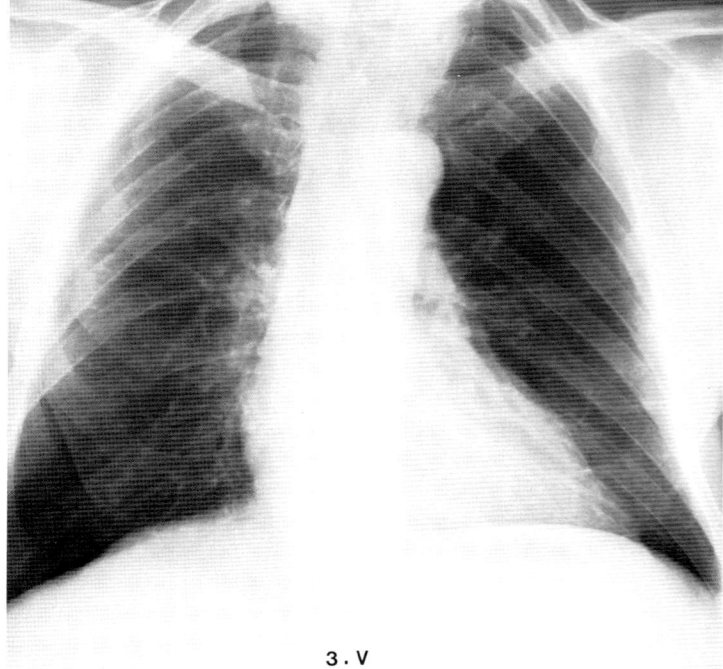

Fig. 2.12 a, b Bilateral pneumonia.
25-year-old woman with Gram-negative pneumonia. Clearing after antibiotic therapy.

Confluent opacities in right upper lobe and lingula. Note obscuration of left heart border.

Fig. 2.**13** **Bronchopneumonia.**
74-year-old patient with left ventricular failure.

Right middle and lower lobe consolidation. Distended upper lobe vessels (1) due to cephalization of pulmonary vascular flow.

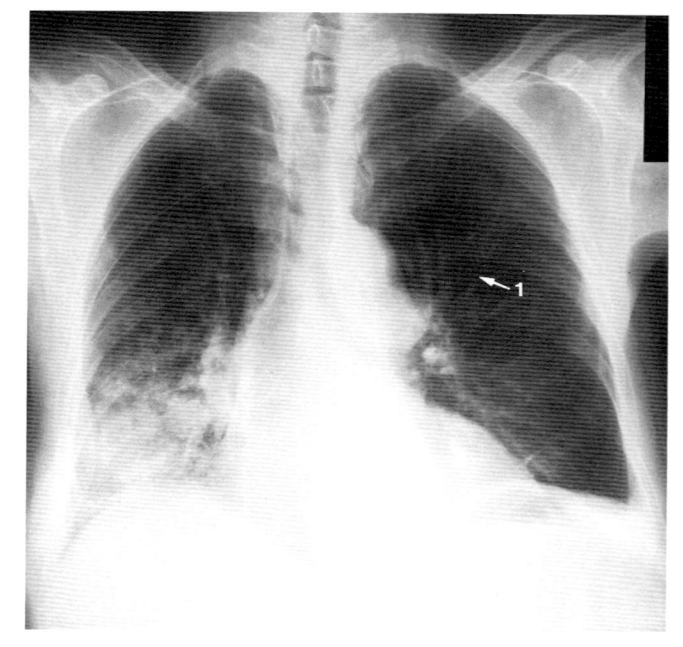

Fig. 2.**14** **Influenza pneumonia.**
24-year-old man with signs and symptoms of influenza.

Diffuse consolidation of entire right lung and of superior segment, left lower lobe, obscuring the left lower lobe pulmonary artery.

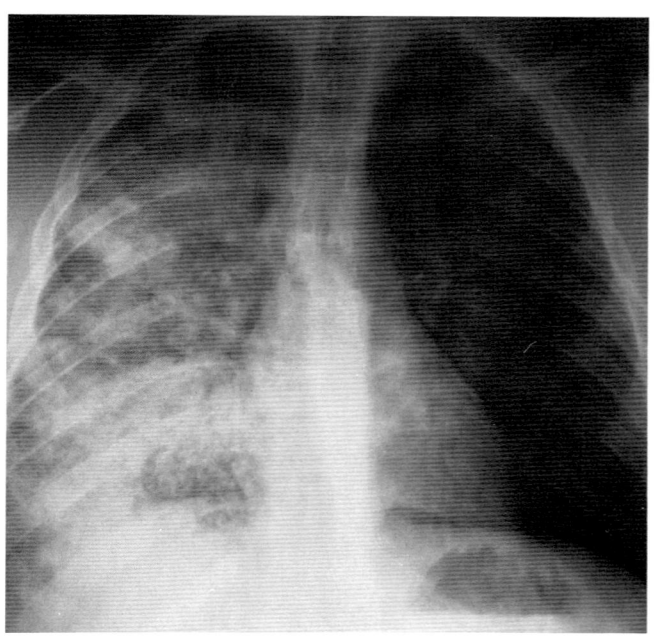

Fig. 2.**15** **Pneumonia.**
65-year-old patient.

Streaky opacification of left mid-lung with slight decrease in aeration of left lung. Right apical fibrosis related to previous postprimary tuberculosis (1).

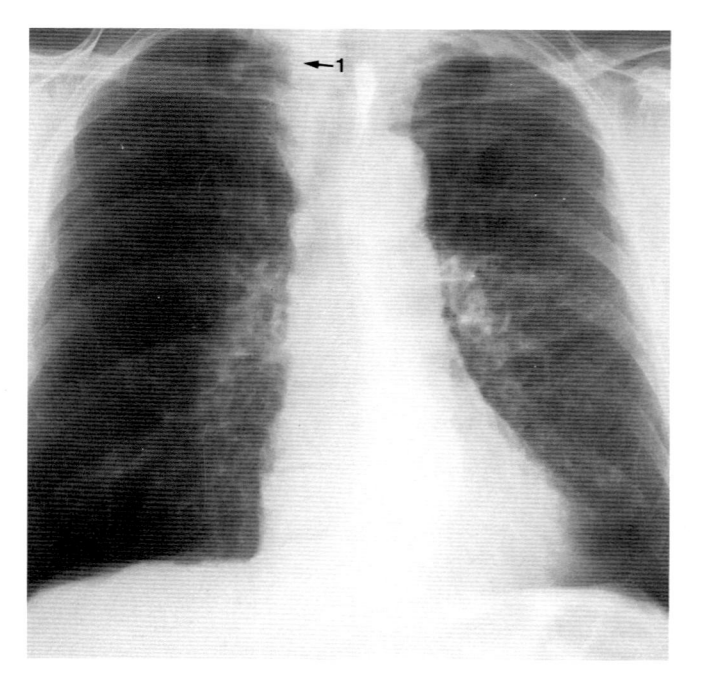

Interstitial Pneumonias

Acute interstitial pneumonias are relatively common and represent transient, reversible, pulmonary, inflammatory processes. The inciting organisms are usually mycoplasma, *Pneumocystis carinii*, viral infections, and rarely rickettsiae. The inflammatory process originates in the bronchial wall and then infiltrates the interlobular septae and the alveoli. The radiologic correlate of these pathologic findings is linear, reticular markings as well as ground glass opacification of the lung, preferentially involving the perihilar regions and the lung bases. A clear differentiation from bronchopneumonia is not always possible on radiological grounds.

References: 131, 142.

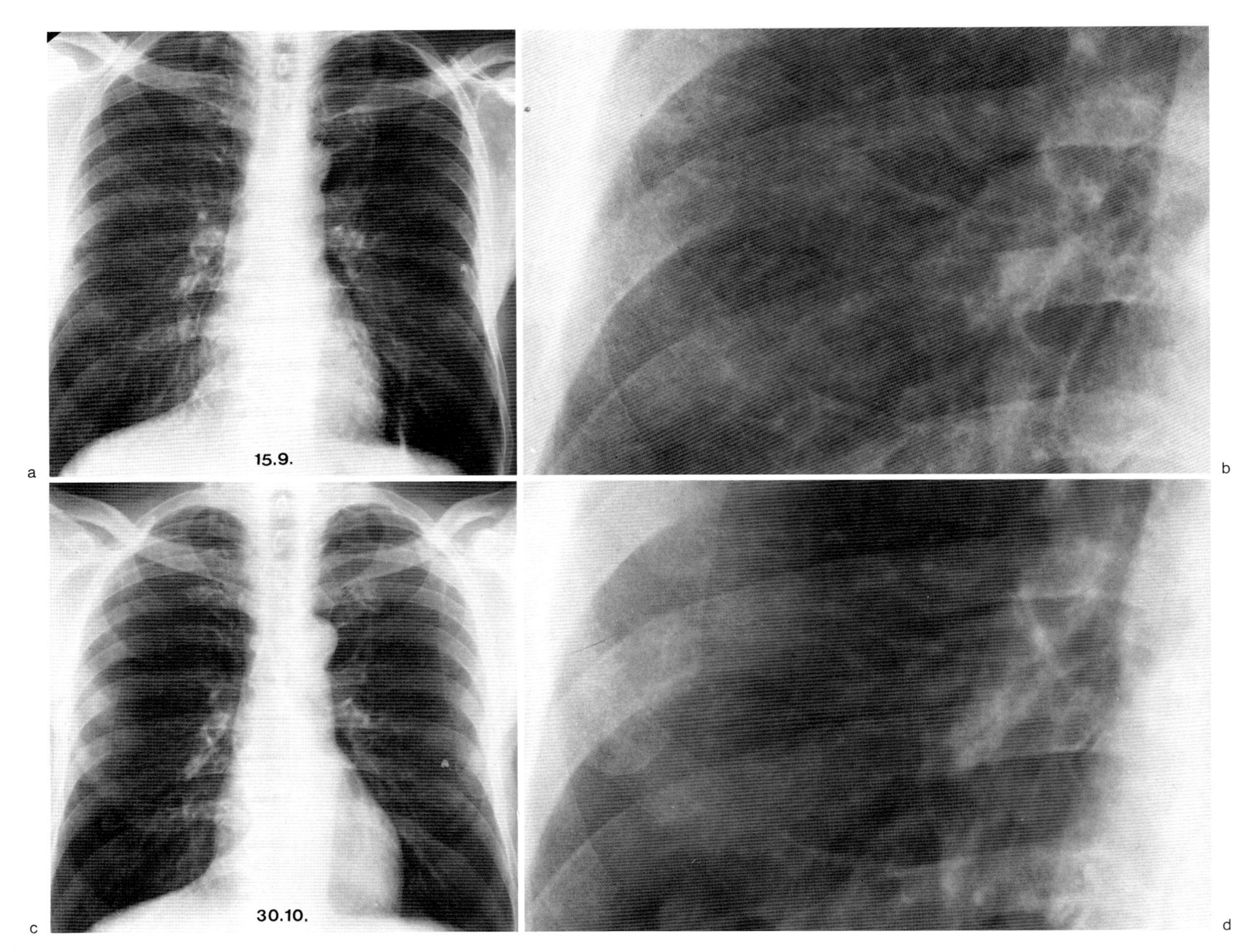

Fig. 2.16 a–d **Interstitial pneumonia.**
59-year-old patient with proven *Mycoplasma* pneumonia. Diffuse reticulonodular opacities throughout both lungs (**a, b**). Follow-up examination 6 weeks later shows complete clearing (**c, d**).

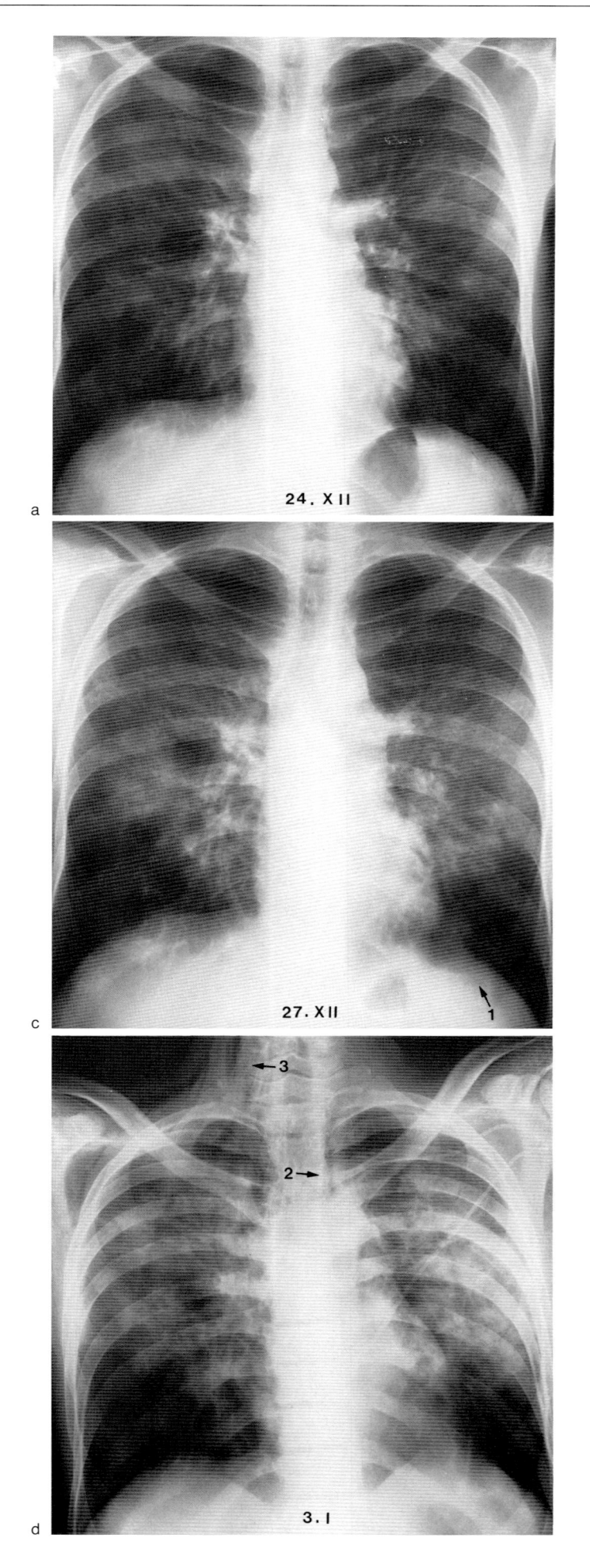

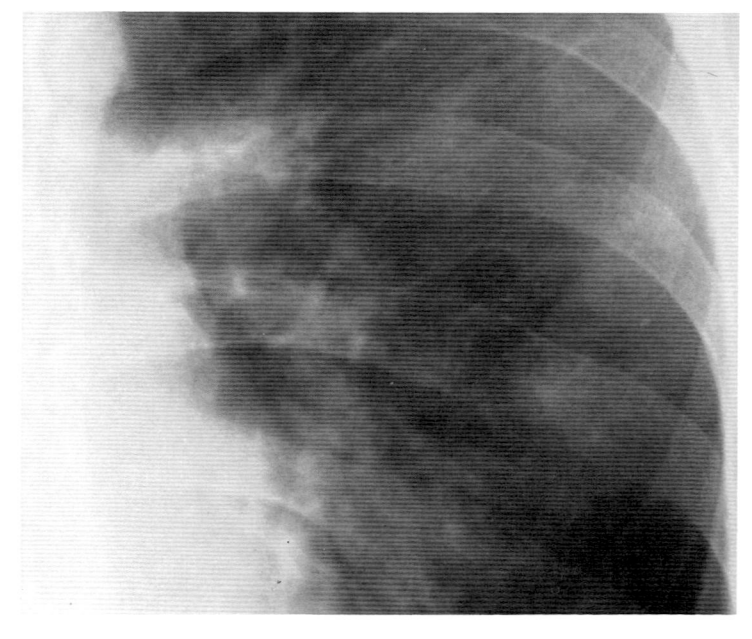

Fig. 2.**17 a–d** *Pneumocystis carinii* **pneumonia.**
23-year-old patient after bone marrow transplant for chronic myelogenous leukemia.

Bilateral, perihilar, ground-glass opacification, sparing the apices and the costophrenic sulci. Progressive obliteration of diaphragmatic contour (1), pneumomediastinum (2), deep cervical emphysema (3), and subcutaneous emphysema.

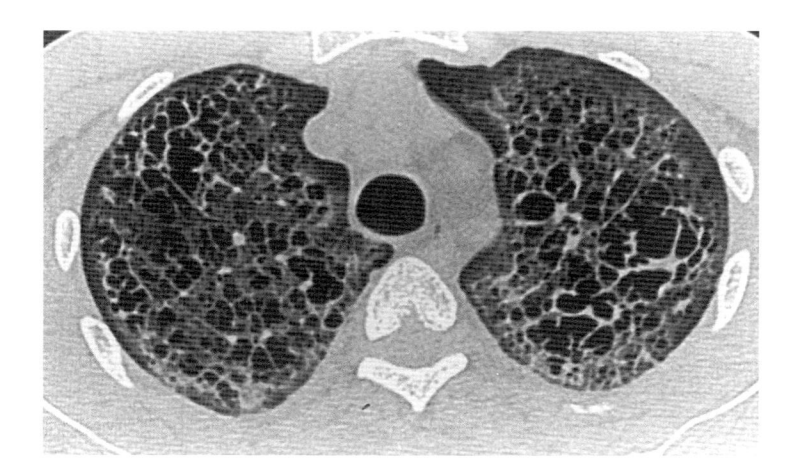

Fig. 2.18 Cystic pneumocystis carinii pneumonia in AIDS patient.
Multiple small cystic spaces representing pneumatoceles and possibly small abscesses as well as premature emphysema are well seen on high-resolution CT. Some of these cysts can resolve spontaneously over time.

Chickenpox Pneumonia

Children with chickenpox develop a pneumonia in less than 1% of cases. In adults with varicella, pneumonia develops in 10% of cases, with a 10% mortality. Pregnant women and immunocompromised patients are at particular risk. The histologic picture consists of an interstitial monocytic infiltration and hemorrhagic alveolar exudate with foci of necrosis. The radiologic picture consists of multiple, ill-defined, so-called acinar nodules 5–10 mm in diameter on a background of reticular opacities. Years later, the necrotic foci can calcify and produce multiple, nodular calcifications in the lung. Multiple calcifications can also be seen in histoplasmosis and rarely in tuberculosis, silicosis, and berylliosis.

References: 89, 102.

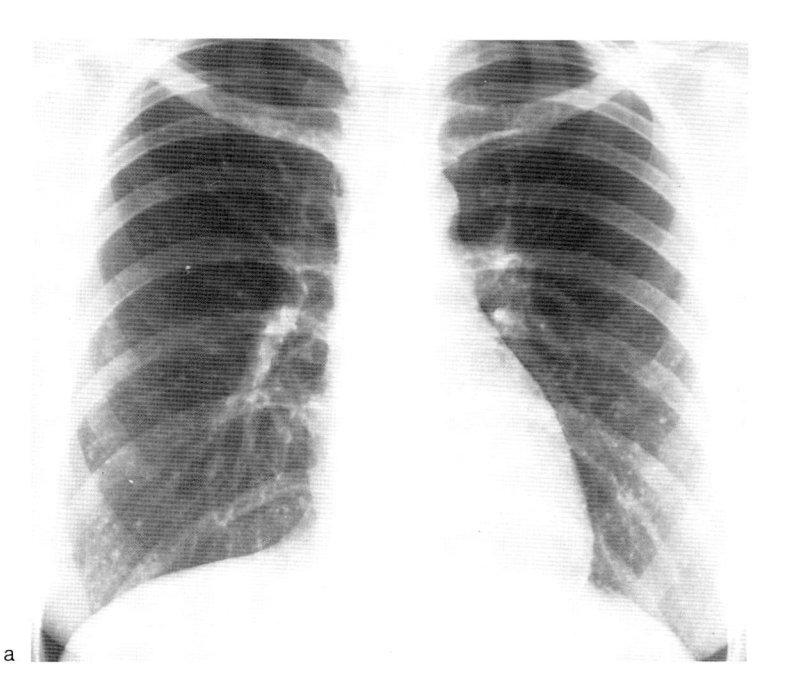

Fig. 2.19 a, b **Healed varicella pneumonia.**
Fourteen years after acute infection. Multiple small pulmonary calcifications.

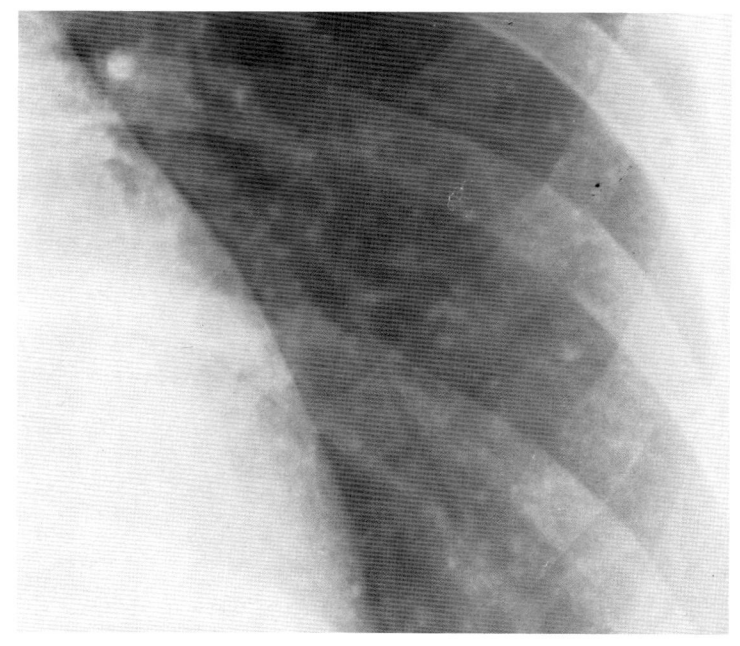

Pneumonia 43

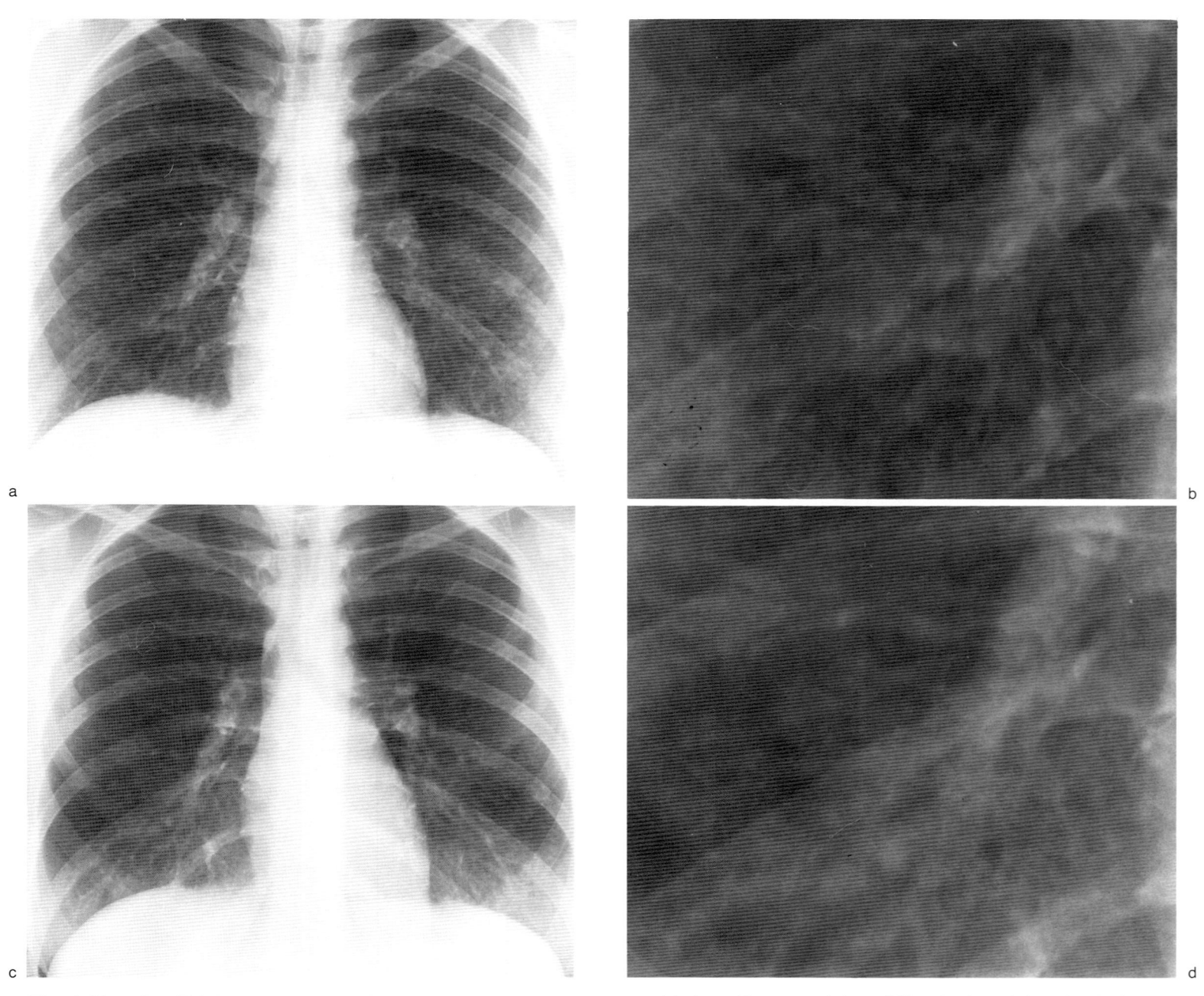

Fig. 2.20 a–d **Chickenpox pneumonia.**
Sequential radiographs of a 33-year-old diabetic patient.
Multiple miliary nodules diffusely involving both lungs. Marked improvement within 3 weeks.

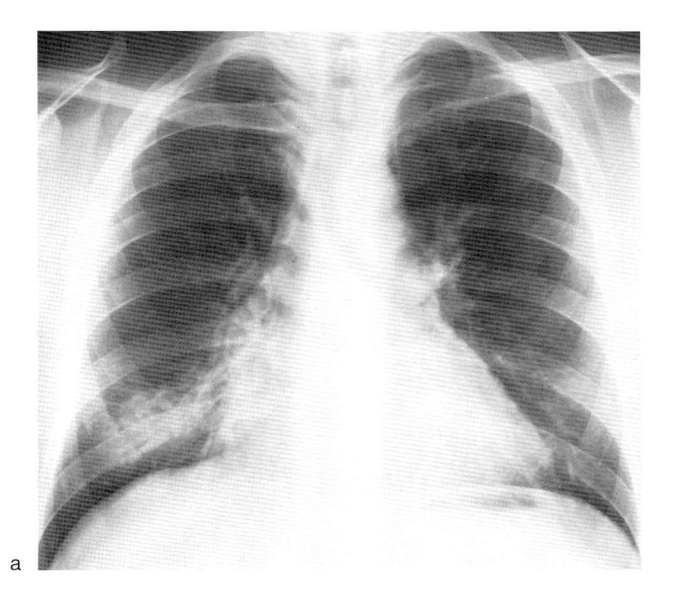

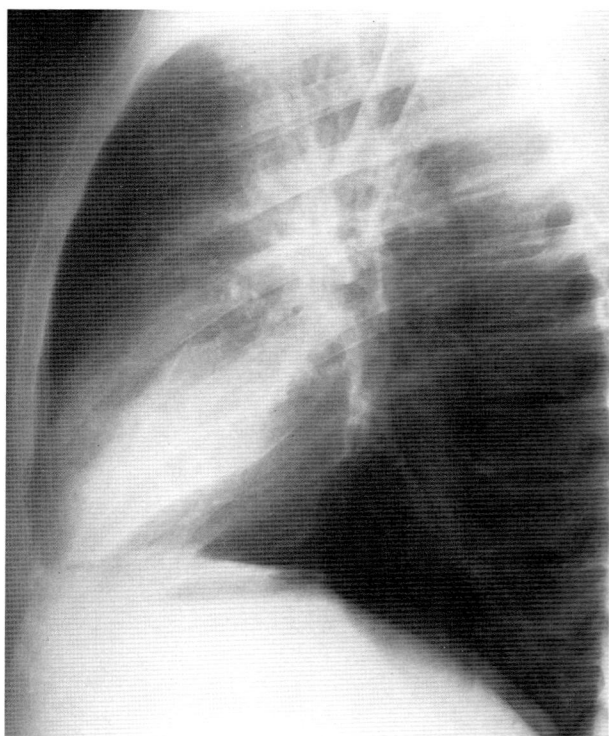

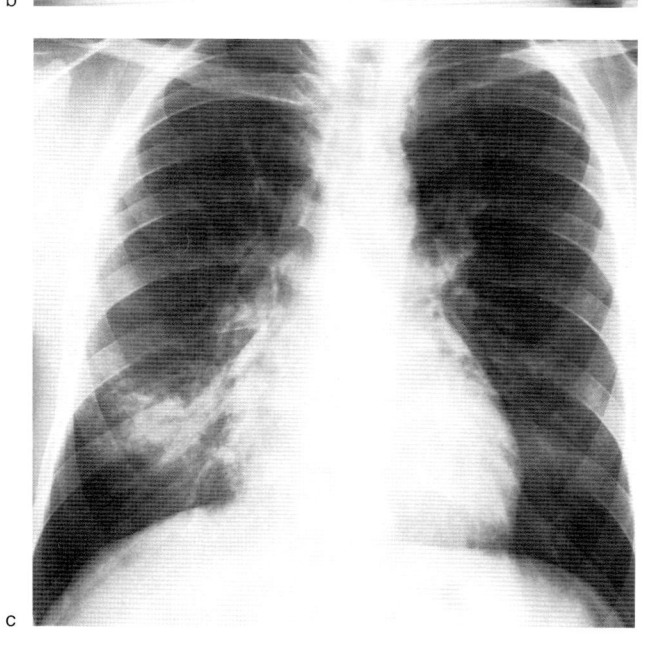

Chronic organizing Pneumonia

In the vast majority of cases, acute pneumonias resolve completely and clear without leaving any residues. Infrequently, the resorption of the exudate occurs incompletely, leading to the organization and eventual fibrosis of the lung parenchyma. Pathological examination reveals a solid, "carnified" lung. Radiologic features include linear, irregular, or even rounded opacities that persist unchanged over many years. Follow-up films are important to exclude an active inflammatory or neoplastic process.

Fig. 2.21 a–c **Chronic organizing pneumonia.**
53-year-old patient. Oval, streaky opacity in right middle lobe, unchanged over 7 years. Residue of an acute pneumonia, 4 years prior to current examination.

Lung Abscess and Necrotizing Pneumonia

Lung abscesses represent a circumscribed, necrotizing, inflammatory process in the lung parenchyma, which lead to pus formation. An abscess cavity forms if the pus is expectorated through a communicating bronchus. Abscesses can result from (1) aspiration of anaerobic mouth flora in persons with poor mouth hygiene, (2) poststenotic pneumonia with necrosis, (3) necrotizing *Staphylococcal* or gram-negative pneumonia, (4) septic embolization. Radiologic features include initially ill-defined, large opacities, with subsequent demarcation towards the adjacent normal lung and eventual cavitation with or without gas-fluid levels. Gas-forming bacteria can occassionally produce small gas bubbles, but these do not usually account for the gas-fluid levels; the latter are proof of communication with the bronchial tree.

The differential diagnosis includes cavitating tumors, tuberculous cavities, and cystic bronchiectases. Lung gangrene is usually the result of Gram-negative or anaerobic infections leading to multiple confluent abscesses with the eventual necrosis of an entire segment of lobe which sloughs off and can produce a mass effect or float within a giant cavity. In such cases, conservative therapy can be attempted, though in some patients surgical resection of the necrotic lung is necessary.

References: 146.

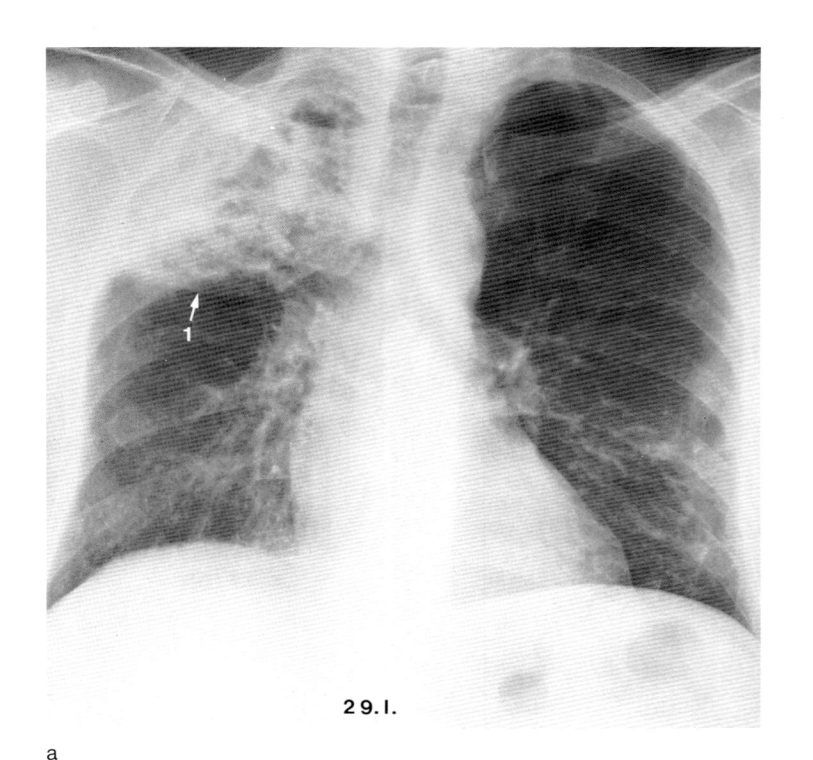

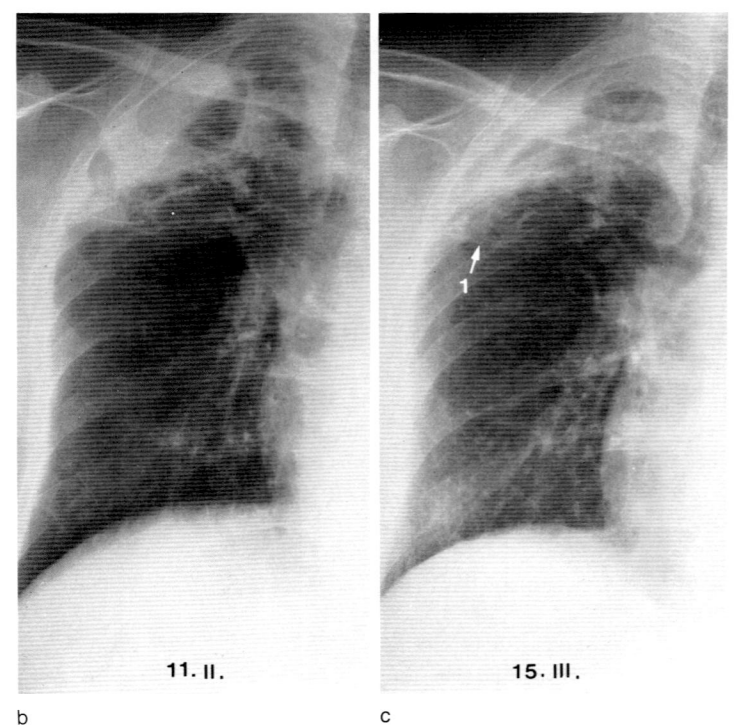

Fig. 2.22 a–c **Necrotizing pneumonia.**
50-year-old patient with *E. coli* in sputum.

Near complete opacification of the right upper lobe with multiple, small cavities (**a**). After 13 days (**b**), confluence of cavities as well as retraction of minor fissure cephalad. After 5 weeks (**c**), cicatrization atelectasis with residual cavity. Minor fissure (1) retracted upwards.

46   2. Infections

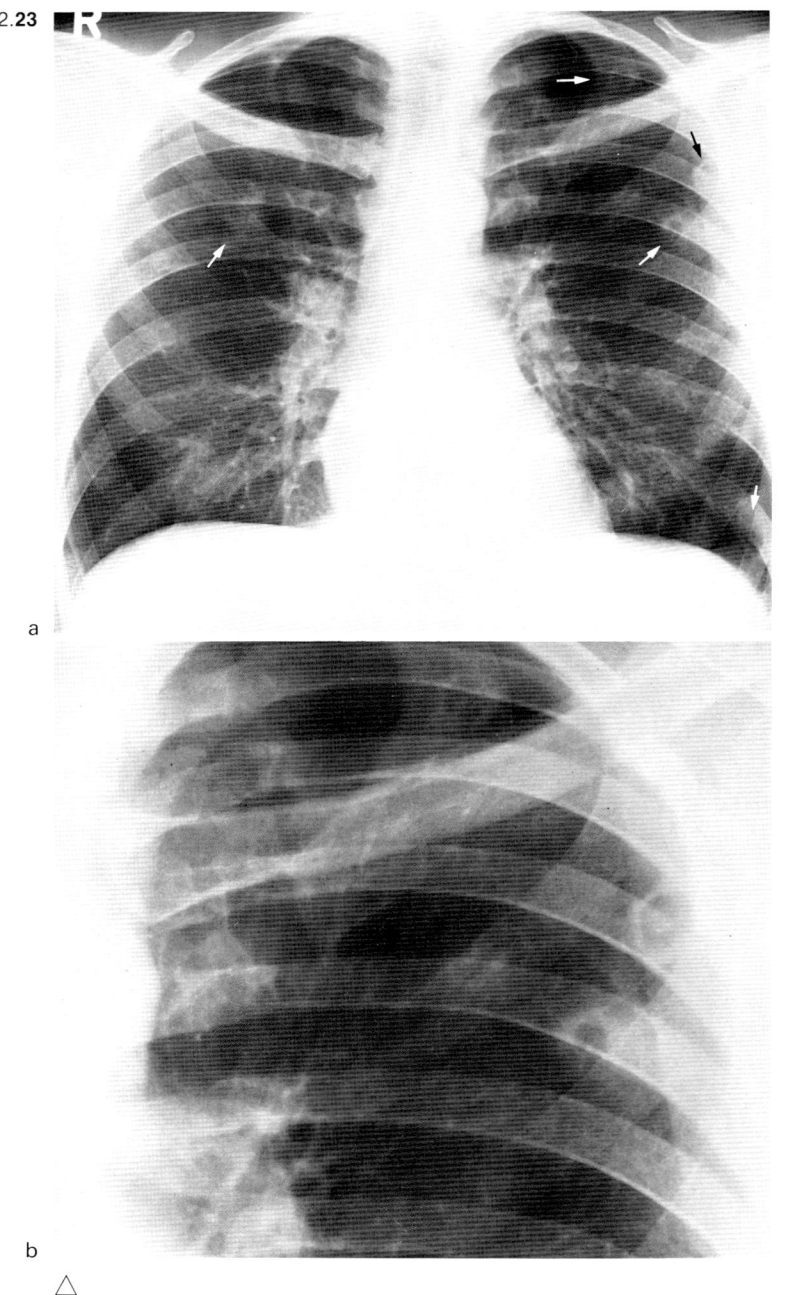

Fig. 2.23a, b   **Septic embolization.**
29-year-old man with postanginal sepsis.

Multiple, bilateral, thin-walled, cavitating, pulmonary nodules.

Fig. 2.24a–c   **Necrotizing pneumonia.**
57-year-old patient with multiple sclerosis and multiple episodes of aspiration.

Multifocal consolidation of both lower lobes, with areas of cavitation. Note gas-fluid level (1) and pleural effusion. Slight improvement after antibiotic therapy. Partial right lower lobe atelectasis accounts for rightward shift of anterior junction line (2).

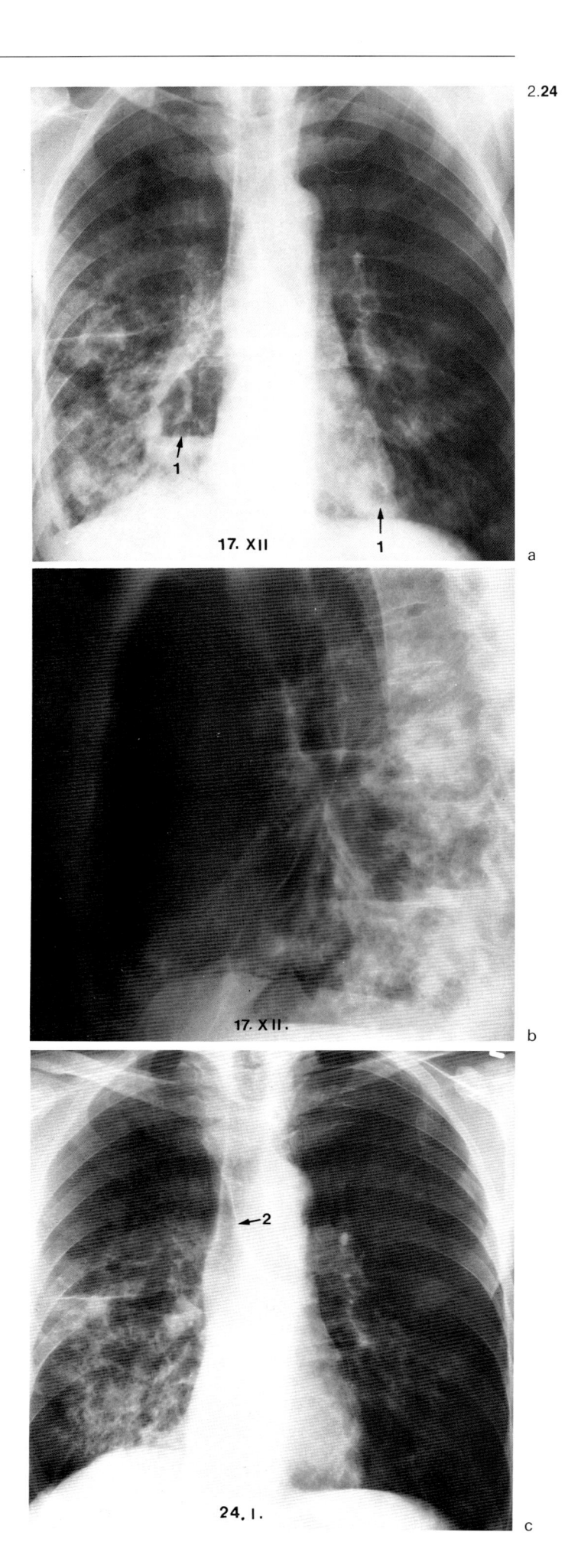

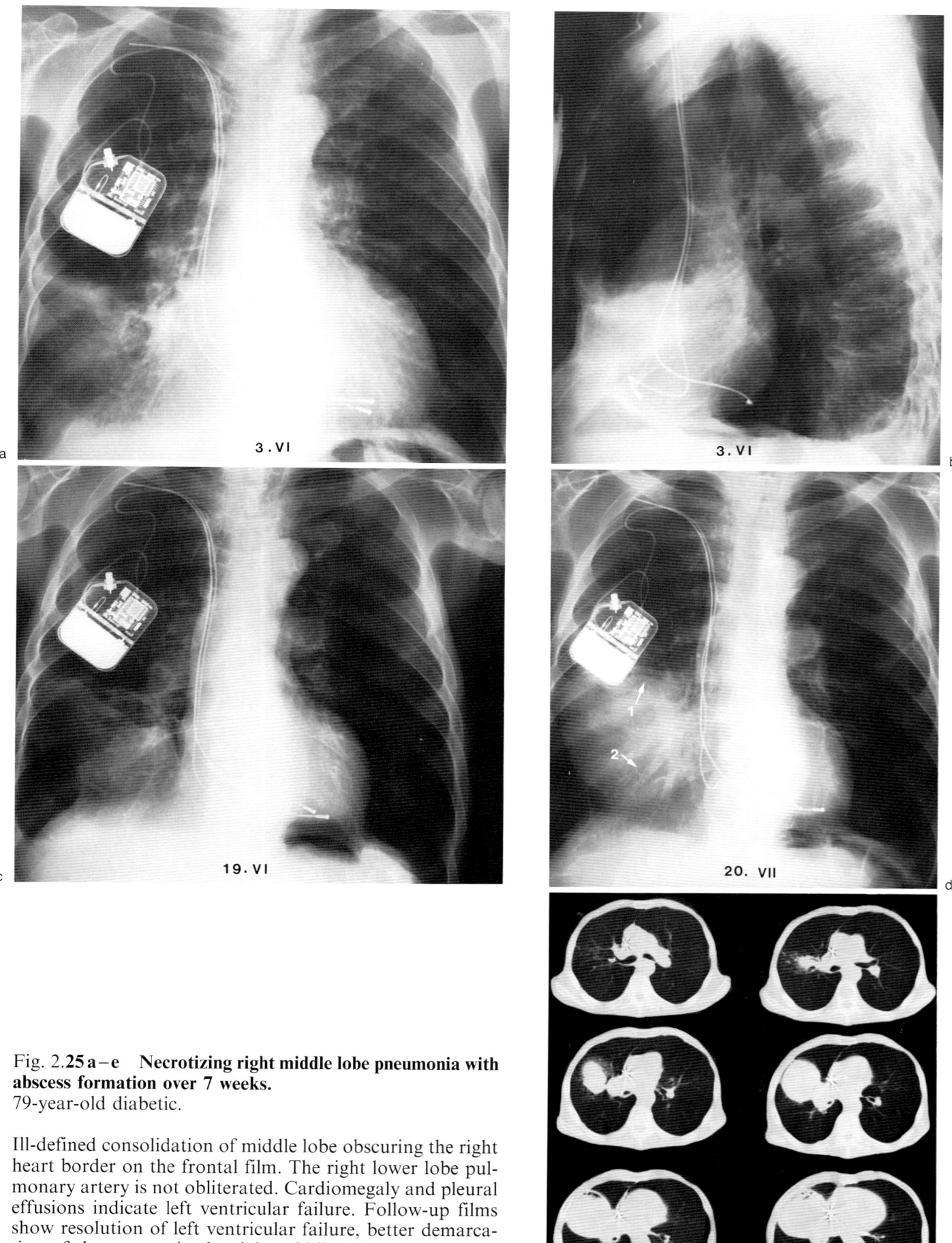

Pneumonia 47

Fig. 2.**25 a–e Necrotizing right middle lobe pneumonia with abscess formation over 7 weeks.**
79-year-old diabetic.

Ill-defined consolidation of middle lobe obscuring the right heart border on the frontal film. The right lower lobe pulmonary artery is not obliterated. Cardiomegaly and pleural effusions indicate left ventricular failure. Follow-up films show resolution of left ventricular failure, better demarcation of the process in the right middle lobe with eventual cavitation and gas-fluid level formation. Abscess cleared after 4 months.

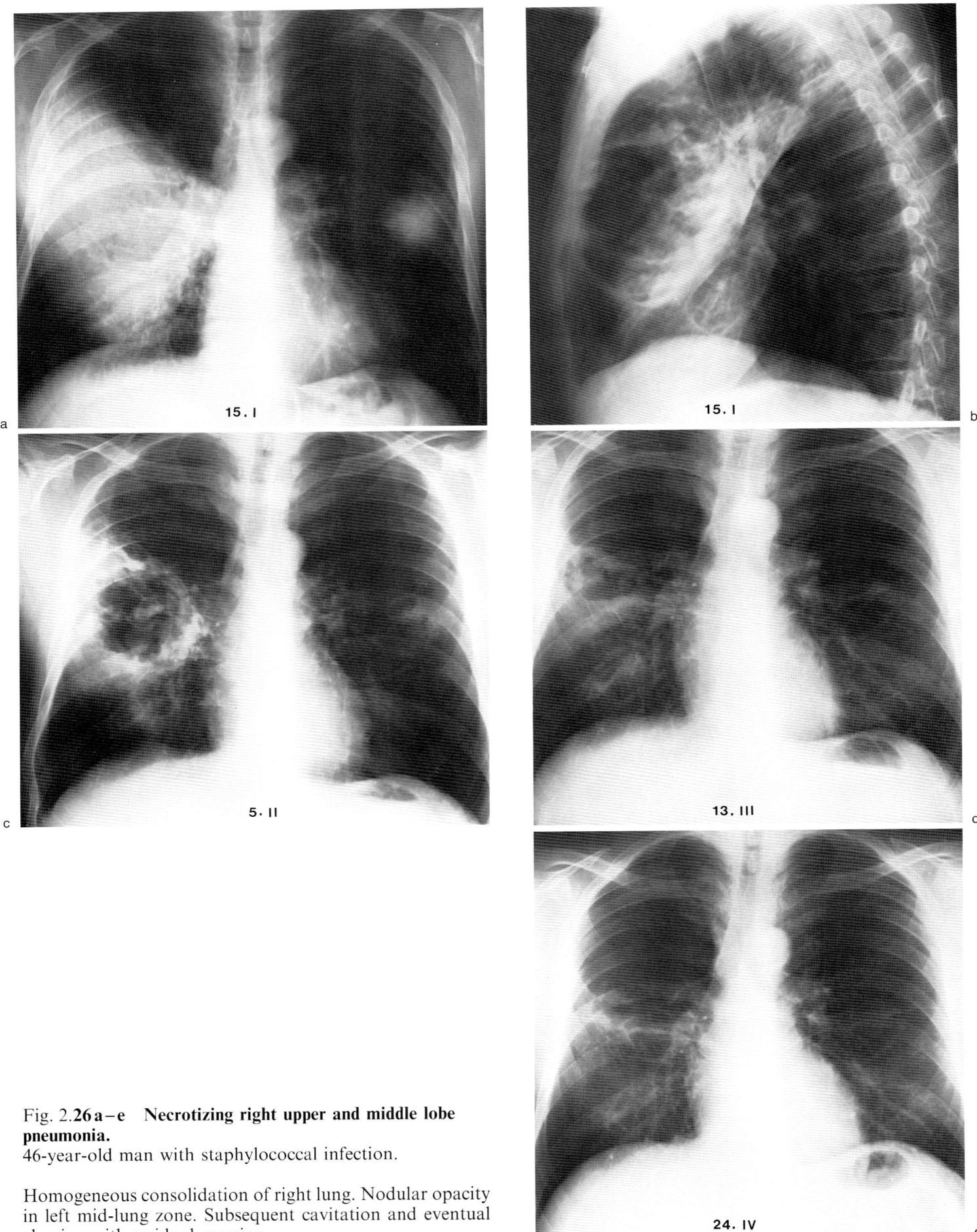

Fig. 2.26 a–e Necrotizing right upper and middle lobe pneumonia.
46-year-old man with staphylococcal infection.

Homogeneous consolidation of right lung. Nodular opacity in left mid-lung zone. Subsequent cavitation and eventual clearing with residual scarring.

Tuberculosis

Tuberculosis results from an infection with *Mycobacterium tuberculosis* and manifests with pulmonary involvement in over 90% of symptomatic cases. The incidence of tuberculosis has dropped continuously in the USA at a rate of 5–7% per year until 1985 when a reversal of this trend was recorded for the first time in 50 years. This is a direct result of an increased incidence of tuberculosis in human immunodeficiency virus (HIV)-infected individuals. Other immuncompromised persons, particularly alcoholics, drug abusers, inmates of prisons or nursing homes, and young physicians are at increased risk of acquiring tuberculosis. In Third World countries, the disease is highly prevalent. Table 2.1 provides the reader with a classification of the different stages of tuberculosis.

References: 6, 10, 19, 41, 81, 97.

Table 2.1 Classification of pulmonary tuberculosis

A. Primary tuberculosis
   Subpleural Ghon focus and Ranke complex including regional lymphadenitis.
B. Hematogemous dissemination
   – Miliary tuberculosis
   – Simon's apical foci
   – Sepsis tuberculosa Landouzy
C. Postprimary (reactivation) tuberculosis
   – Acinous-nodous apical disease
   – Aschoff's coarse nodules in apices
   – Infraclavicular consolidation
   – Cavitary tuberculosis
   – Fibrocalcific, cicatrizing, destructive form

Primary Tuberculous Complex

After aerogenous infection, a subpleural, nonspecific alveolitis ensues, followed by a caseous focus (primary focus). Lymphangitis and lymphadenitis follow. This primary complex remains asymptomatic and heals without residues in well over 90% of cases. In children, the primary complex can lead to a persistent, symptomatic lymphadenitis. A primary tuberculous pneumonia can also develop and lead to early cavitation.

Tuberculous Pleurisy

Following the primary infection, a pleural effusion can form either due to subpleural tuberculous focus or due to hematogenous dissemination with granulomatous studding of the pleura. A large, unilateral, pleural effusion in a mildly symptomatic patient is typical. In only 30% can mycobacteria be cultured from the effusion. Pleural biopsy yields positive results in 60% of patients. These tuberculous pleural effusions can clear spontaneously, but these patients have a 60% chance of developing postprimary tuberculosis within 5 years, if not recognized and treated.

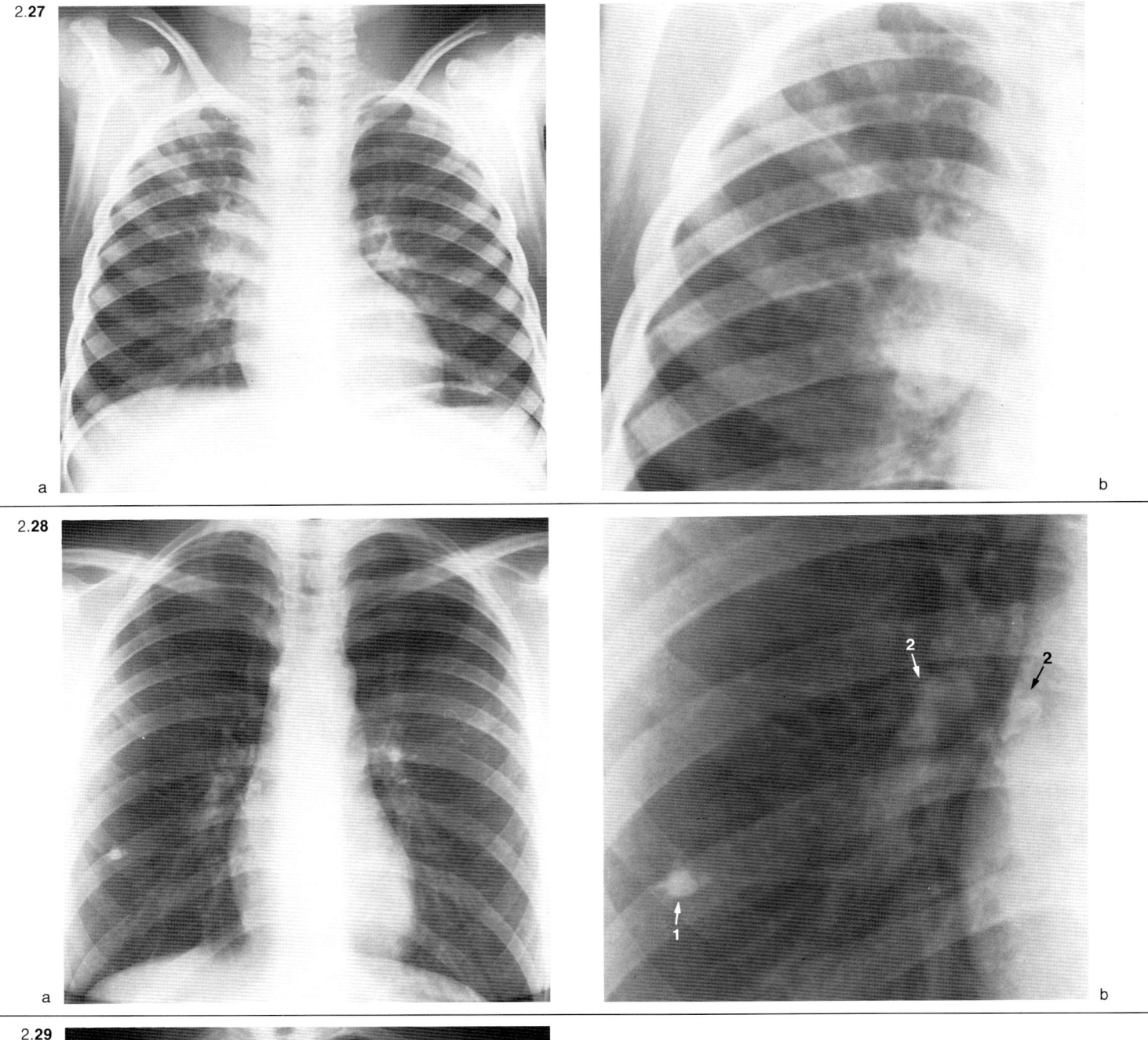

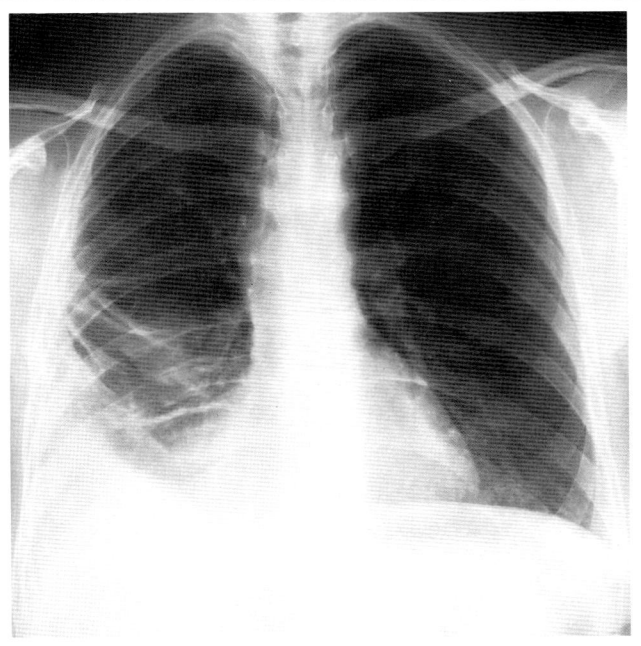

Fig. 2.27 a, b **Primary complex in asymptomatic child.**
Ill-defined opacity in right upper lobe with adjacent right hilar and right paratracheal lymph node enlargement.

Fig. 2.28 a, b **Calcified primary complex.**
Incidental finding in asymptomatic person. Calcified peripheral granuloma (1) and calcified hilar lymph nodes (2).

Fig. 2.29 **Tuberculous pleurisy.**
46-year-old man with fever. Right pleural effusion obliterating the right hemidiaphragm and the right costophrenic sulcus. Scar-like curvilinear opacities represent residues from previous thoracoscopy.

Miliary Tuberculosis

Miliary tuberculosis accounts for 1–2% of all cases of tuberculosis. Half of all patients are either children under 1 year of age or patients over 60 years of age. Close to 50% of cases of miliary tuberculosis as determined by autopsy were not suspected clinically. Pathologically, multiple, small, rounded opacities, 1–3 mm in diameter, permeate the entire lung. Due to complete or incomplete superimposition of shadows, the radiograph will show a micronodular or reticulonodular pattern.

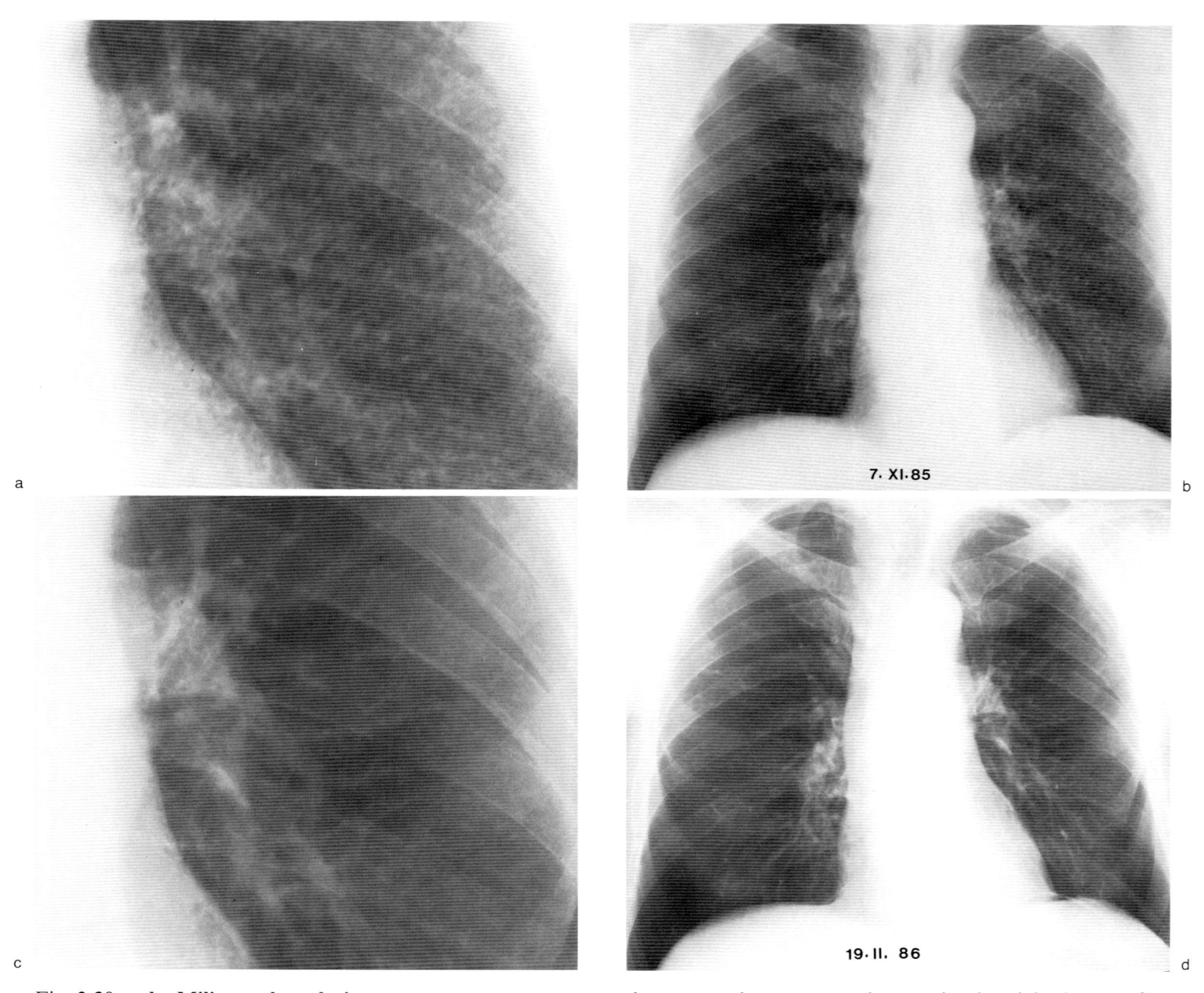

Fig. 2.30 a–d **Miliary tuberculosis.**
69-year-old man with worsening cough for 6 weeks. Micronodular and reticular pattern with asymmetric involvement due to emphysematous changes in the right lung. After 3 months of antituberculous chemotherapy, clearing of the miliary nodules is visible.

52   2. Infections

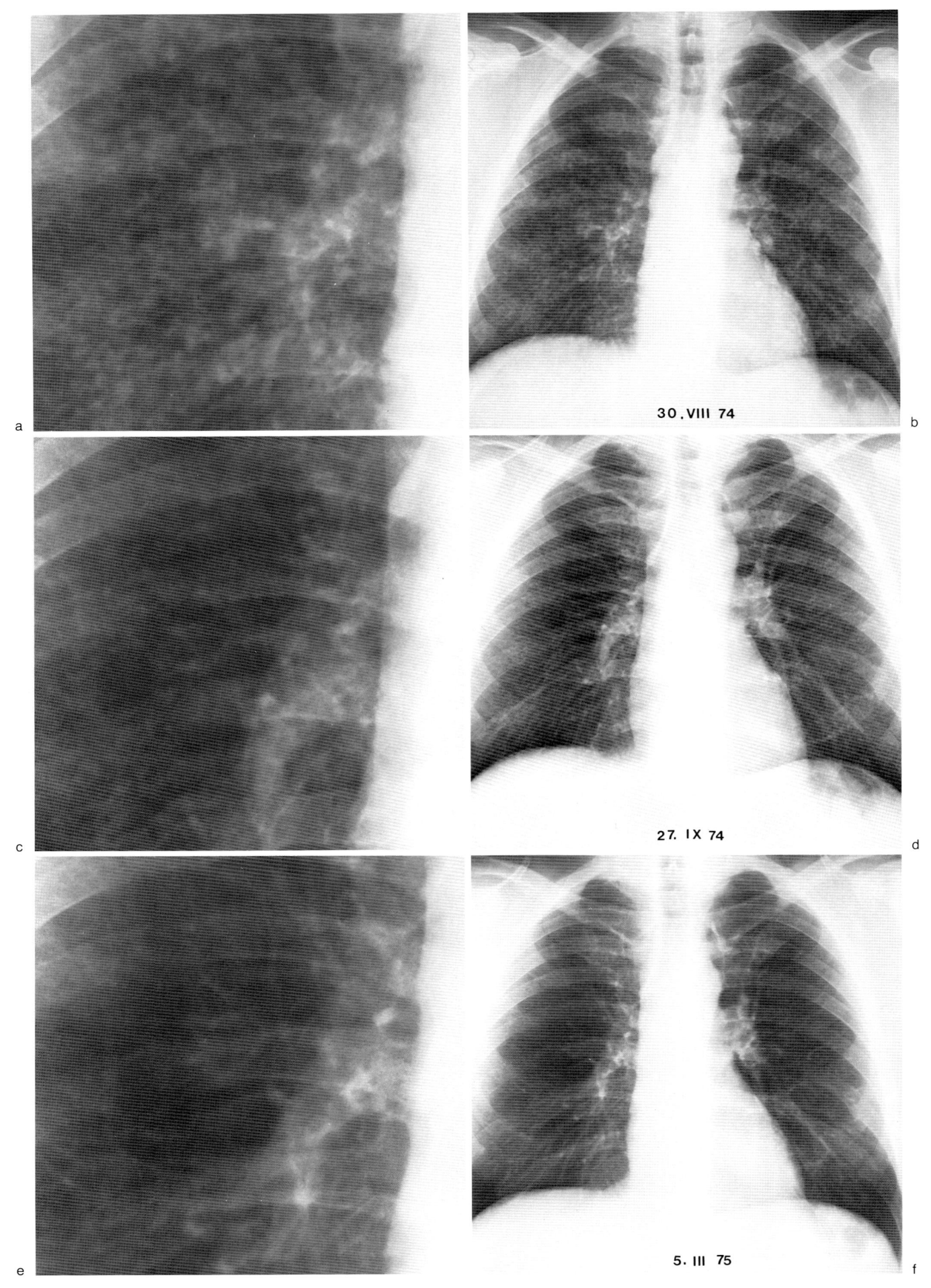

30. VIII 74

27. IX 74

5. III 75

Fig. 2.**31a–f**

◁ Fig. 2.**31 a–f Miliary tuberculosis.**
43-year-old woman complaining of weight loss and night sweat.

Disseminated miliary nodules scattered throughout both lungs, eventually clearing slightly after 1 month of chemotherapy and completely after 7 months of therapy.

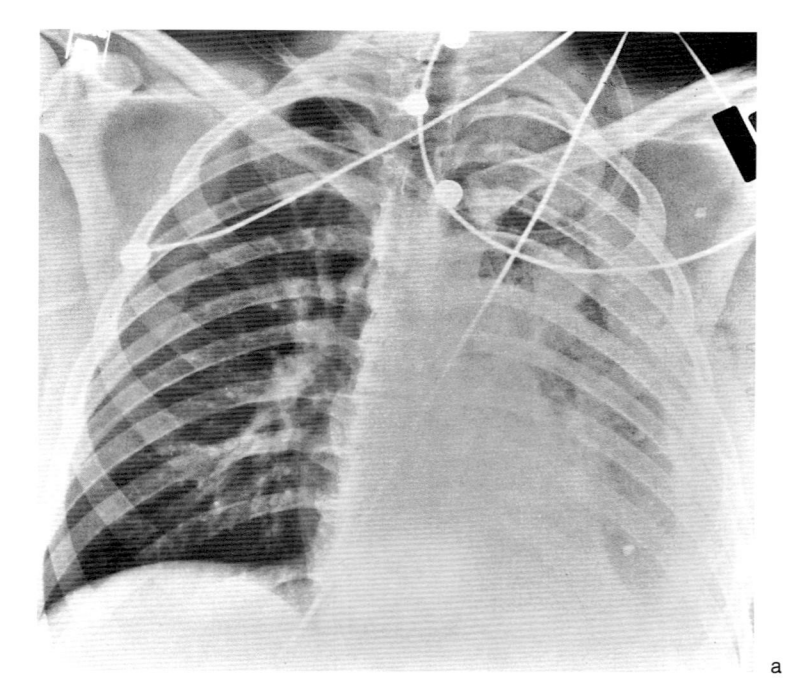

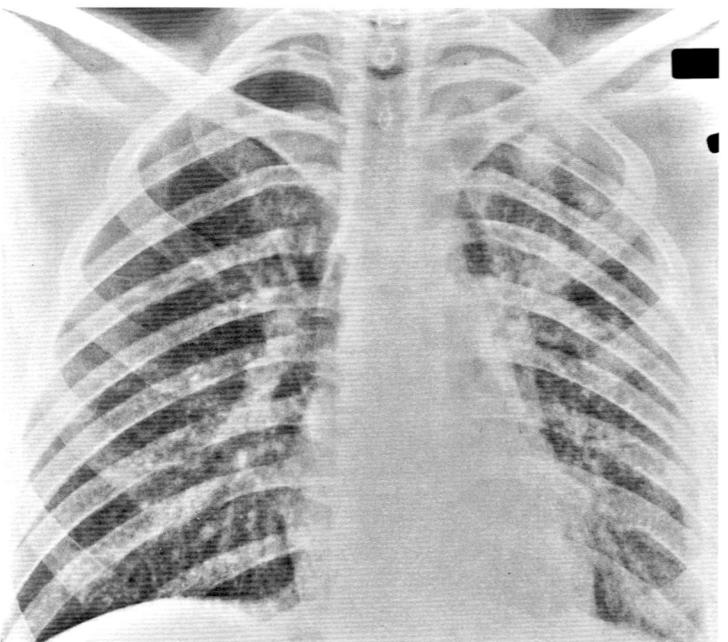

Fig. 2.**32 a, b** Tuberculous pleural effusion, mistaken for ▷ posttraumatic hemothorax, progressing to miliary tuberculosis. **a** Initial chest radiograph, taken after car accident shows left pleural effusion. **b** Six weeks later, multiple miliary nodules are visible throughout both lungs.

Tuberculous Pneumonia

Tuberculous pneumonia can develop either during the primary or postprimary phase of the disease. It can coexist with granulomas, with caseous necrosis, with cavities, and with fibrocalcific manifestations of tuberculosis. The radiographic features include confluent opacities. These can be located in the lower lobes if they occur during the primary stage or after bronchogenic spread. Tuberculous pneumonia in the postprimary phase of the disease involves the apical and posterior aspects of the upper lobes and the superior segment of the lower lobe.

Upper lobe pneumonia which persists in spite of conventional antibiotic therapy should lead to a workup for tuberculosis. Fungal pneumonias, bronchoalveolar cell carcinoma, pulmonary lymphoma, and pseudolymphoma can also produce persistent lung parenchymal consolidations.

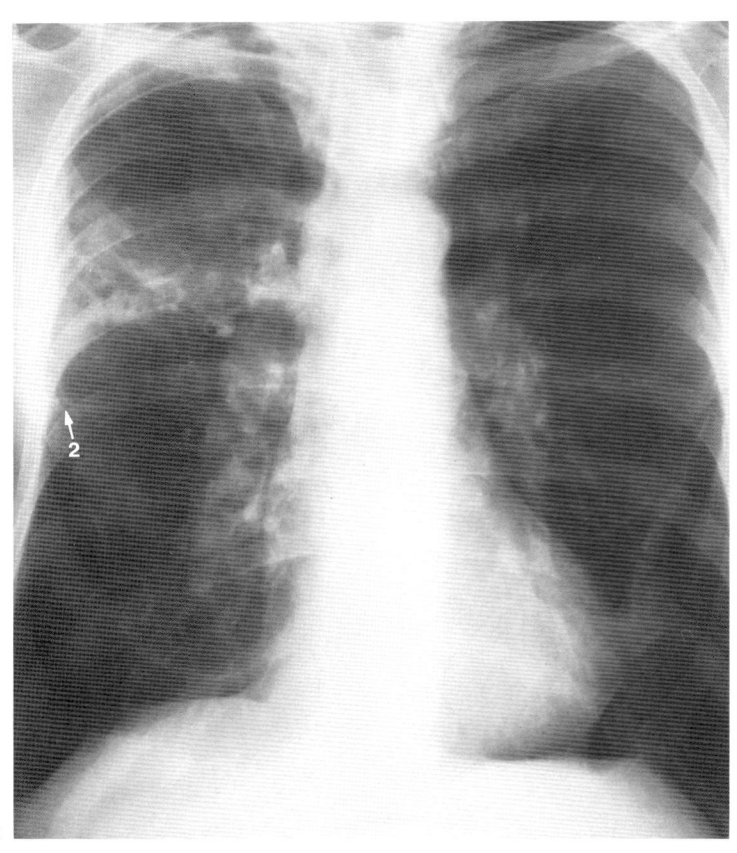

Fig. 2.**33 a, b Tuberculous pneumonia.**
68-year-old man with cough, fever, positive purified protein derivative (tuberculin) (PPD) test result, and sputum positive for *Mycobacteria*.

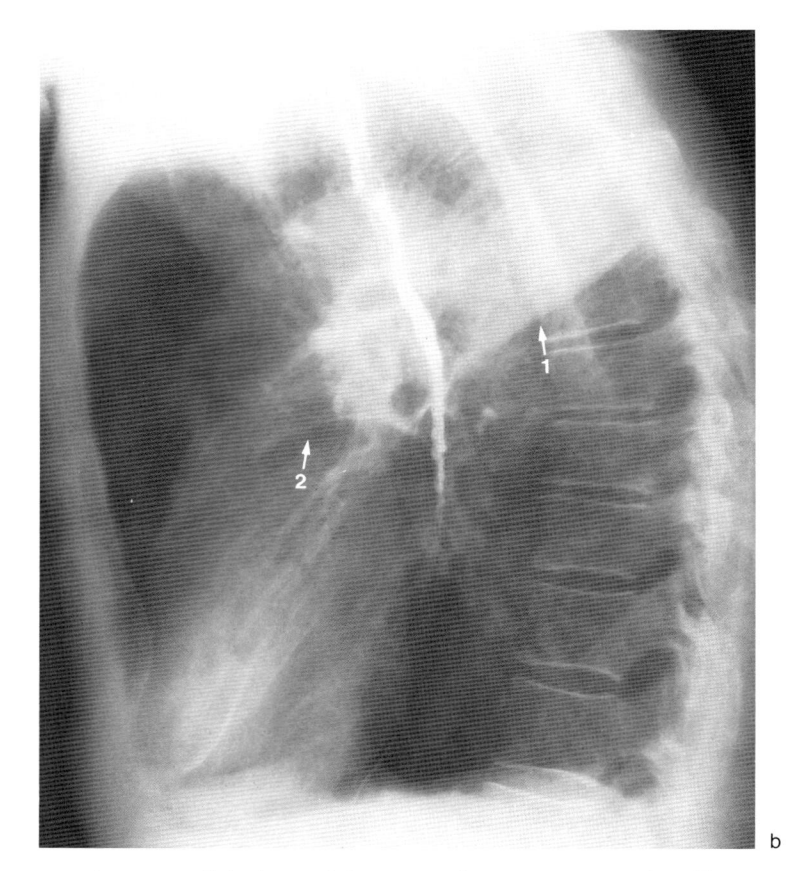

Patchy consolidation of the posterior segment and axillary subsegment of the right upper lobe. Major fissure (1), minor fissure (2).

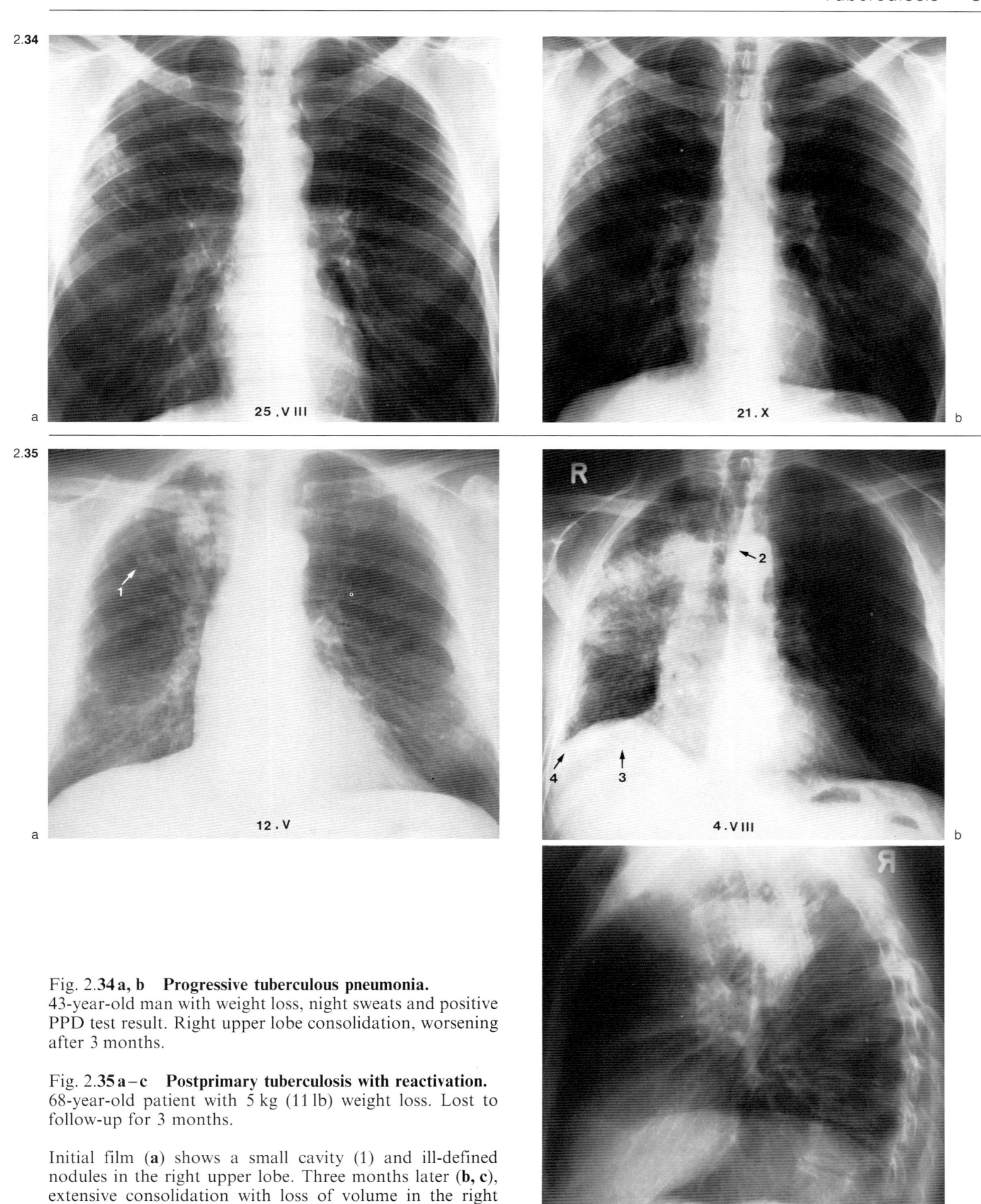

Tuberculosis

Fig. 2.**34 a, b** **Progressive tuberculous pneumonia.**
43-year-old man with weight loss, night sweats and positive PPD test result. Right upper lobe consolidation, worsening after 3 months.

Fig. 2.**35 a–c** **Postprimary tuberculosis with reactivation.**
68-year-old patient with 5 kg (11 lb) weight loss. Lost to follow-up for 3 months.

Initial film (**a**) shows a small cavity (1) and ill-defined nodules in the right upper lobe. Three months later (**b, c**), extensive consolidation with loss of volume in the right lung. Tracheal shift to the right (2), elevation of the right lung base (3), pleural thickening (4).

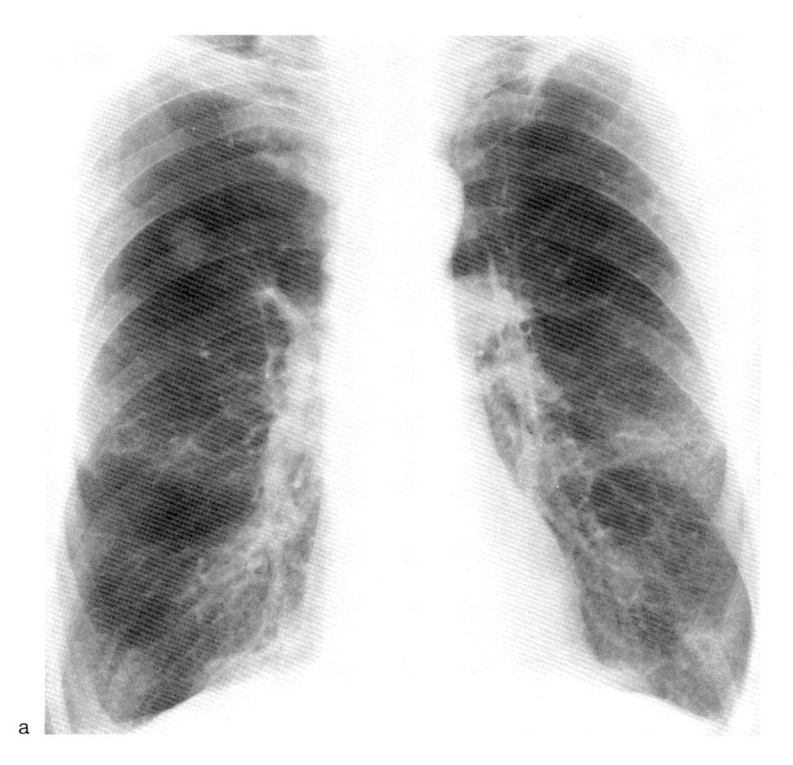

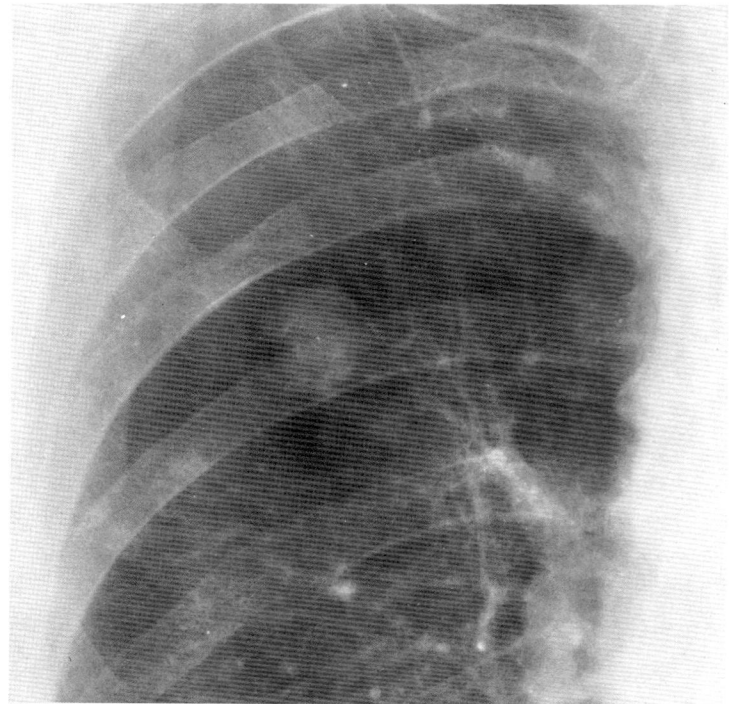

Granulomatous Form-Tuberculomas

Tuberculous granulomas are formed by conglomerates of epithelioid cells and reach a diameter of 1–2 mm. They can grow and reach a diameter of 1–3 cm. Tuberculomas constitute a walled-off collection of caseous material surrounded by connective tissue and granulation tissue. Radiologically, they appear as solitary pulmonary nodules. If they contain benign calcifications and are surrounded by satellite nodules, the correct diagnosis is easy to reach. In the absence of these features, a diagnosis can only be secured by comparison with previous films, which prove size stability over 2 years, or by means of a closed or open biopsy.

Fig. 2.36 a, b **Tuberculoma.**
Solitary pulmonary nodule in right upper lobe with excentric stippled calcifications. Resection showed a walled-off caseous focus. Old films were not available for comparison.

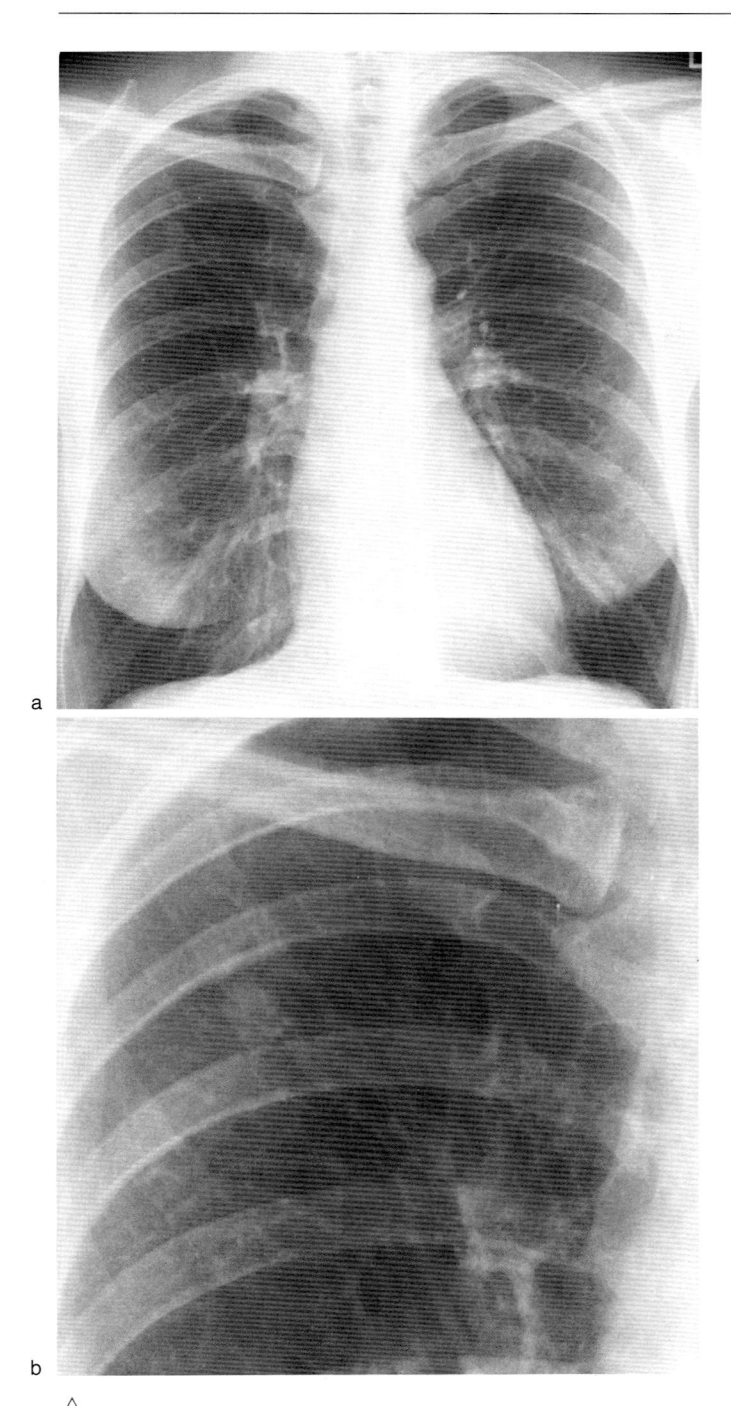

Fig. 2.37 a, b Tuberculoma.
38-year-old smoker.
Small, solitary, pulmonary nodule in right upper lobe. Resection yields walled-off caseous focus.

Fig. 2.38 a–c Calcified tuberculous granulomas in right upper lobe.
Asymptomatic 61-year-old man with known history of tuberculosis early in life.

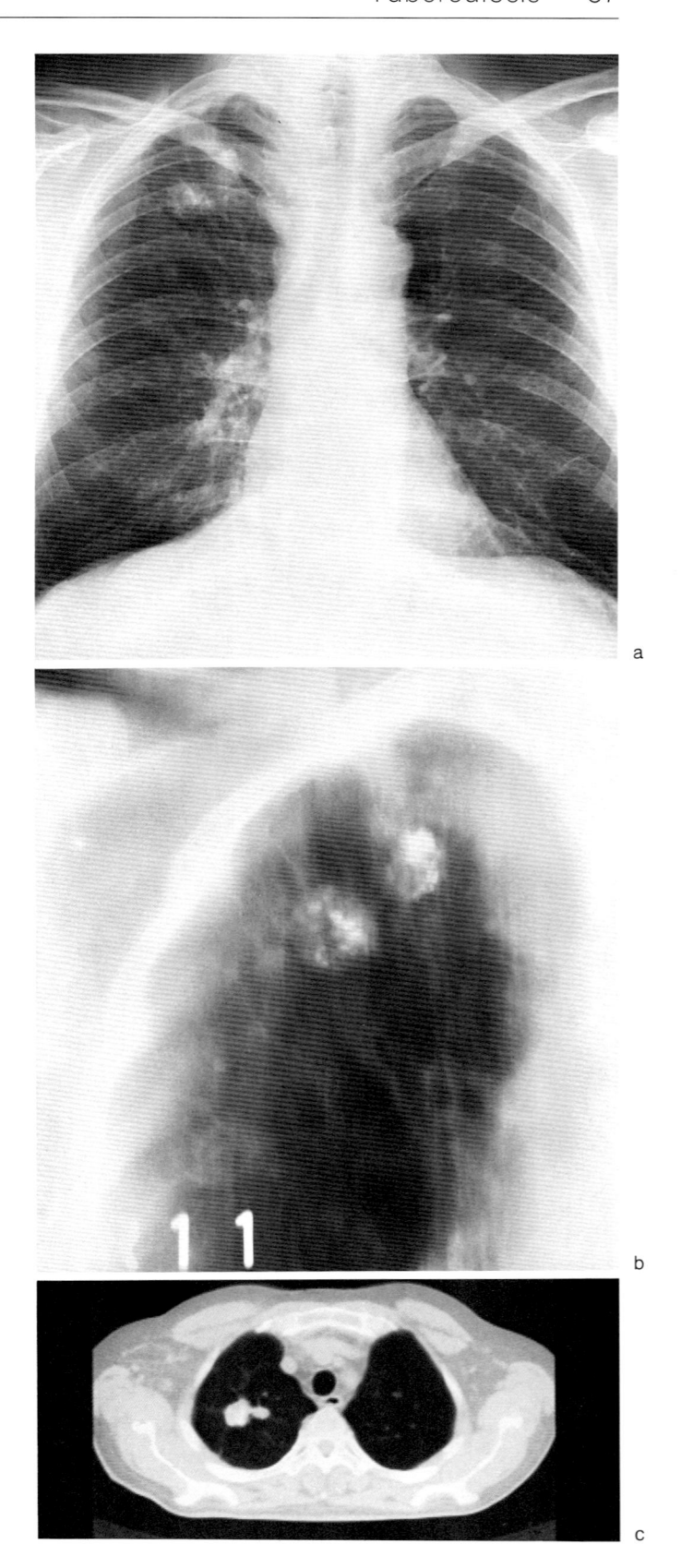

Cavitary Tuberculosis

Cavities result after the expectoration of caseous, necrotic material through a bronchial communication. Cavitation can occur within a tuberculous pneumonia or within a tuberculoma, provided a bronchial connection is formed. The highly infectious material can also spread to other parts of the lung, the so-called bronchogenic spread of tuberculosis. It leads to the formation of acinar-nodose foci. Radiologic features include relatively thin-walled cavities with occasional gas-fluid levels.

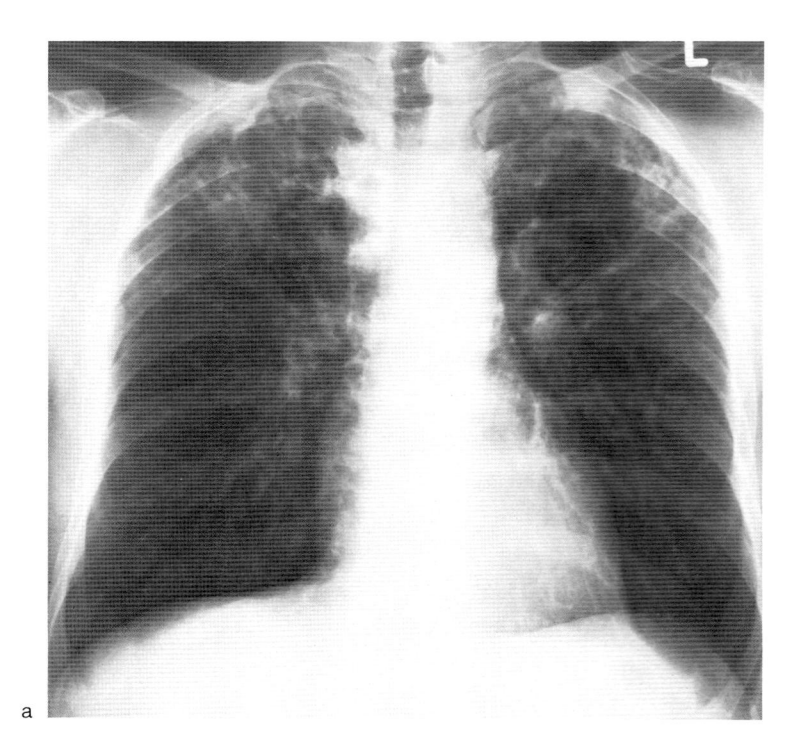

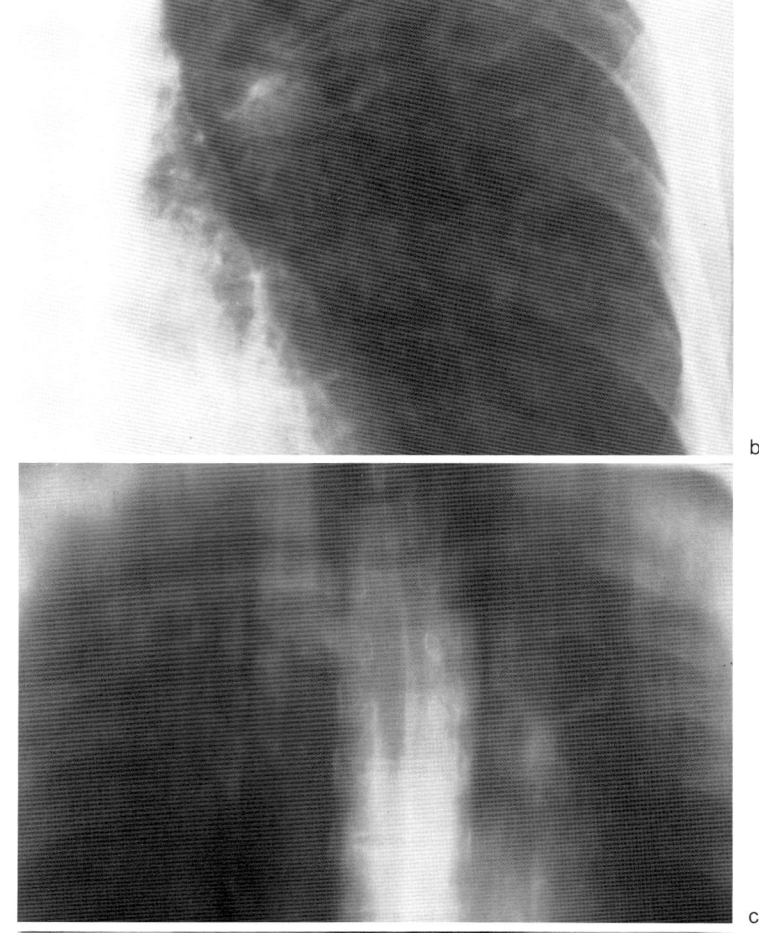

Fig. 2.39 a–d **Cavitary tuberculosis.**
55-year-old man with hoarseness due to laryngeal tuberculosis.

Multiple, bilateral cavities surrounded by multiple acinar nodules as a result of bronchogenic spread.

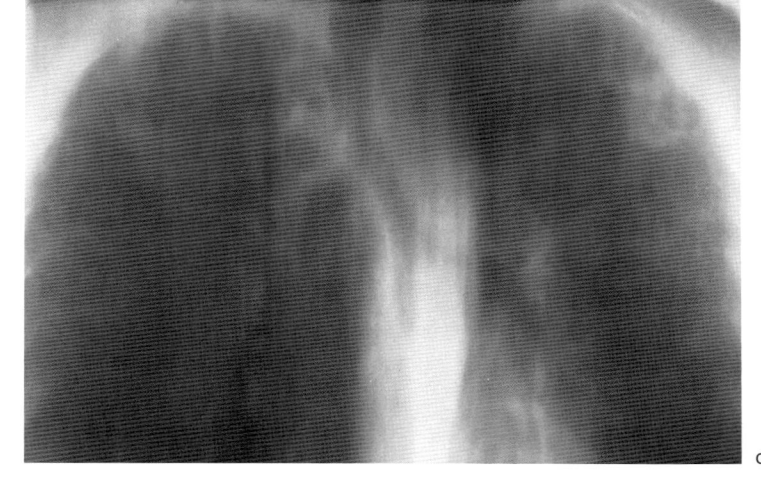

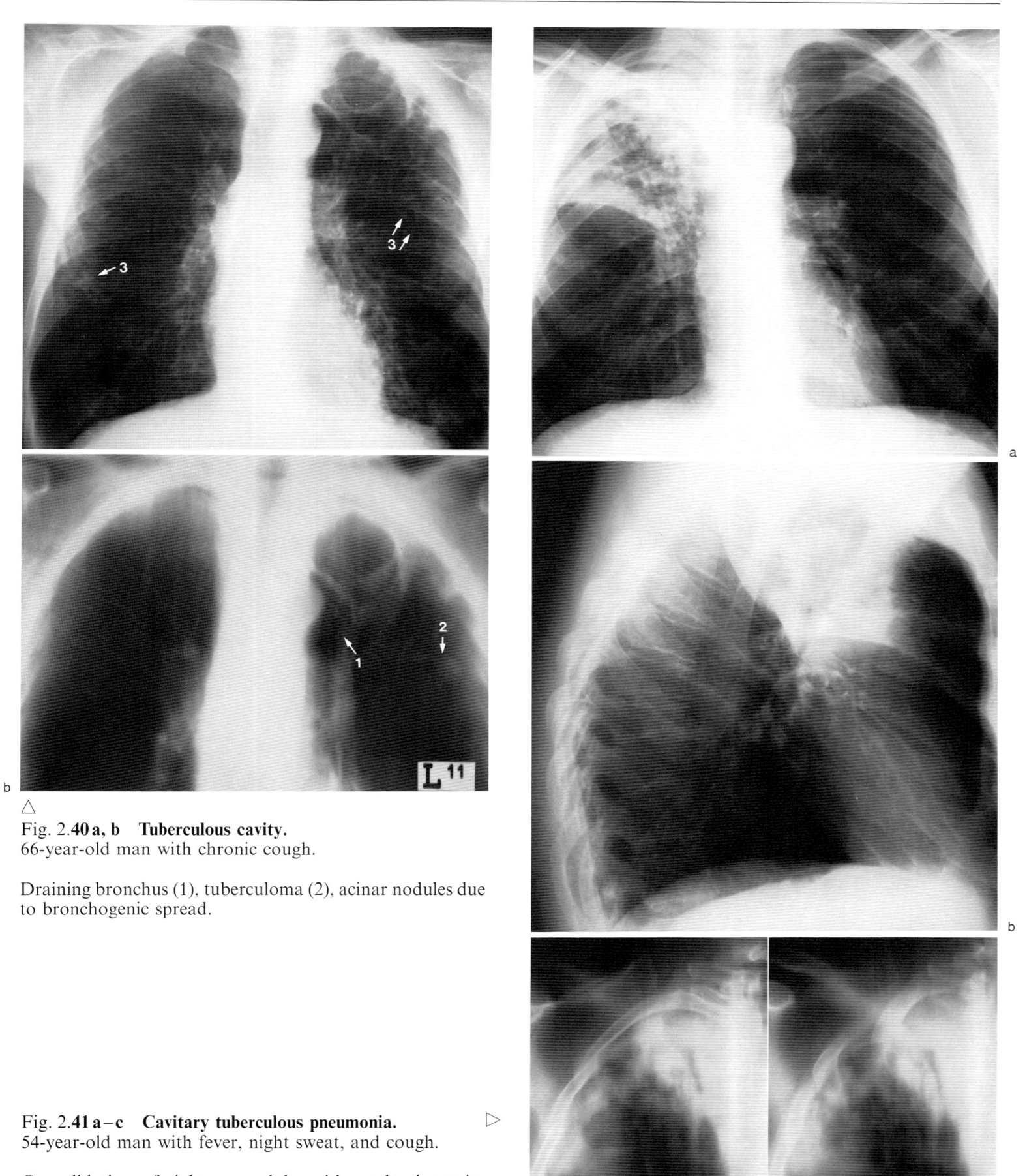

Fig. 2.**40 a, b Tuberculous cavity.**
66-year-old man with chronic cough.

Draining bronchus (1), tuberculoma (2), acinar nodules due to bronchogenic spread.

Fig. 2.**41 a–c Cavitary tuberculous pneumonia.**
54-year-old man with fever, night sweat, and cough.

Consolidation of right upper lobe with predominant involvement of apical segment. Cavities and air bronchogram are visible.

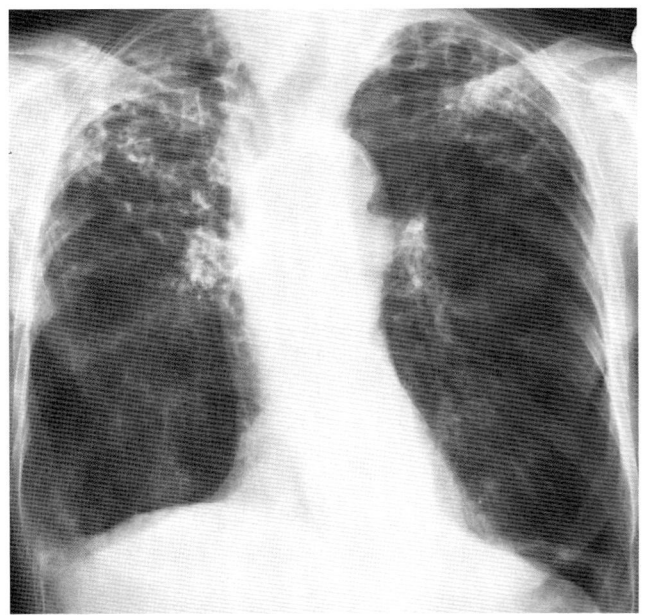

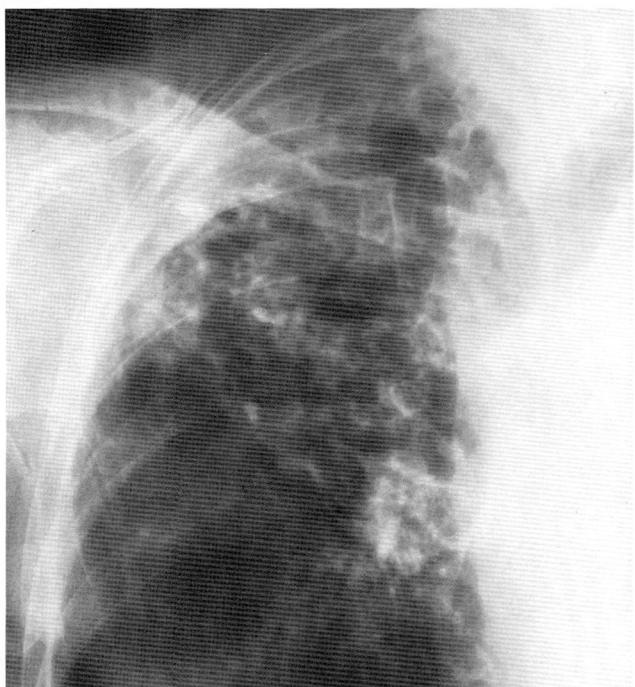

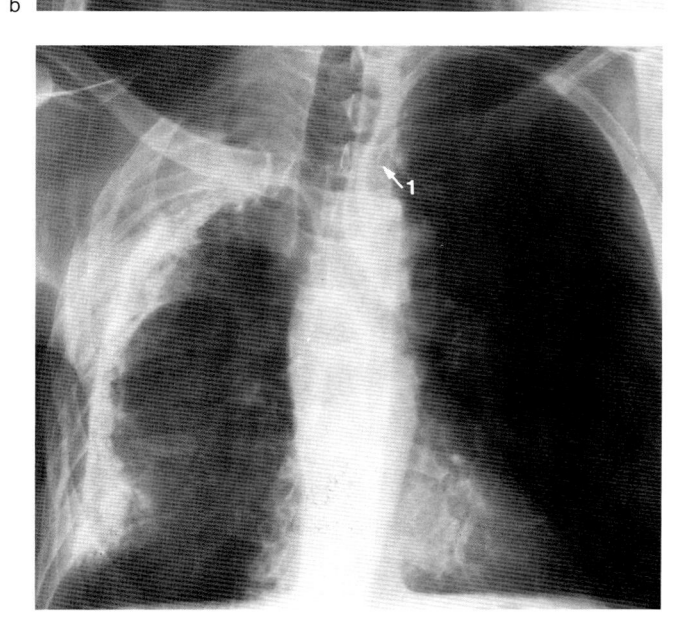

Fibrous, Postprimary Tuberculosis

Cicatrization of lung parenchyma can lead to extensive distortion and displacement of the vascular structures, resulting in traction bronchiectases and pericicatricial emphysema. A decrease in the number of small pulmonary vessels as well as hypoxic vasoconstriction with ventilation-perfusion mismatch lead to increased pulmonary vascular resistance, pulmonary arterial hypertension, cor pulmonale, and eventual respiratory failure. Radiologic findings include apical pleural and parenchymal scars with vertical stranding, cephalad retraction of hilar structures, bulla and bronchiectasis formation, ipsilateral cardiomediastinal shift, scoliosis, and a small ipsilateral hemithorax.

◁ Fig. 2.**42 a, b Fibrous pulmonary tuberculosis.**
88-year-old woman treated in her youth for tuberculosis and now asymptomatic. Scars, bullae in both upper lobes, cephalad hilar retraction, right basilar pleural scarring, and compensatory bibasilar hyperexpansion.

◁ Fig. 2.**43 Calcified right pleural peel with thoracogenic scoliosis.**
52-year-old patient decades after pneumothorax therapy of cavitary tuberculosis and now asymptomatic. Calcified pleural peel is 5 cm in thickness. Traction tracheomegaly and tracheal deviation. Air-filled esophagus to left of trachea (1).

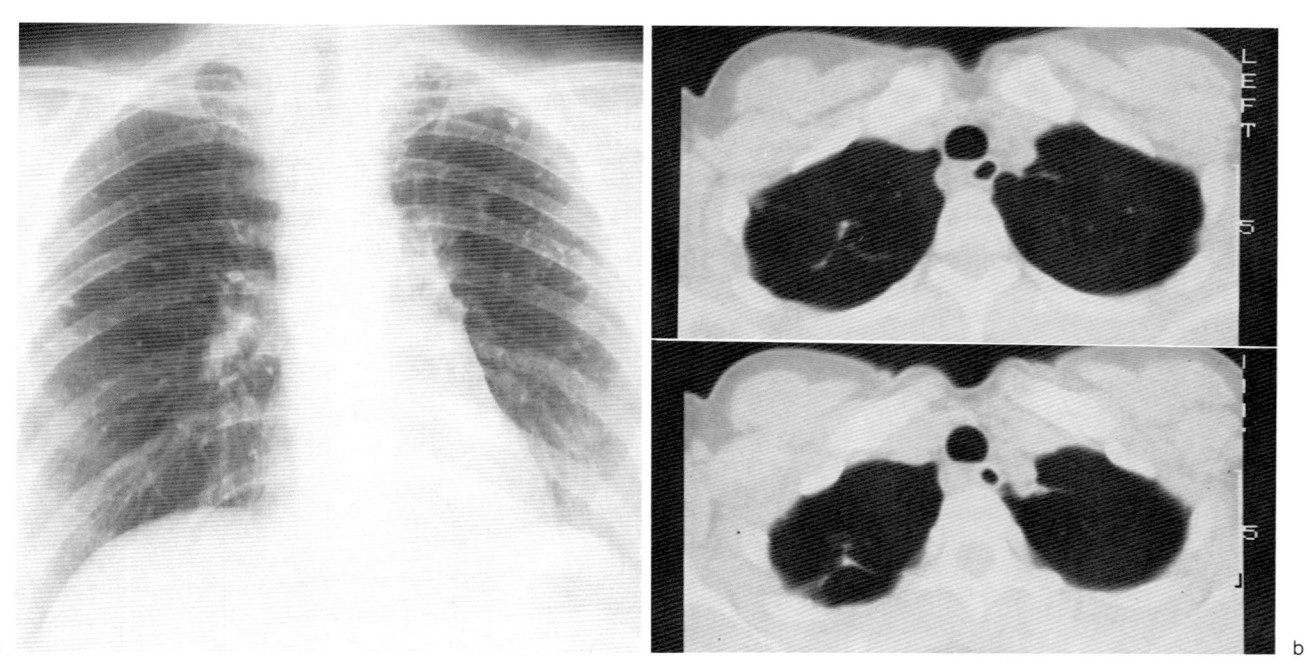

Fig. 2.**44 a, b Multiple calcified tuberculous granulomas.**
41-year-old, asymptomatic patient. Multiple, small, calcified, nodular opacities in both upper lung zones. Cephalad retraction of left hilar structures. CT scan shows bilateral stellate scars.

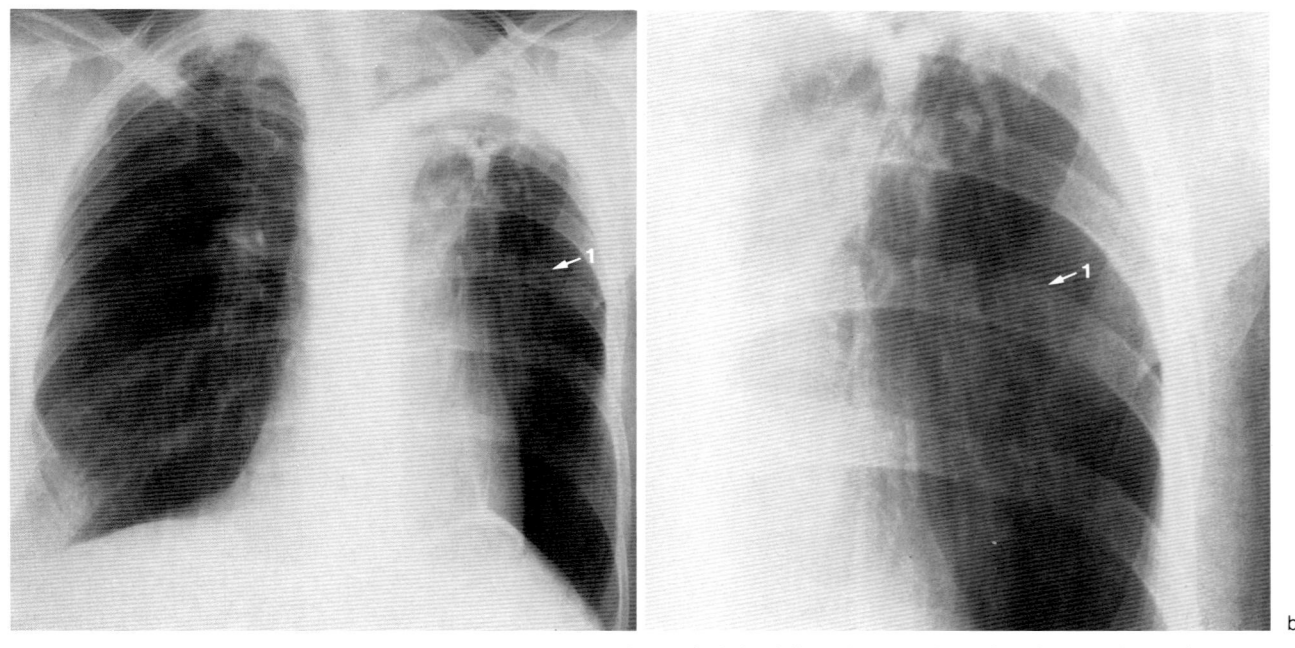

Fig. 2.**45 a, b Extensive tuberculous scarring.**
Bilateral, apical, pleuroparenchymal scarring with extreme elevation of right hilus due to cicatrization atelectasis. Vertical orientation of elevated lower lobe vessels (1).

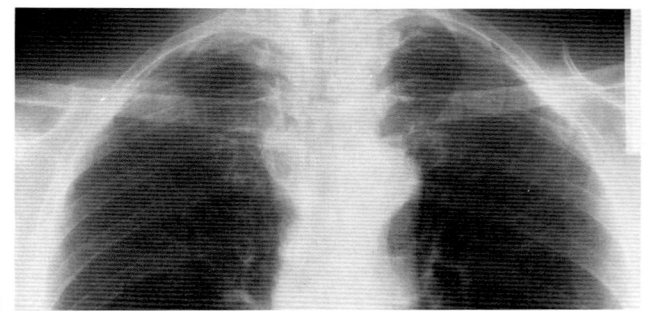

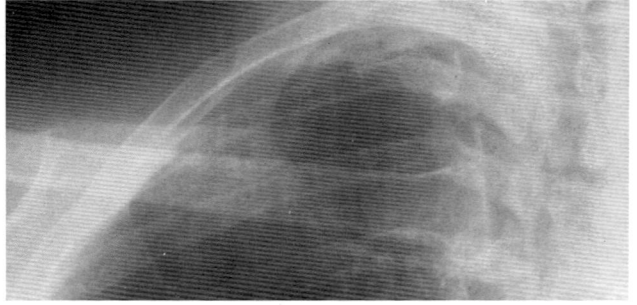

Fig. 2.**46 a, b Bilateral, apical, pleural caps without obvious parenchymal scarring.**
78-year-old, asymptomatic person. These pleural changes are not of tuberculous etiology, rather they represent reactive visceral pleural fibrosis due to gravitational stress on the lung apices.

Intrapulmonary Calcifications

Pulmonary calcifications can be dystrophic, metastatic, or secretory in nature. Dystrophic calcifications occur in necrotic tissue like caseous material in granulomas, in hamartomas with chondroid matrix, and in pneumoconiotic nodules. Metastatic calcifications occur in hypercalcemic states, particularly in chronic renal failure, when the $Ca \times P$ product exceeds 70. Calcifications can be seen in 1% of bronchogenic carcinomas on plain films and in 6% on CT. Broncholithiasis represents calcified lymph node material which has gained access to the bronchial tree by eroding the wall. Patients complain of recurrent pneumonias distal to the obstruction, bronchiectasis formation, and rarely lithoptysis (expectoration of stones). Alveolar microlithiasis is a rare familial disease of unknown etiology. The alveoli are filled with calcospherites, containing calcium phosphate deposits. Patients can be asymptomatic over many years or can develop recurrent pneumothoraces and eventually pulmonary fibrosis with restrictive physiology.

References: 12, 33, 87.

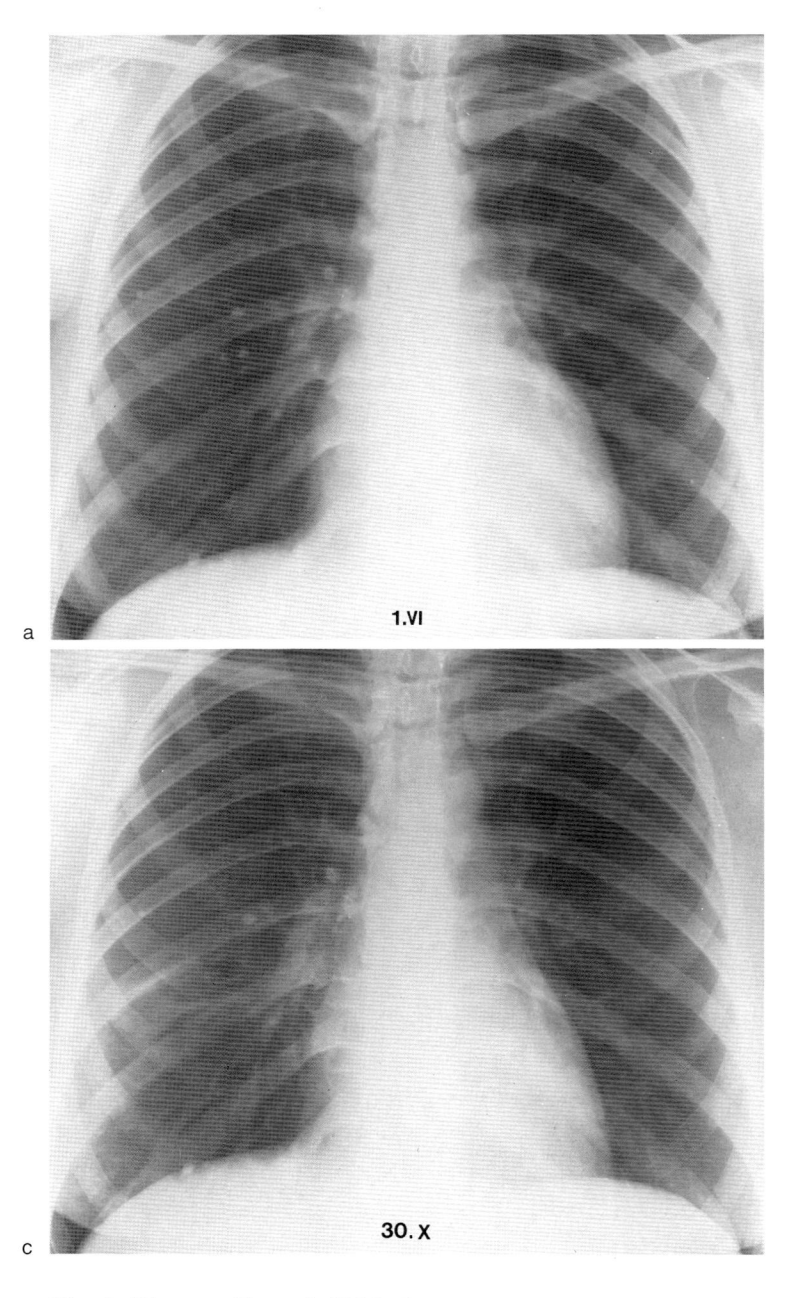

Fig. 2.47 a–c **Broncholithiasis.**
Multiple, calcified nodules in right lung (**a**). Partial right middle lobe atelectasis (**b**). At bronchoscopy, several broncholiths were extracted (**c**).

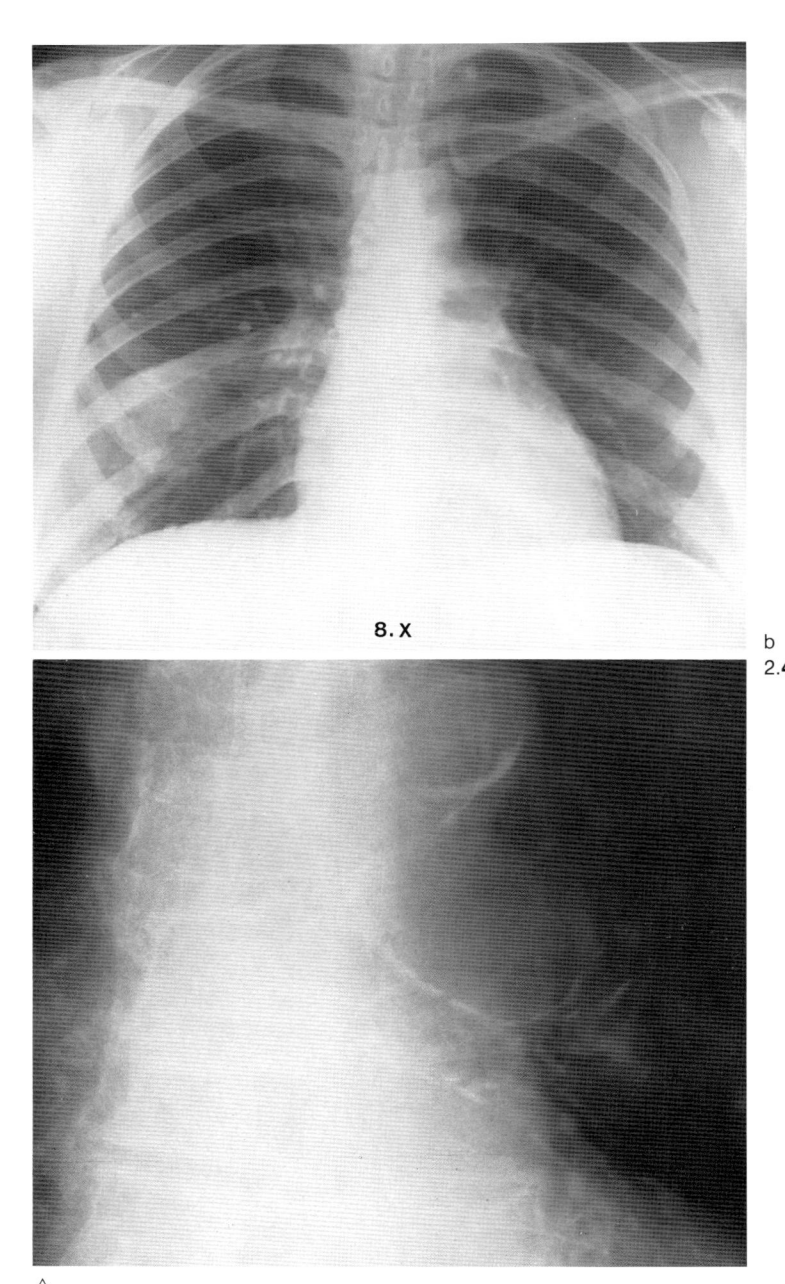

Fig. 2.48 **Calcification of tracheobronchial cartilages.**
It is seen primarily in elderly women and has no pathological significance. Note calcified aortic arch.

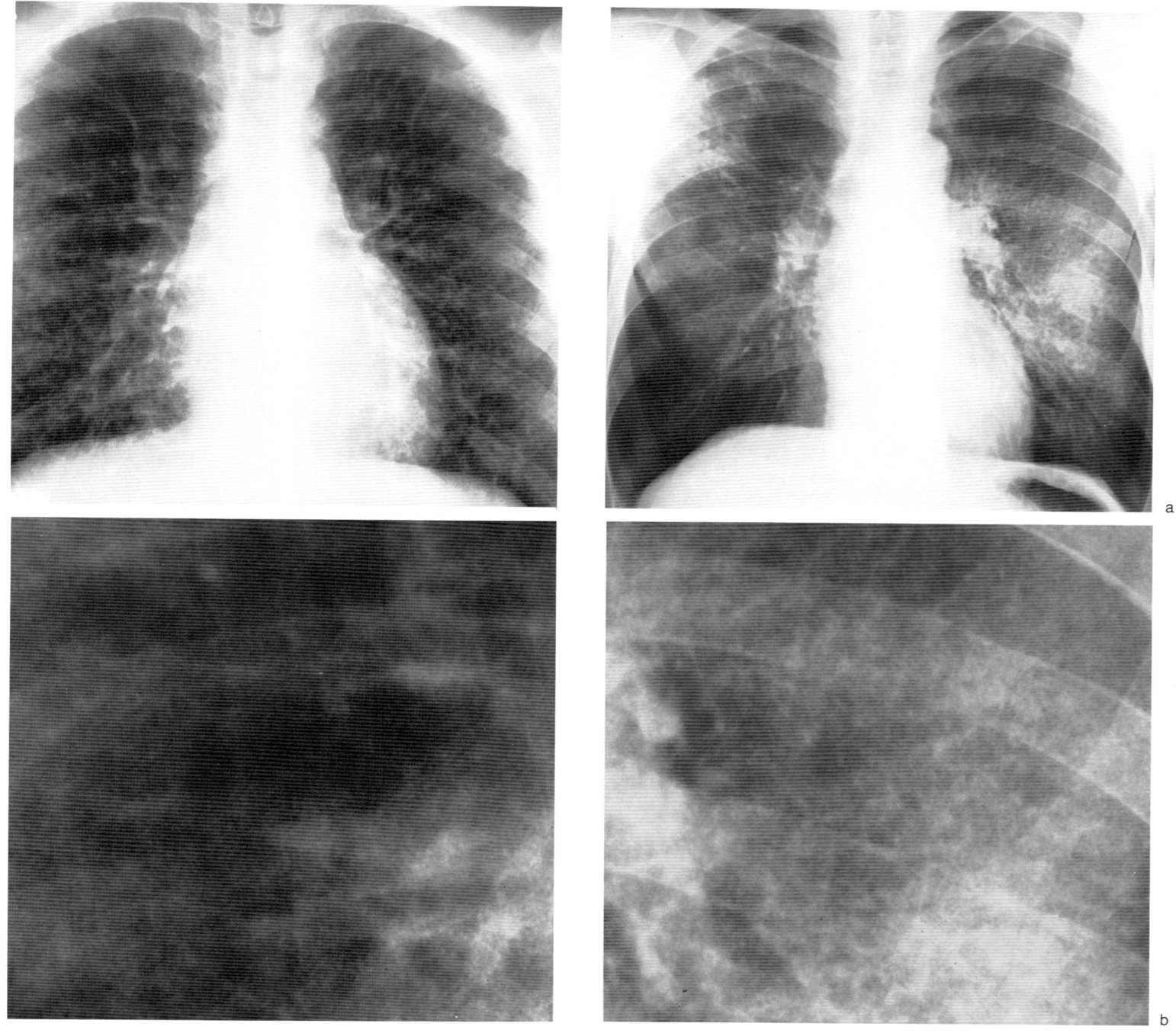

Fig. 2.**49 a, b Alveolar microlithiasis.**
10-year-old, asymptomatic boy. Reticulonodular opacities scattered diffusely throughout both lungs.

Fig. 2.**50 a, b Alveolar microlithiasis.**
Asymmetric, bilateral, micronodular pattern. Right upper lobe shows sequelae of postprimary tuberculosis.

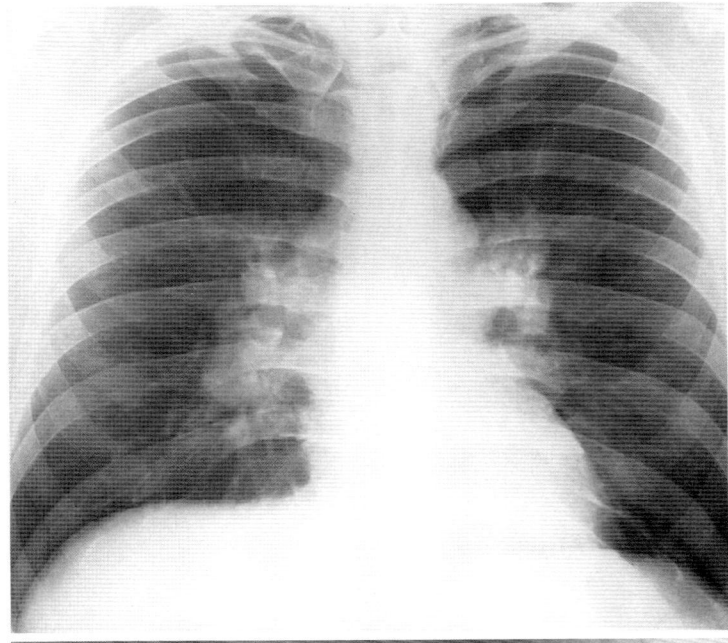

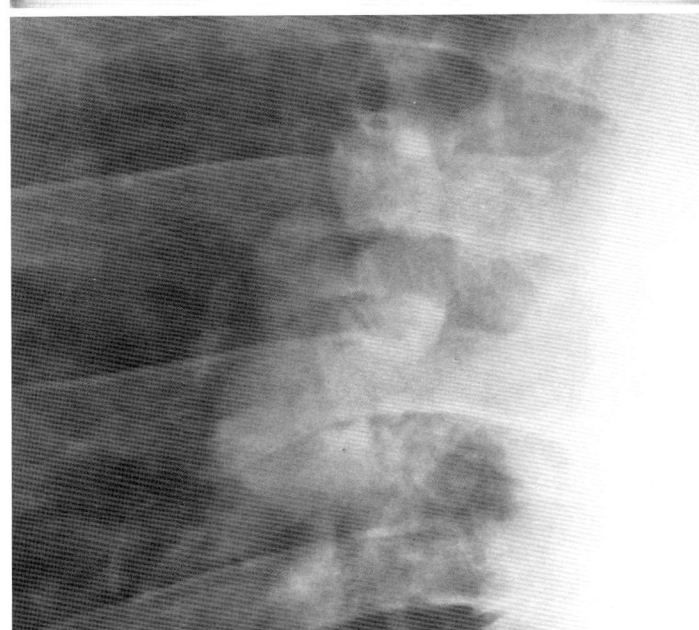

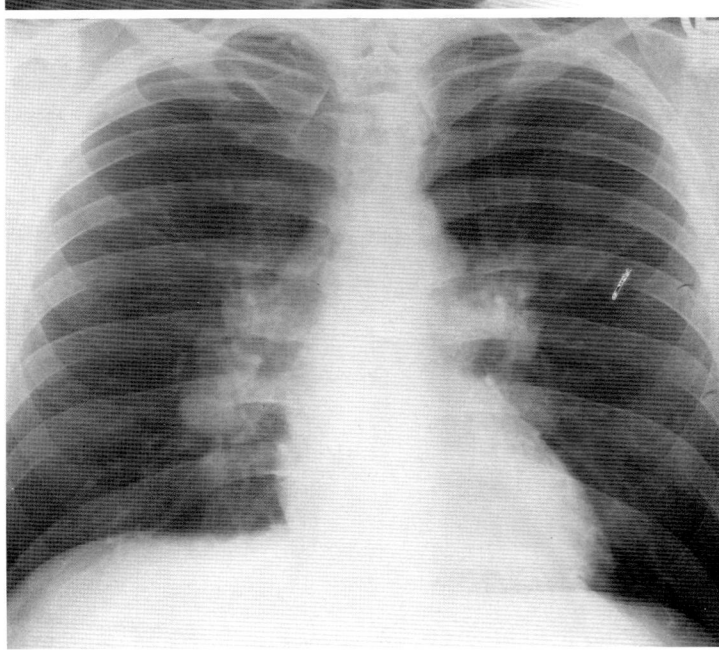

Sarcoidosis

Sarcoidosis is a generalized granulomatous disorder of unknown etiology. Four stages have been described.

Stage I patients present with bilateral hilar and paratracheal lymph node enlargement. About 50% of patients are seen at this stage. They have a favorable prognosis, and the lymph nodes regress in 80% within 5 years. The remaining 20% can progress to stages II, III, and IV.

Stage II consists of hilar, mediastinal lymph node enlargement and visible lung parenchymal involvement. Some 20% of patients are discovered at this stage. About 60% of these patients improves within 5 years.

Stage III sarcoidosis is defined as diffuse lung parenchymal disease without obvious lymph node involvement. About 15–20% of patients present at this stage. Some 30% of these patients can recover their normal radiographic appearance.

Stage IV implies irreversible lung disease with pulmonary fibrosis, upper lobe scarring, cyst formation, bronchiectases and cor pulmonale. Less than 10% of patients reach this stage.

Over half or about 60% of patients with sarcoidosis are asymptomatic at presentation and are discovered incidentally. Extrathoracic signs like uveitis, parotitis (uveoparotid fever of Heerfordt), lupus pernio of the skin, or cystic bone changes can predominate. Lofgren syndrome, described in young women, consists of fever, arthralgia, erythema nodosum, and an abnormal chest radiograph. Bronchoalveolar lavage will demonstrate a high number of lymphocytes in the sputum. A PPD test will usually be negative, and a Kveim test is only of historical importance. The diagnosis is suspected from the characteristic radiologic picture and is usually substantiated by biopsy, which shows epithelioid cell containing noncaseating granulomas.

Fig. 2.51 a–c **Sarcoidosis stage I.**
20-year-old patient with uveitis. Marked bilateral, hilar, right paratracheal and aortic-pulmonic window lymph node enlargement (**a, b**) persisting unchanged over 1 year (**c**).

Fig. 2.**52 a, b** **Sarcoidosis stage I.**
26-year-old patient with erythema nodosum. Bilateral, enlarged, hilar regions, right paratracheal lymph nodes (2), prevascular lymph nodes (1), subcarinal lymph nodes (3).

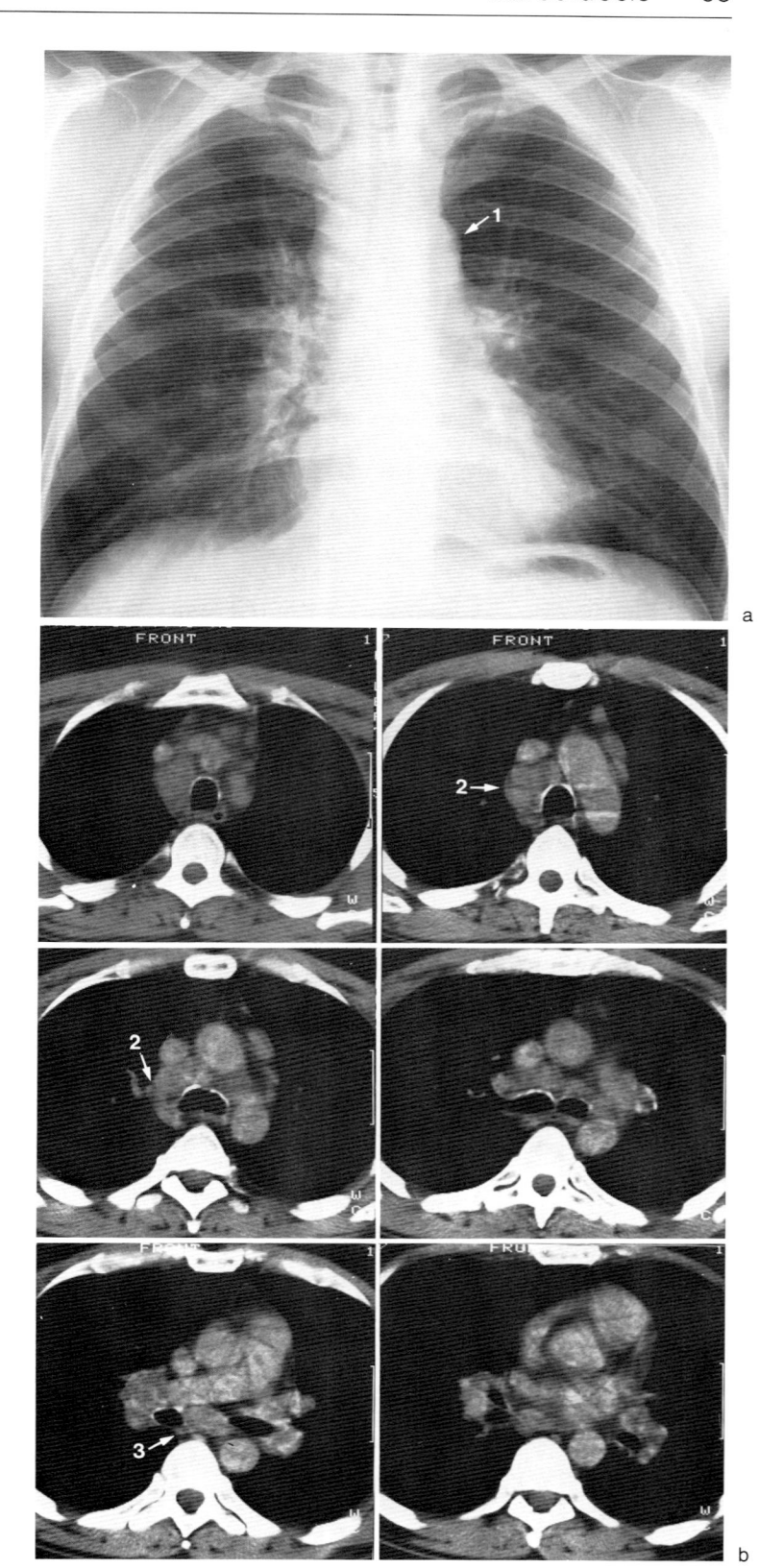

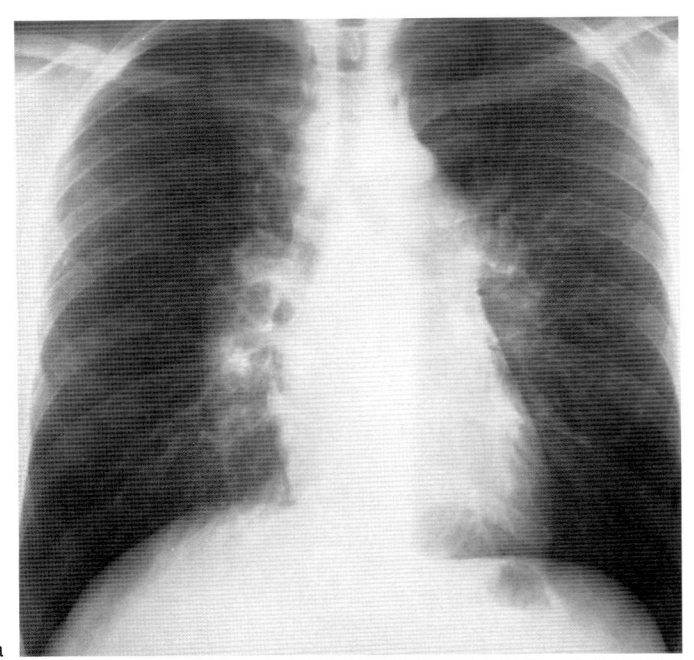

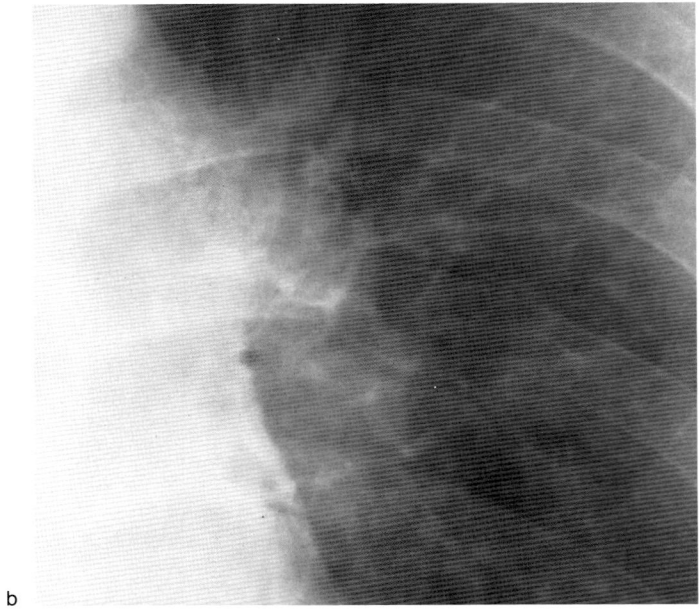

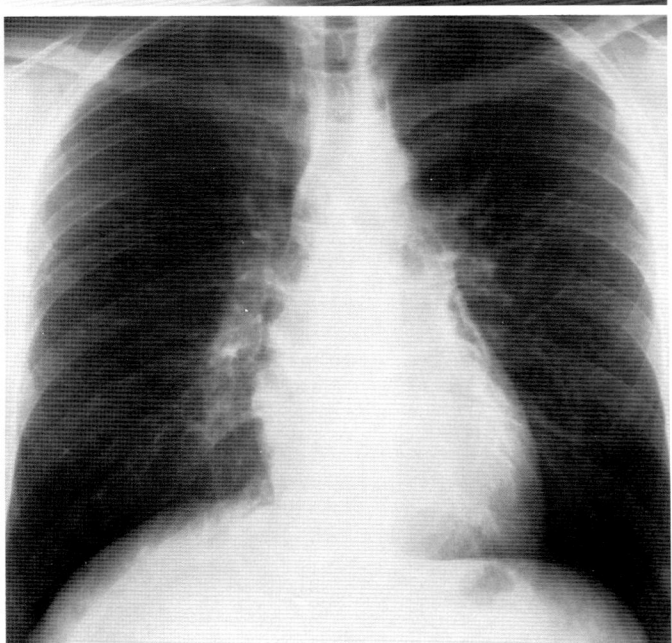

Fig. 2.53 a–c Sarcoidosis stage II.
38-year-old patient with swelling. Bilateral hilar and paratracheal lymph nodes with reticulonodular changes particularly on the left (**a, b**). Marked improvement after corticosteroid therapy (**c**).

Fig. 2.**54a, b Sarcoidosis stage II.**
37-year-old patient with fever of unknown origin. Faint perihilar miliary pattern.

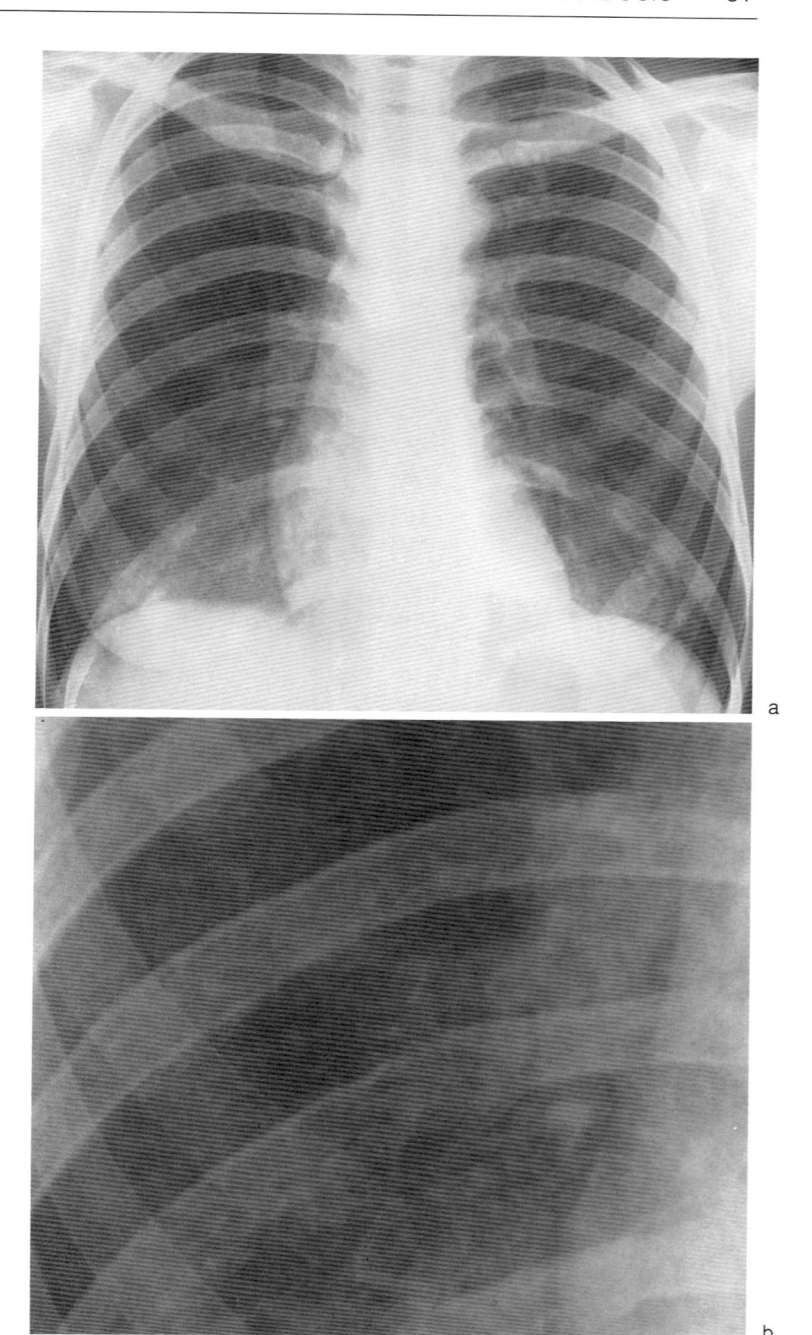

68 2. Infections

2.55

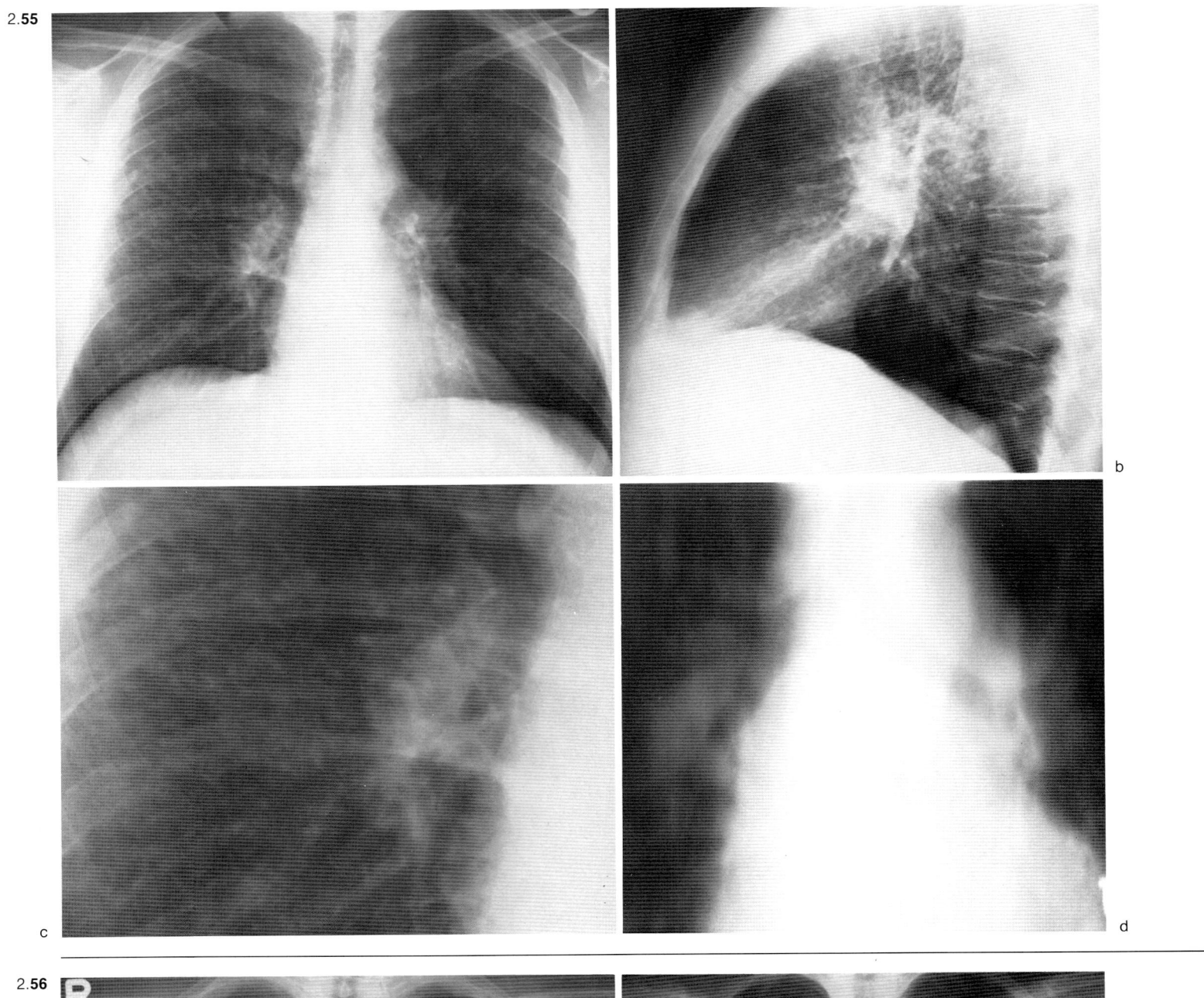

a

b

c

d

2.56

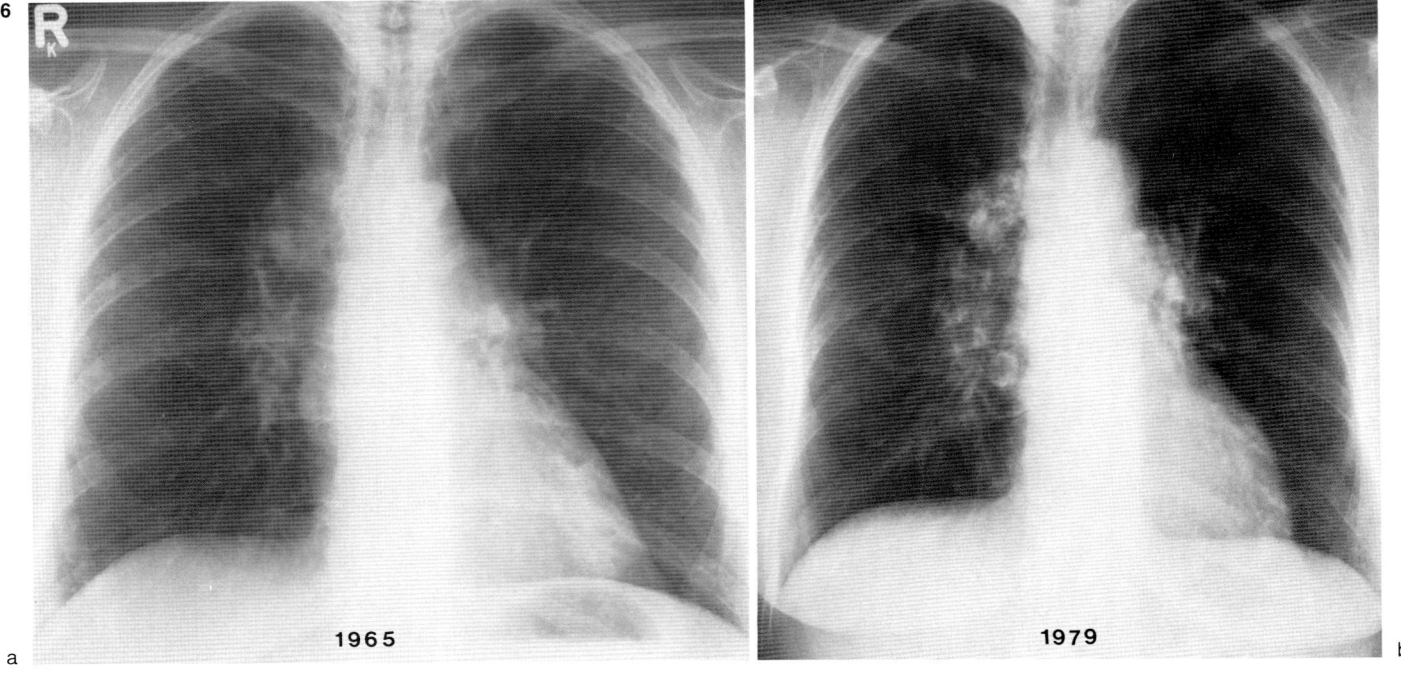

a 1965

b 1979

◁ Fig. 2.55 a–d **Sarcoidosis stage II.**
28-year-old man presents with dyspnea. Bilateral, hilar, paratracheal, aortic-pulmonic window lymph node enlargement and reticulonodular lung parenchymal changes.

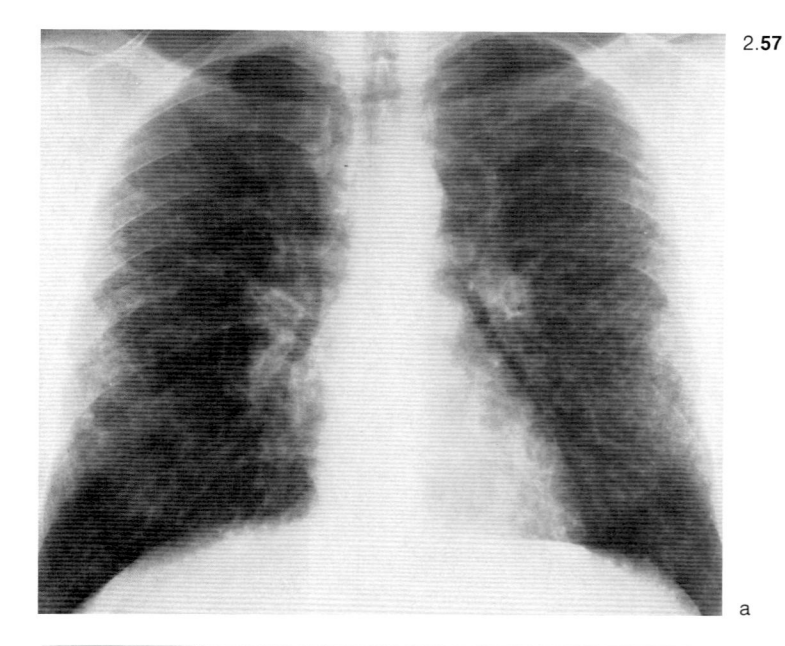

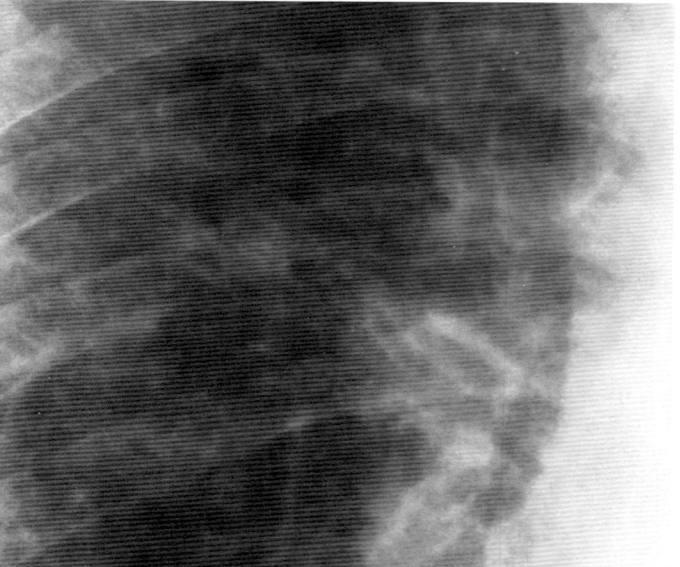

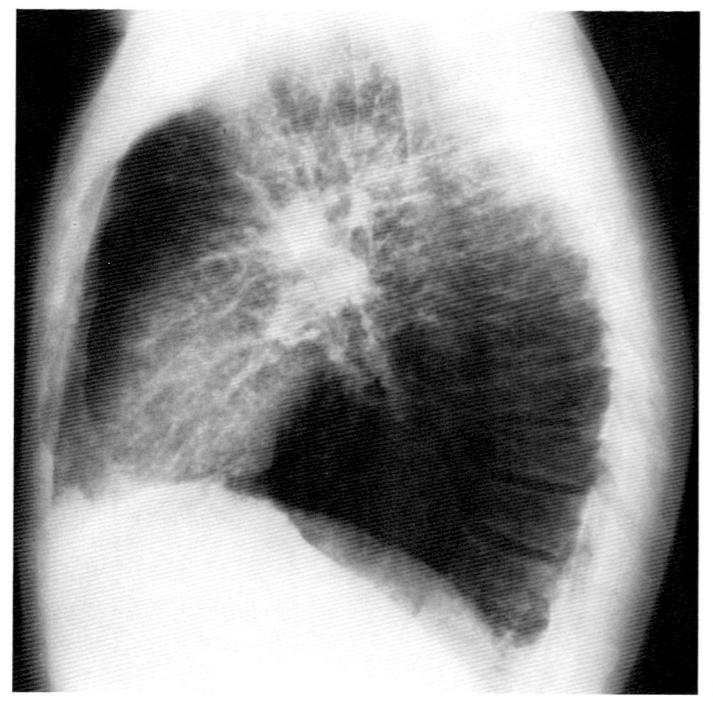

◁ Fig. 2.56 a, b **Sarcoidosis.**
57-year-old, asymptomatic patient. Follow-up over 15 years. Enlarged hilar and mediastinal lymph nodes eventually calcify. Note typical eggshell pattern of calcification.

Fig. 2.57 a–c **Sarcoidosis stage III.** ▷
60-year-old patient with a 20-year history of sarcoid and progressive exertional dyspnea. Diffuse reticulonodular opacification of both lungs.

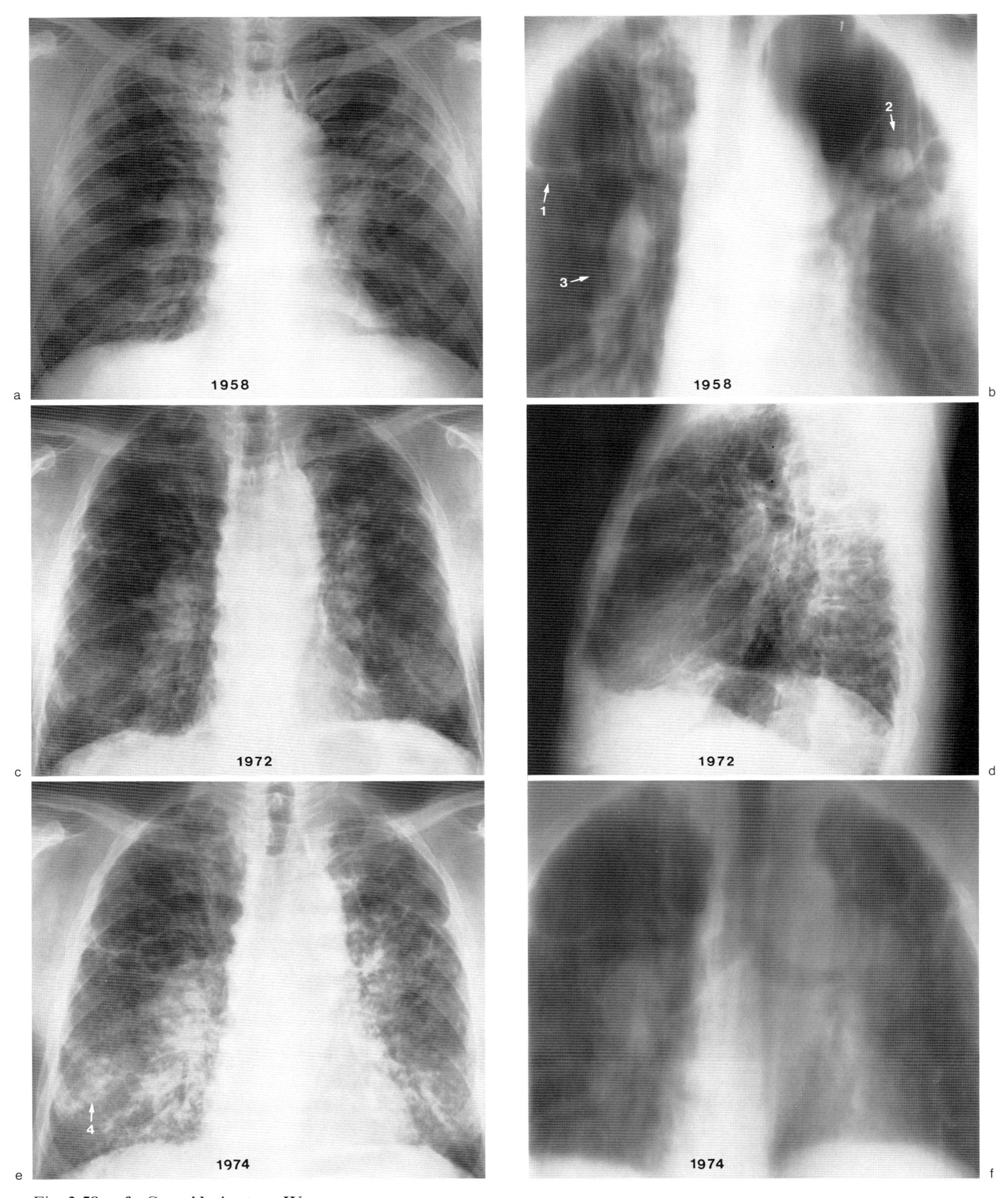

Fig. 2.58 a–f Sarcoidosis stage IV.
50-year-old patient with a 20-year history. Upper lobe bullous emphysema (1), fungus ball (mycetoma) due to *Aspergillus* (2), dilated central pulmonary arteries indicative of pulmonary arterial hypertension and cor pulmonale.

Fungal Diseases

Fungal diseases can be subdivided into endemic and opportunistic infection (Tables 2.2, 2.3). Endemic fungi include *Histoplasma, Sporothrix, Blastomyces, Coccidioides,* and *Cryptococcus*. These infections occur either on a global scale or have their epidemiologic niche. They usually affect immunocompetent patients. Opportunistic fungi include *Candida albicans, Aspergillus, Mucor,* and *Cryptococcus*. They affect immunocompromised hosts. Cryptococcosis is listed with both groups since only 50% of affected patients are immunocompromised.

Actinomycosis and nocardiosis are bacterial infections caused by variants of *Mycobacteria*. The radiological picture and the clinical behavior are similar to that of fungal diseases.

Recently, *Pneumocystis carinii* was reclassified as a fungal organism.

Table 2.2 Classification of fungi

A. Dimorphic fungi
  – Mycelial phase in nature
  – Yeast phase in tissue
  – *Histoplama capsulatum, Coccidioides immitis, Sporothrix schenckii, Blastomyces dermatitidis*
B. Budding yeast with Pseudomycelia in tissue phase
   Candida albicans
C. Unimorphic fungi
   Same form in nature and in tissue
   Cryptococcus neoformans (budding yeast), *Aspergillus, Mucor* (mycelia in tissue)

Table 2.3 Clinical classification of fungi

A. Epidemic or endemic fungi
  1. Worldwide distribution (*Cryptococcus, Sporothrix*)
  2. Selective ecological niches (*Blastomyces, Histoplasma, Coccidioides*)
B. Opportunistic fungi
   Aspergillus, Mucor, Candida, Cryptococcus, Torulopsis glabrata

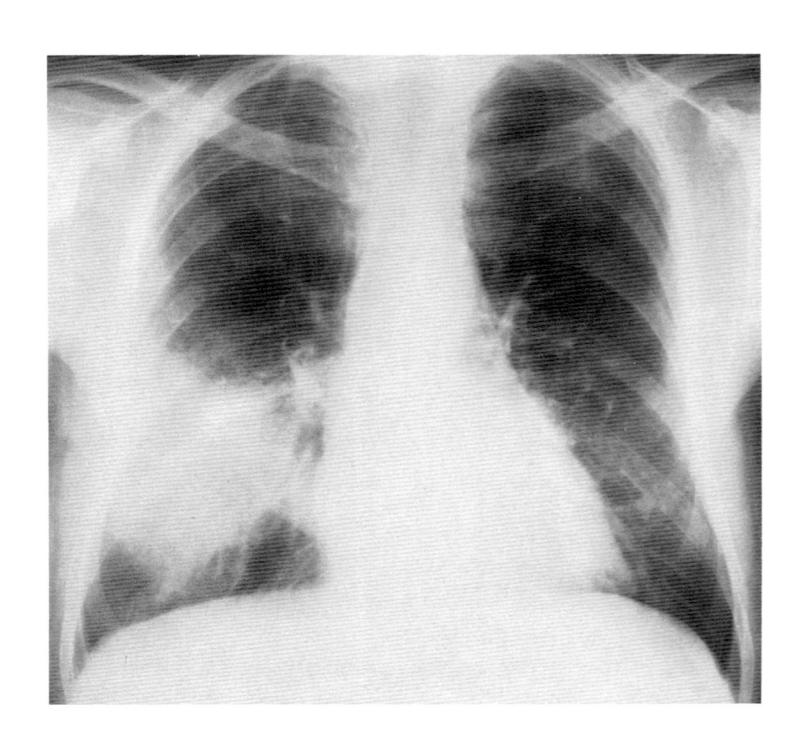

Fig. 2.59 **Invasive Aspergillosis in a leukemia patient.** Extensive consolidation of the right lower lung. Pneumonia caused by *Aspergillus fumigatus*. Autopsy proof.

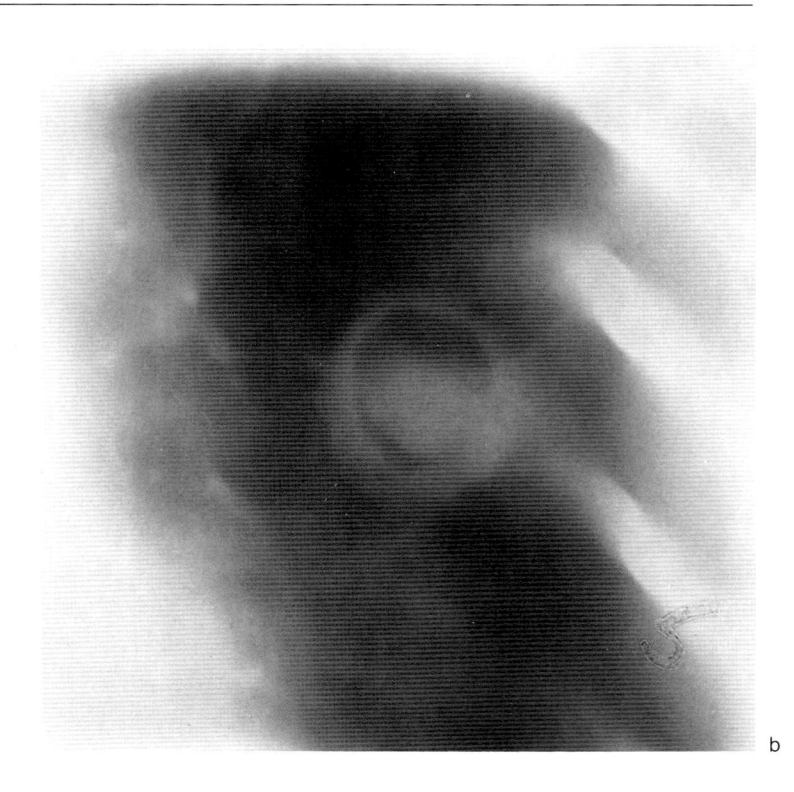

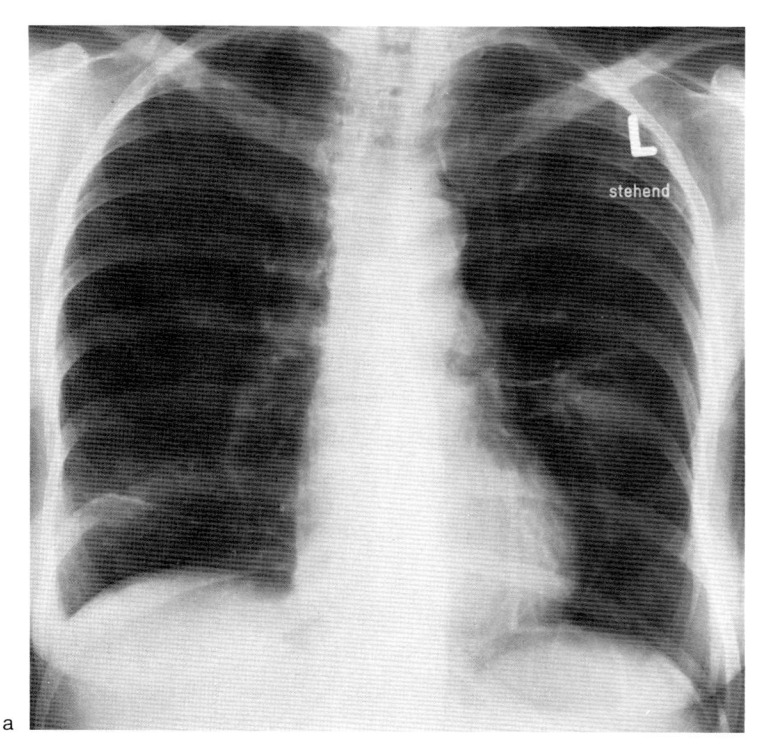

Fig. 2.60 a, b Aspergilloma.
55-year-old patient with chronic destructive pulmonary disease. Pulmonary nodules in left midlung and right lower lobe. The left-sided nodule is surrounded by a rind of air. Left lesion was resected because of recurrent hemoptysis and proved to represent a fungus ball in a bulla with slightly thickened wall.

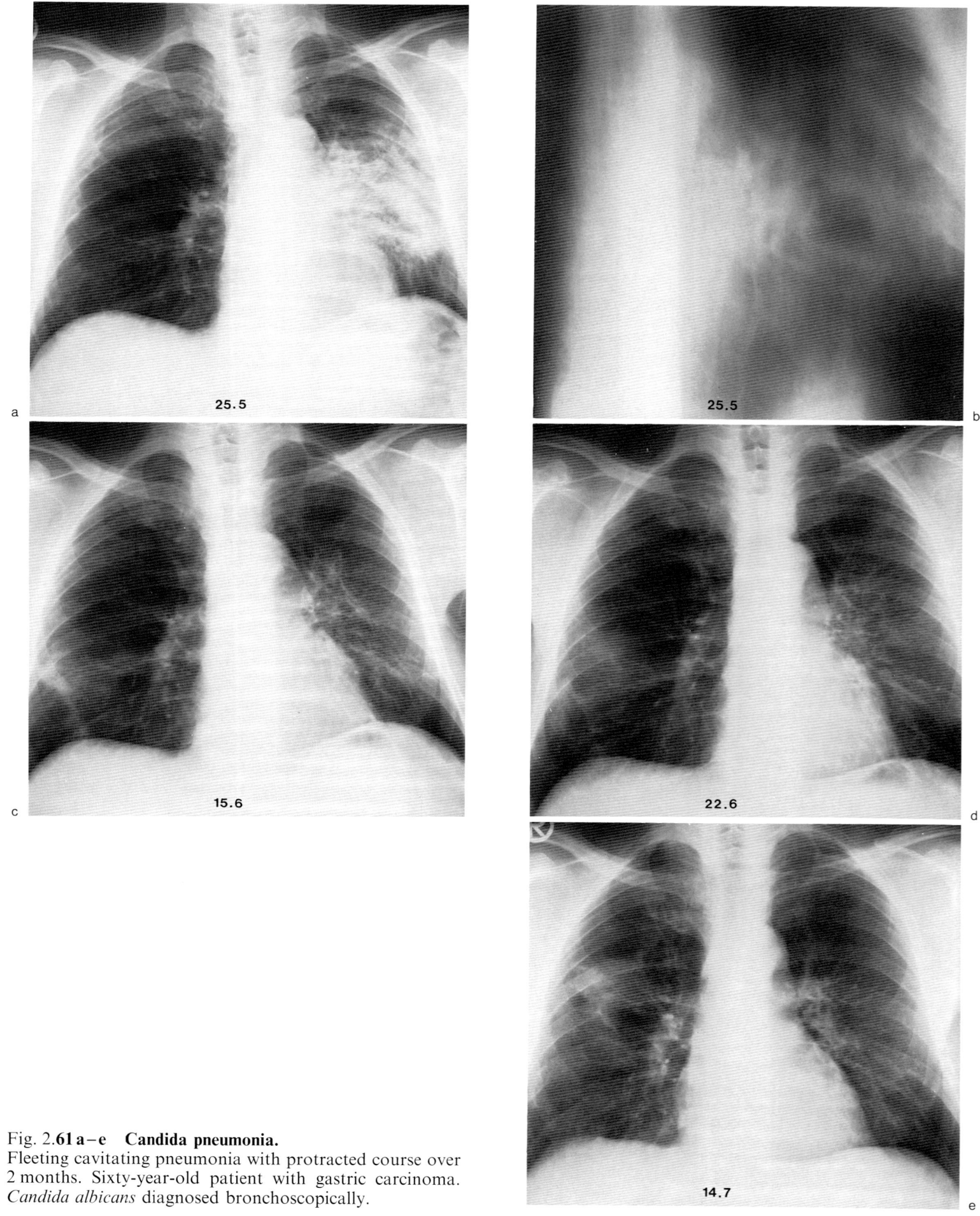

Fig. 2.61 a–e Candida pneumonia.
Fleeting cavitating pneumonia with protracted course over 2 months. Sixty-year-old patient with gastric carcinoma. *Candida albicans* diagnosed bronchoscopically.

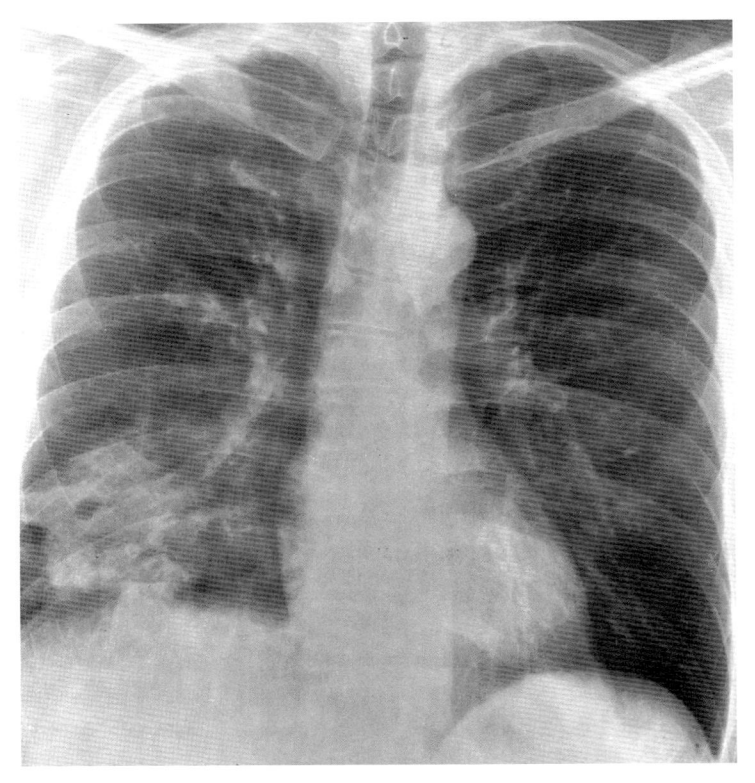

74 2. Infections

Fig. 2.62 **Cryptococcosis.**
Asymptomatic 37-year-old patient who spent time on an animal farm. Chest radiograph shows large right lower lobe mass with air bronchograms as well as smaller right upper lobe nodules.

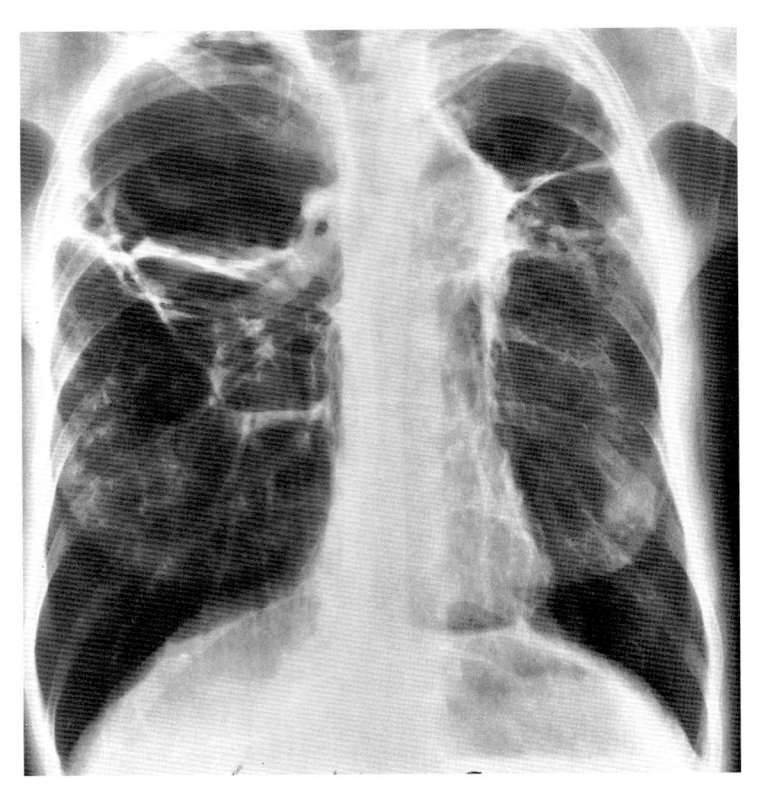

Fig. 2.63 Sporotrichosis, in a gardener, infected most likely percutaneously after thorn puncture. Frontal chest radiograph shows bilateral, upper lobe, thin-walled cavities, loss of volume, retraction of hilar regions cephalad, distortion of remaining lung parenchyma, and tracheal deviation to the left.

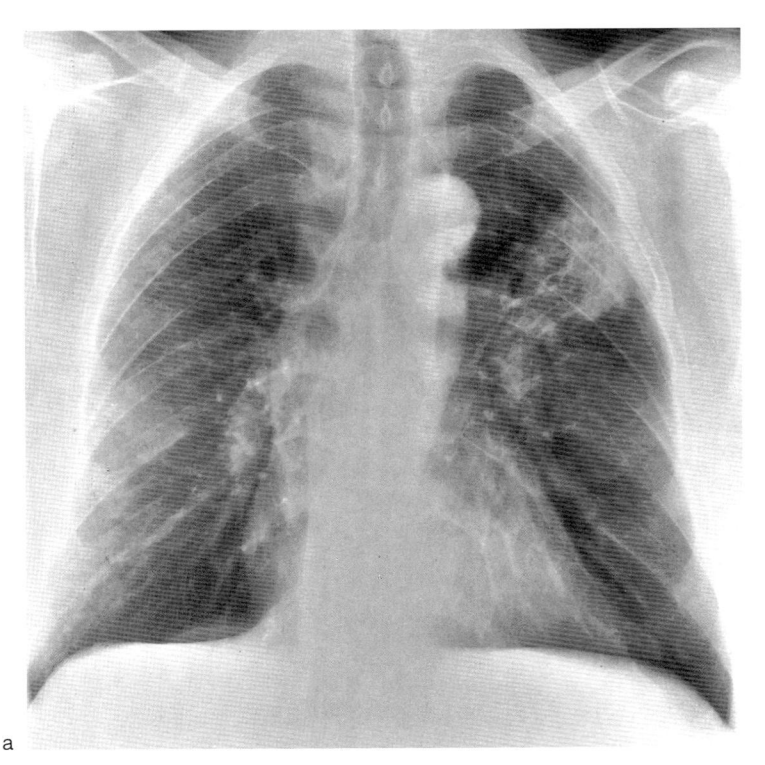

Fig. 2.64 a–c **Mucormycosis in a diabetic patient.**
Initial chest radiograph shows consolidation of left upper lobe with several small cavities and adjacent pleural thickening (**a**). A week later, a large cavity in the left upper lobe has formed and a second nodular focus in the lingula becomes visible (**b**). A frontal view of the paranasal sinuses reveals opacification of the right maxillary sinus, due to mucor involvement (**c**).

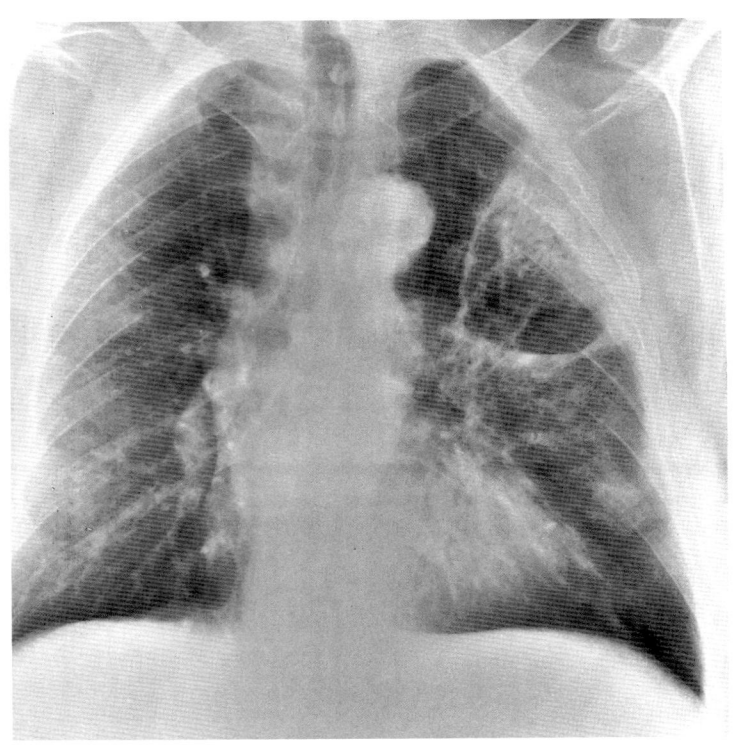

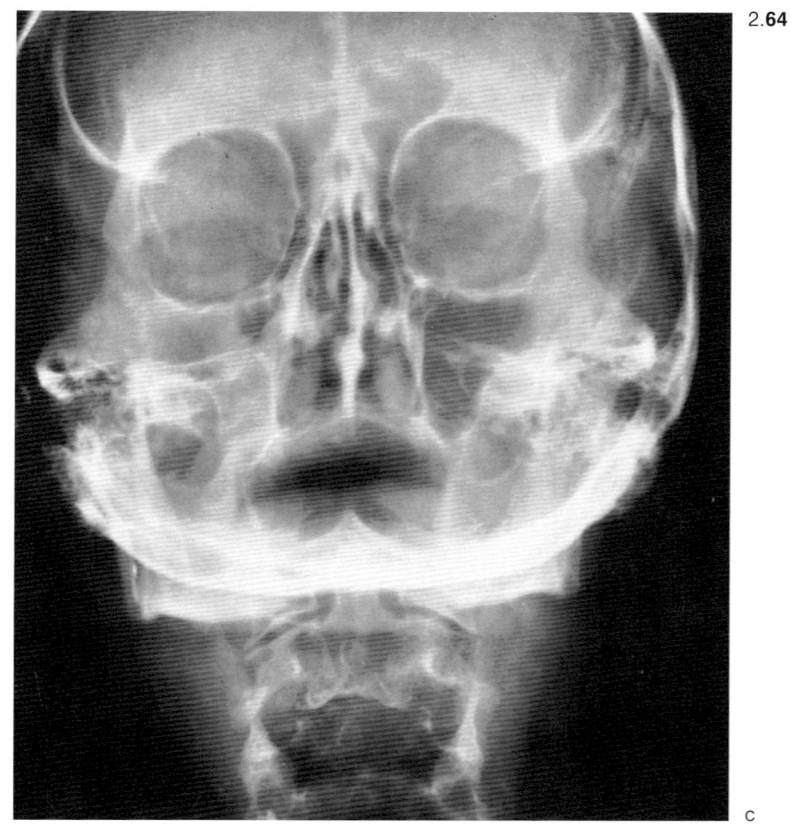

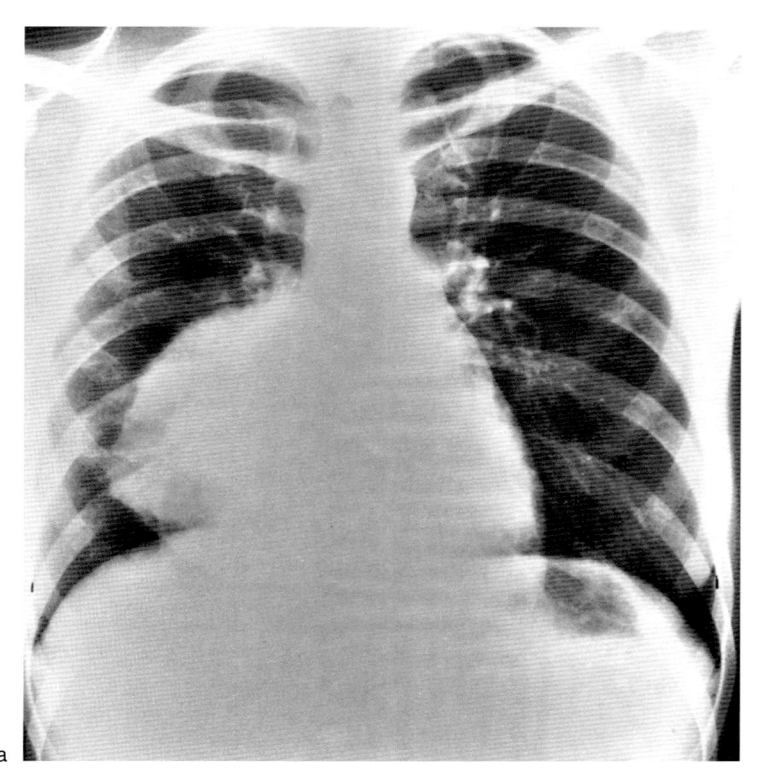

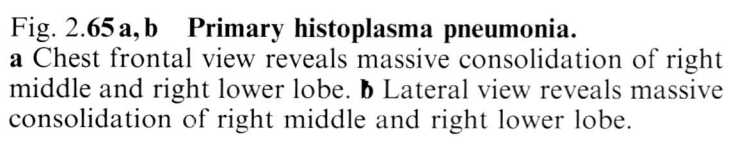

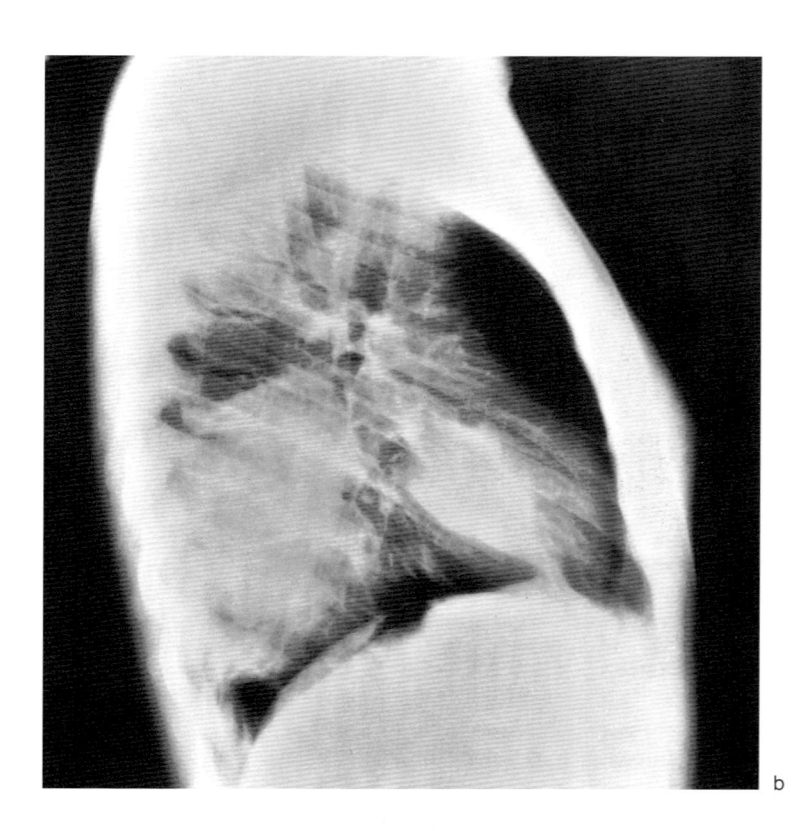

Fig. 2.**65 a, b Primary histoplasma pneumonia.**
a Chest frontal view reveals massive consolidation of right middle and right lower lobe. b Lateral view reveals massive consolidation of right middle and right lower lobe.

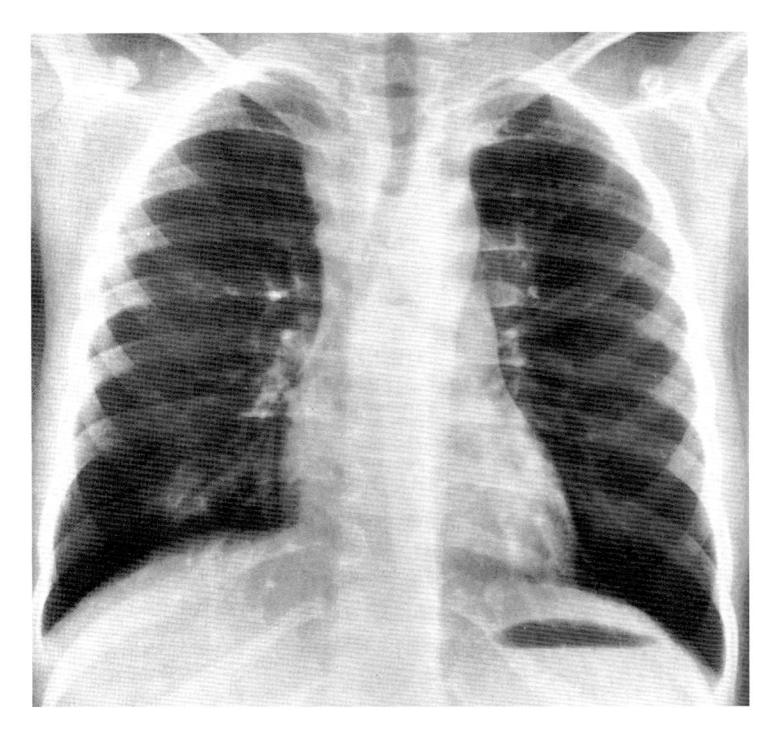

Fig. 2.66 **Primary histoplasmosis in an 8-year-old child.**
Ill-defined focus of consolidation in right lower lobe with marked enlargement of paratracheal and aortic-pulmonic window lymph nodes, accounting for superior mediastinal widening.

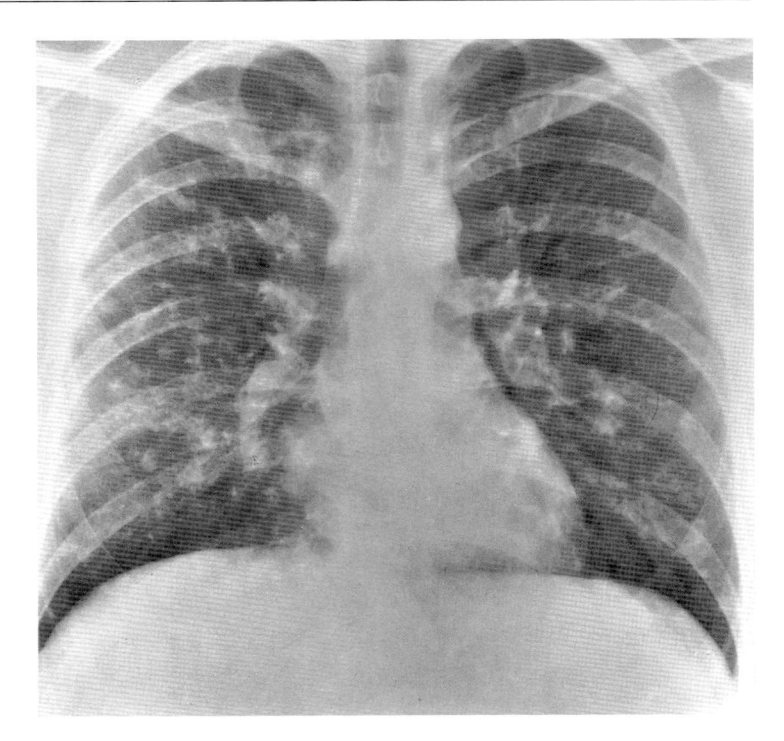

Fig. 2.67 Primary histoplasmosis in a young man who became ill after exploring a cave in Mexico and most likely inhaled fungal spores from contaminated bats. Chest radiograph reveals multiple, ill-defined, patchy, bilateral foci of consolidation in the lungs, typical of massive aerogenous infection.

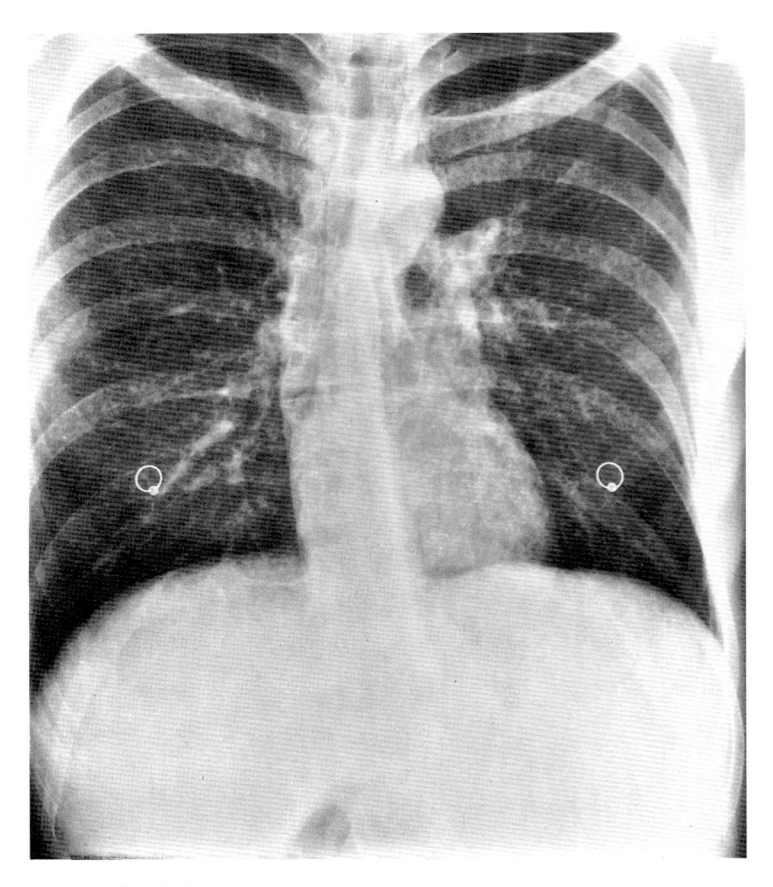

Fig. 2.68 **Miliary histoplasmosis in AIDS patient.**
Chest radiograph reveals multiple, small, rounded opacities measuring 1–3 mm in diameter, typical of hematogenous dissemination. Note bilateral nipple rings.

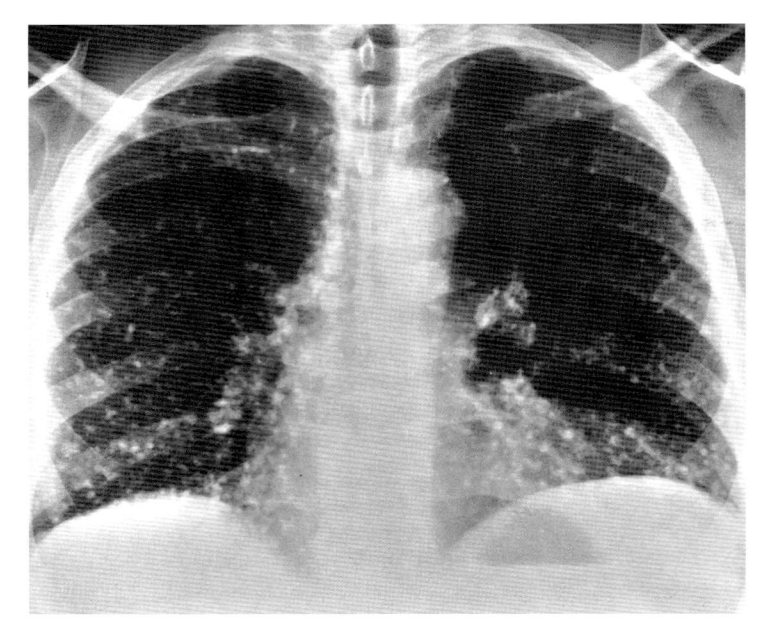

Fig. 2.69 **Healed histoplasmosis.**
Multiple calcific nodules are scattered throughout both lungs, most likely representing sequelae of remote massive aerogenous infection.

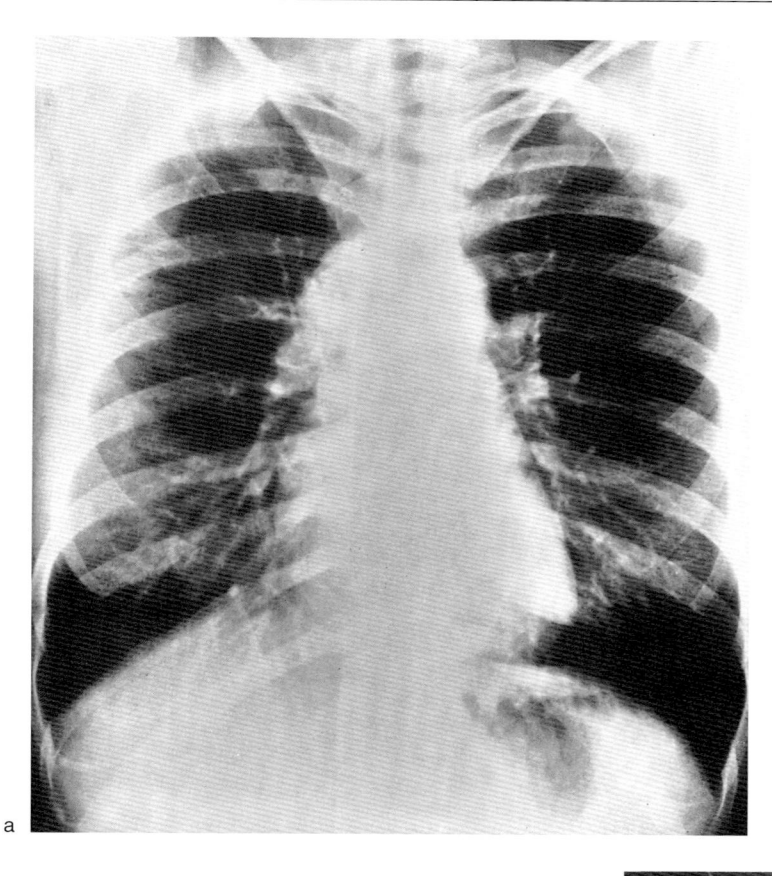

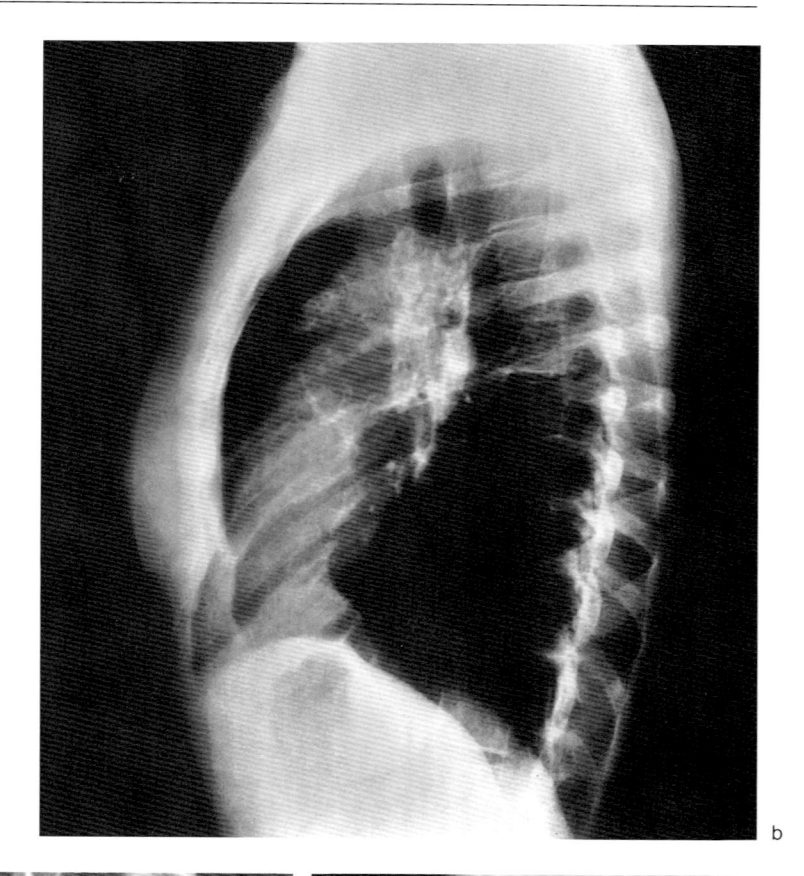

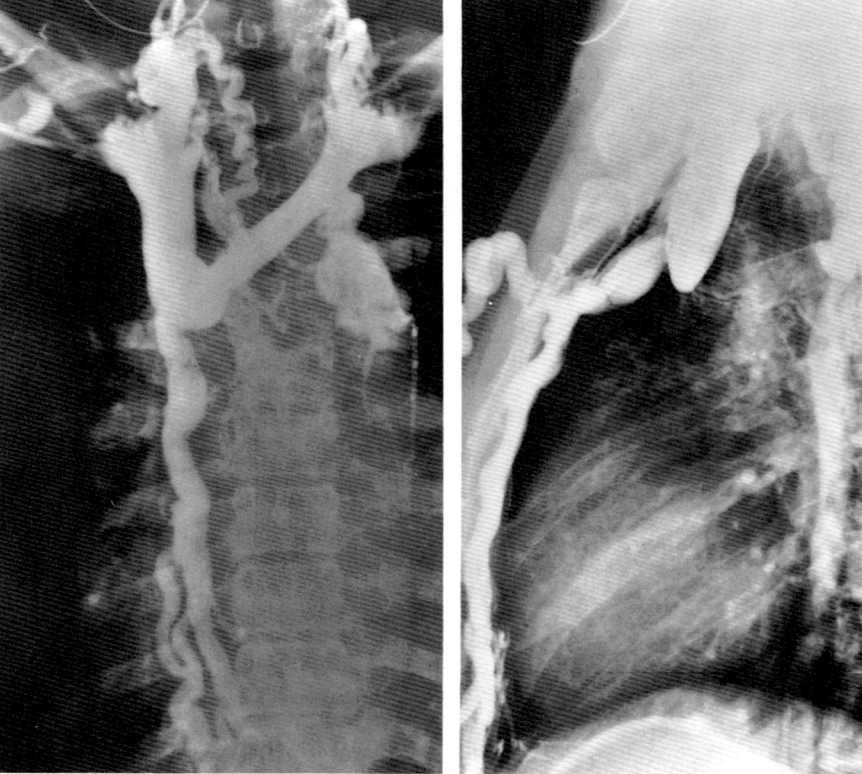

Fig. 2.70 a–d Chronic mediastinal granuloma due to histoplasmosis resulting in superior vena cava obstruction. **a** Chest frontal. **b** Lateral radiograph reveals a calcified right hilar and paratracheal mass in juxtaposition to the superior vena cava. **c** Frontal view of a venogram demonstrates occlusion of superior vena cava with dilatation of both brachiocephalic veins and collateral flow in internal mammary and azygos veins. **d** Lateral view of same venogram.

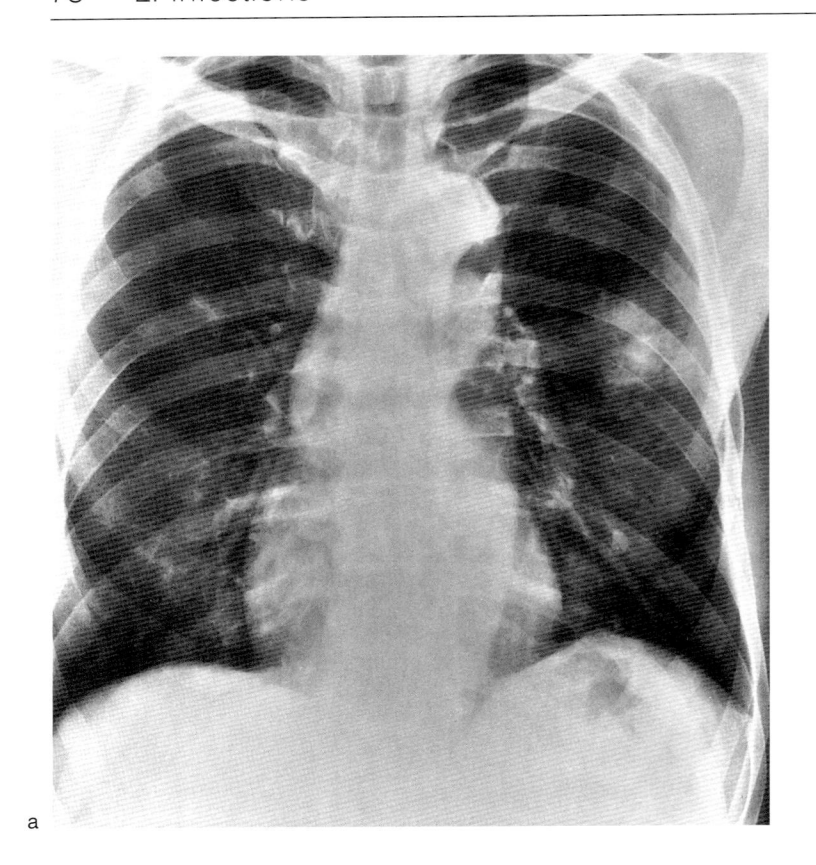

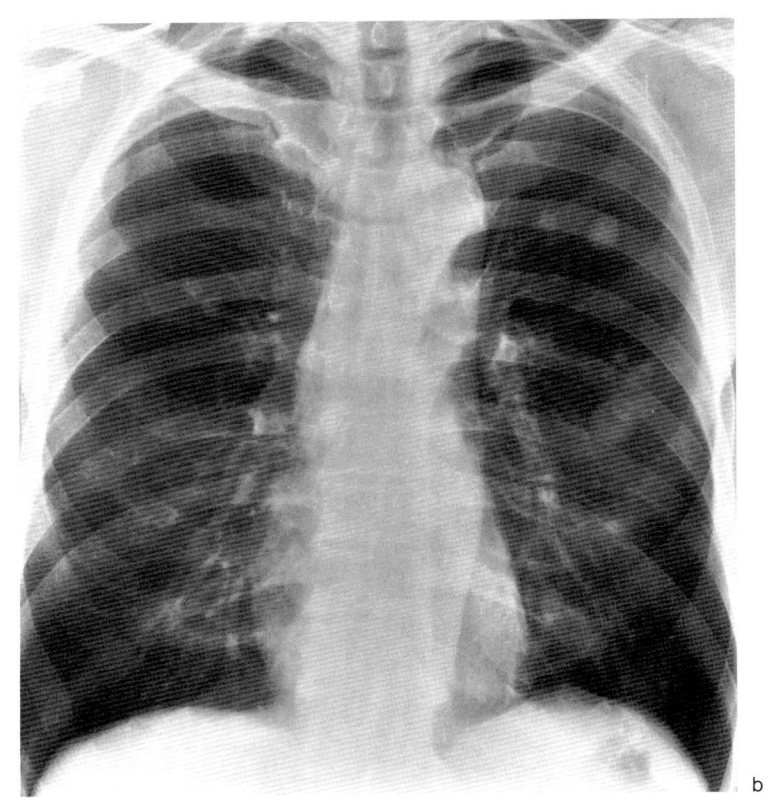

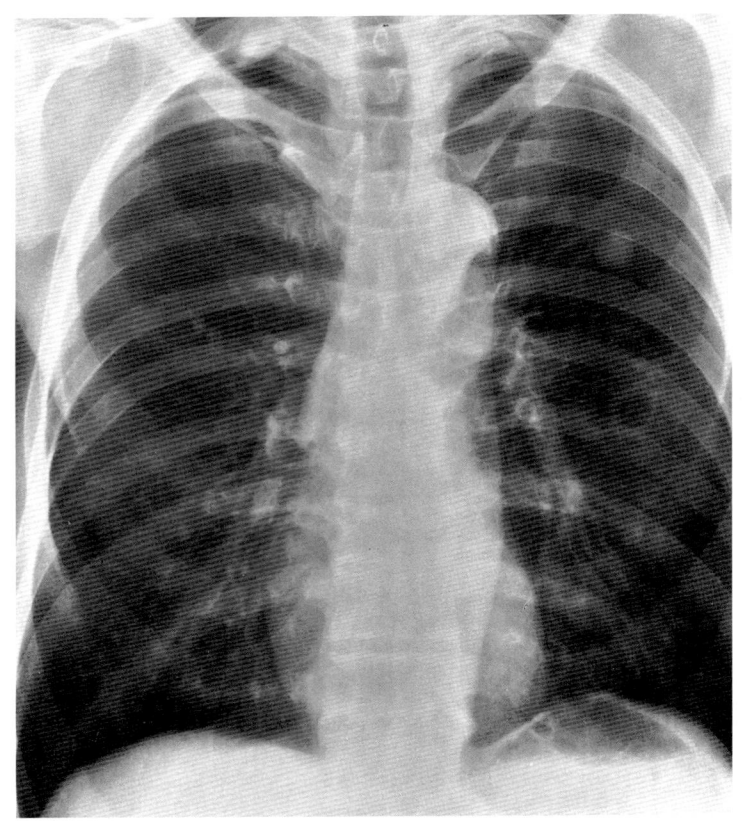

Fig. 2.71 a–c Coccidioidomycosis.
a Initial chest radiograph shows a dominant left upper lobe pneumonic focus. **b** Three years later, several left-sided nodules remain. Six years later (**c**), a thin-walled cavity has formed in the left mid-lung zone.

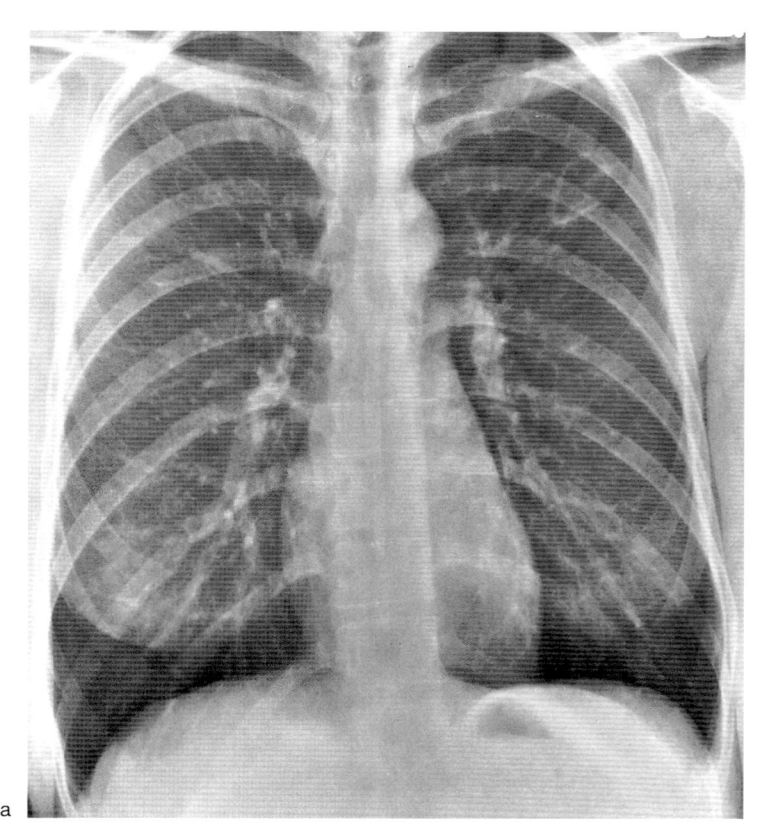

Fig. 2.**72 a, b** **Coccidioidomycosis.**
a Chest radiograph shows typical thin-walled left upper lobe cavity. Two years later (**b**), the cavity has enlarged.

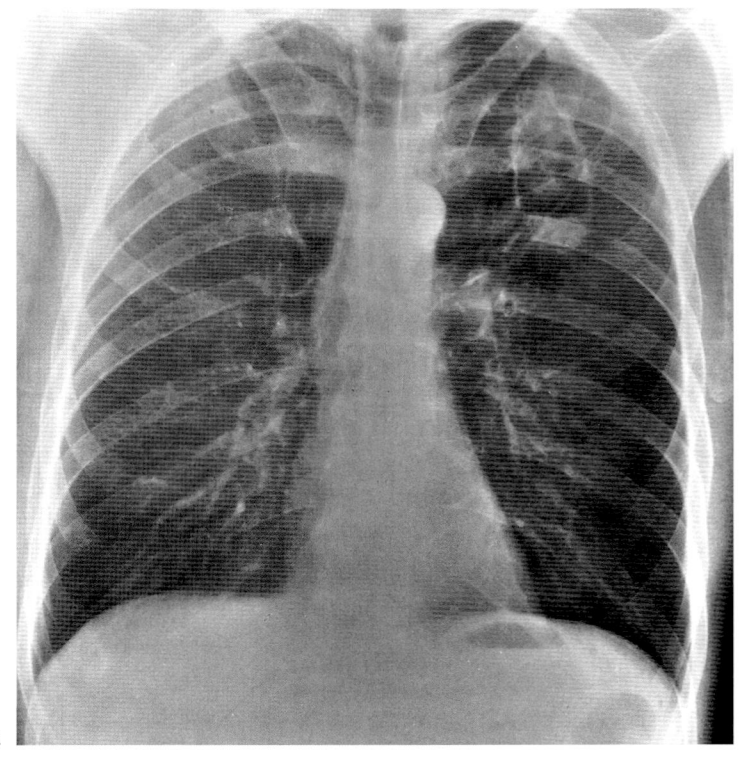

Fig. 2.**73 a, b** **Coccidioidomycosis.**
a Progressive, destructive form, thin-walled cavity with air-fluid level. **b** Follow-up chest film 1 year later shows large cavity with near-complete destruction of left upper lobe.

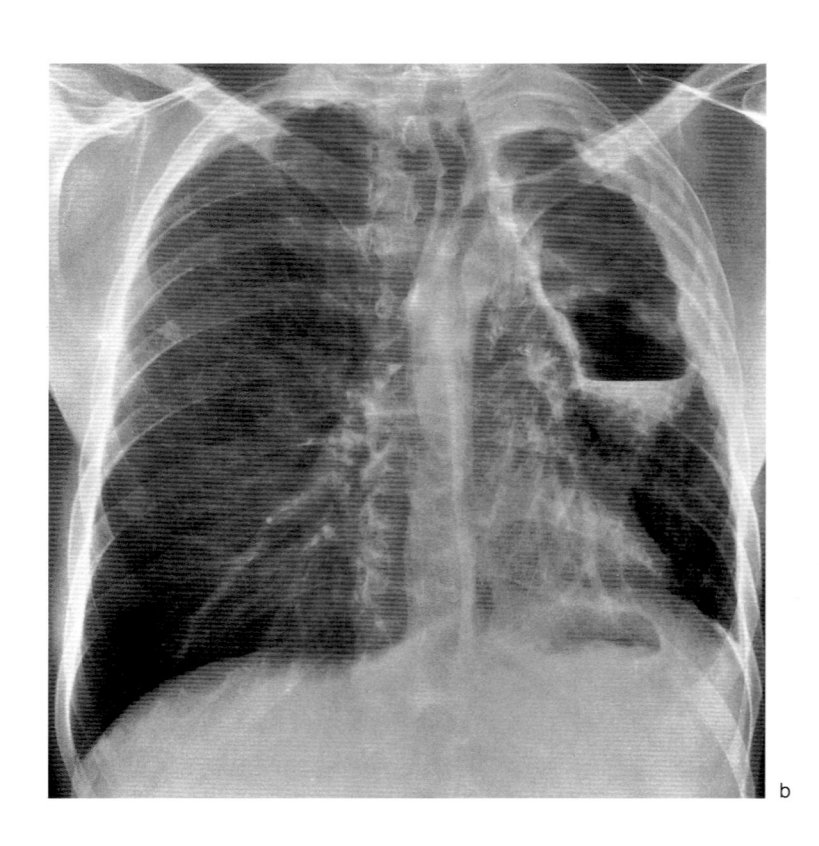

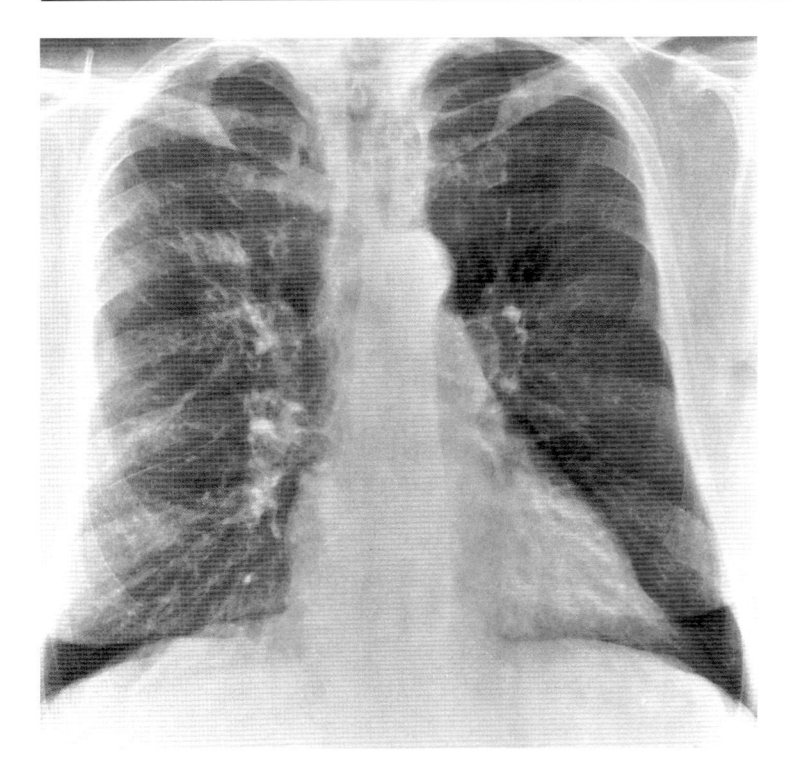

Fig. 2.74 **Coccidioidomycosis.**
Primary infection in 56-year-old smoker. Chest radiograph reveals ill-defined mass in right upper lobe with adjacent right hilar lymph node enlargement. Patient mistakenly operated on for presumed bronchogenic carcinoma.

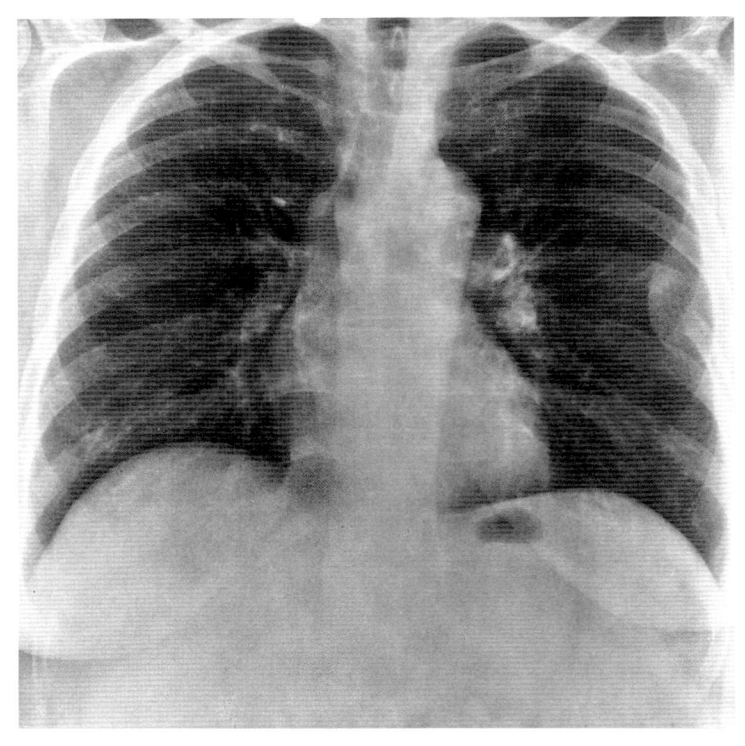

Fig. 2.75 **Coccidioidomycosis of rib.**
Chest radiograph reveals an expansile, destructive, lytic lesion of the left seventh posterior rib with a pathologic fracture.

Echinococcal Disease

This disease is endemic in southern Europe, the Middle East, and other regions with large populations of sheep. Human beings represent accidental intermediate hosts. The natural intermediate hosts are the sheep; the definitive hosts, the dogs. They ingest the worm eggs with contaminated food. The eggs hatch in the bowel, the larvae penetrate the bowel mucosa, and eventually cysts form, primarily in the liver, lung, brain, and bones. These cysts are filled with fluid and small daughter cysts. They consist of a fibrous pericyst produced by the host, an ectocyst, and an endocyst. The ecto- and endocyst contain chitin and are fused. If the cyst connects to the bronchial tree, air can dissect between the pericyst and the endocysts, producing a crescent sign. If the endocyst ruptures, it floats on a gas-fluid level, forming the so-called waterlily sign.

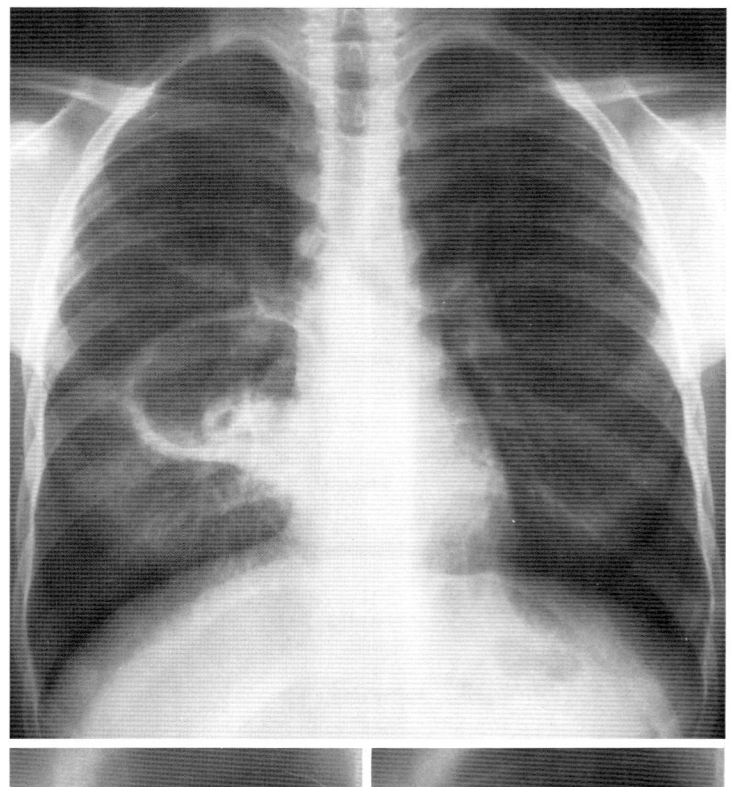

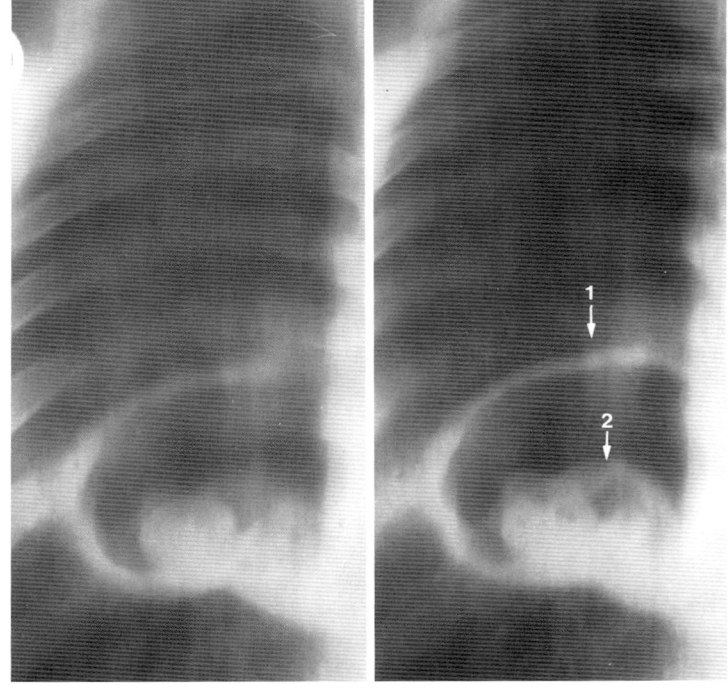

Fig. 2.76 a–d **Echinococcal cyst.**
15-year-old Turkish girl. Gas-containing cavity in superior segment of right lower lobe. Pericyst (1), endocyst (2). Bronchogram shows how superior segmental bronchial branches are splayed by the cyst, which is drained by a superior segmental bronchial branch.

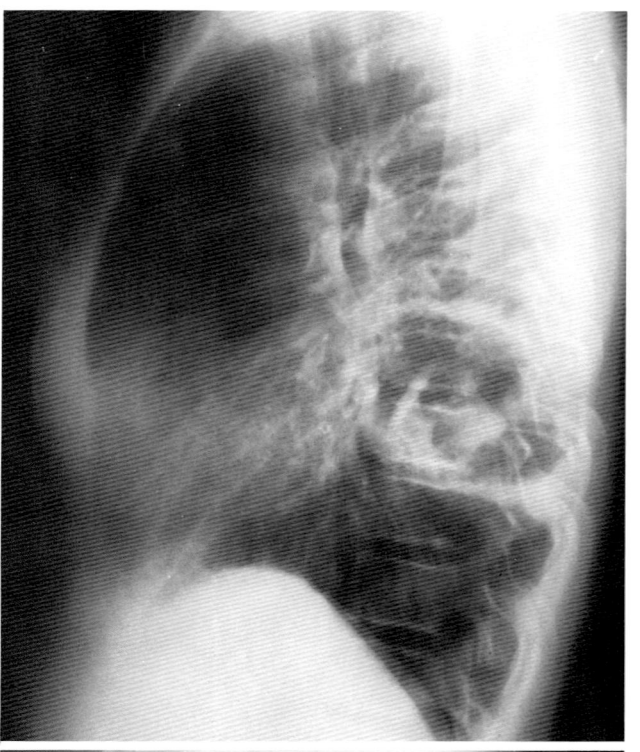

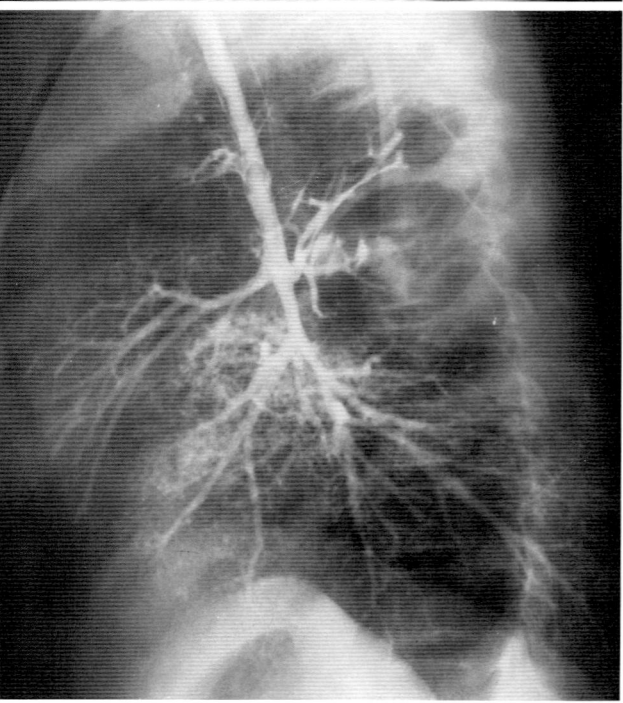

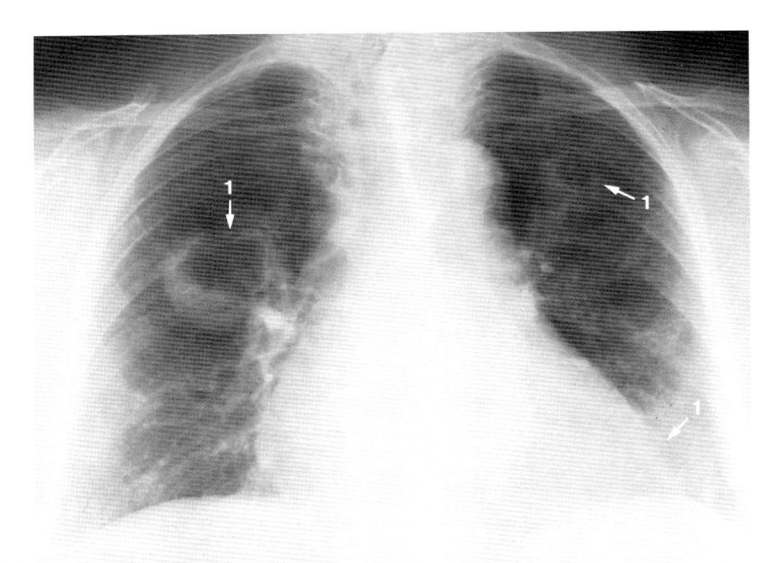

Fig. 2.77 a–b **Echinococcal disease.**
71-year-old patient admitted for left ventricular failure. Sputum contained scoleces. Multiple cavitary lesions scattered throughout both lungs (1). Differential diagnosis includes cavitating metastases, Wegener granulomatosis, and multiple septic emboli with abscess formation.

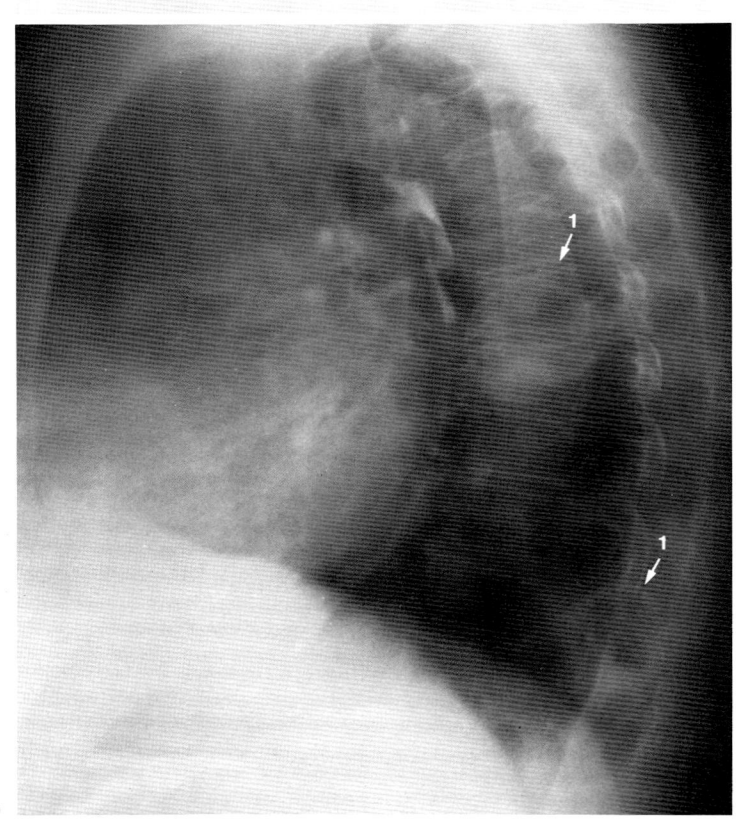

Collagen Vascular Diseases

These diseases are due to an autoimmune process. The lung, pleura, pericardium, and pulmonary vessels can be affected. Usually, interstitial pneumonitis can lead to diffuse interstitial fibrosis. Vasculitis can result in cavitating nodules and pulmonary hemorrhage. Pleural and pericardial effusions are also common. Pulmonary fibrosis is most likely in scleroderma (30%). Polyserositis is a hallmark of lupus erythematosus. Cavitating, necrobiotic nodules occur primarily in rheumatoid arthritis.

References: 32, 78, 131.

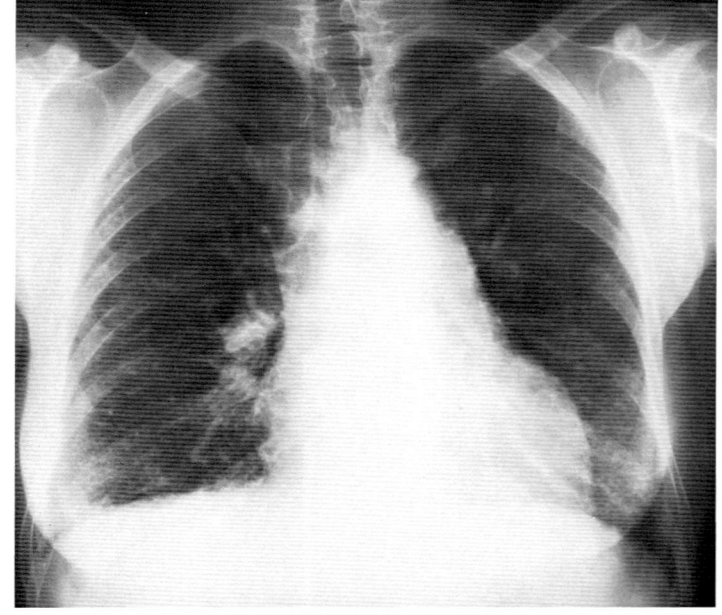

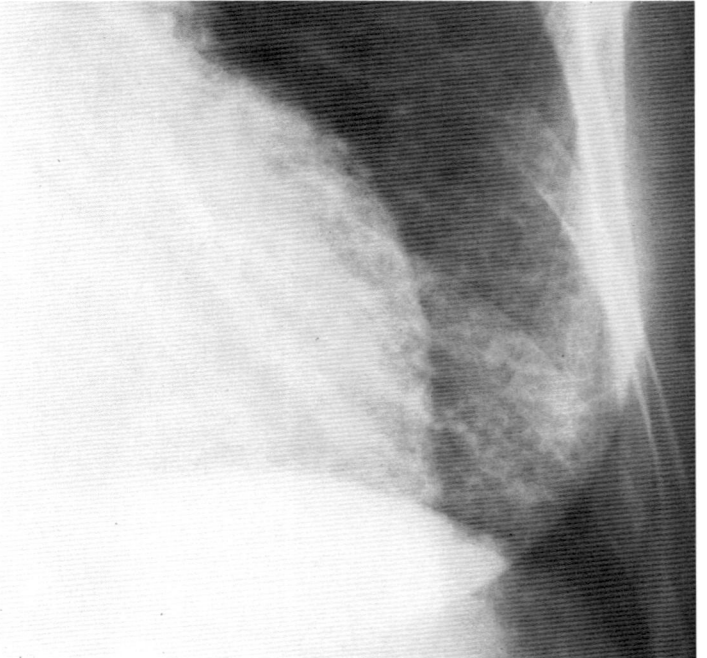

Fig. 2.**78 a, b   Scleroderma.**
66-year-old patient with reflux esophagitis. Abnormal linear and reticular opacities in both middle and lower lung zones. Moderate cardiomegaly with dilatation of central pulmonary arteries, indicating pulmonary arterial hypertension.

84 2. Infections

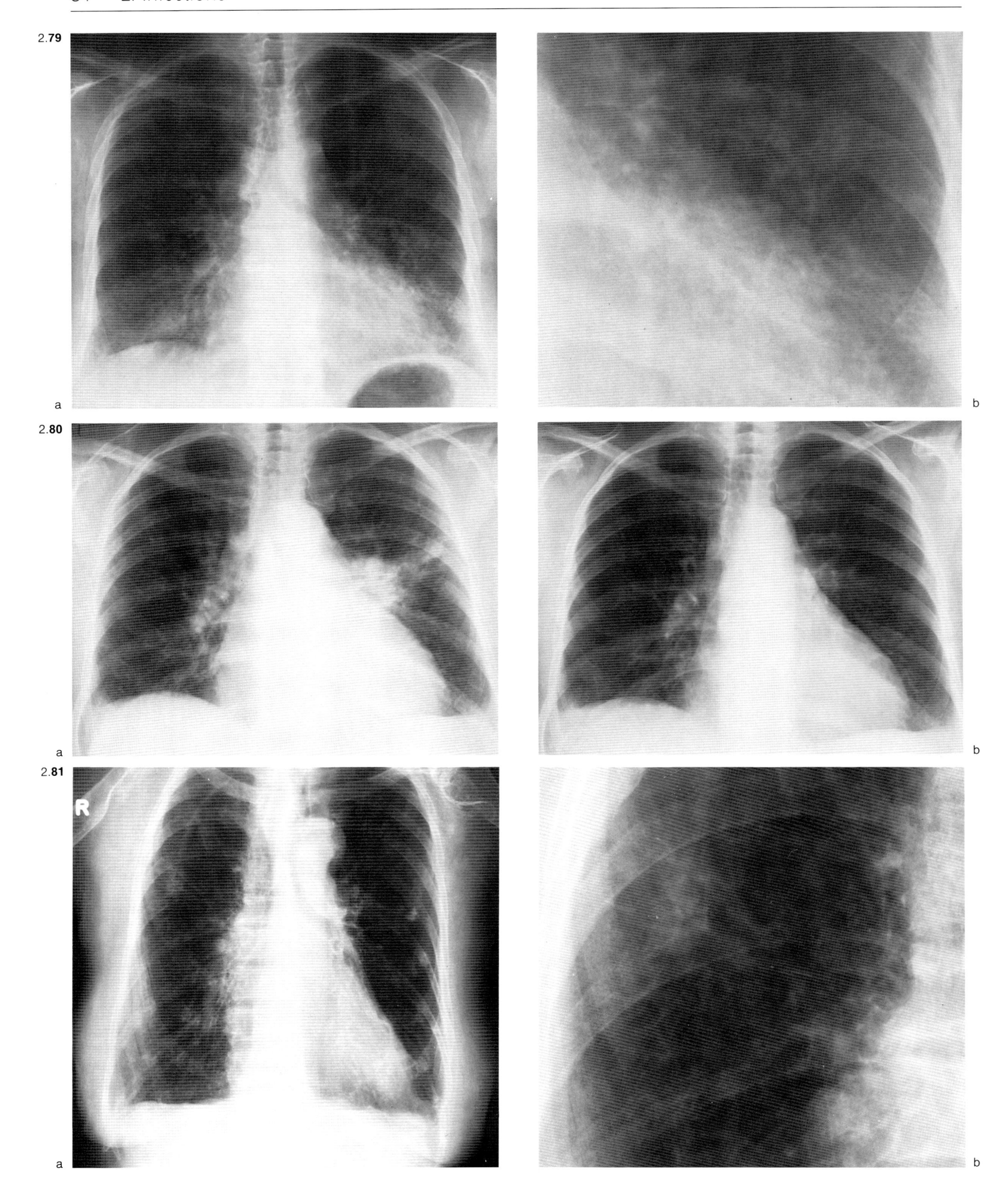

Wegener Granulomatosis

This autoimmune disorder consists of a vasculitis with glomerulonephritis and necrotizing granulomas in the paranasal sinuses, nasal cavity, upper airways, and lungs. Chest radiography reveals multiple pulmonary nodules which cavitate in at least 30% of cases, ill-defined segmental consolidation, or diffuse pulmonary hemorrhage.

Fig. 2.**82 a–c Wegener granulomatosis.**
37-year-old man with maxillary sinusitis and proteinuria. Multifocal areas of pulmonary consolidation with early cavitation in left lung.

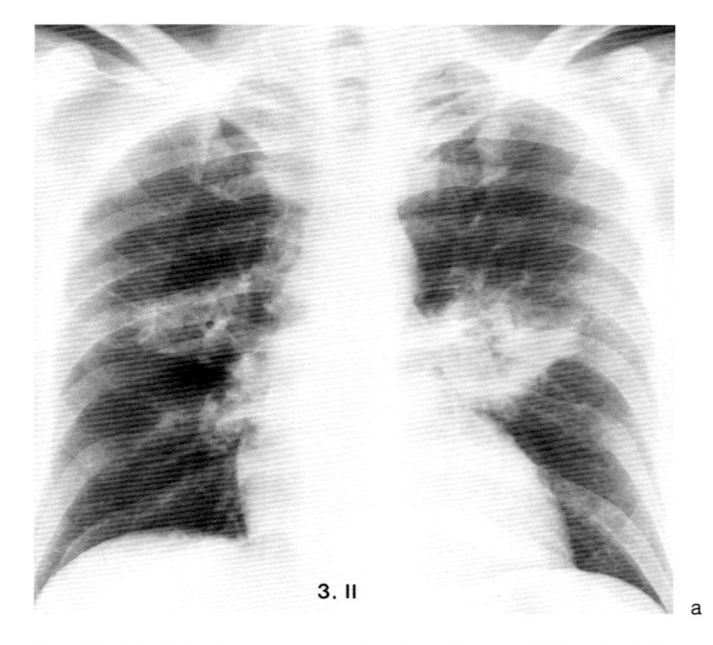

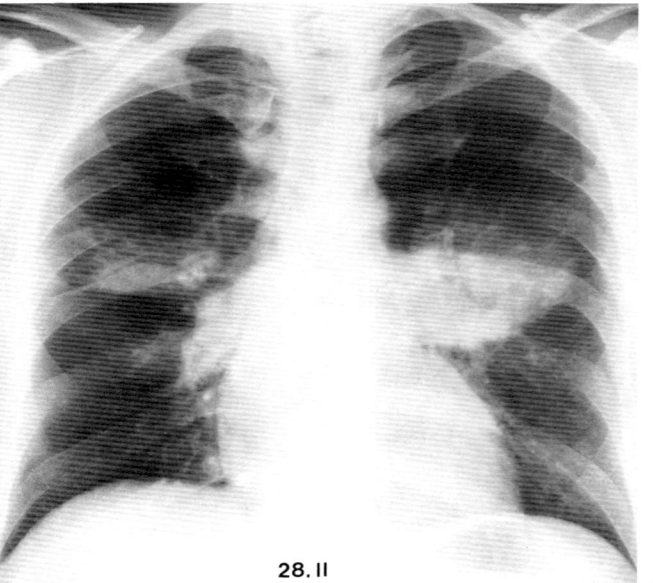

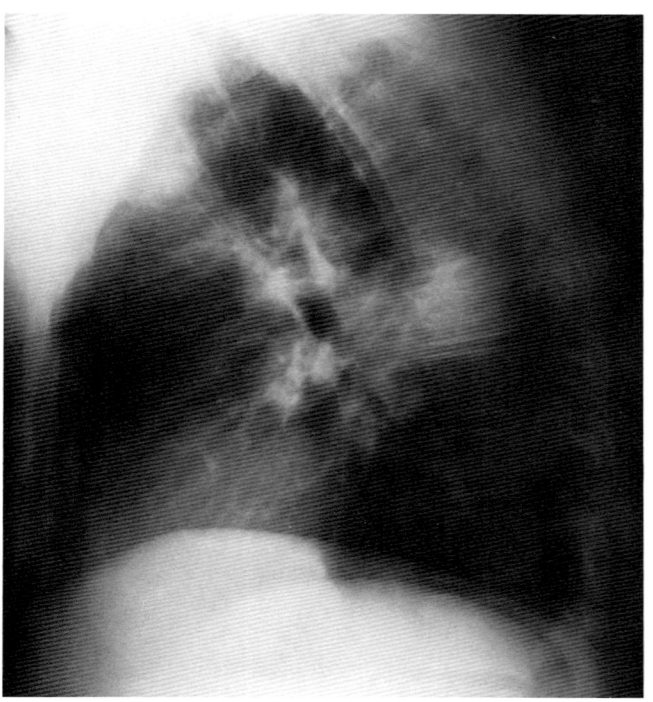

Fig. 2.**79 a, b Systemic lupus erythematosus.**
57-year-old patient with polyarthritis. Bibasilar, small, linear and reticular opacities and enlarged cardiac silhouette.

Fig. 2.**80 a, b Systemic lupus erythematosus.**
Enlarged cardiac silhouette, small, bilateral, pleural effusions, consolidation of superior segment left lower lobe. Marked improvement after corticosteroid therapy.

Fig. 2.**81 a, b Rheumatoid nodules with biopsy proof.**
50-year-old patient with long-standing history of rheumatoid arthritis. Multiple, peripheral nodules are visible in both lungs.

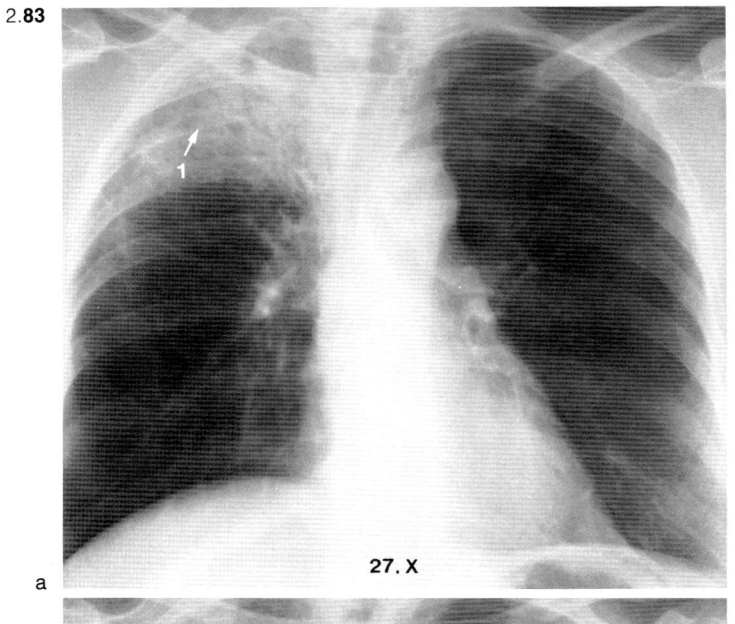

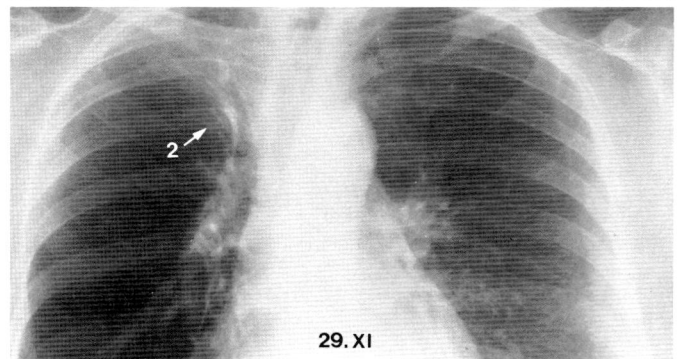

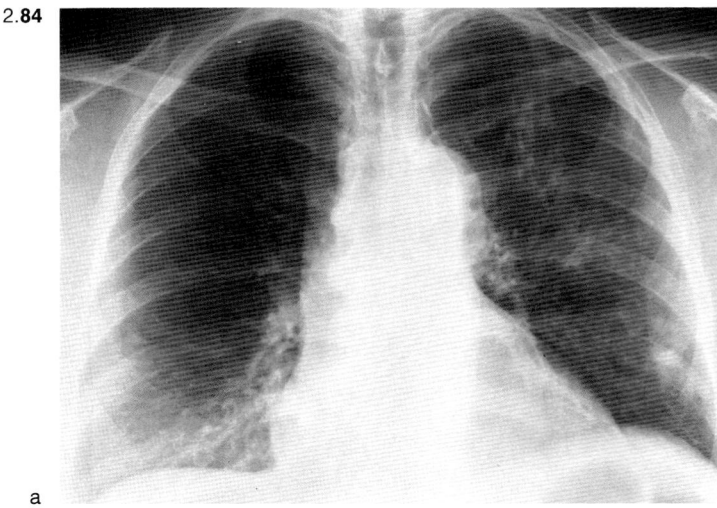

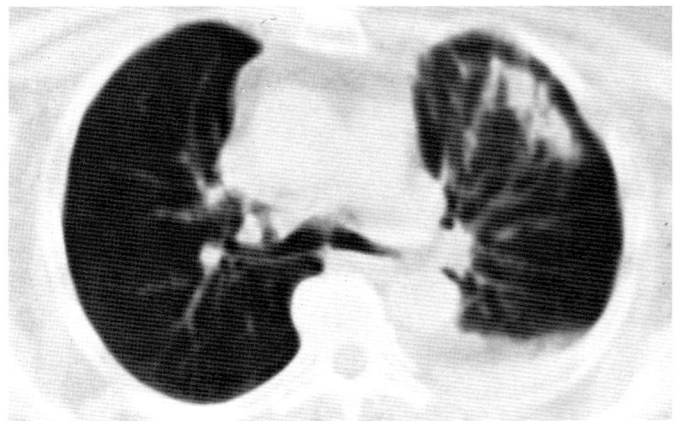

Radiation Pneumonitis

Ionizing radiation induces lung damage, depending on the total dose, the fractionation, and the volume of tissue irradiated. The tolerance dose for the entire lung is 15–20 Gy (1500–2000 R). If a smaller volume is irradiated, the tolerance dose increases to 35–40 Gy (3500–4000 R). As a rule, radiation pneumonitis becomes visible 8 weeks after the completion of 40 Gy (4000 R) given over 4 weeks in fractions of 2 Gy (200 R) per day. For every additional 10 Gy (1000 R) total dose, the pneumonitis will appear a week earlier (e.g., 6 weeks after 60 Gy).

The initial damage occurs at the capillary level, with subsequent leakage of fibrinous material into the alveoli. Over the next 10–12 months, radiation fibrosis develops, due to obliteration of the capillaries and subsequent ischemic damage. Radiologically, the initial consolidation is patchy, then homogeneous, with an air bronchogram. A straight-edge effect contributes to the nonsegmental, nonanatomical distribution of the consolidation and is characteristic of radiation damage. In later stages, cicatrization atelectasis with loss of lung volume and traction bronchiectasis is visible.

Fig. 2.**83 a, b** Acute radiation pneumonitis (**a**) evolving to fibrosis after 9 months.
63-year-old female patient irradiated for carcinoma of the breast up to a dose of 60 Gy. Confluent opacification of right upper lobe with air bronchograms (1). Oblique, linear, scarlike opacities (2) with cephalad hilar retraction.

Fig. 2.**84 a, b**   **Radiation pneumonitis.**
71-year-old patient treated with tangential fields for chest wall recurrence. Streaky opacification of the left upper lung zone. CT scan reveals subpleural, anterolateral location of consolidative process as well as a left pleural effusion.

Fig. 2.85 a–c **Pneumonitis after radiation for bronchogenic carcinoma.**
72-year-old smoker unwilling to undergo surgery. Right-sided tumor irradiated with 60 Gy. Solitary pulmonary nodule in right upper lobe (**a**). Consolidation conforms to radiation portal (**b**). Air bronchogram (1). Radiation fibrosis (**c**) with right upper lobe volume loss, deviation of trachea to the right, narrow intercostal spaces, and slight elevation of right hemidiaphragm.

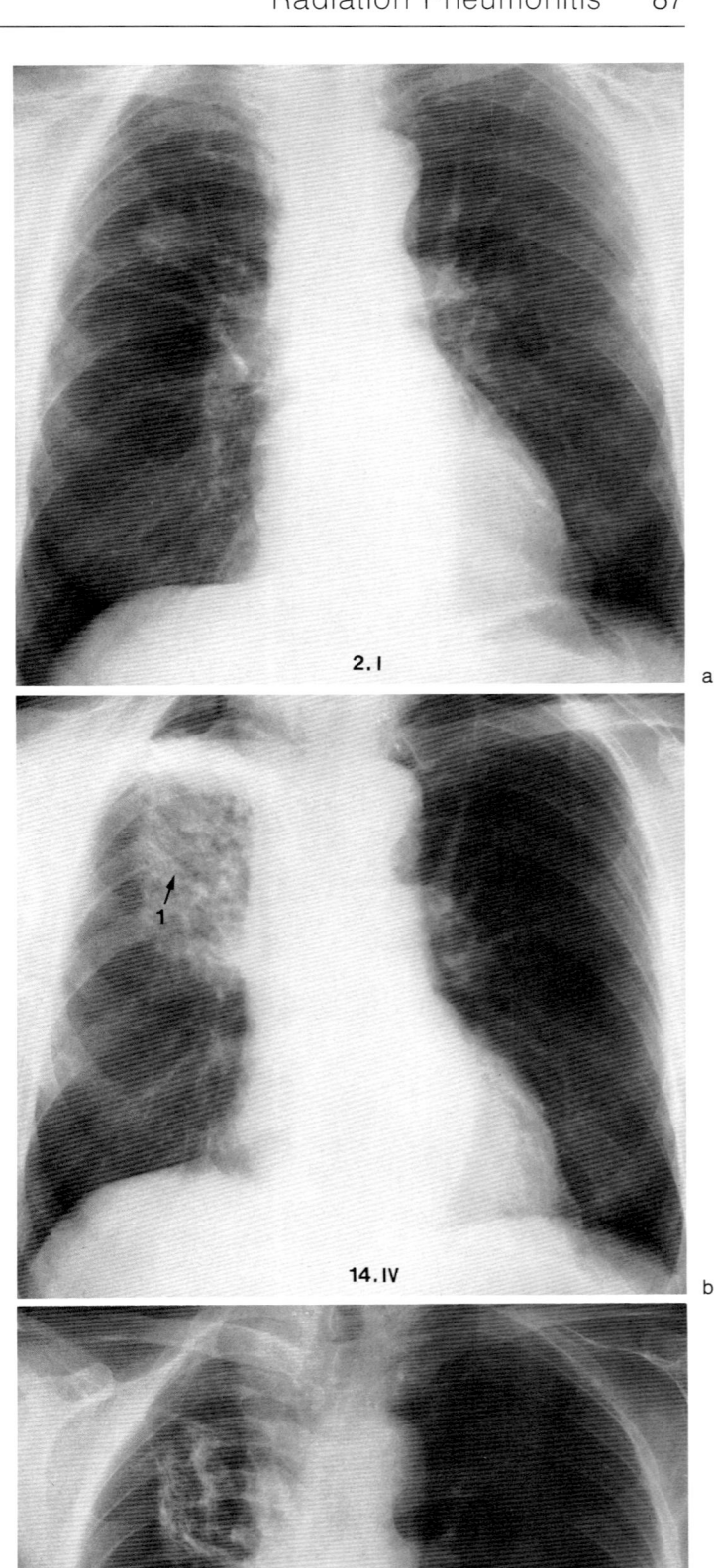

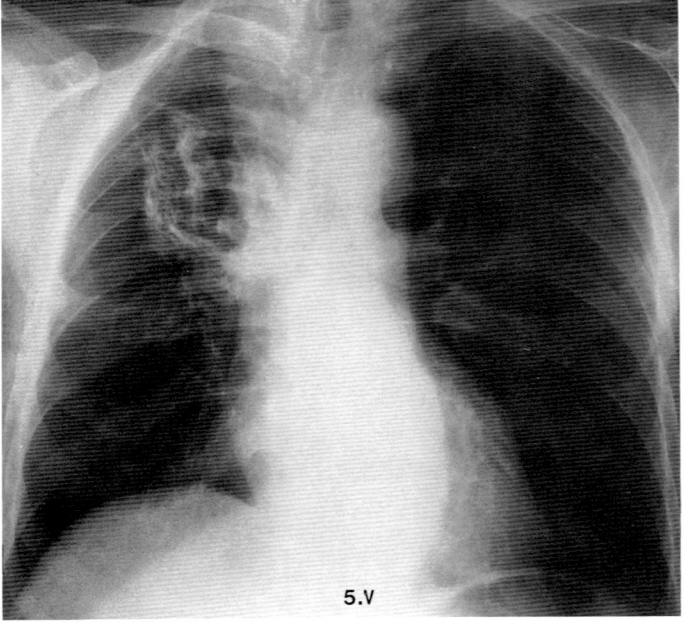

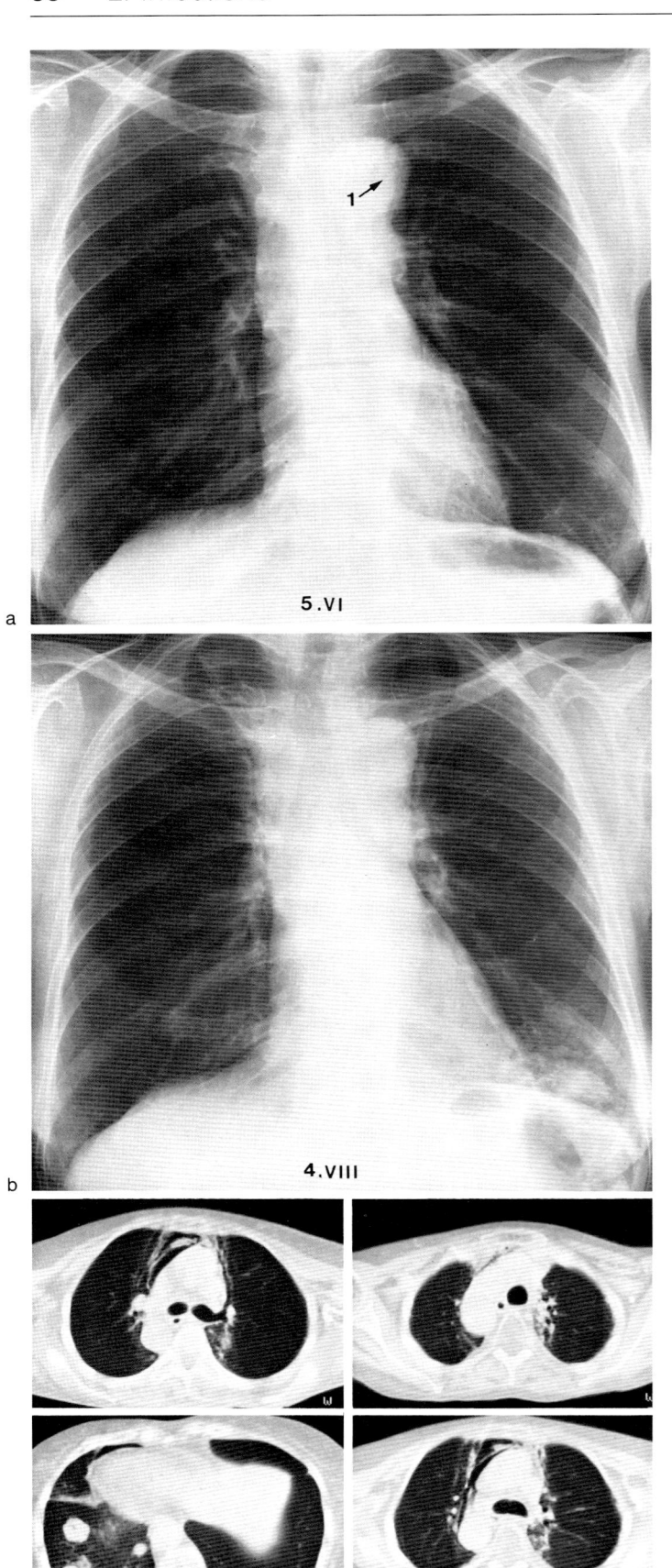

Fig. 2.86 a–c **Paramediastinal radiation fibrosis.**
Patient irradiated for non-Hodgkin lymphoma.
Superior mediastinal widening. Aortic arch (1) not obscured by mass. Paramediastinal, vertical, streaky opacities, bilateral hilar superomedial retraction (**b**). Ill-defined left lower lobe nodules (**b**), better delineated on CT scan (**c**).

Histiocytosis of Langerhans

Eosinophilic granuloma or histiocytosis of the lung accounts for 3% of all chronic infiltrative pulmonary diseases. In 60% of cases, only the lung is involved; in 20%, additional lytic bone lesions are present, and in 20%, systemic disease develops with involvement of other organ systems. Smokers are more likely to develop pulmonary histiocytosis.

Radiologically, the upper and middle lung zones are primarily involved. In the early stages, small nodules form; later, reticulonodular changes and honeycombing develop. A higher incidence of spontaneous pneumothorax has been recorded. The disease can progress slowly and can be reversible. High-resolution CT scanning displays characteristic thin-walled cysts throughout the lung parenchyma.

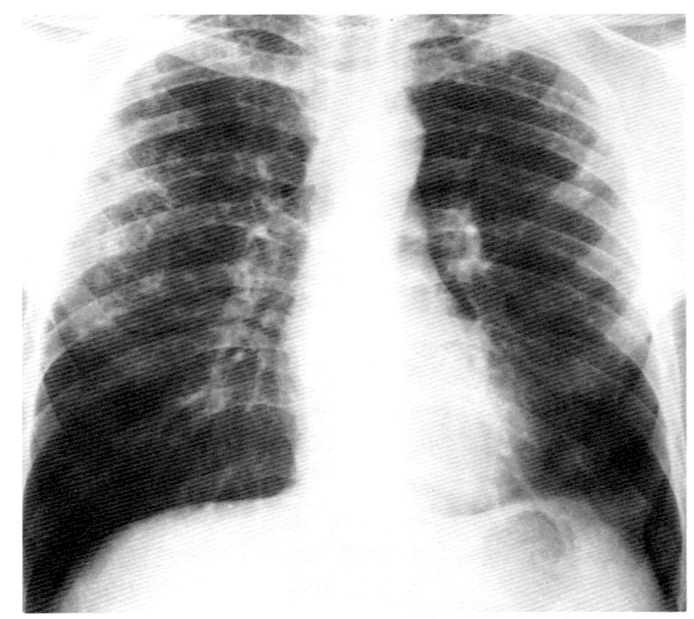

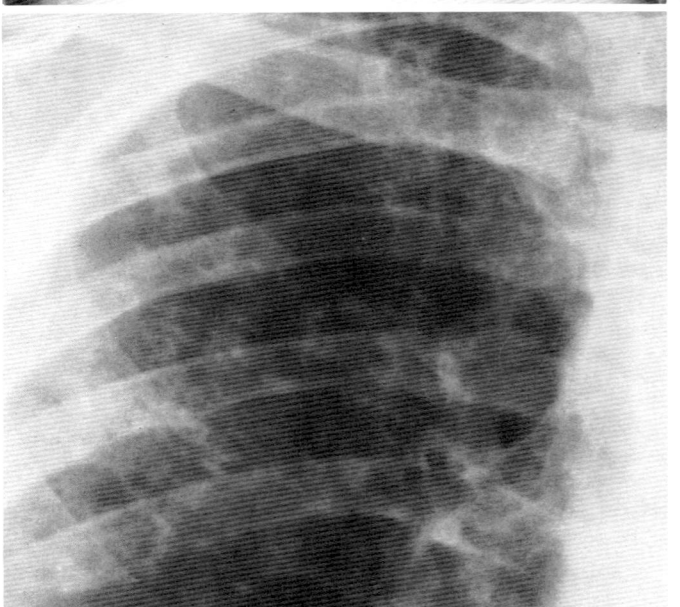

Fig. 2.**87 a, b Histiocytosis X, Hand-Schüller-Christian disease.**
21-year-old patient with a 7-year history of diabetes insipidus, osteolytic skull lesions, and mild dyspnea. Biopsy-proven granulomas containing Langerhans cells.

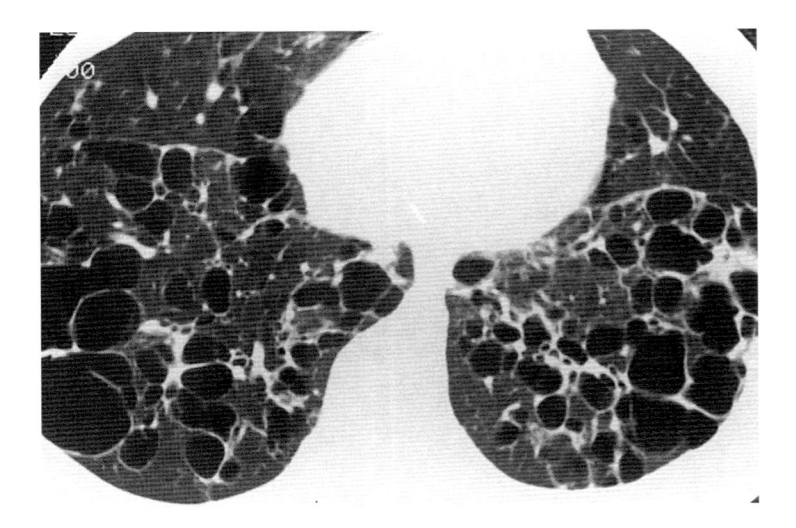

Fig. 2.**88** 8-year-old child with eosinophilic granuloma (histiocytosis) of the lungs. CT scan reveals multiple cysts scattered throughout both lungs; the thicker wall allows differentiation from bullae.

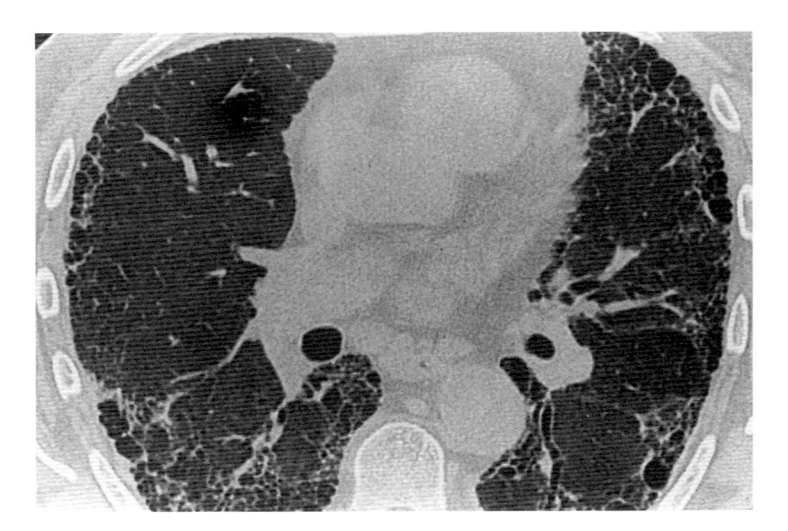

Fig. 2.**89** Patient with biopsy-proven usual interstitial pneumonitis and idiopathic pulmonary fibrosis. High-resolution CT scan shows focal subpleural honeycombing and bronchiolectasis with intervening normal lung in between abnormal areas.

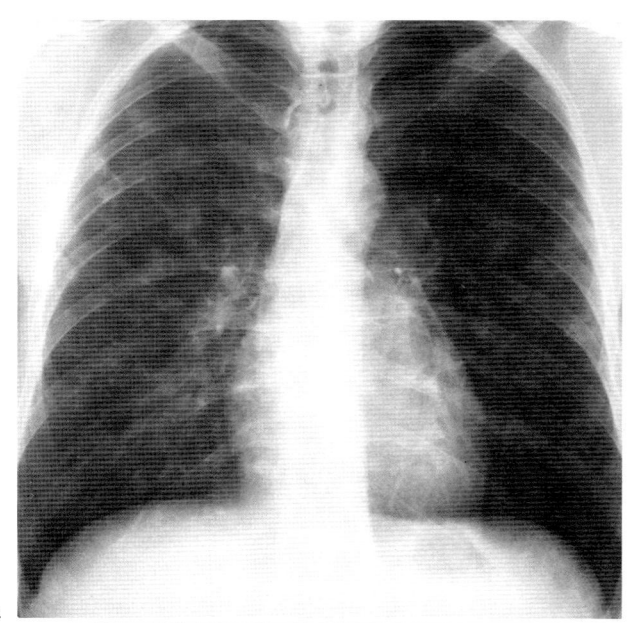

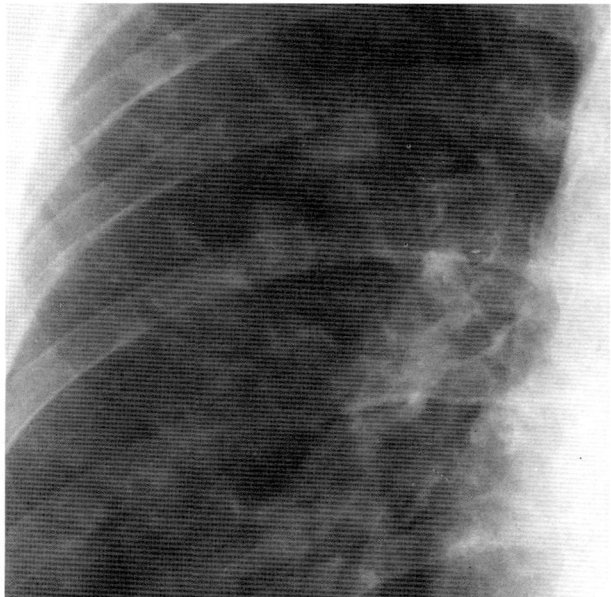

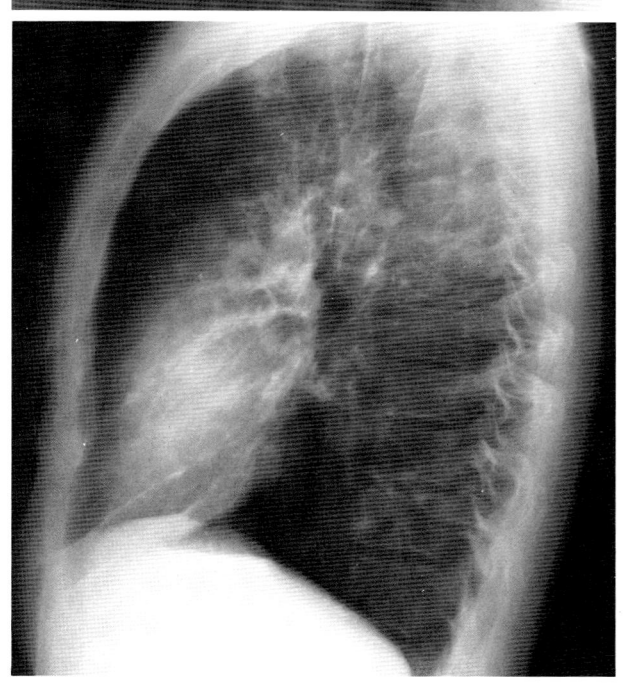

Fig. 2.**90 a–c****Histiocytosis X.**
32-year-old asymptomatic man. Incidental finding of multiple reticulonodular opacities scattered throughout the upper and middle lung zones.

3. Chronic Obstructive Lung Diseases

Emphysema

Emphysema is characterized by irreversible dilatation of the airspaces distal to the terminal bronchioles, without accompanying pulmonary fibrosis. Four types are differentiated pathologically:

1. Centriacinar emphysema occurs in smokers and is seen primarily in the upper lobes.
2. Panacinar emphysema occurs in the upper and lower lobes and is seen in smokers and elderly people as senile emphysema or due to α_1-antitrypsin deficiency.
3. Paraseptal or distal acinar emphysema is found in subpleural location and is the precursor or apical blebs or subpleural bullae.
4. Pericicatriceal emphysema is seen in the immediate vicinity of a scar.

Compensatory hyperexpansion seen after a loss of volume in adjacent parts of the lung should not be called emphysema since it is reversible in most cases. In general, emphysema is considered to be the result of uninhibited protease activity originating from polymorphonuclear leukocytes in the lung parenchyma. Emphysema results in ventilation-perfusion mismatch with subsequent hypoxic vasoconstriction, pulmonary arterial hypertension, respiratory failure, and cor pulmonale.

Radiologic findings include signs of external and internal hyperexpansion. External hyperexpansion relates to a decrease in the elastic recoil of the lung and results in flattening of the diaphragm, increase in the retrosternal clear space to a depth exceeding 3.5 cm, increased sagittal diameter of the chest, lung length over 30 cm, more than 7 anterior ribs and more than 10 posterior ribs visible above the dome of the diaphragm in the medioclavicular line. Signs of internal hyperexpansion relate to destruction of the lung parenchyma and include disorganization of the vascular pattern, increase of the vascular angle of bifurcation greater than 80°, and frank bulla formation.

Patients with chronic obstructive lung disease and or pulmonale can display the so-called increased markings emphysema. These findings include bronchial wall thickening, mild cylindrical bronchiectases, dilated central pulmonary arteries, and small airways disease. The decreased markings emphysema correlates with bullous changes. These patients are less likely to have ventilation-perfusion mismatch and cor pulmonale.

In daily practice, these two types of emphysema produce a combination of radiographic findings. High-resolution CT is the most sensitive method for analyzing the different types of emphysema. Cor pulmonale implies right ventricular hypertrophy due to pulmonary disease. It does not always lead to enlargement of the cardiac silhouette, but it frequently leads to dilatation of the main pulmonary artery segment and the central pulmonary arteries with concomitant pruning of the peripheral vascular structures.

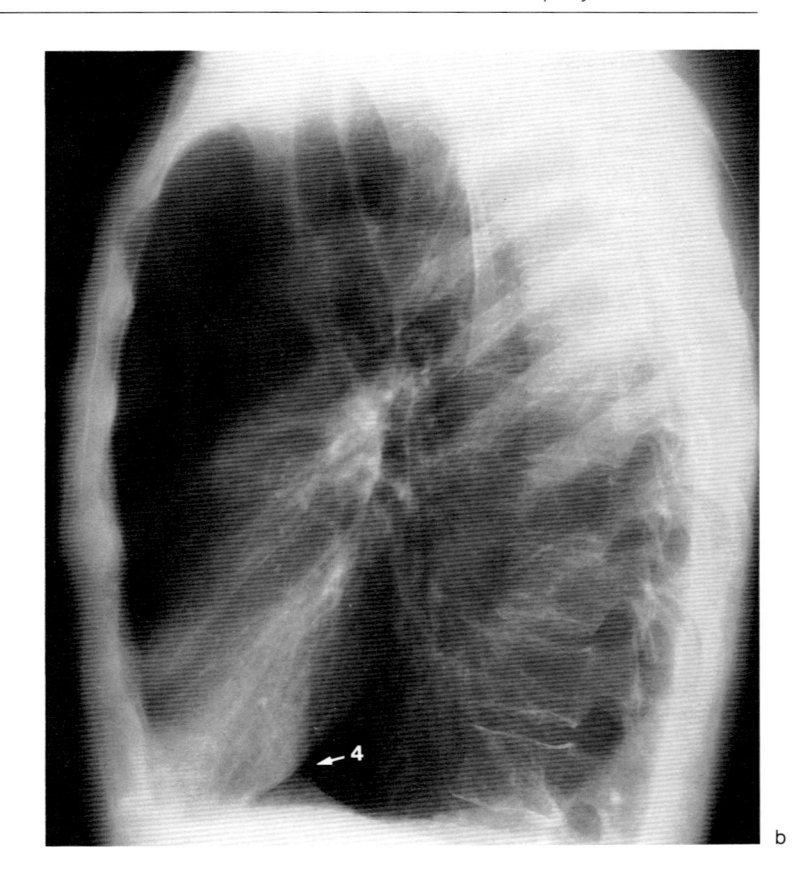

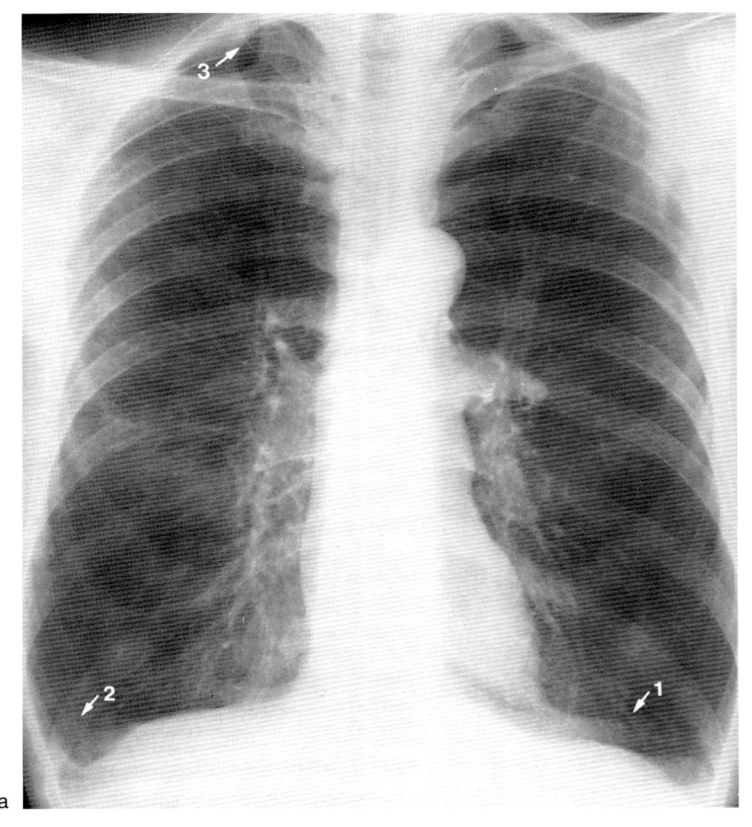

Fig. 3.1 a, b **Emphysema.**
55-year-old smoker with barrel chest. Wide intercostal spaces, flattened diaphragm, diaphragmatic muscle slips (1), blunted costophrenic sulcus due to diaphragmatic inversion (2), apical bulla (3), inferior vena cava (4).

3. Chronic Obstructive Lung Diseases

Emphysematous Bullae

Bullae represent emphysematous spaces that exceed 1 cm in diameter. The bullae are usually multiple but can occasionally be solitary. They result from the confluence of paraseptal or panacinar emphysema. The bullae can perforate into the pleural space and lead to spontaneous pneumothorax. They can become infected and sometimes obliterate spontaneously.

The radiologic features of bullae include areas of vascular rarefaction with a very thin wall. Sometimes such a sharp delineation of a bulla is not present. Large bullae with increased compliance allow the normal lung to retract away from it. The effect is that of an "intrapulmonary tension pneumothorax." Differentiation of a bulla from a pneumothorax can occasionally create problems. Bullae have an inner border which is convex towards the mediastinum, whereas a pneumothorax is delineated by a visceral pleural line that is straight or convex towards the rib cage. CT can display bullae well and in complicated cases facilitates the differentiation from pneumothorax.

Fig. 3.2 a, b **Emphysema.**
65-year-old patient with barrel chest with anterior convexity of sternum and deep retrosternal space. Left descending pulmonary artery (1), left mainstem bronchus (2), right pulmonary artery (3), anterior segmental artery, and bronchus (4).

Fig. 3.3 a–d **Emphysema in patient with chronic cyanosis and dyspnea.**
Abnormal pulmonary markings (1), minor fissure (2), segmental bronchi seen end on (3,5), prominent left first costochondral junction (4), left pulmonary artery (6). CT demonstrates multiple bullae interspersed with preserved lung parenchyma.

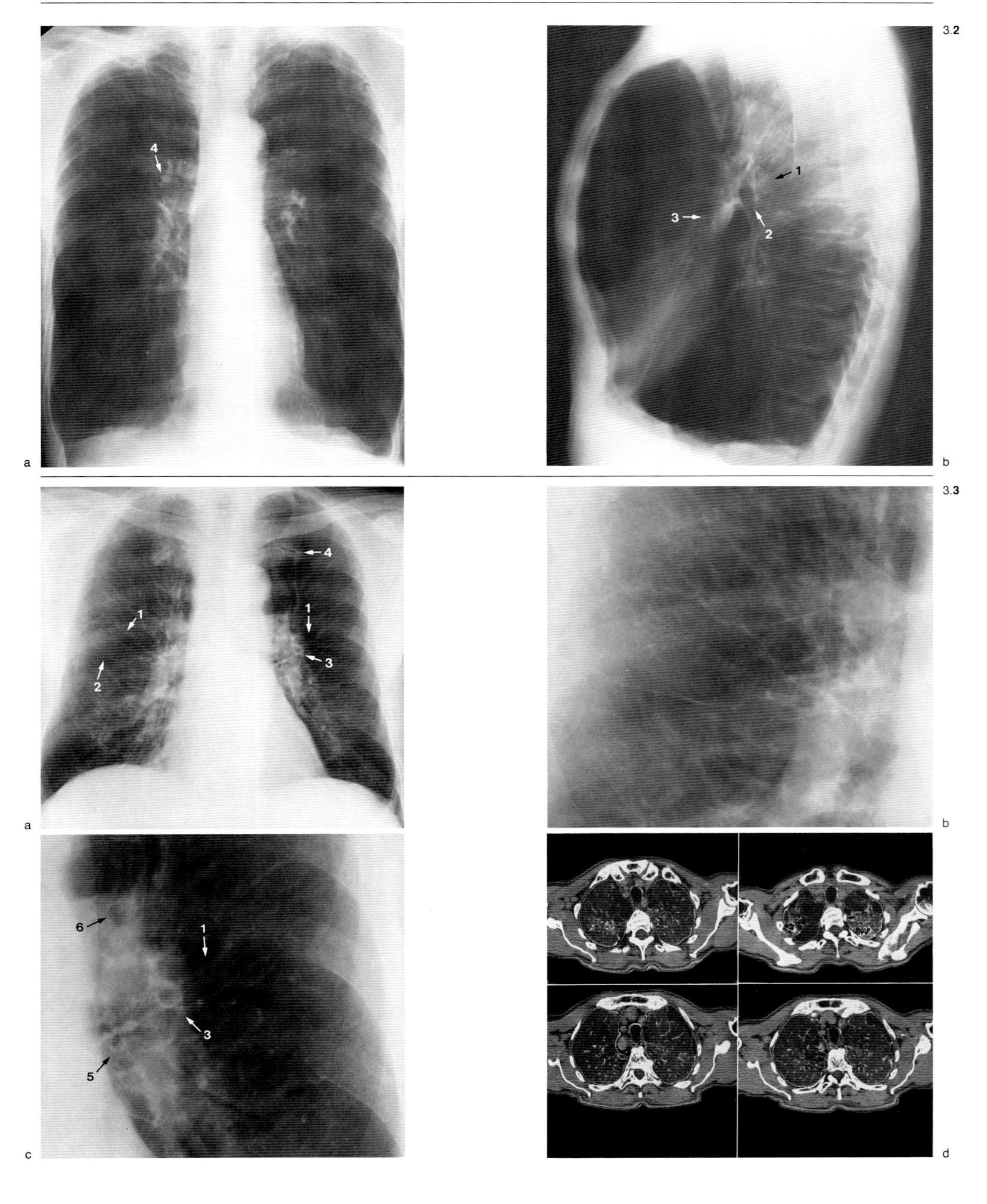

Emphysema 95

3. Chronic Obstructive Lung Diseases

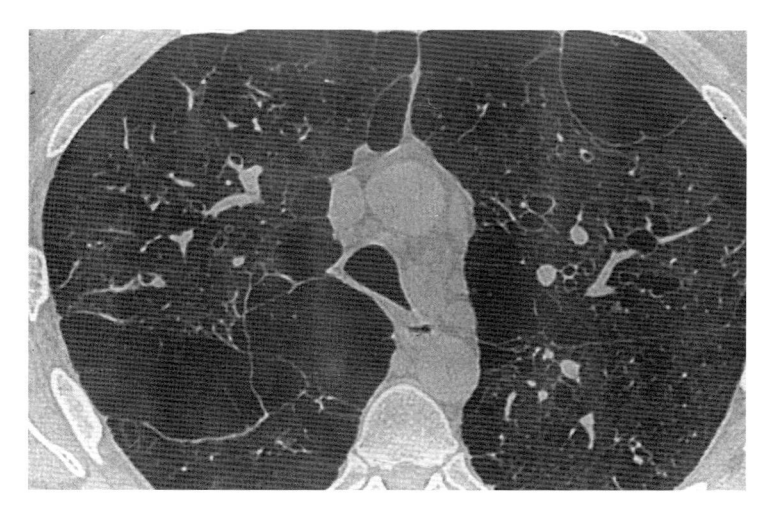

Fig. 3.4 **Severe emphysema.**
High-resolution CT scan demonstrates multiple bilateral bullae and paraseptal emphysema in subpleural location and along right major fissure.

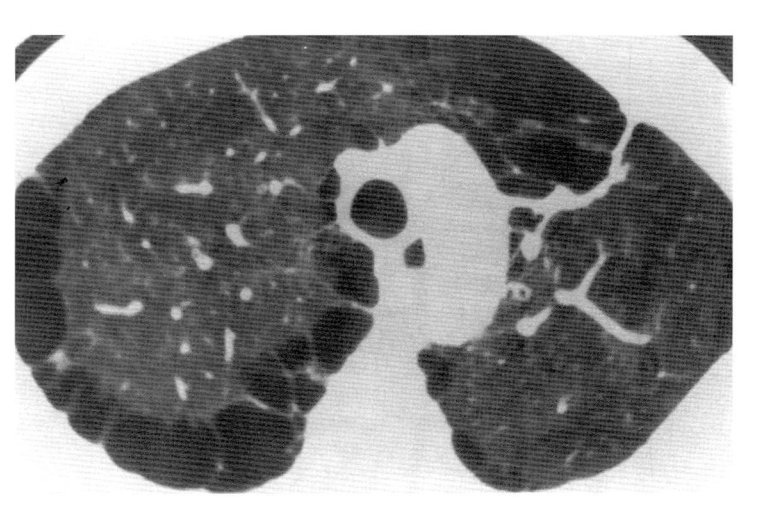

Fig. 3.5 **Paraseptal emphysema in smoker.**
CT scan shows multiple subpleural emphysematous spaces smaller than 1 cm in diameter. This type of emphysema is the precursor of subpleural bullae and intrapleural blebs.

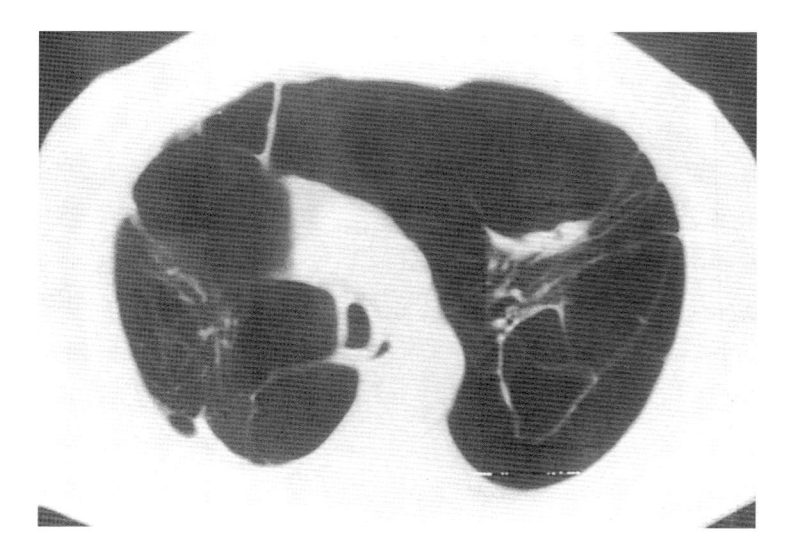

Fig. 3.6 **Heavy smoker with severe emphysema.**
CT scan displays severe bullae replacing both upper lobes.

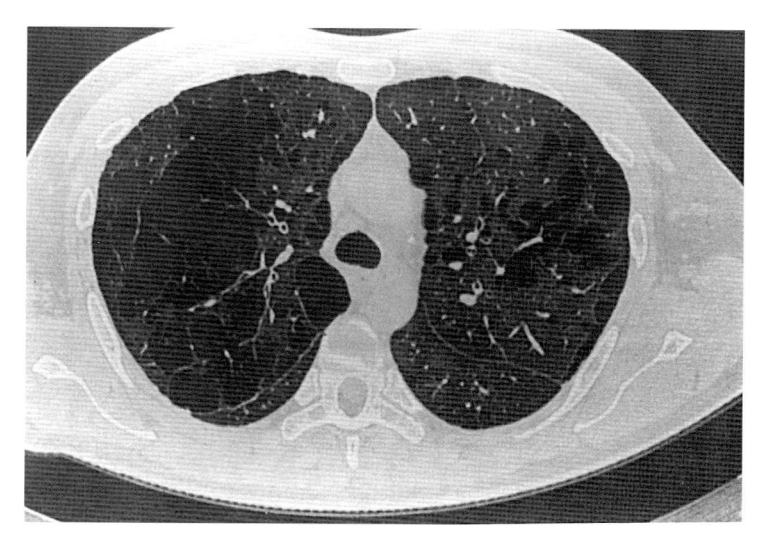

Fig. 3.7 **A 37-year-old patient with AIDS and premature emphysema.**
High-resolution CT scan shows severe centrilobular emphysema and bullae.

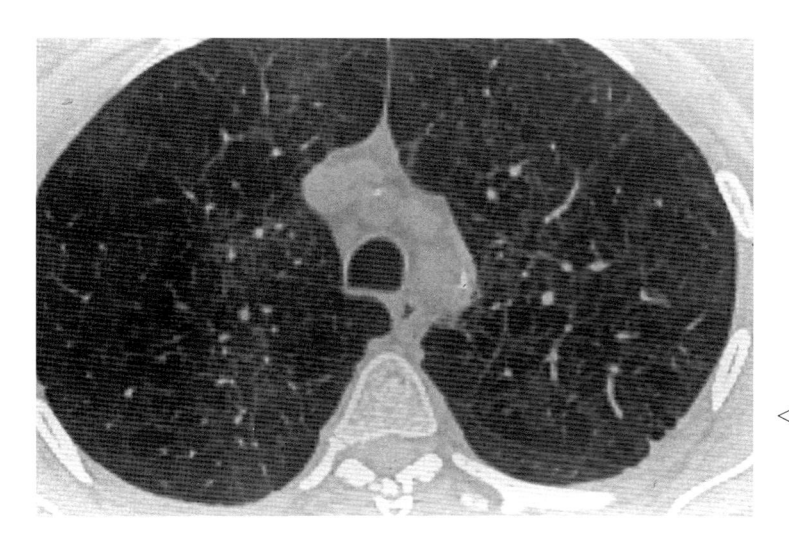

Fig. 3.8 **Smoker with emphysema.**
High-resolution CT scan shows multiple cystic lucencies with imperceptible walls, permeating and destroying the lung.

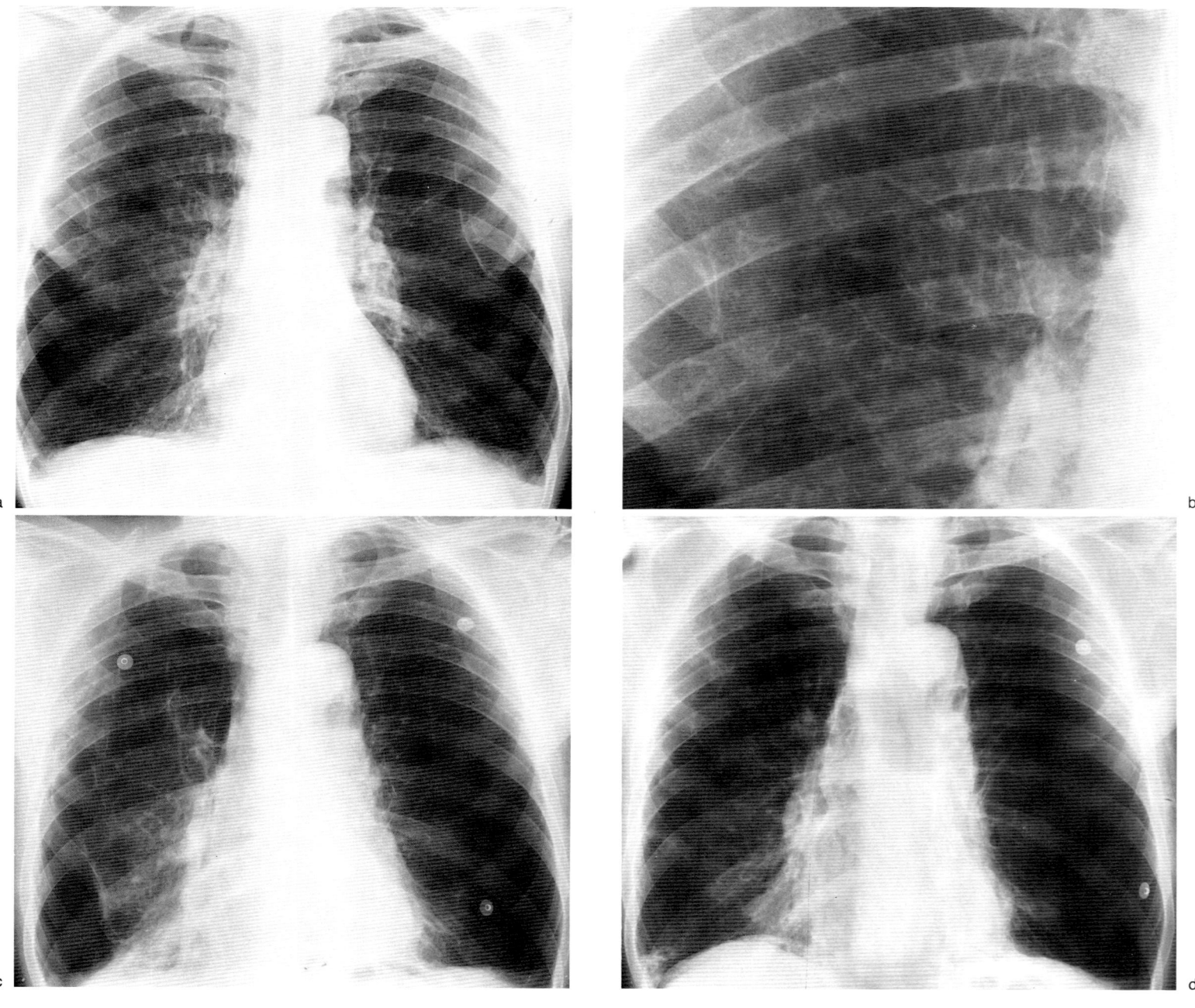

Fig. 3.9 a–d **Emphysema with bullae.**
53-year-old patient with chronic respiratory failure and recurrent spontaneous pneumothoraces.

Hyperexpanded lungs with disorganized peripheral pulmonary vessels. Multiple small bullae in right middle lung zone (**a**). Four years later (**c**), further progression of emphysema with vascular attenuation in left lung and right basilar pneumothorax, drained with chest tube (**d**).

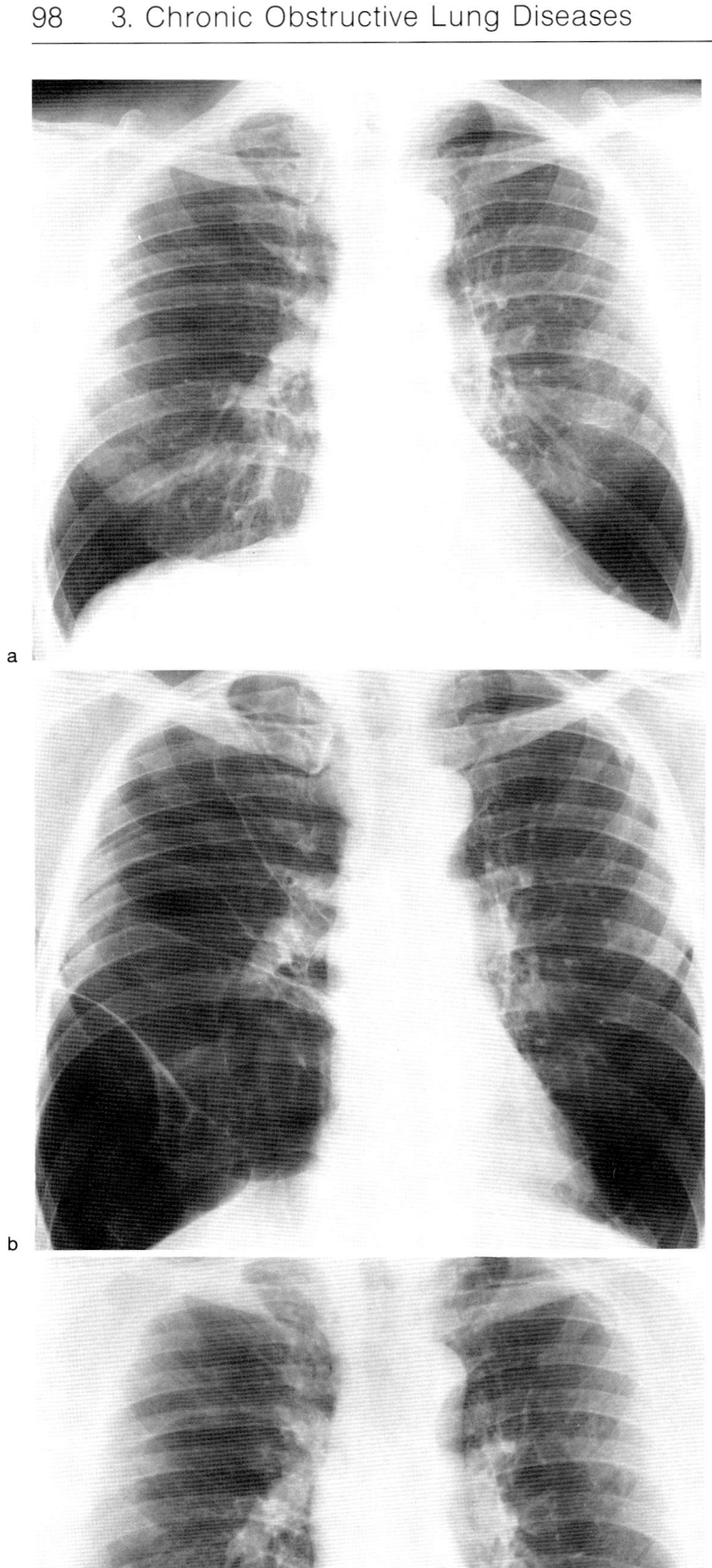

Fig. 3.10 a–c Emphysema with large bullae.
57-year-old patient with chronic bronchitis and recurrent spontaneous pneumothorax.

Initial chest radiograph in 1975 shows hyperexpansion and paucity of vascular structures in the right upper lobe and at both lung bases (**a**). Four years later, right basilar pneumothorax and pleural adhesions are visible (**b**). After another 4 years, the central pulmonary arteries have enlarged, indicating pulmonary arterial hypertension.

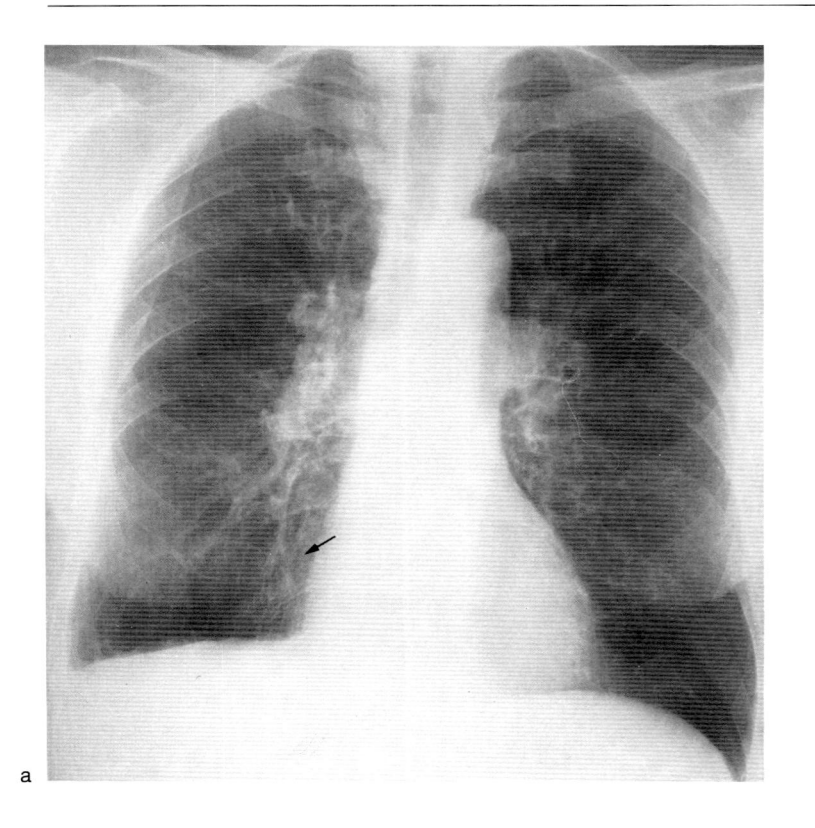

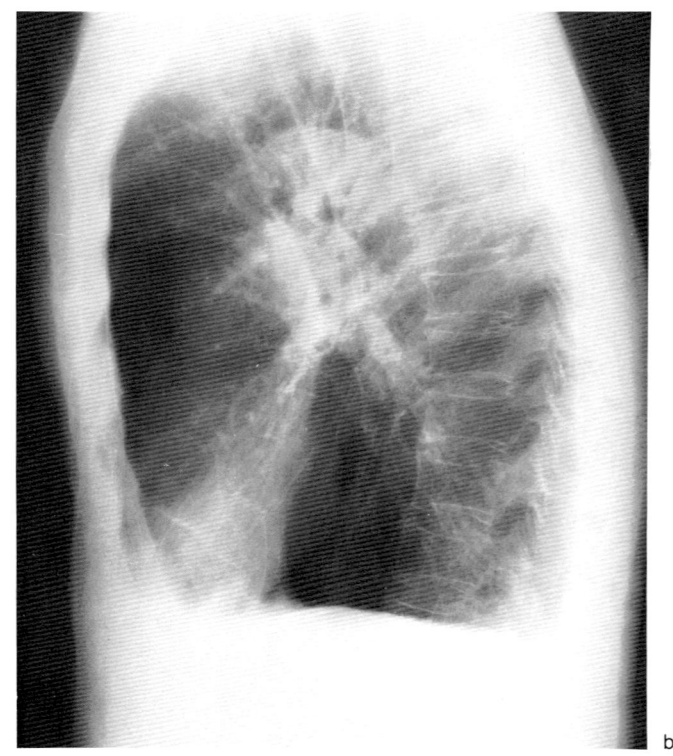

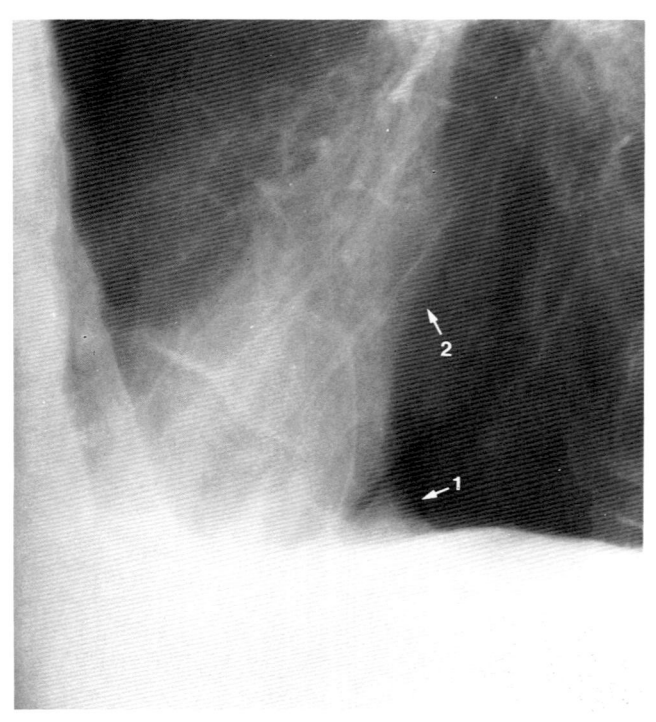

Fig. 3.11 a–c Emphysema.
Central pulmonary arteries are dilated. Peripheral pulmonary vessels are attenuated. Right retrocardiac bulla, 5 cm in diameter, inferior vena cava (1), major interlobar fissure (2).

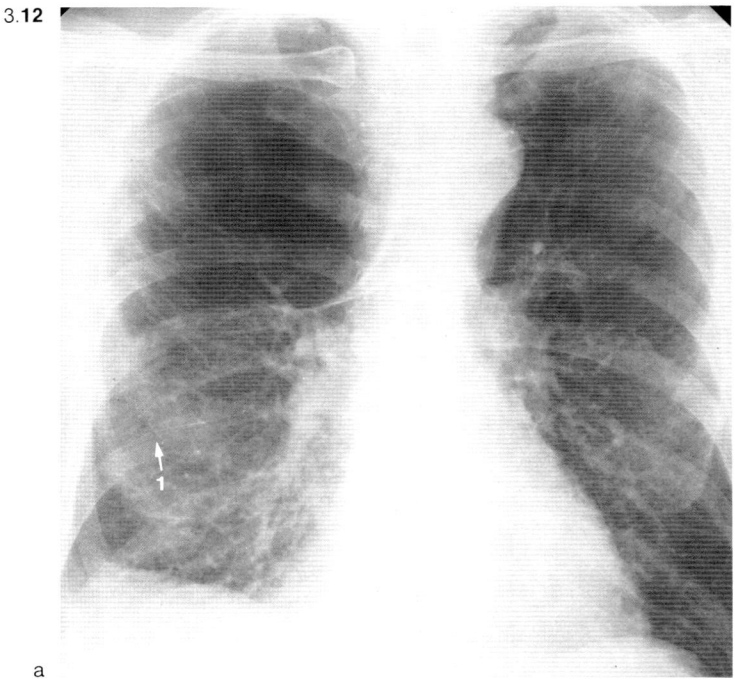

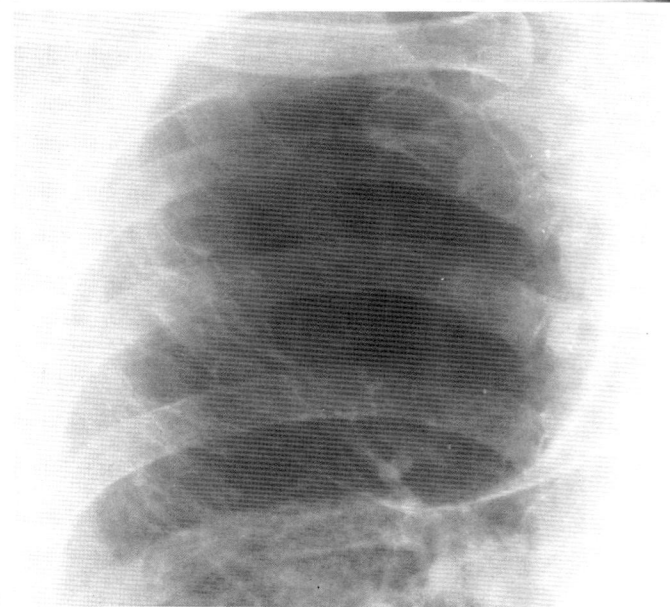

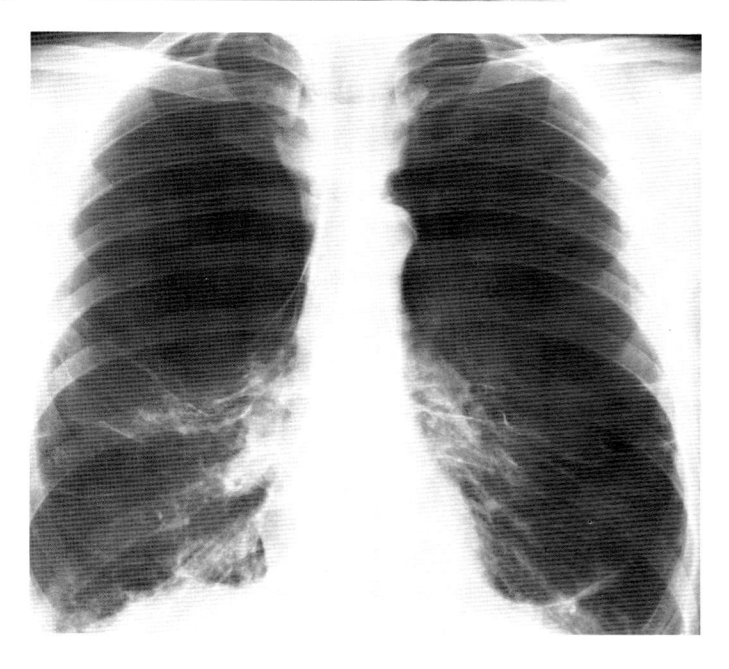

Vanishing Lung

This is a particularly severe form of emphysema encountered even in young people, usually either heavy smokers or persons with α_1-antitrypsin deficiency.

Antiprotease deficiency (α_1-antitrypsin deficiency derives from an inherited gene defect; the deficient gene has been recently identified, cloned, and sequenced, making replacement therapy possible; 0.05% of the population is homozygous and 5% heterozygous for the disease.

These people are extremely susceptible to smoking damage and develop premature, predominantly basilar, emphysema. The destruction of lung parenchyma results from the uninhibited lysosomal activity of polymorphonuclear leukocytes.

Fig. 3.12 a, b **Severe emphysema in right upper lobe.**
63-year-old smoker. Right upper lobe bulla. Abnormal basilar markings due to peribronchial thickening and crowding of vessels. Minor fissure (1), displaced caudad.

Fig. 3.13 **Vanishing lung.**
39-year-old patient with progressive dyspnea over 5 years. Emphysematous destruction of both upper lobes with displacement of both hila caudad.

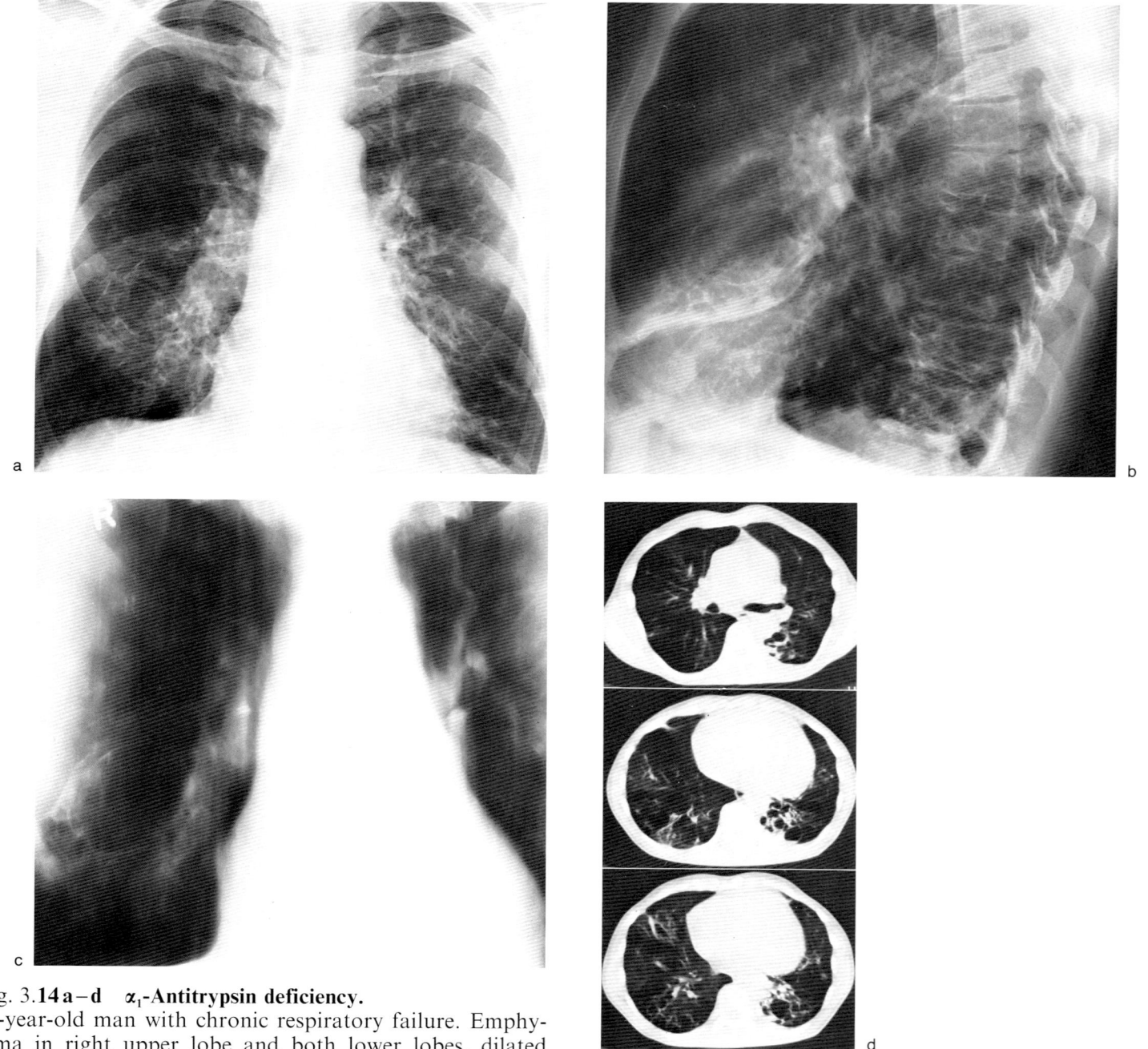

Fig. 3.**14 a–d** α₁-**Antitrypsin deficiency.**
45-year-old man with chronic respiratory failure. Emphysema in right upper lobe and both lower lobes, dilated central pulmonary arteries indicative of pulmonary arterial hypertension and cor pulmonale. Bronchiectases are visible in right middle lobe and in left lower lobe, most likely resulting from recurrent infections.

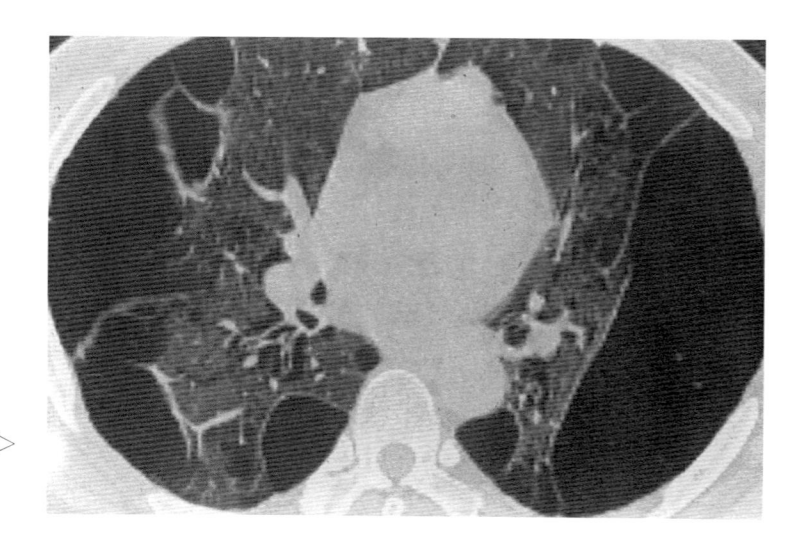

Fig. 3.**15 Patient with α₁-protease deficiency.**
High-resolution CT scan shows multiple peripheral bullae; remaining normal lung retracts towards the mediastinum.

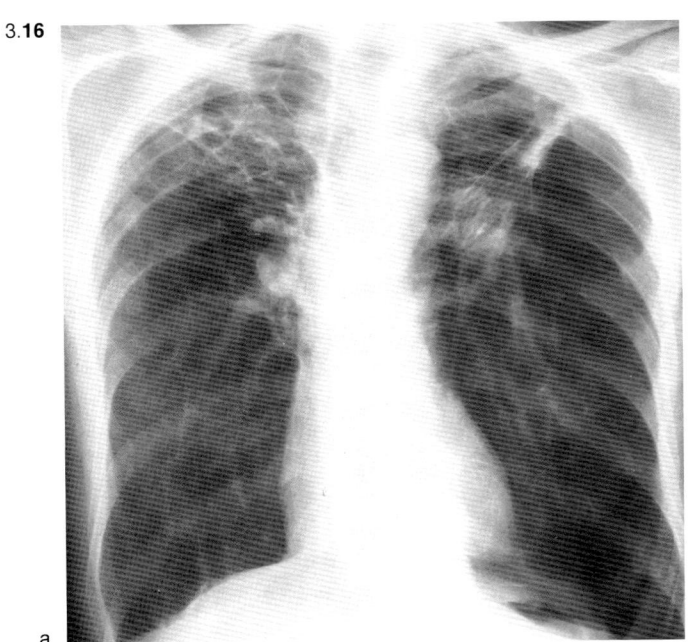

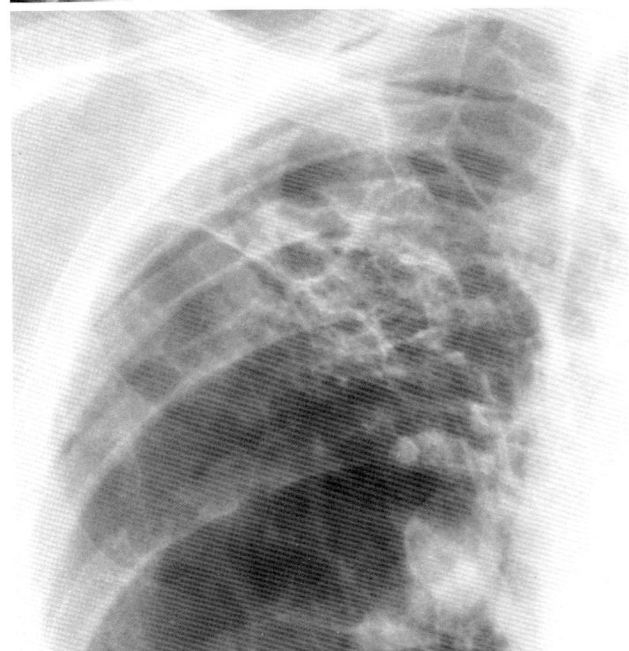

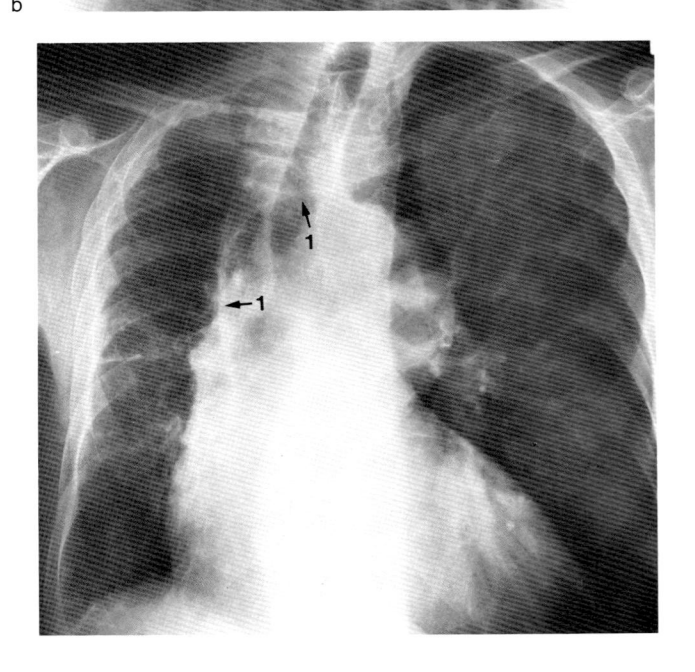

Pericicatriceal Emphysema

This arises in the vicinity of scars, which distort the neighboring bronchi and thus lead to air-trapping and compensatory hyperexpansion of the adjacent lung.

Fig. 3.16 a–b **Cicatrizing tuberculous changes with pericicatriceal emphysema.**
73-year-old patient with a history of remote postprimary tuberculosis. Marked bilateral cephalad retraction of both hila with distortion of the central pulmonary vessels. Pericicatriceal emphysema adjacent to scars and compensatory hyperexpansion of both lower lobes.

Fig. 3.17 **Right pleural peel with restriction of right lung and compensatory hyperexpansion of left lung.**
Displaced anterior junction line (1) by hyperexpanded anterior segment of left upper lobe. Enlarged cardiac silhouette and tortuous aorta.

Swyer-James Syndrome

This syndrome is the result of an early childhood broncholitis obliterans affecting an entire lung or occasionally only a lobe. The infection inhibits the retrograde alveolarization with compensatory hyperexpansion of the remaining alveoli. Radiologically, the involved lung is small and hyperlucent on inspiration but shows air-trapping with contralateral mediastinal shift on expiration. On perfusion scanning, the affected lung reveals a marked diminution of blood flow – this finding can be confirmed angiographically.

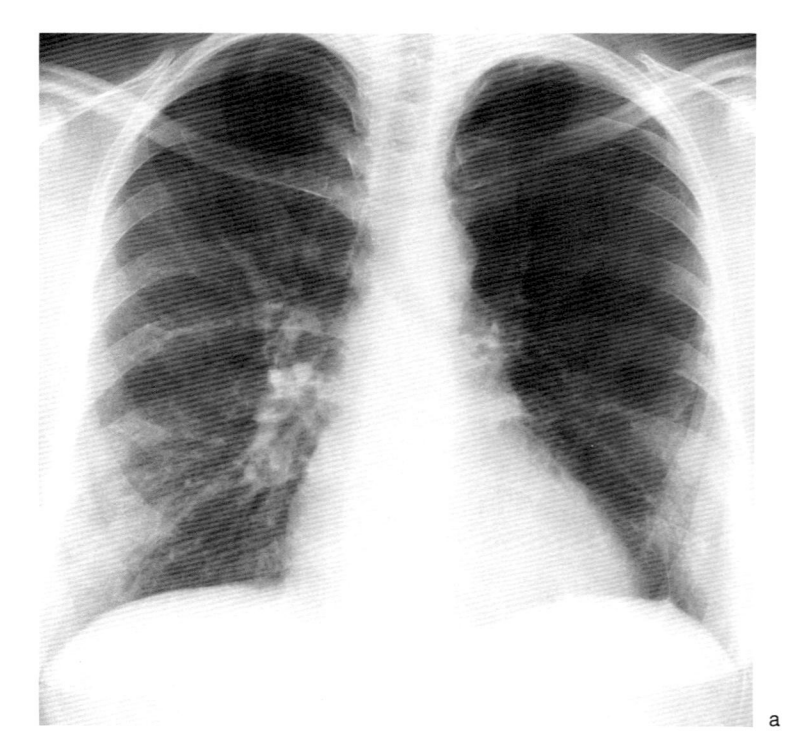

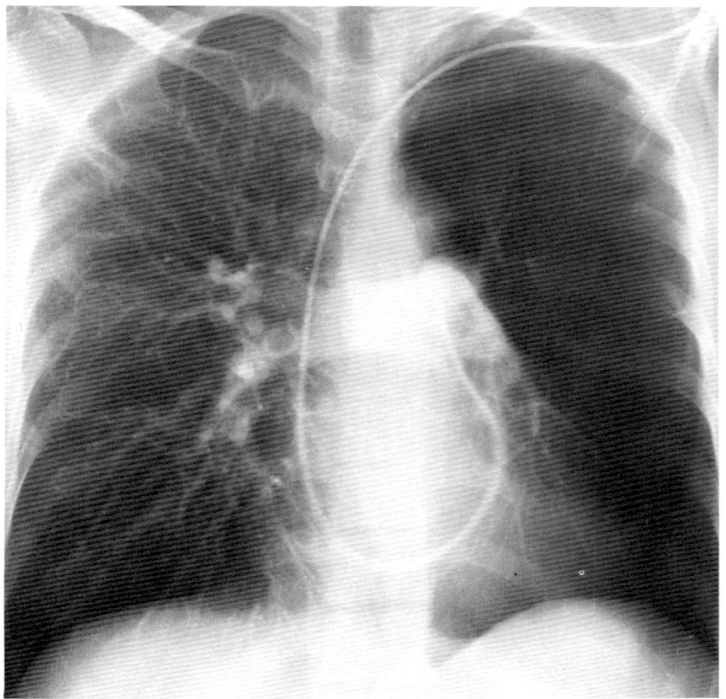

Fig. 3.**18a, b** **Swyer-James syndrome.**
Asymptomatic, 35-year-old woman with history of bronchiolitis in infancy. Hyperlucent left lung. Pulmonary angiogram shows paucity of vascular structures in the left lung.

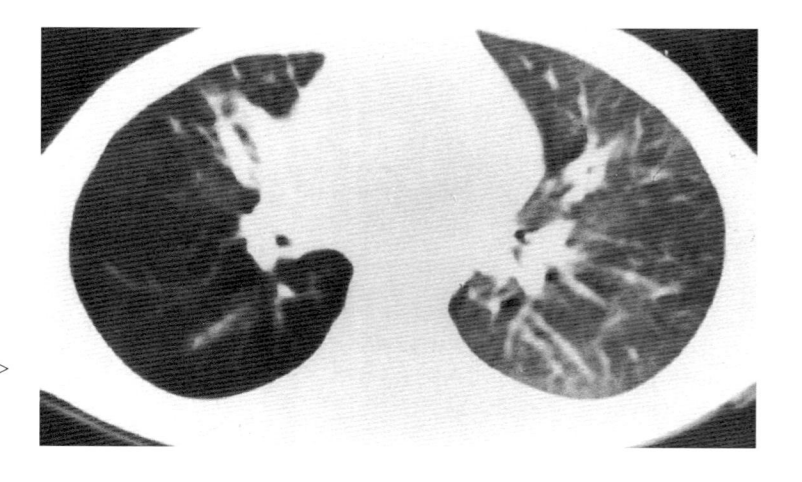

Fig. 3.**19** **Swyer-James syndrome.**
4-year-old child with recurrent respiratory infections. CT scan shows a small, hyperlucent right lung.

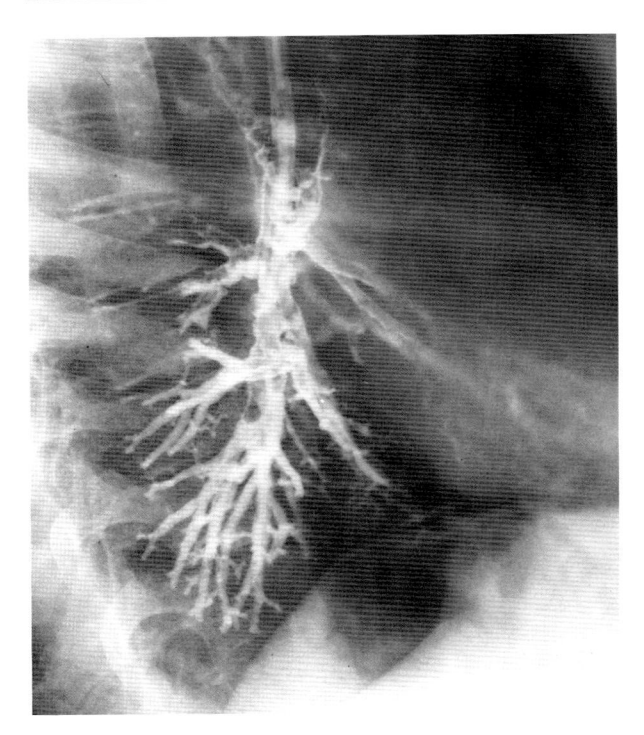

Fig. 3.20 **Cylindrical bronchiectases.**

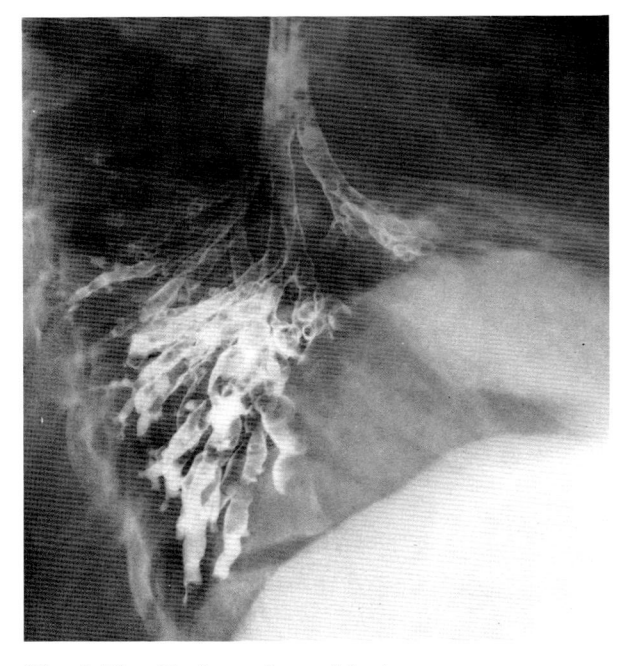

Fig. 3.21 **Varicous bronchiectases.**

Bronchiectases

Classic bronchiectases are the result of early childhood pneumonia or bronchiolitis. Immunization against pertussis and measles as well as antibiotic therapy for pneumonias have led to a marked decrease in the incidence of bronchiectases. The inflammatory process results in damage to the bronchial walls, irreversible dilatation of bronchi, and frequently in destruction of the adjacent subtended lung parenchyma. Traction bronchiectases are the result of adjacent scarring, e.g., radiation fibrosis, tuberculosis. Obstructive bronchiectases are rare sequelae of bronchial obstruction by slowly growing tumors such as carcinoids or chronic aspirated foreign bodies.

Only rarely do congenital defects result in bronchiectases: Cystic fibrosis, immotile cilia, immunoglobulin A (IgA) deficiency, Ehlers-Danlos syndrome or Williams-Campbell syndrome (congenital cartilage deficiency of the tracheobronchial tree) are some possible causes. The pathologic classification includes: (1) cylindrical, (2) varicose, and (3) cystic or saccular forms.

Radiological features include the visualization of dilated bronchi and their thick walls as "double tracks" or "tram tracks," cystic lucencies, mucoid impactions, or air-fluid levels. The adjacent lung shows a loss of volume, occasionally leading to complete lobar collapse.

CT can display subtle bronchiectases, particularly with the high-resolution or spiral technique. In cross-section, ring shadows become visible, accompanied by the respective pulmonary artery branch; together, they form the "signet ring" configuration. Bronchography used to represent the gold standard for the diagnosis of bronchiectases and the determination of their extent. In recent years, CT has all but replaced bronchography in the work-up of patients with bronchiectases.

References: 80, 115.

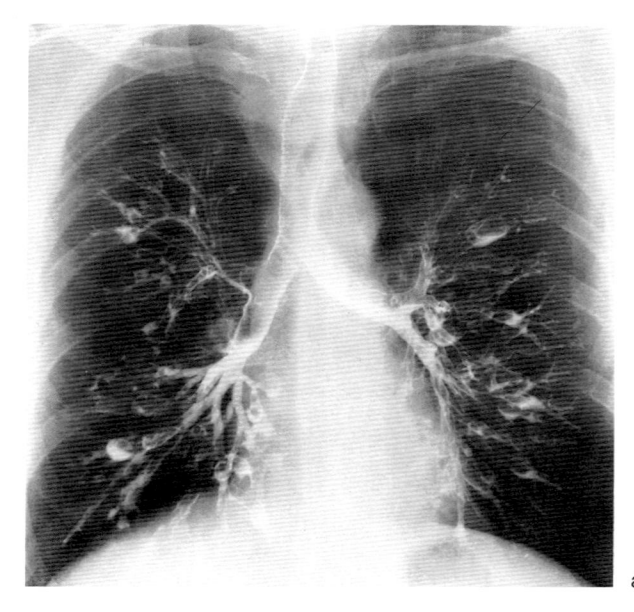

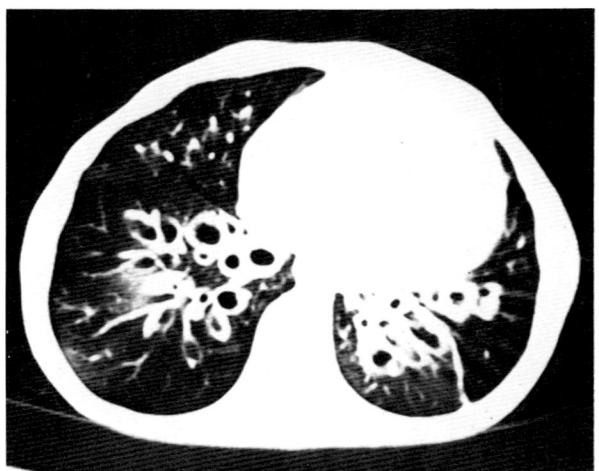

Fig. 3.**22 a, b** Saccular bronchiectases.

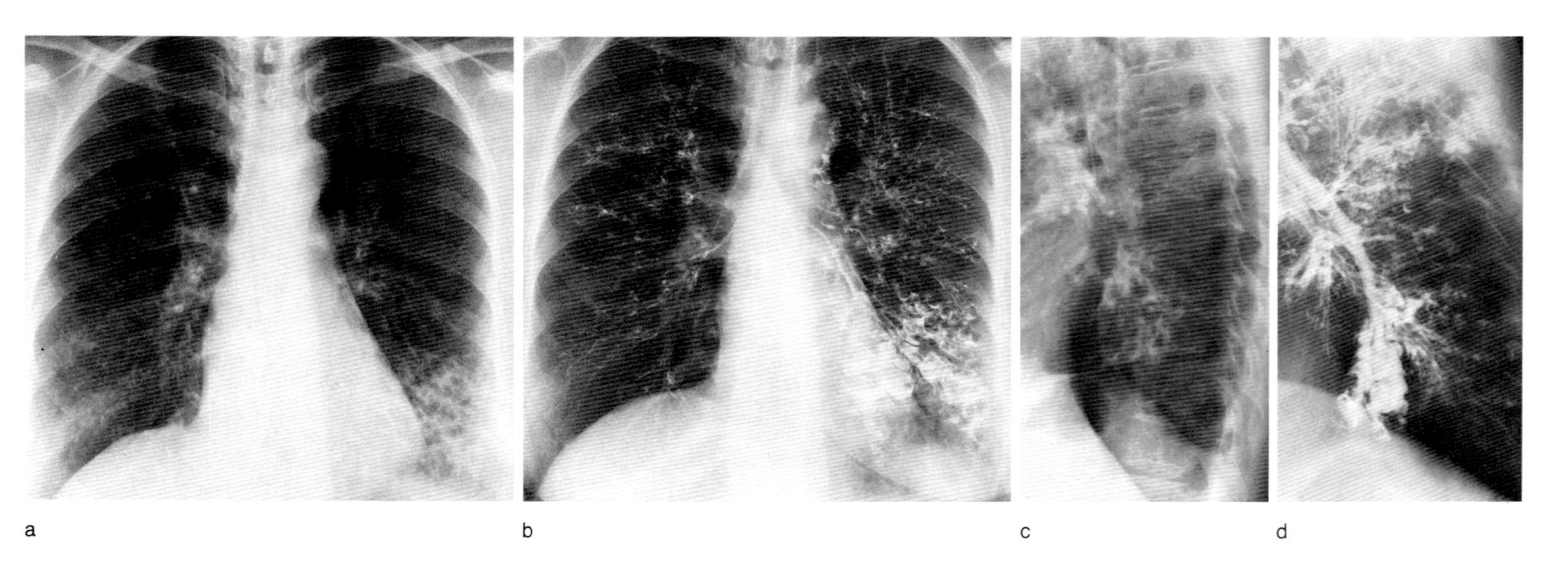

Fig. 3.**23 a–d** **Left lower lobe saccular bronchiectases.** 32-year-old woman with recurrent pneumonia. Ill-defined left lower lobe consolidation with cystic lucencies. Bronchogram confirms saccular bronchiectases.

3. Chronic Obstructive Lung Diseases

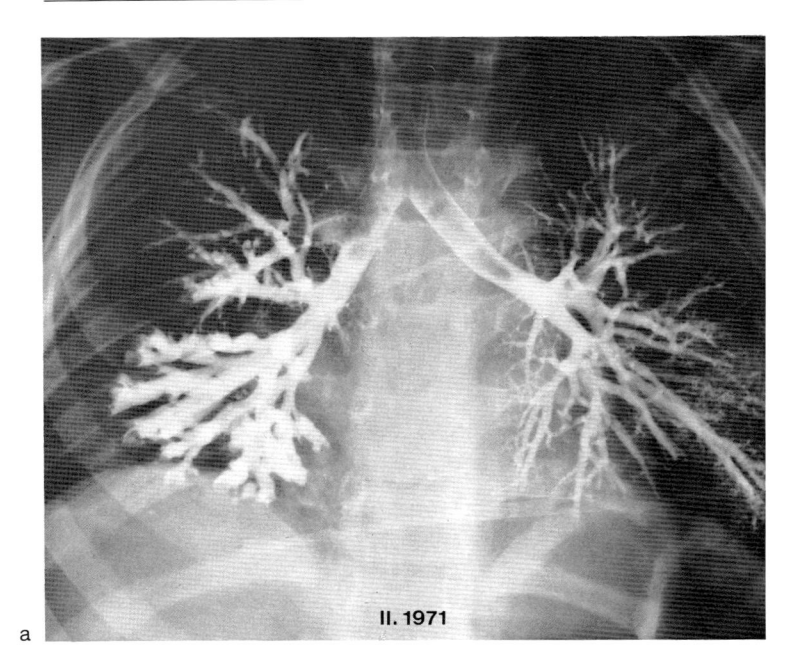

Fig. 3.**24 a–c** **Cylindrical bronchiectases in right lung.**
5-year-old child. Due to severe recurrent pneumonia unresponsive to antibiotics and postural drainage, a pneumonectomy was performed. Postoperative chest film shows hydropneumothorax. Delayed chest film shows marked herniation of contralateral lung and mediastinum into vacant right hemithorax.

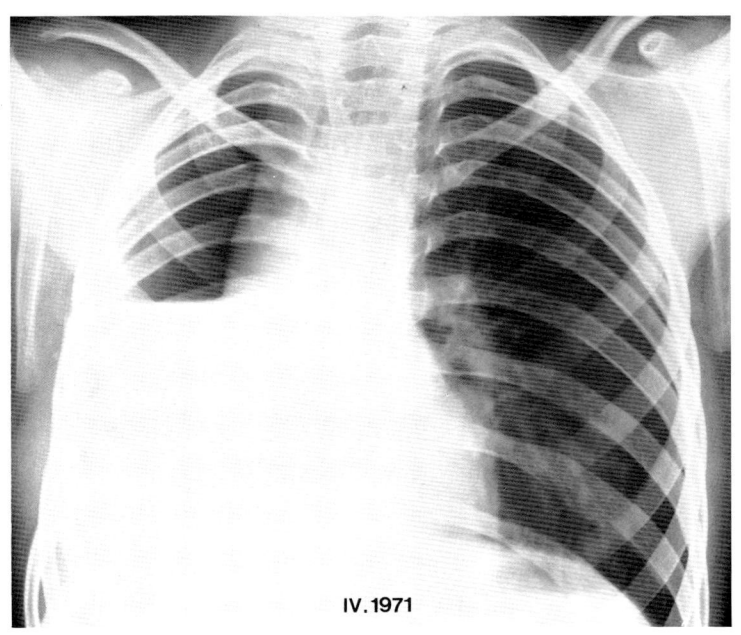

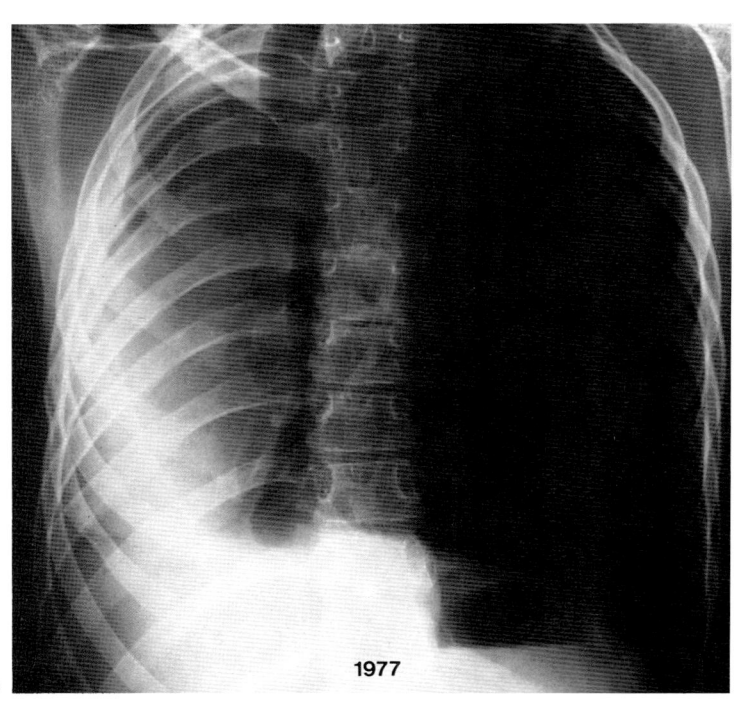

Fig. 3.25 **Patient with chronic cough.**
CT scan shows cystic bronchiectases in a completely atelectatic right middle lobe and left lower lobe.

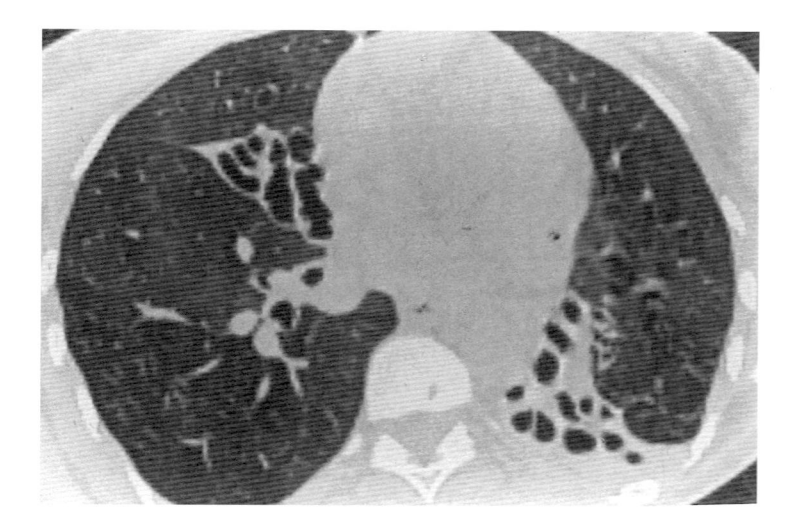

Fig. 3.26 **Cystic bronchiectases.**
Patient with long-standing productive cough. CT scan shows right lower lobe cystic bronchiectases and a right lower lobe abscess in a bronchiectatic cavity accounting for the basilar gas-fluid level.

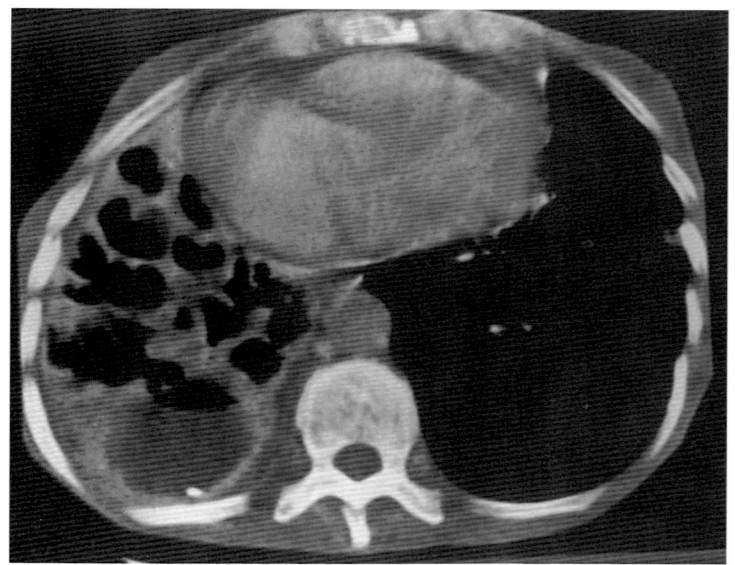

Chronic Bronchitis

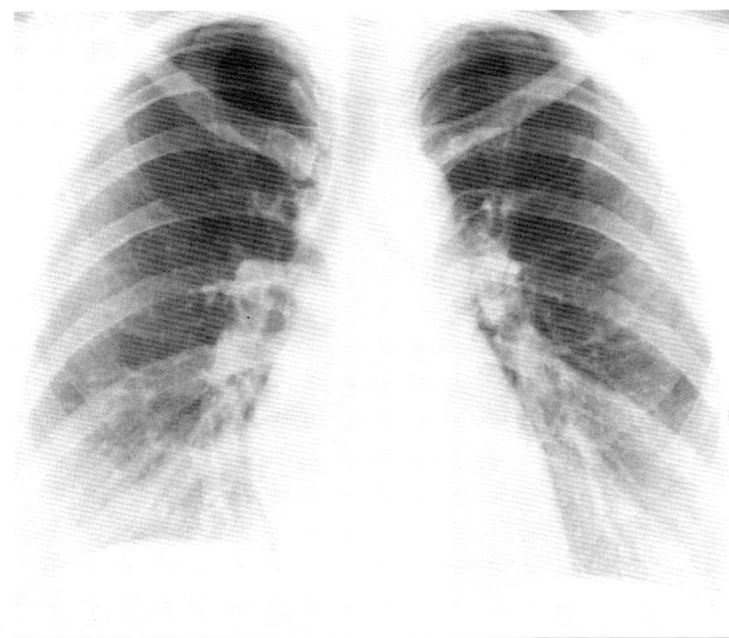

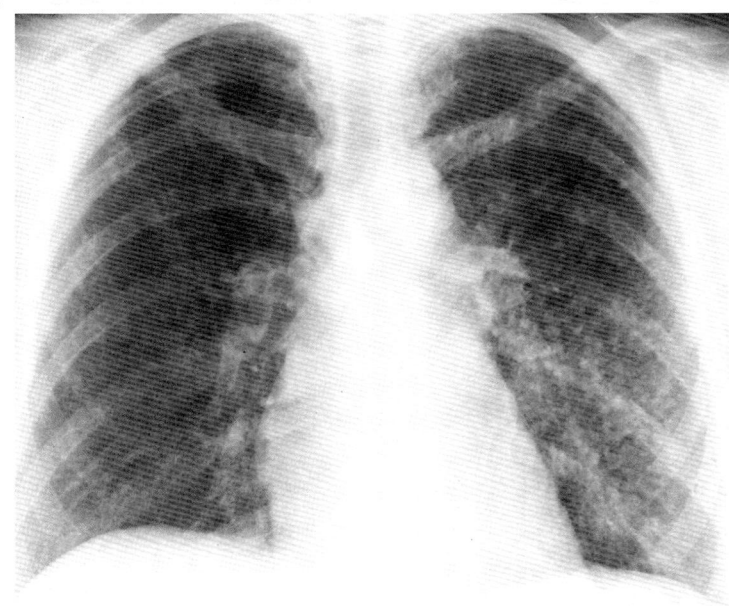

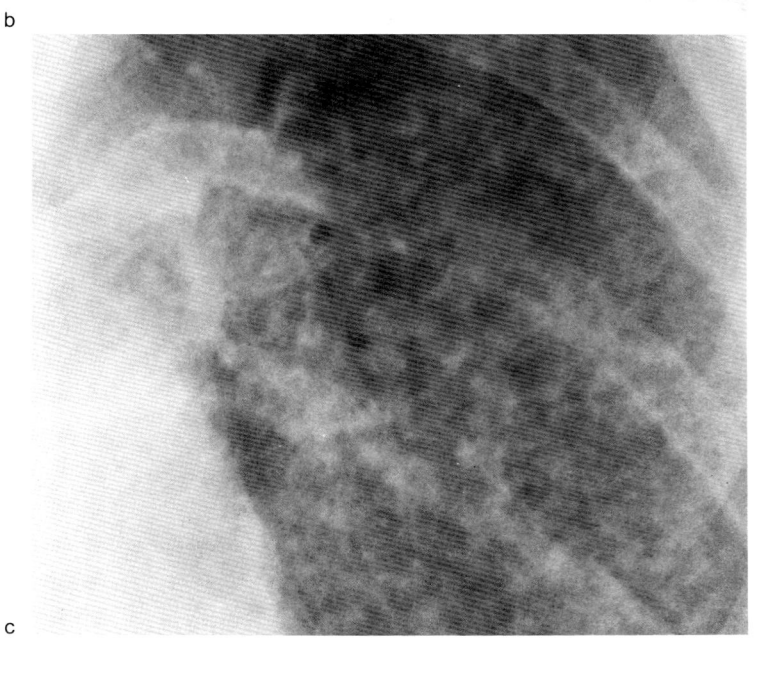

Chronic bronchitis is defined as sputum production over at least 3 months in 2 consecutive years. Radiologic findings can be absent, yet slight bronchial wall thickening, peribronchial thickening, and abnormal peripheral irregular markings can be visible. Bronchography can demonstrate glandular filling and multiple mucus plugs.

Broncholitis Obliterans

This can lead to hyperexpansion of the lungs; multiple, small, rounded opacities can be present and produce a miliary pattern. Broncholitis obliterans can be either idiopathic, related to viral infections or inhalation of noxious fumes or can occur after organ transplantation. The idiopathic variety can be associated with organizing pneumonia (BOOP). In such cases, a multifocal peripheral consolidation is present. These findings regress with corticosteroid therapy.

Cystic Fibrosis

This is the most common inherited disease in whites and occurs with a frequency of 1 in 2000 births. Patients produce a thick, tenacious mucus which leads to the formation of mucoid impaction, bronchiectases, and recurrent bronchopneumonia, particularly with *Pseudomonas aeruginosa*.

Radiologic findings include bronchiectases, hyperexpanded lungs, hilar enlargement due to enlarged reactive lymph nodes or dilated pulmonary arteries, pneumonia, atelectasis, mucoid impaction, spontaneous pneumothorax. Complications include cor pulmonale, massive hemoptysis, and respiratory failure.

Fig. 3.**27 a–c   Broncholitis obliterans.**
36-year-old woman who succumbed to this acute inflammatory process proven at autopsy. Previous film was normal (**a**). One year later, a miliary pattern is evident (**b**). Differential diagnosis includes miliary tuberculosis and extrinsic allergic alveolitis.

Chronic Bronchitis 109

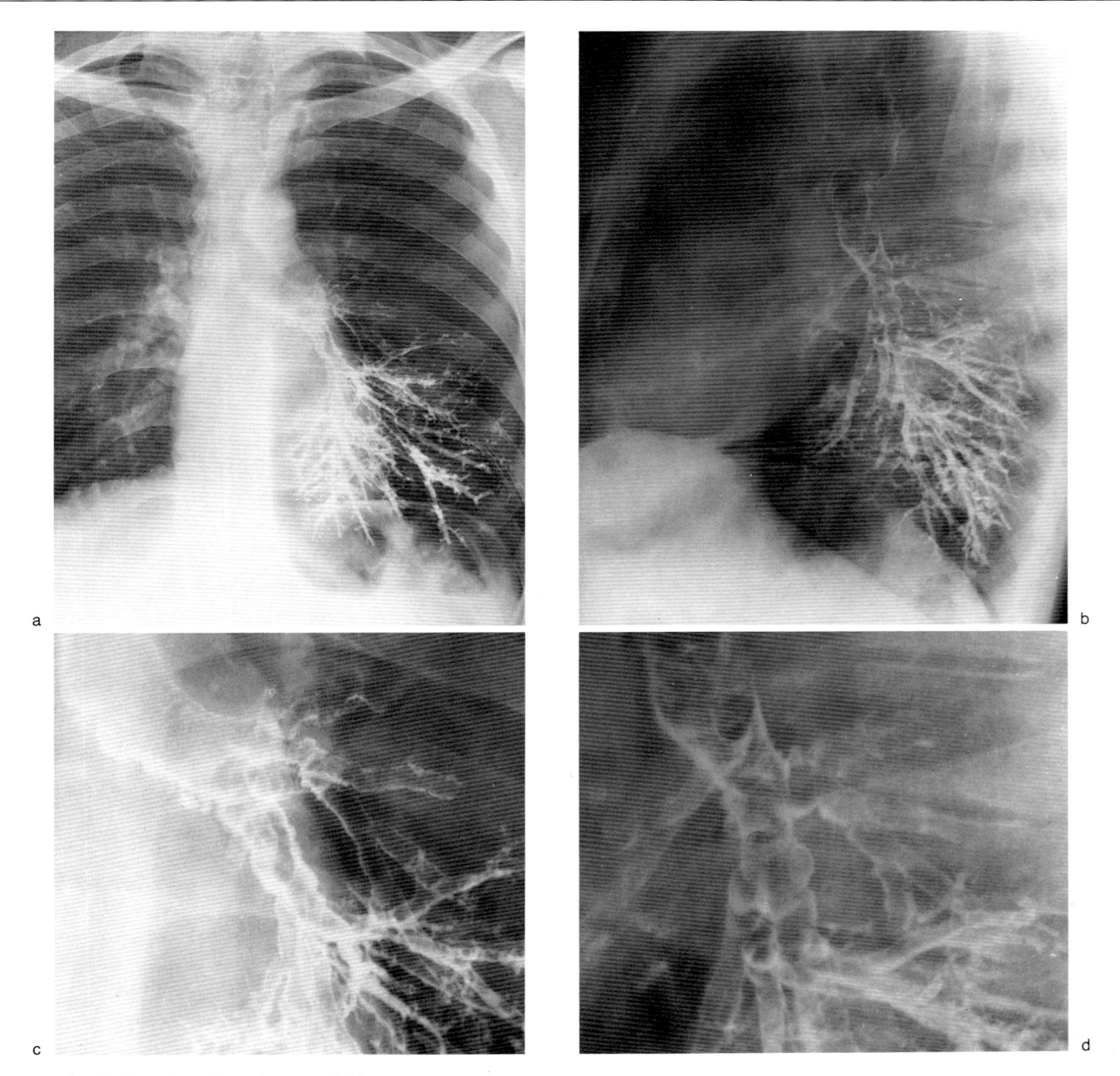

Fig. 3.28 a–d **Chronic bronchitis.**
Bronchogram showing slight dilatation and contour irregularity of lobar, segmental, and subsegmental bronchi. Glandular filling seen in mainstem bronchi.

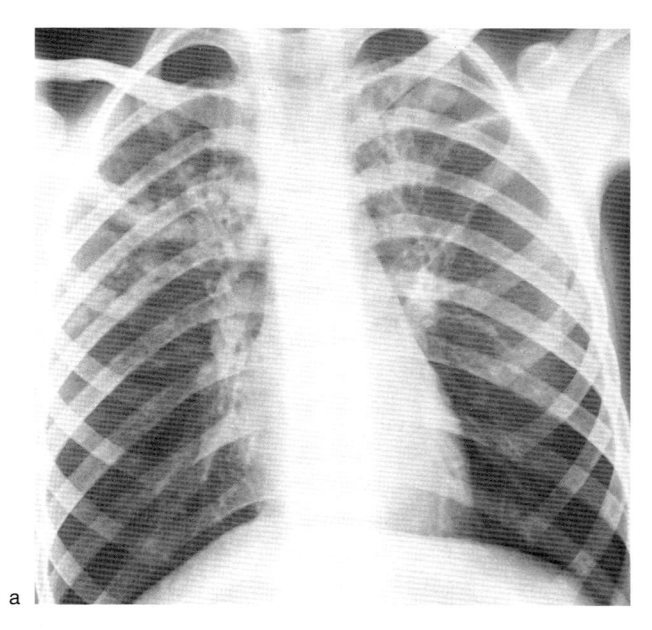

Fig. 3.29 a, b   Cystic fibrosis.
Progression of the disease over an interval of 12 years.

Initial film at age 10 years shows bilateral upper lobe and right middle lobe peribronchial thickening, bronchiectases, mucoid impaction, and pneumonic residues. (**a**) Twelve years later, a marked increase in size and distribution of the bronchiectases has occurred: Cystic and nodular opacities are distributed throughout both lungs. Dilatation of the main pulmonary artery segment indicates pulmonary arterial hypertension and cor pulmonale.

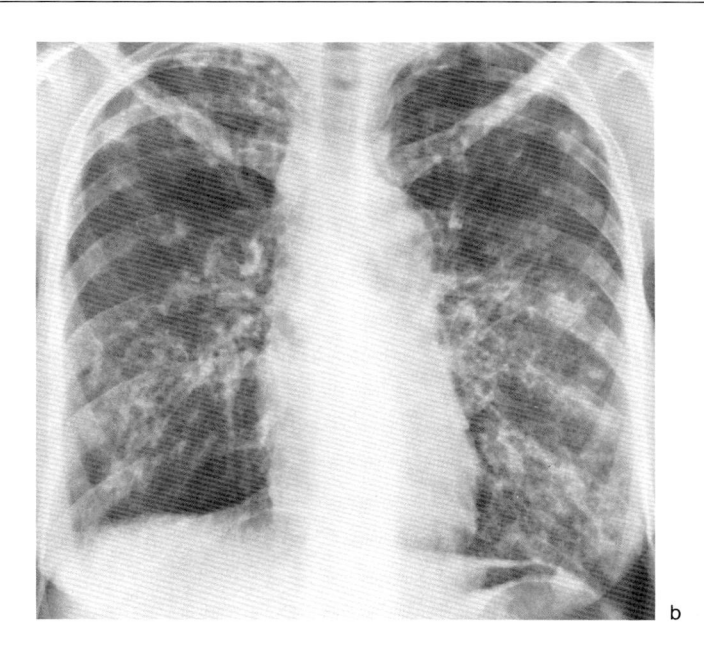

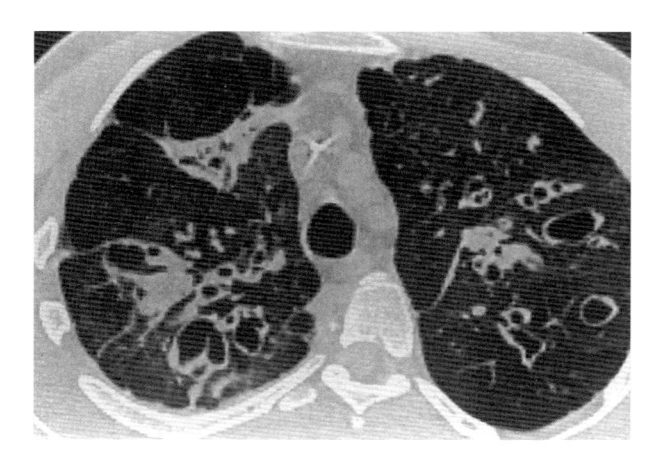

Fig. 3.30   Cystic fibrosis in a 30-year-old man.
High-resolution CT scan shows cystic bronchiectases, mucoid impactions, peribronchiectatic pneumonia, and scarring as well as bullae.

4. Pneumoconiosis

Types of Pneumoconiosis

These diseases are the result of chronic inhalation of inorganic dust. Particles or fibers are deposited in the alveoli and incite a foreign body reaction. Eventually, diffuse fibrosis or a nodular granulomatous response ensues with restrictive and occasionally obstructive changes on pulmonary function tests. In advanced stages of the disease, pulmonary arterial hypertension and cor pulmonale supervene.

Silicosis, coal workers' pneumoconiosis, and asbestosis are the most common inorganic pneumoconiosis. Silicosis and coal workers' pneumoconiosis produce multiple, small, rounded opacities with a predilection for the upper and middle lung zones. These small opacities can become confluent and lead to the formation of large opacities called conglomerate shadows or progressive massive fibrosis. In 5% of affected workers, eggshell calcifications of the marginal lymph node sinuses occur.

The radiologic manifestations of pneumoconioses are categorized according to the ILO (International Labor Office) classification. It takes into account the size, shape, distribution, and profusion of opacities. Standard films for every described abnormality are available and are mandatory for the graphic description and interpretation of such cases.

References: 23, 24, 25, 66.

Types of Pneumoconiosis 113

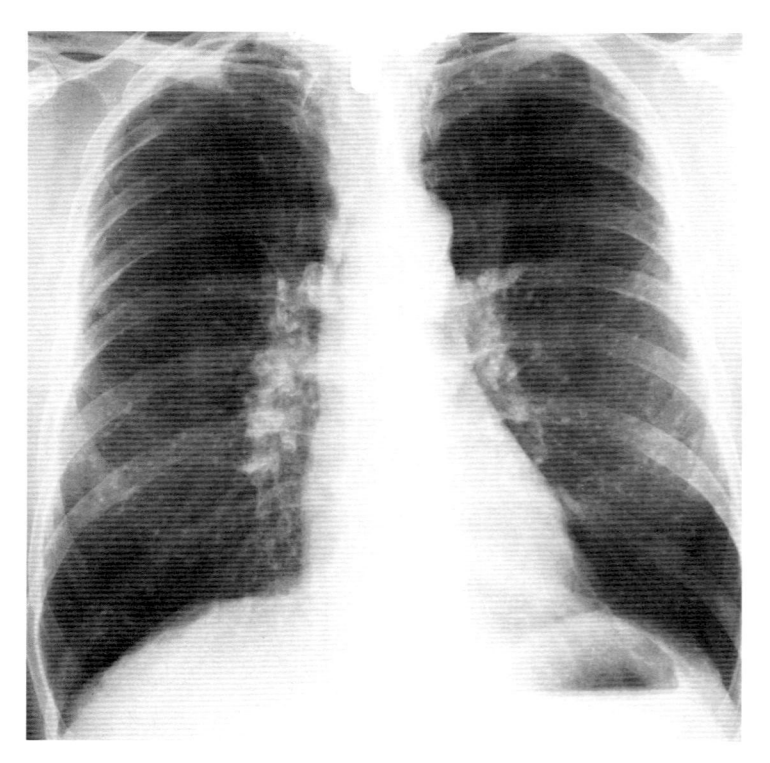

Fig. 4.1 **Simple silicosis.**
Multiple, small, rounded nodules with diameter of 1.5–3 mm scattered throughout both lungs.

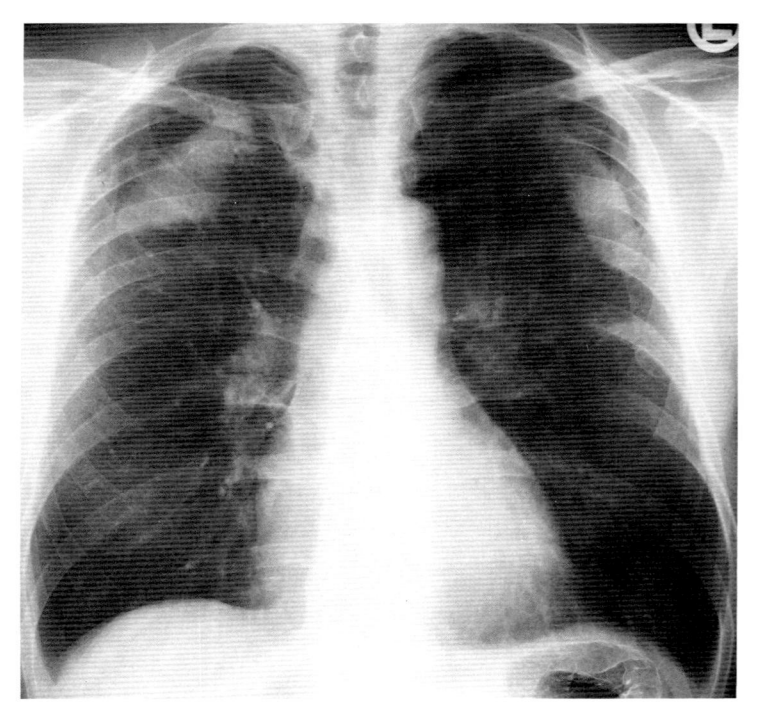

Fig. 4.2 **Complicated silicosis.**
Conglomerate masses producing bilateral upper lobe large opacities.

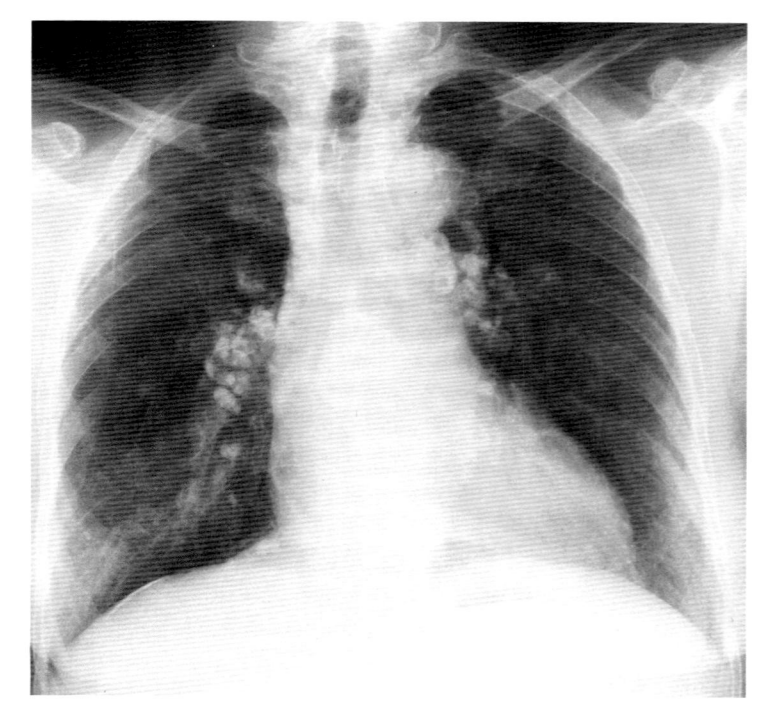

Fig. 4.3 **Silicosis with eggshell calcifications.**
Calcifications are located in the marginal sinus of the hilar and mediastinal lymph nodes. Calcifications of diaphragmatic pleura on the right side indicate additional exposure to asbestos fibers.

Round Opacities

The ILO classification subdivides round opacities according to their size, profusion, and distribution:

Size

p: diameter up to 1.5 mm
q: diameter between 1.5 and 3 mm
r: diameter between 3 and 10 mm

Profusion

Category 0: no definite round opacities seen
Category 1: scattered, round opacities present
Category 2: multiple, round opacities present, lung markings visible
Category 3: multiple, round opacities obliterating lung markings

A further subdivision into 12 subgroups allows for more flexibility: 0/−, 0/0, 0/1, 1/0, 1/1, 1/2, 2/1, 2/2, 2/3, 3/2, 3/3, 3/+. For instance, 2/3 implies a higher profusion than category 2 but slightly less than category 3.

Classification of round opacities according to their size and profusion can be further refined in terms of location. For this purpose, the lung is subdivided into upper, middle, and lower zones. The overall profusion results from visual integration of the individual zonal profusions.

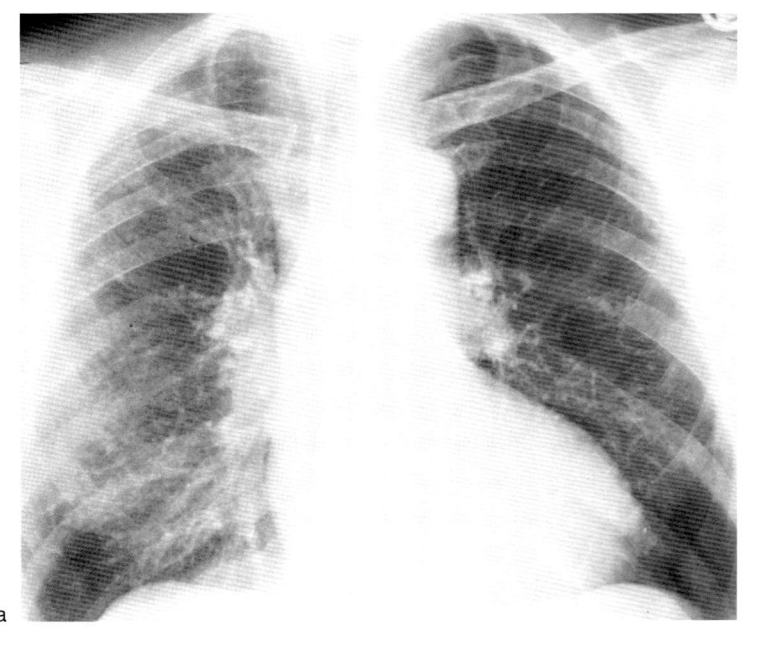

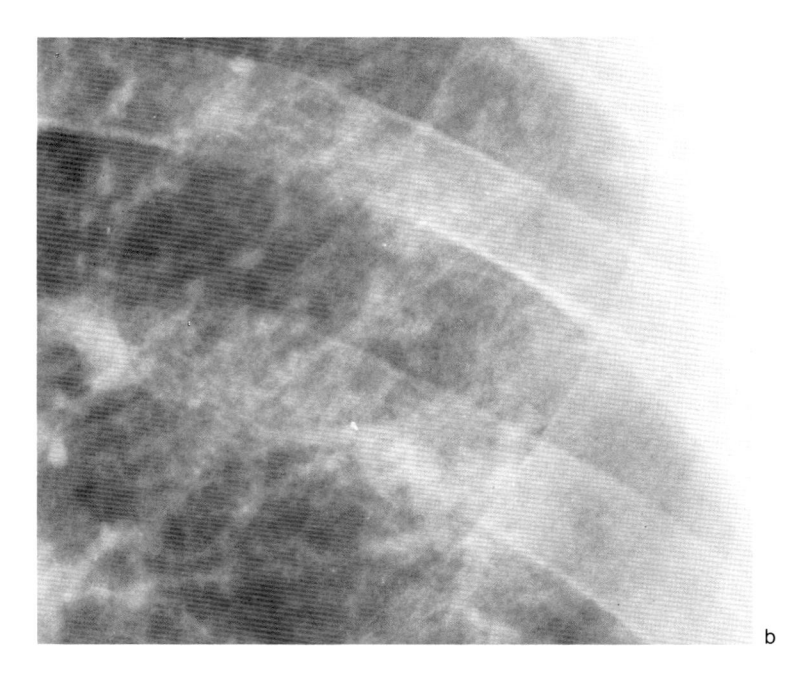

Fig. 4.4 a, b **Pneumoconiosis p 2/2**

	right	left
Upper zone	2/2	1/2
Middle zone	1/2	2/2
Lower zone	1/1	1/2

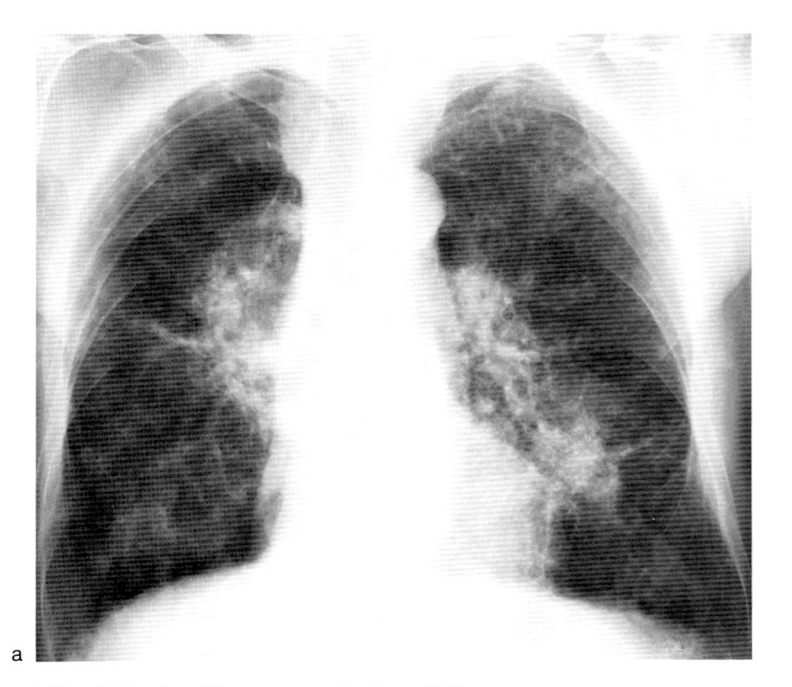

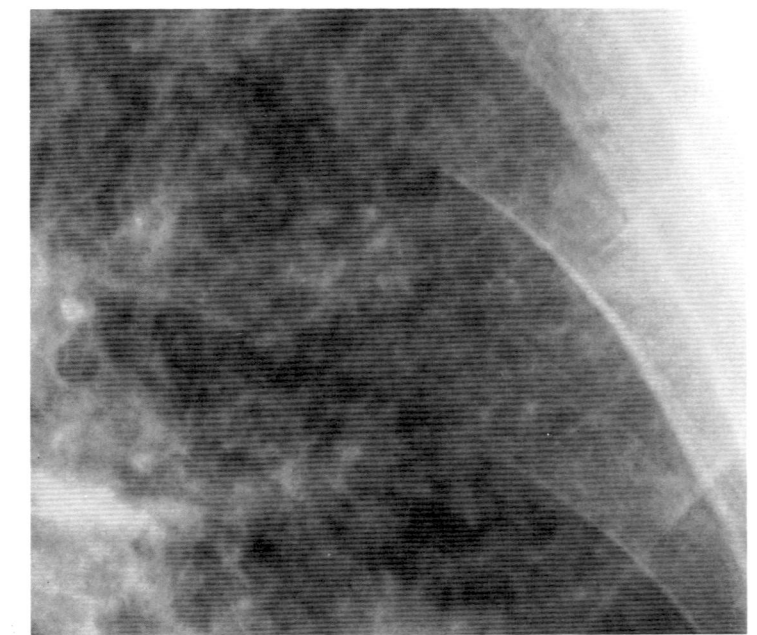

Fig. 4.5 a, b   Pneumoconiosis q 2/2

	right	left
Upper zone	1/0	2/2
Middle zone	1/1	2/2
Lower zone	1/1	1/1

Additional large opacities are also present.

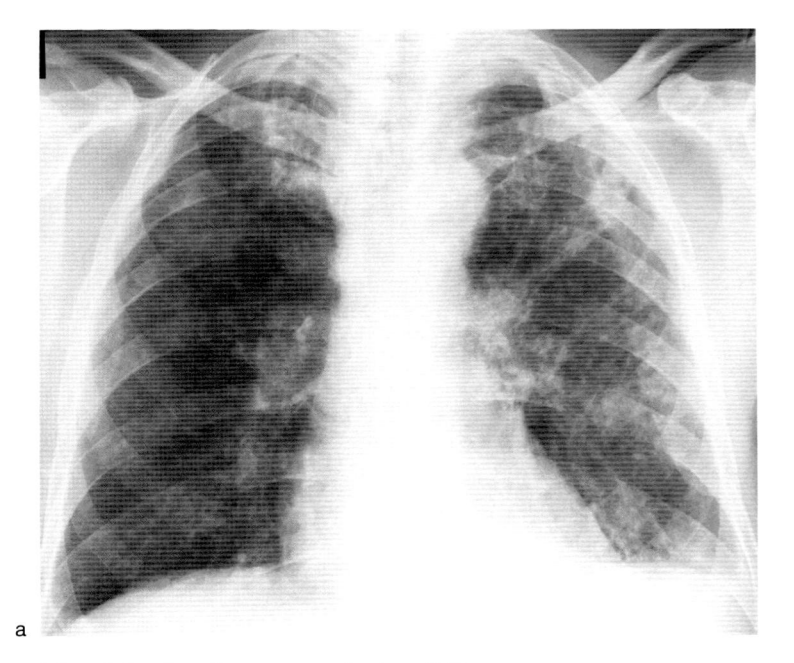

Fig. 4.6 a, b   Pneumoconiosis r 2/2

	right	left
Upper zone	1/1	2/2
Middle zone	1/2	2/2
Lower zone	1/2	1/2

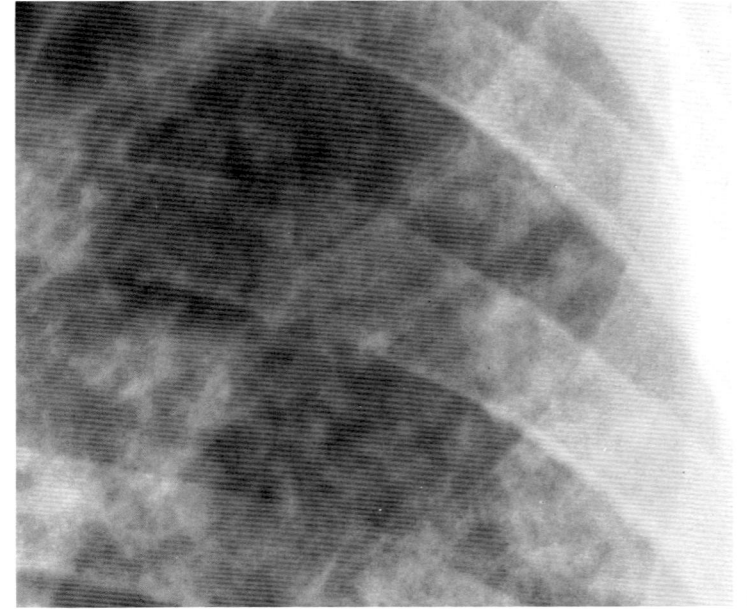

Small, Irregular Opacities

These opacities are characterized by their size, profusion, and distribution.

Size

s: small, irregular, or linear (1.5 mm or smaller)
t: medium-sized, irregular (1.5–3 mm)
u: large, irregular (3–10 mm)

Comparison with standard films is important for the determination of size and profusion.

Profusion

Category 0: no irregular opacities seen
Category 1: few irregular opacities present
Category 2: many irregular opacities present and lung markings visible
Category 3: multiple, irregular opacities obscuring normal lung markings

Further subdivision into a 12-scale system is identical to that used for round opacities.

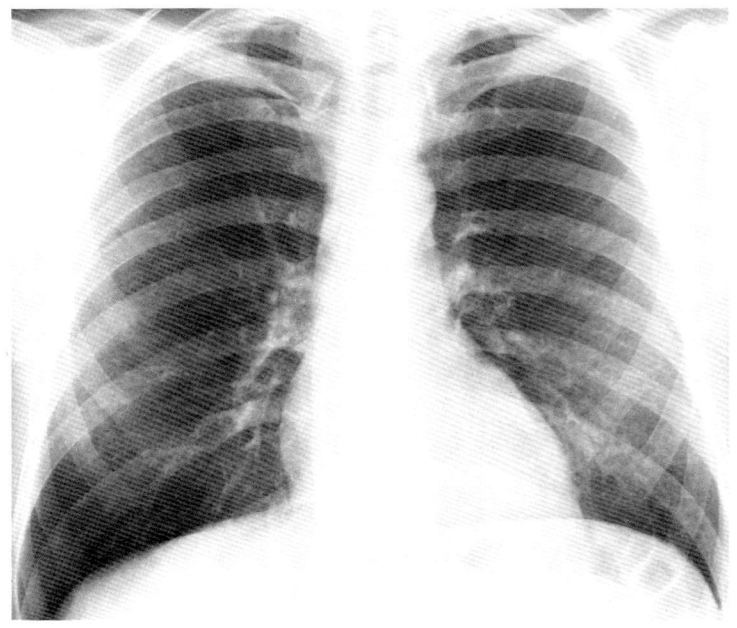

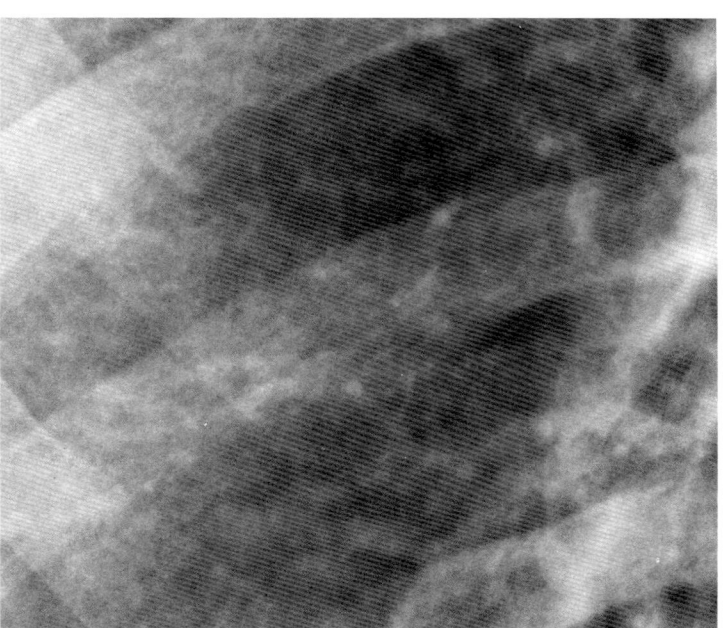

Fig. 4.7 a, b   Pneumoconiosis s 2|1

Types of Pneumoconiosis 117

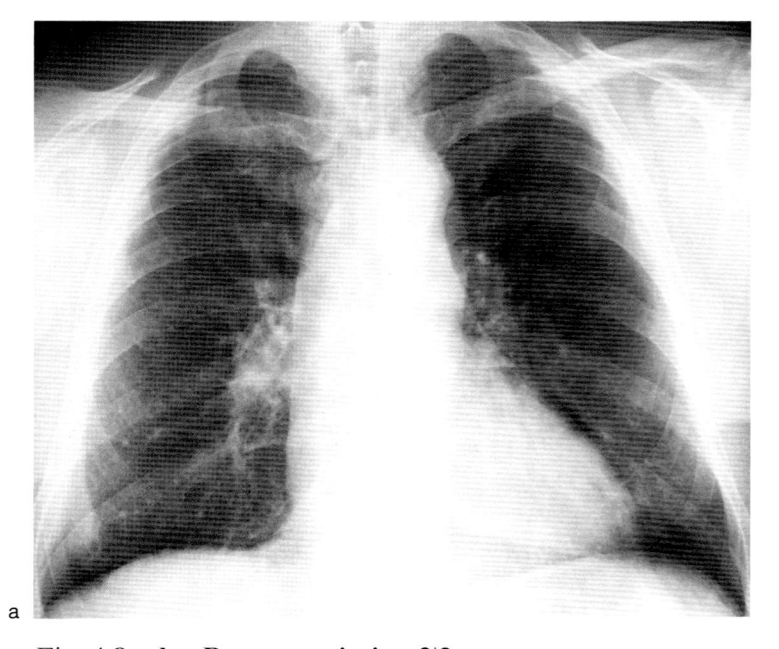

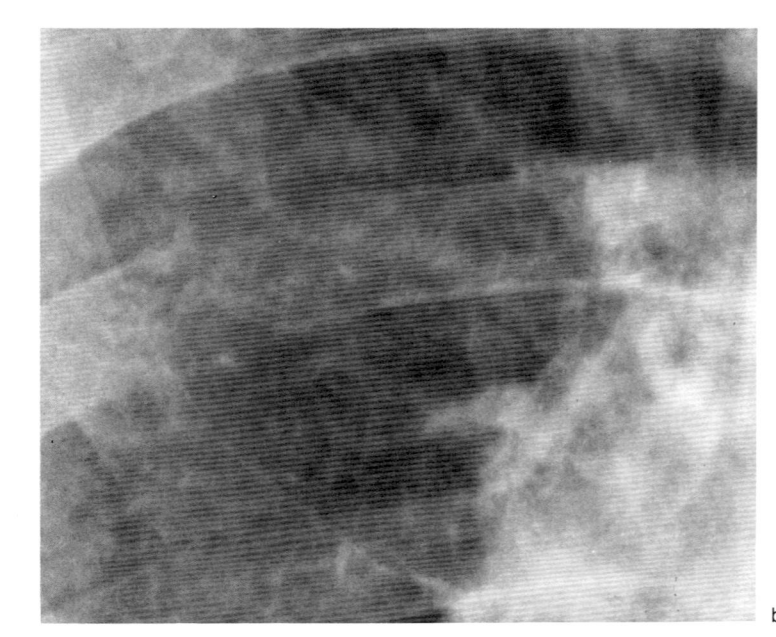

Fig. 4.8 a, b   Pneumoconiosis t 2|2

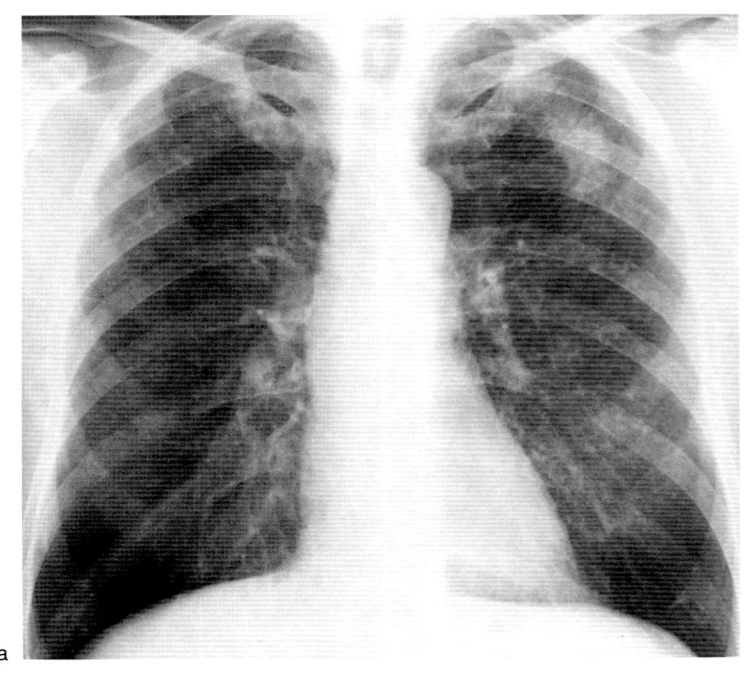

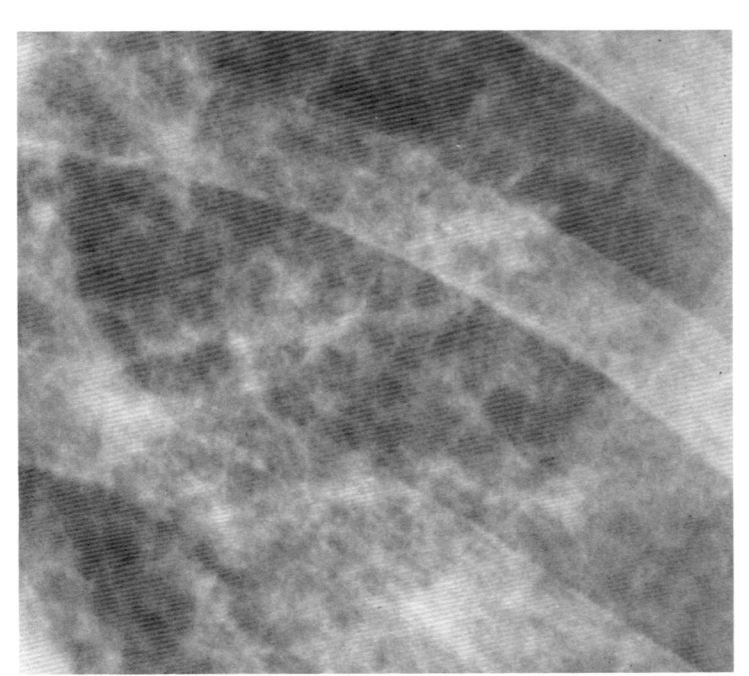

Fig. 4.9 a, b   Pneumoconiosis u 2|2.
Large opacity visible in left upper lung zone.

Large Opacities (Conglomerate Shadow, Progressive Massive Fibrosis)

The ILO classification distinguishes three types of large opacities, according to their size:

Category A: Large opacity 1–5 cm in diameter

Category B: One or more large opacities whose combined surface area does not exceed the area of the right upper lobe

Category C: One or more opacities whose combined surface area exceeds the area of the right upper lobe.

The character of the margin is also recorded:

wf: well-defined opacity
id: ill-defined opacity

Fig. 4.10 **Pneumoconiosis category A.**
Large opacity in left upper lung zone (4 cm in diameter)

Fig. 4.11 **Pneumoconiosis category B.**
Large opacities in both upper lung zones. The sum of both opacities exceeds 5 cm but is smaller than the entire right upper lobe.

Fig. 4.12 **Pneumoconiosis category B.**
Large opacities whose combined surface area does not equal that of the right upper lobe.

Fig. 4.13 **Pneumoconiosis category C.**
Conglomerate shadows whose sum exceeds the surface area of the right upper lobe. Basilar emphysema is present.

Fig. 4.14 **Pneumoconiosis category C.**
Marked emphysema with adjacent scarring and distortion of the lung parenchyma. Displaced anterior junction line (1) indicates herniation of right lung across midline into left hemithorax.

Fig. 4.15 **Pneumoconiosis category C with evidence of previous postprimary tuberculosis.**
Multiple opacities with conglomeration exceeding surface area of right upper lobe. Marked apical pleuroparenchymal scarring due to documented previous open tuberculosis. Note distortion and rightward shift of trachea and esophagus.

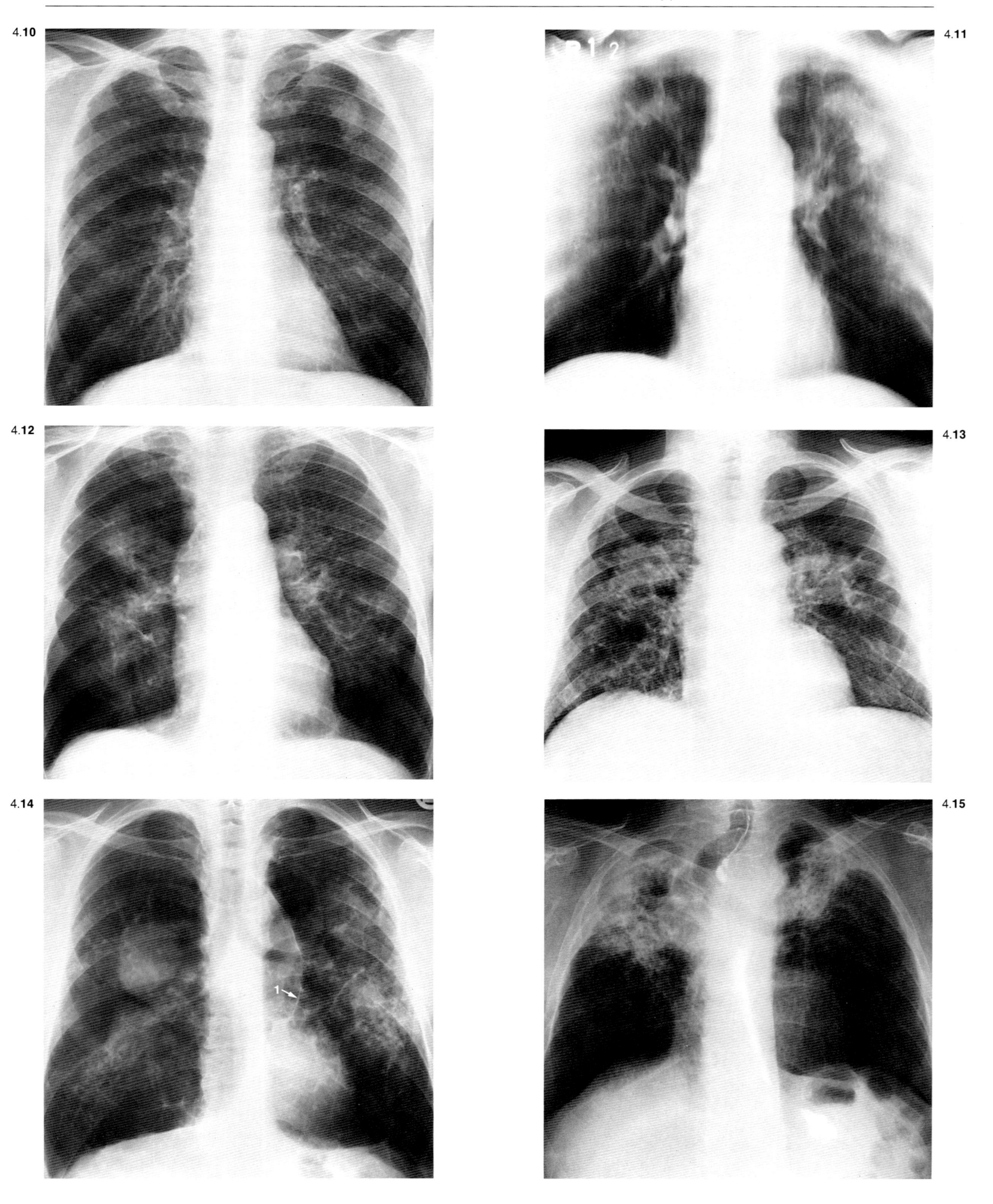

Types of Pneumoconiosis   119

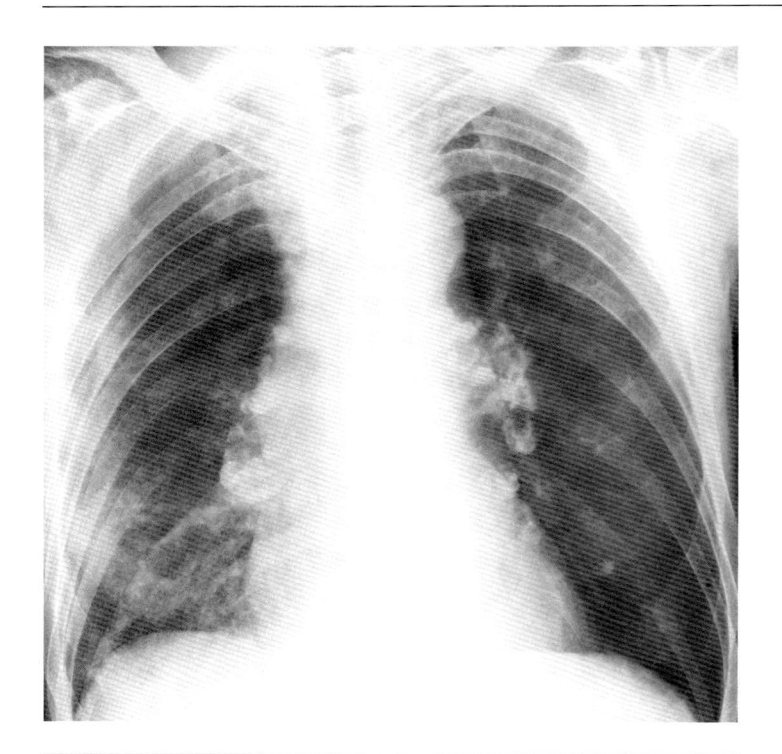

Silicosis

Fig. 4.16 Eggshell calcifications of lymph nodes.
Calcium deposits are present in the marginal sinus region of the affected lymph nodes.

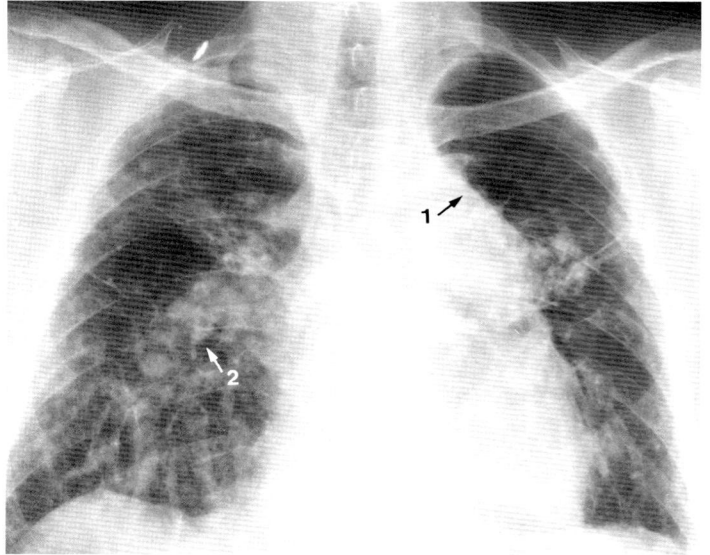

Fig. 4.17 Scarring, conglomerate shadows, and eggshell calcification of lymph nodes.
Dilated main pulmonary artery segment (1), dilated central pulmonary arteries (2) indicating pulmonary arterial hypertension. Emphysematous changes in both upper lobes.

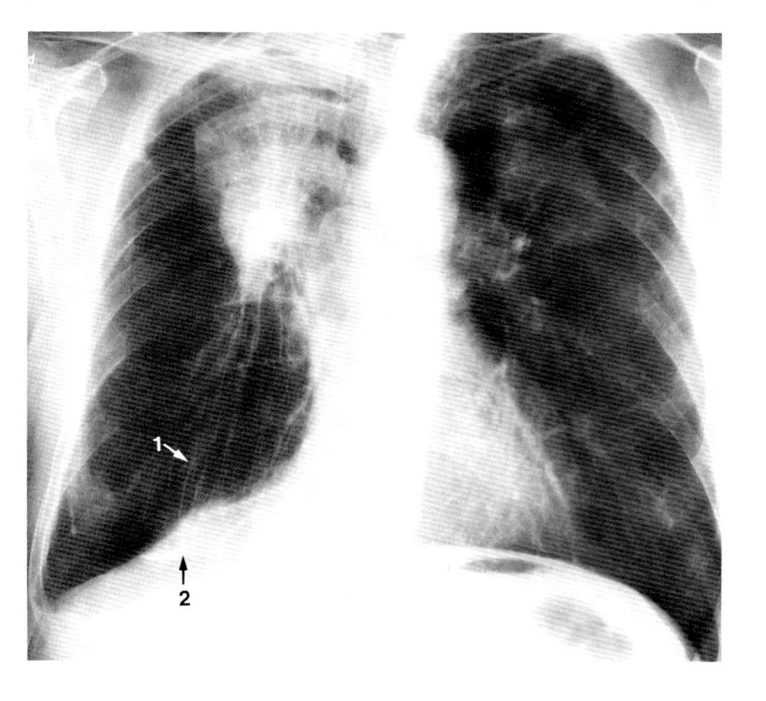

Fig. 4.18 Conglomerate shadows with marked scarring and right upper lobe volume loss.
Stretched right lower lobe pulmonary artery branches (1), pleural calcifications over right hemidiaphragm (2).

Fig. 4.19 a–f Silicosis.
Course of disease over 9 years. A 60-year-old miner, retired in 1959 due to progressive dyspnea; clinical symptomatology worsened over the ensuing years. Small round opacities of size q (1959 **a, b**). Round opacities of size r (1959 **c, d**), diffuse infiltrative lung disease with conglomerate shadows in both upper lung zones. Note progressive overall loss of lung volume from 1959 to 1968.

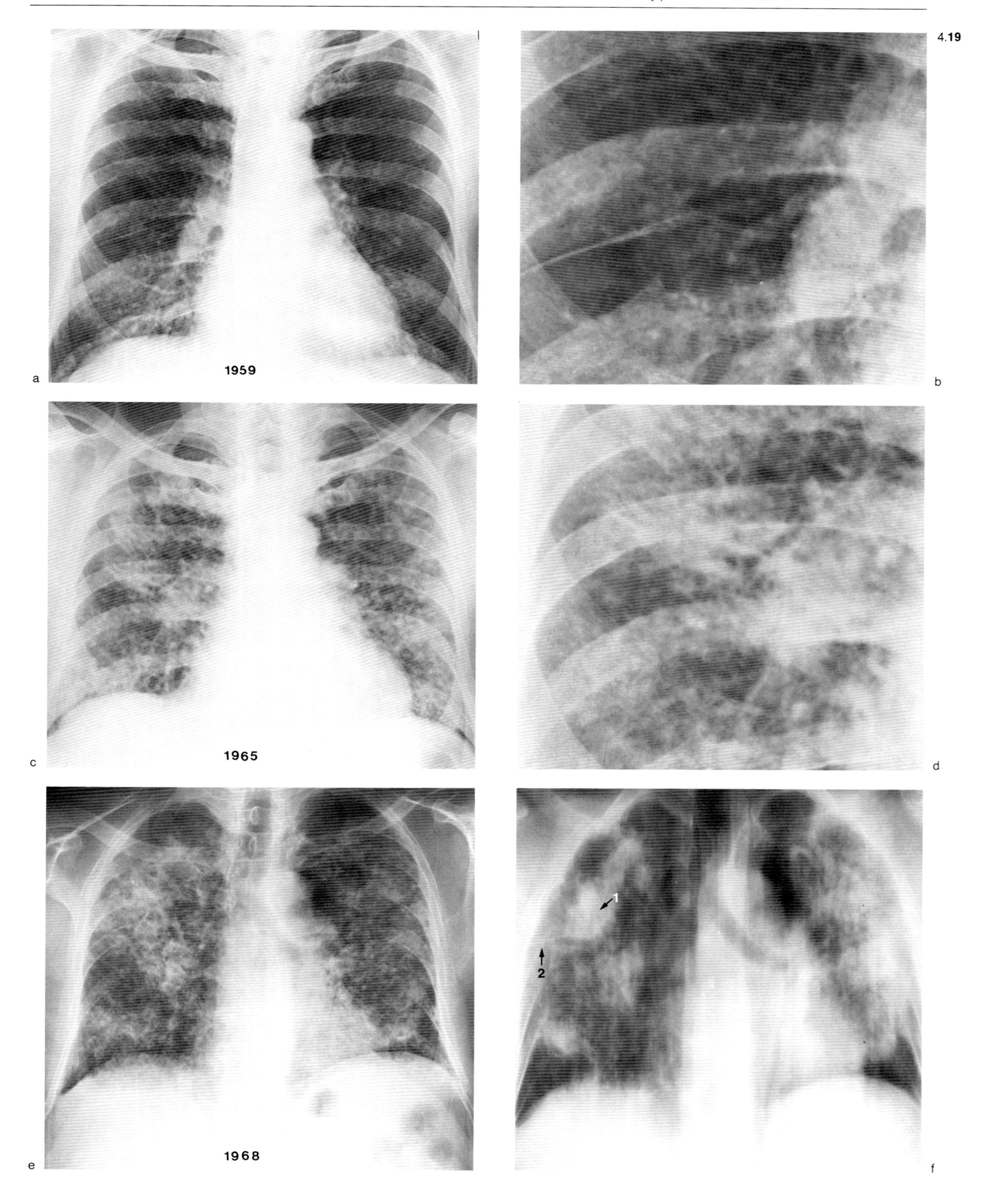

Types of Pneumoconiosis   121

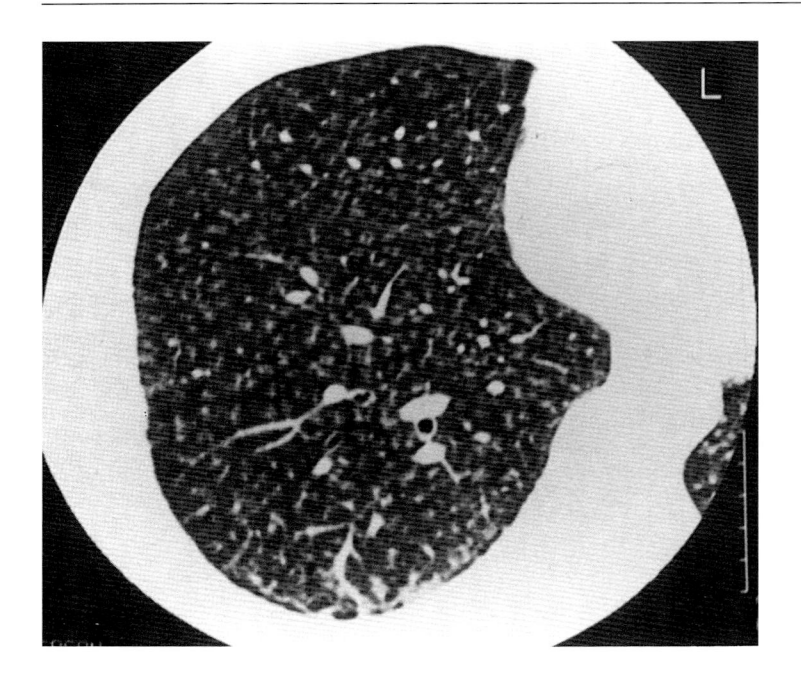

Fig. 4.20 Coal worker's pneumoconiosis in asymptomatic, 45-year-old miner.
High-resolution CT scan shows multiple, small, rounded opacities corresponding to coal macules throughout the lung. (Courtesy Dr. Robert Pugatch)

Asbestosis

Asbestos-containing dust is found in industries dealing with the processing of asbestos fibers, e.g., pipefitting, shipyard work, insulation, textile and plastic material industries. Asbestos fibers are less than 5 µm in diameter and can reach the alveoli even though their length exceeds 150 µm.

Reactive pulmonary fibrosis and parietal pleural plaques result from the interaction of the fibers with the lung and pleura. Plaques contain subpleural hyalin collagen and can calcify in up to 60% of patients examined with CT. The radiographic features of pleural plaques include focal pleural thickening along the midaspect of the chest, more marked along the course of ribs. Diaphragmatic pleural plaques are common, while the costophrenic sulci and the apices are usually spared.

Pulmonary fibrosis involves primarily the lower lung zones. It can lead to honeycombing and obliteration of the cardiac and diaphragmatic contour. Asbestos exposure increases the incidence of bronchogenic carcinoma and malignant mesothelioma.

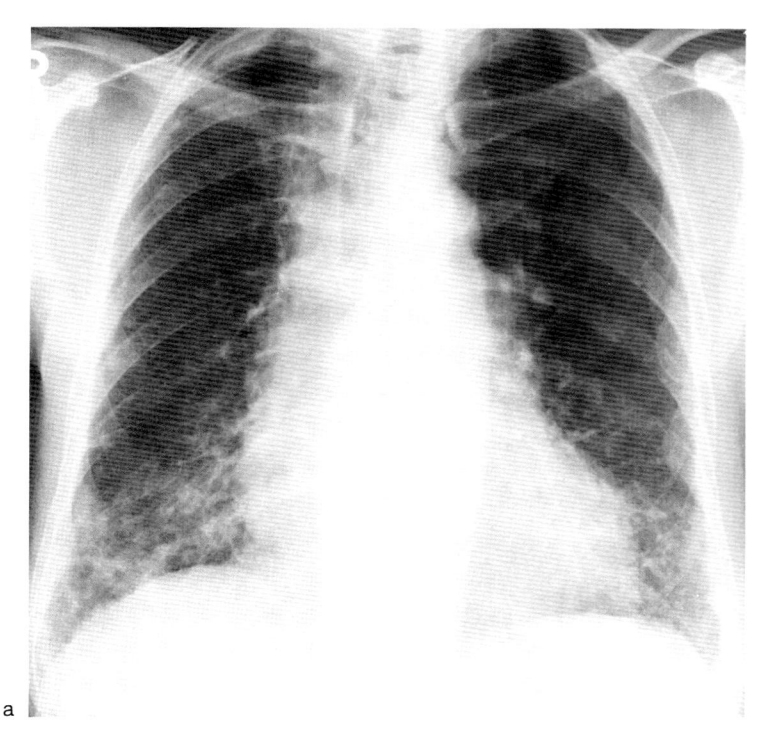

Fig. 4.21 a, b **Asbestosis.**
71-year-old insulation worker. Abnormal linear and reticular markings at both lung bases. "Shaggy" heart.

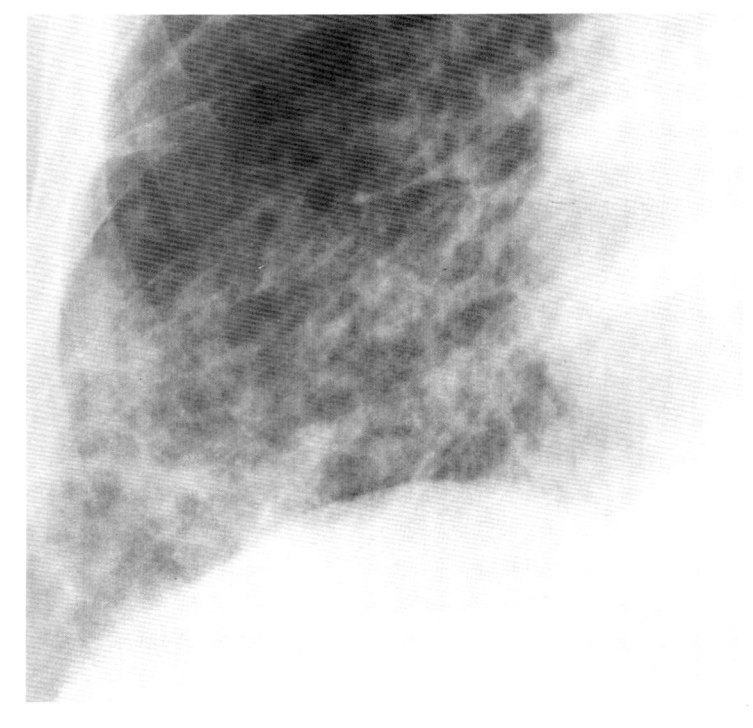

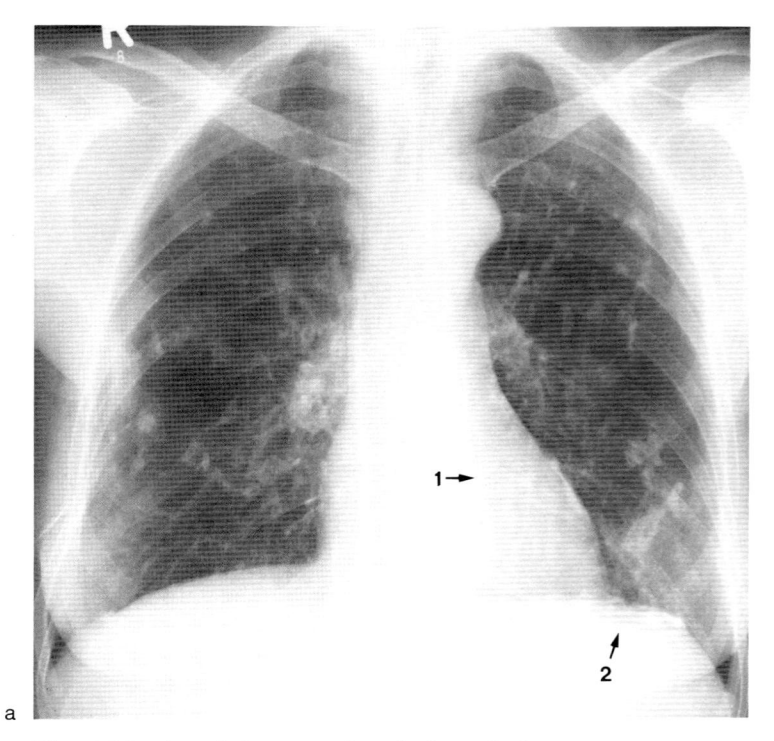

Fig. 4.**22 a, b Asbestos-related pleural plaques.**
Irregular, partially calcified opacities project on the lung.

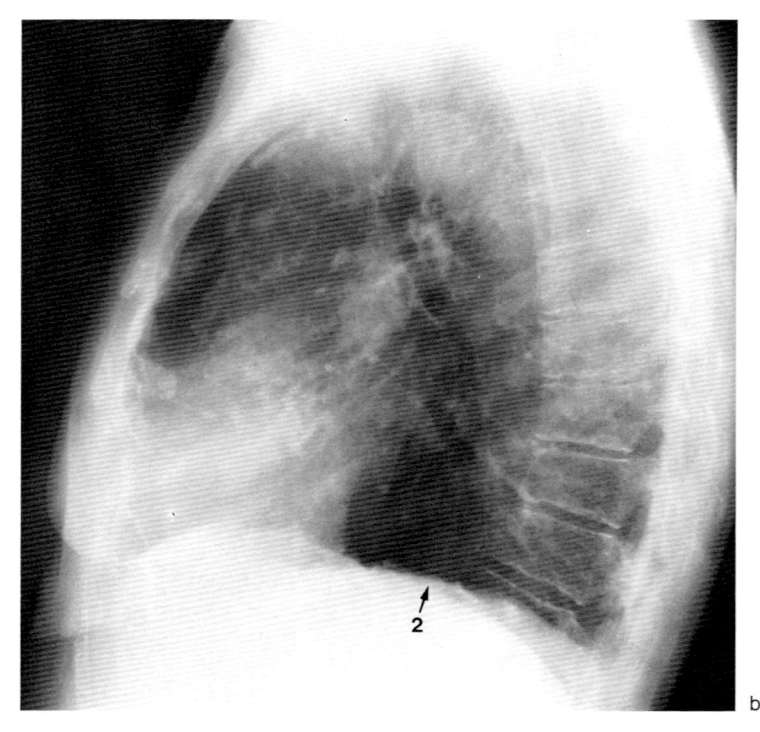

Curvilinear calcification of the mediastinal (1) and diaphragmatic (2) pleura.

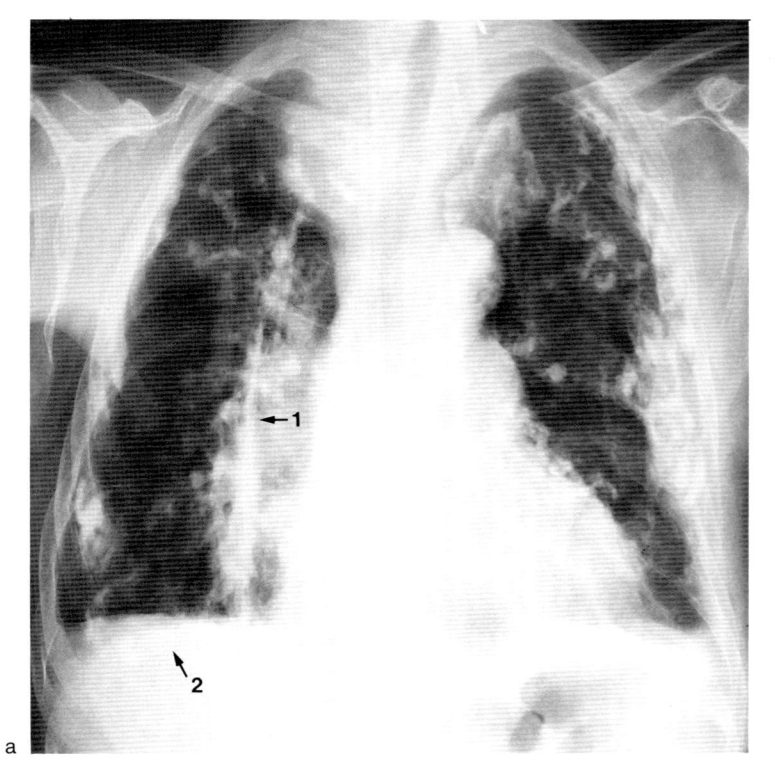

Fig. 4.**23 a, b Asbestos-related pleural plaques.**
84-year-old patient with known occupational exposure to asbestos. Extensive pleural calcifications (1) clearly visible due to the thoracic dextroscoliosis, calcified diaphragmatic pleura (2), dilated main pulmonary artery segment. Large goiter in the superior mediastinum.

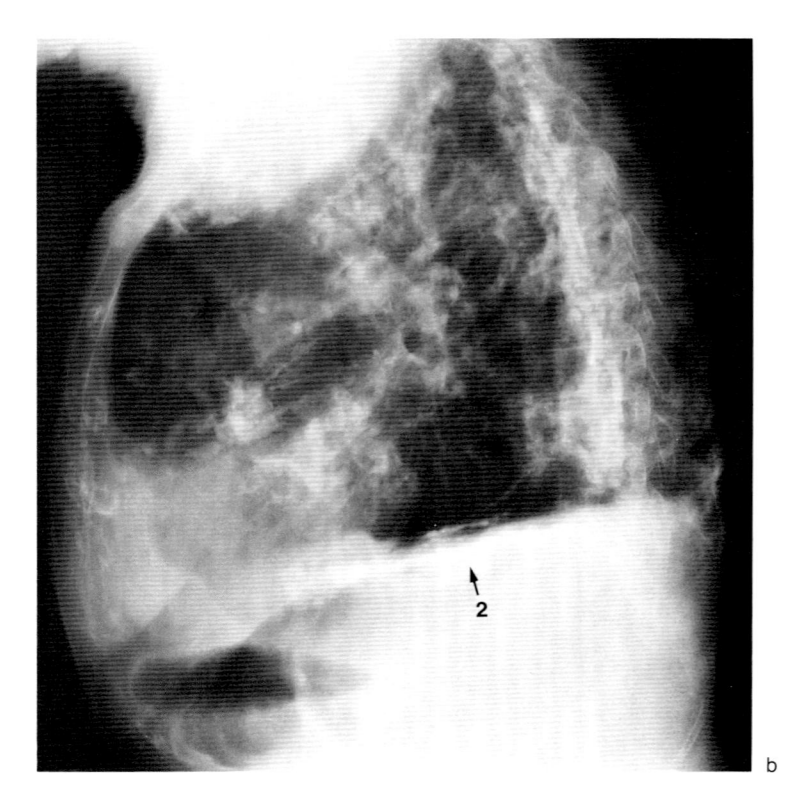

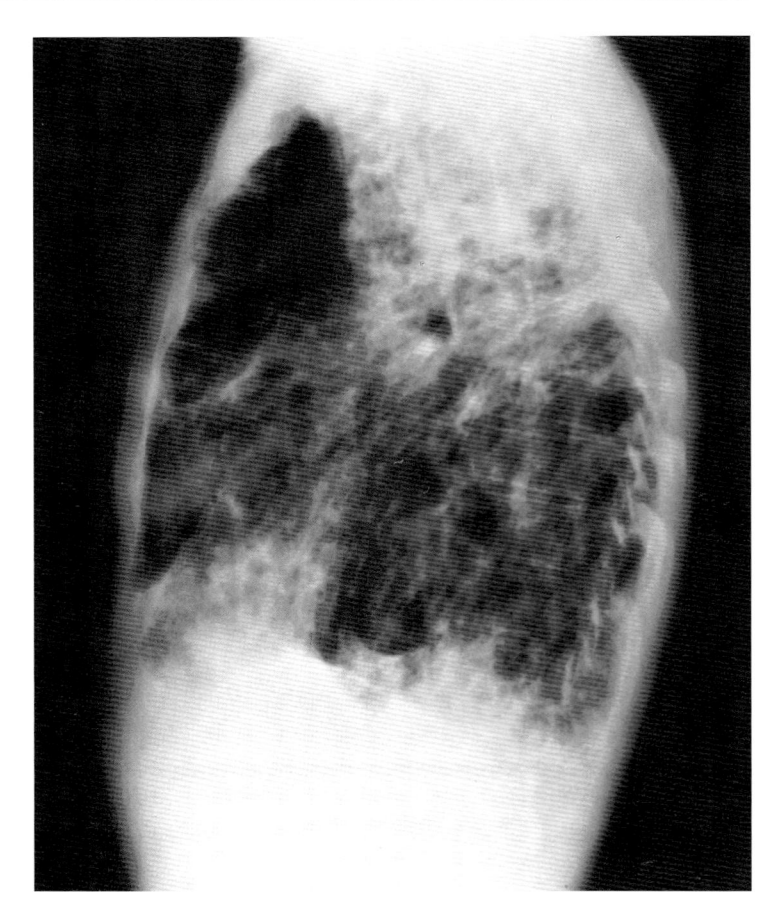

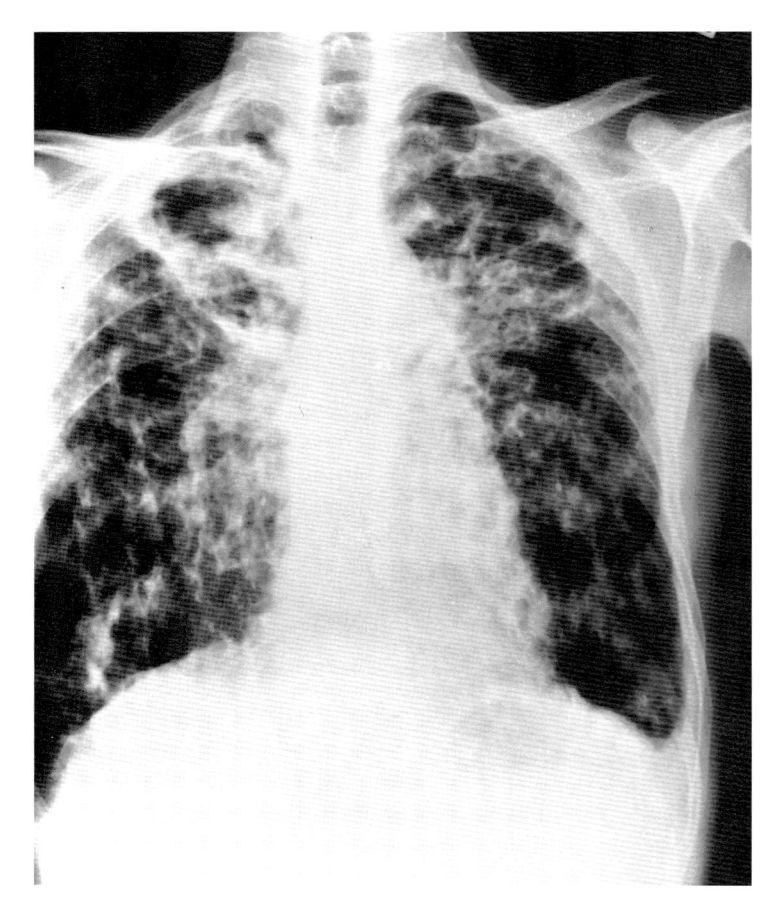

Fig. 4.24 **Vineyard sprayer's lung disease.**
Chest frontal and lateral views reveal marked upper lobe scarring with coarse reticulonodular opacification, honeycombing, traction bronchiectases, and conglomerate masses. Patient sprayed vineyards over many years with a mixture of copper sulfate and lime.

5. Neoplasms

Bronchogenic Carcinoma

Carcinoma of the lung has become the most common malignant tumor in the industrialized world. In the past 50 years, the incidence of this lethal cancer has increased tenfold, paralleling the increase in cigarette consumption. In 1990, the American Cancer Society predicted over 140 000 deaths due to bronchogenic carcinoma.

The World Health Organization (WHO) classifies bronchogenic carcinomas into four histologic groups:

- Squamous cell carcinoma
- Small cell carcinoma
- Large cell carcinoma
- Adenocarcinoma.

Mixed histologic types can occur. Therapy planning is contingent on differentiating only between small cell and non-small cell carcinoma. The histologic type cannot be predicted reliably from the radiographic features, even though cavitation is more likely in squamous cell carcinoma, large hilar and mediastinal masses are suggestive of small cell carcinoma, and peripheral nodules are more typical of adenocarcinoma. Air bronchograms within a nodule make a bronchoalveolar cell carcinoma, a variant of adenocarcinoma, likely. The TNM Staging System (Table 5.1) is important in evaluating the extent, resectability, and prognosis of non-small cell carcinomas.

Imaging procedures are crucial in the preoperative staging of tumors, in conjunction with bronchoscopy and mediastinoscopy. Bronchogenic carcinomas are usually unifocal. They form in the bronchial mucosa and spread centrally along the bronchial wall and through lymphatics.

Central bronchogenic carcinomas, like squamous cell and small cell cancers, originate in the segmental bronchi and extend toward the hilus. Peripheral cancers presenting as solitary pulmonary nodules originate in the subsegmental or even more peripheral bronchi. Central tumors can either have an endobronchial component and lead early to lobar atelectasis or can grow transbronchially and produce a large central hilar or mediastinal mass.

The following illustrated examples will focus on:
1. Peripheral bronchogenic carcinomas with and without hilar metastases
2. Bronchoalveolar or pneumonic form of carcinoma
3. Central tumors with endobronchial or transbronchial growth
4. Invasive tumors with invasion of chest wall or mediastinal structures.

Table 5.1 TNM Classification of Lung Cancer

Primary Tumor (T)
- Tx – Tumor proven by presence of malignant cells in sputum
- T0 – No evidence of primary tumor
- Tis – Carcinoma in situ
- T1 – A tumor that is 3.0 cm or less in diameter surrounded by lung or visceral pleura
- T2 – A tumor more than 3.0 cm in greatest dimension, or one that invades visceral pleura or involves bronchus at least 2 cm distal to carina
- T3 – A tumor of any size with direct extension into chest wall, diaphragm, mediastinal pleura, pericardium; tumor within 2 cm of carina without involving carina
- T4 – A tumor of any size with invasion of the mediastinum or involving heart, great vessels, trachea, esophagus, vertebral body, or carina, or presence of malignant pleural effusion

Nodal Involvement (N)
- N0 – No demonstrable metastasis to regional lymph nodes
- N1 – Hilar lymph node involvement
- N2 – Metastasis to ipsilateral mediastinal and subcarinal lymph nodes
- N3 – Metastasis to contralateral mediastinal lymph nodes, contralateral hilar lymph nodes, ipsilateral or contralateral scalene or supraclavicular lymph nodes

Distant Metastasis (M)
- M0 – No known distant metastasis
- M1 – Distant metastasis present

Stage Grouping of TNM Subsets

Occult carcinoma:	Tx	N0	M0
Stage 0:	Tis	N0	M0
Stage I:	T1	N0	M0
	T2	N0	M0
Stage II:	T1	N1	M0
	T2	N1	M0
Stage IIIa:	T3	N0	M0
	T3	N1	M0
	T1–3	N2	M0
Stage IIIb:	Any T	N3	M0
	T4	Any N	M0
Stage IV:	Any T	Any N	M1

Stages I–IIIa are resectable; stages IIIb and IV are non-resectable.

Peripheral Lung Cancer

Peripheral bronchogenic carcinomas present as solitary pulmonary nodules or masses. This represents the most common radiologic finding in lung cancer. The tumor is either found incidentally or becomes symptomatic because of distant metastases. Peripheral nodules smaller than 3 cm in diameter, distal to a lobar bronchus, and without lymph node or distant metastases have a relatively good prognosis in operable patients: If resected, a 5-year survival of up to 50% can be expected.

Radiographic criteria for a malignant, solitary, pulmonary nodule:
- Diameter greater than 2 cm
- Ill-defined, lobulated contour
- Corona radiata
- Notch sign
- Pleural tail
- Volume doubling time between 1 and 16 months on CT scans

Only 1% of lung cancers are calcified on plain films. Yet in 6% of tumors, calcifications are visible on CT scans. These malignant calcifications are excentric, punctate, reticular, or amorphous. Benign calcifications are either central, diffuse, lamellated, target-like, or coarse, popcornlike.

Calculation of the tumor volume doubling time is possible on semilogarithmic paper. A graphic representation of time on the x-axis and volume on the y-axis allows for an easy read-out of values. Figure 5.1 shows an example assuming a diameter of 1.2 cm on January 29, 1974: $V = 0.21 \times 4/3 \times \pi = 0.86$ cm^3. The diameter of the lesion has increased to 2.2 cm on February 3, 1975: $V = 1.3 \times 4/3 \times \pi = 5.23$. On the semilogorithmic scale, the doubling time is 148 days. Since the volume of a sphere is $4/3 \times \pi \times r^3$ or $4.18 \times r^3$, the volumes can be easily calculated and compared. For a given diameter, multiplication by 1.24 will yield the diameter corresponding to volume doubling.

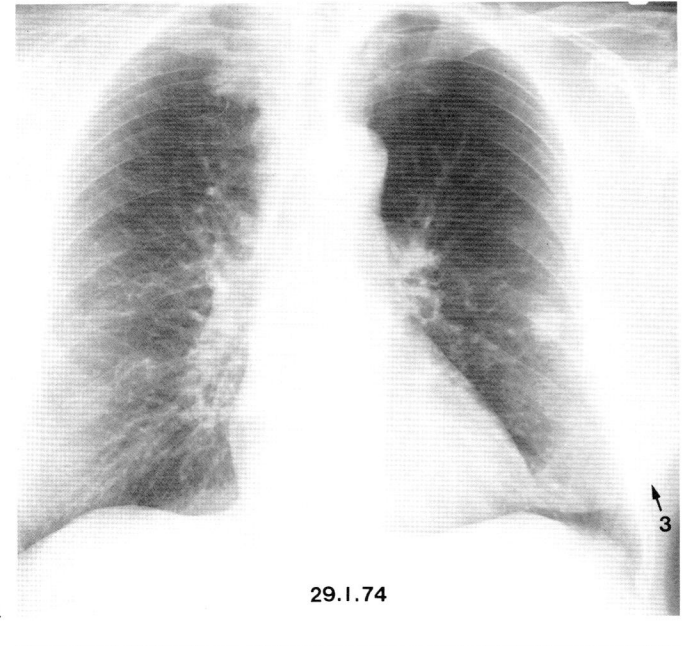

128   5. Neoplasms

Fig. 5.1 a–e   Solitary nodule in left mid-lung zone.
61-year-old patient. Incidental discovery. Patient initially refused a further work-up. Eventual transbronchial biopsy yields squamous cell carcinoma. Increase in size of nodule on sequential films taken at 12 months and 21 months. Pleural tail (1), subsegmental atelectasis (2), gynecomastia (3).

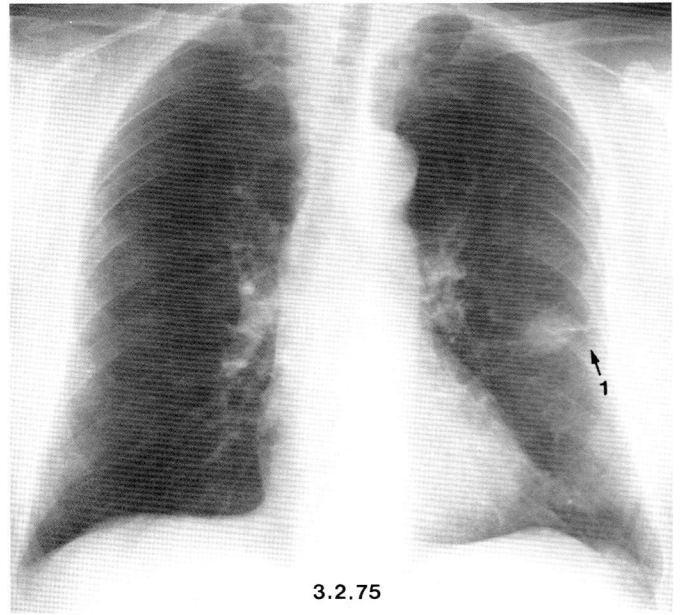

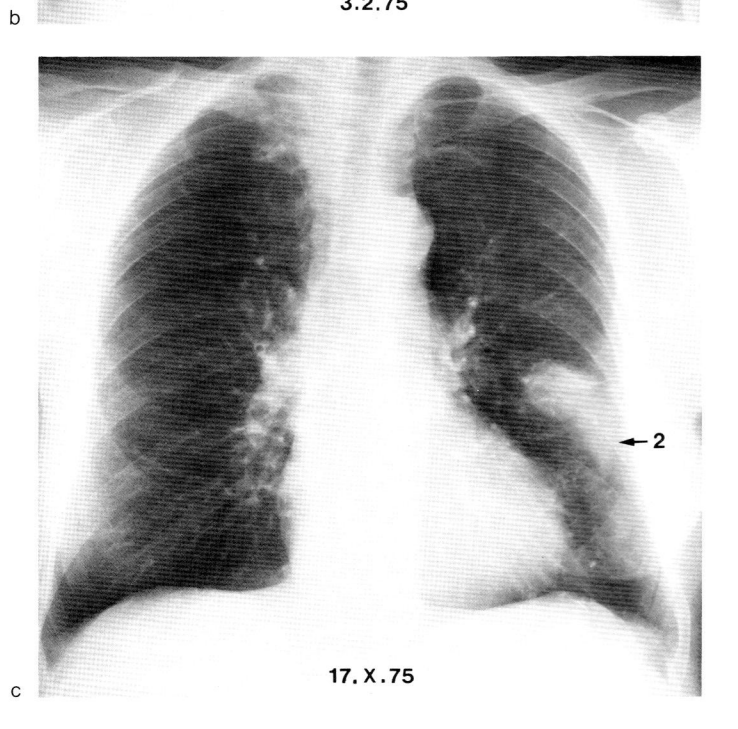

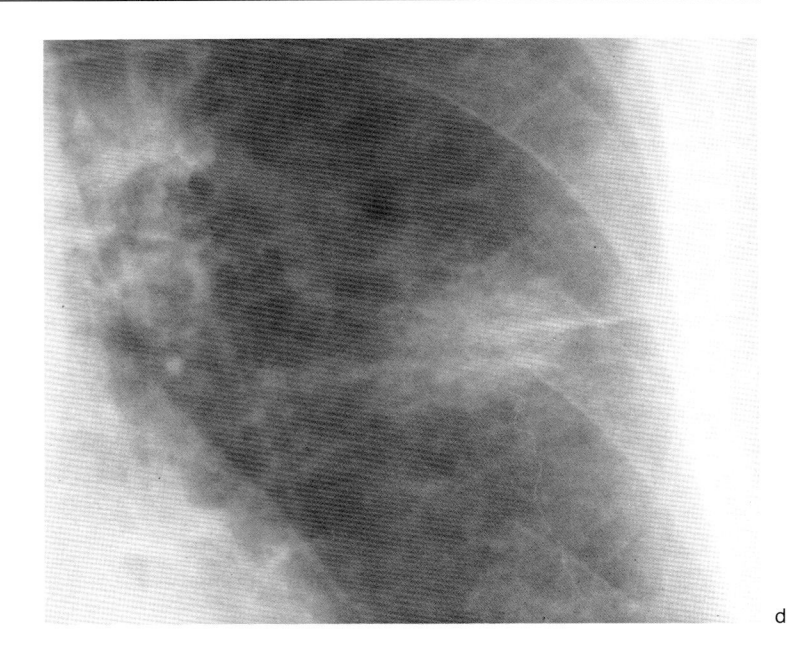

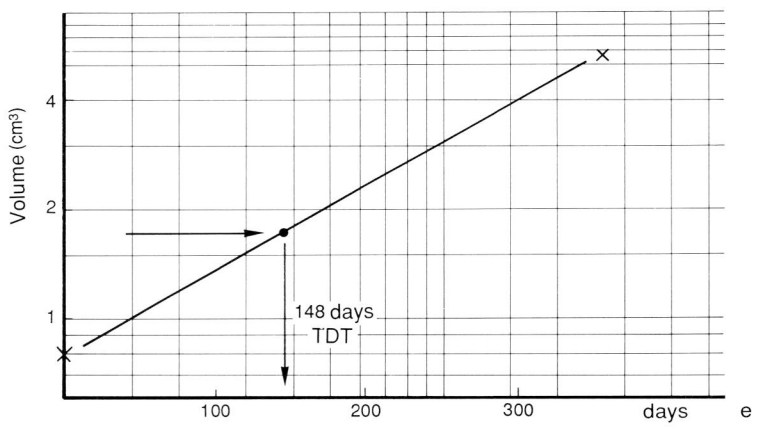

TDT = Tumor doubling time

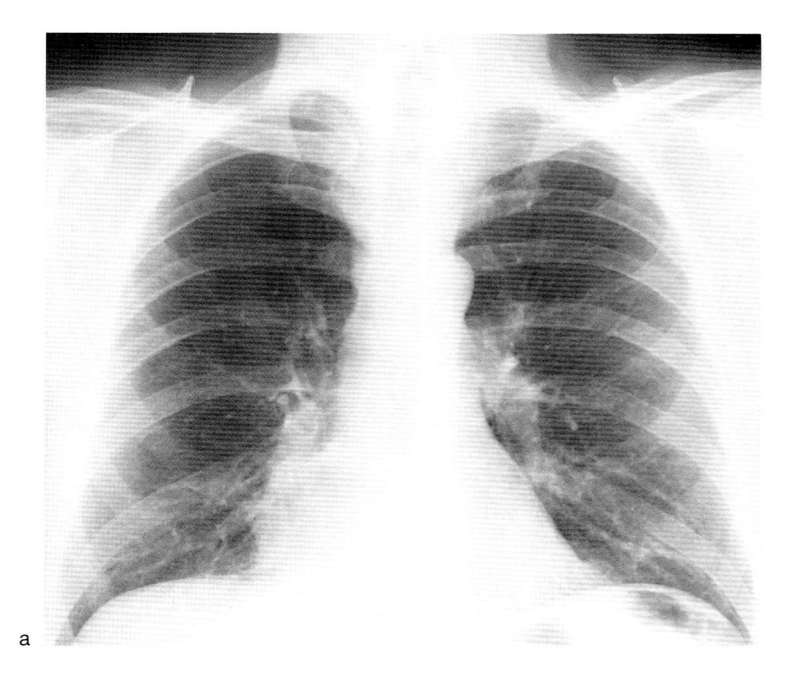

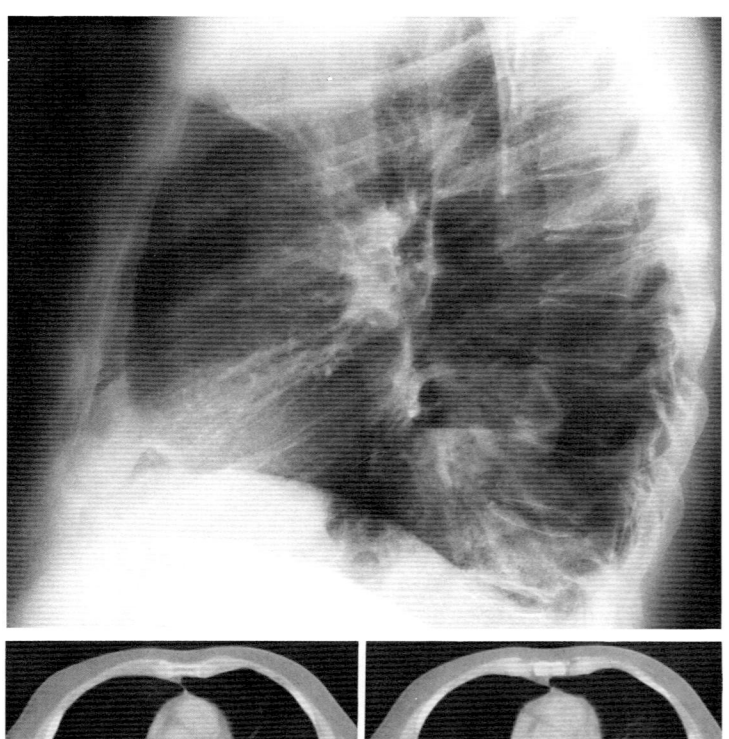

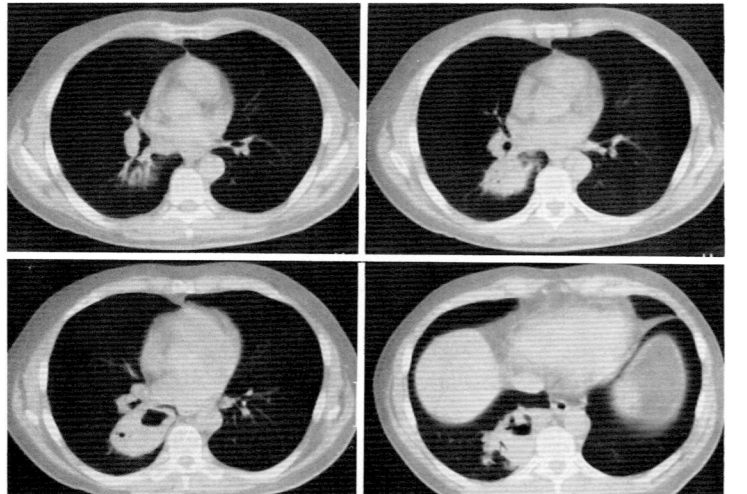

Fig. 5.**2a–c** **Peripheral squamous cell carcinoma.**
70-year-old patient with weight loss and sputum production. Mass in mediobasal and posterobasal segment, right lower lobe with cavitation and gas-fluid level (**a**, **b**) and filiform extensions into the surrounding parenchyma.

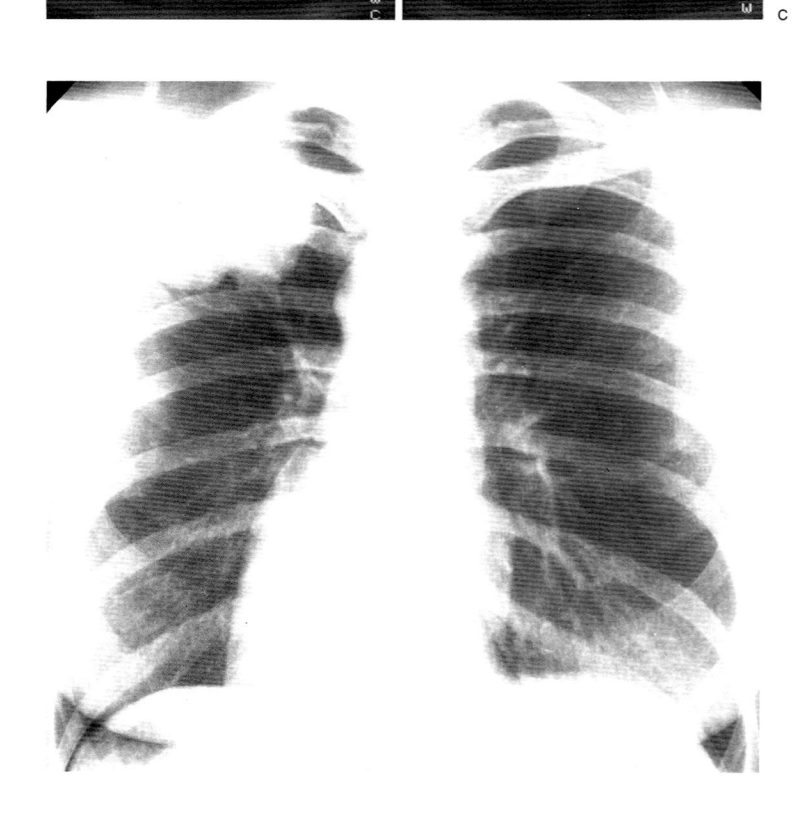

Fig. 5.**3** **Peripheral left upper lobe bronchogenic carcinoma.**
Lobular mass in apical posterior segment with linear extension to left hilus.

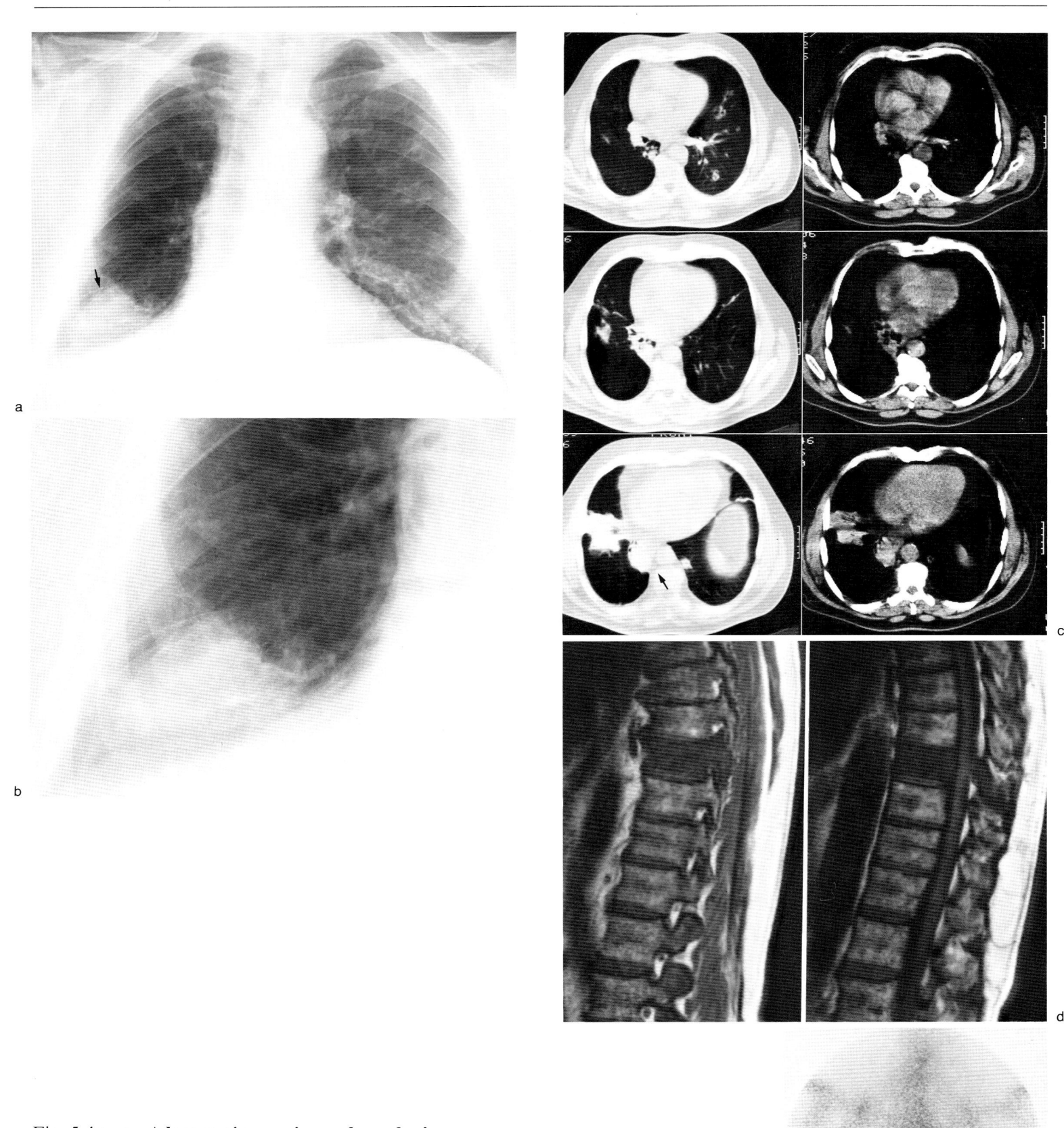

Fig. 5.4a–e Adenocarcinoma in coal worker's pneumoconiosis.
Patient presented with back pain. Coarse linear opacities in left lung. Right lower lobe shows complete atelectasis due to occlusion of right lower lobe bronchus. Middle lobe consolidation with air bronchogram on CT scan represents biopsy-proven adenocarcinoma. MR scan and bone scan demonstrate destroyed thoracic vertebra.

Bronchoalveolar Cell Carcinoma

This variant of adenocarcinoma can present as an ill-defined, solitary, pulmonary nodule or mimic a pneumonic consolidation. Tumor cells use the alveolar walls as scaffolding and spare the bronchial lumen. Bronchioloalveolar cell carcinomas originate from type II pneumocytes and from surfactant-producing Clara cells in the wall of bronchioles.

They account for 2–4% of all bronchogenic carcinomas. The characteristic radiologic feature is the well-preserved air bronchogram. Initially, it can be mistaken for an inflammatory process. In 10–30% of cases, a multifocal origin is likely. Pulmonary dissemination occurs either by way of bronchogenic spread or hematogenous metastases. Multiple nodules or confluent opacities become visible.

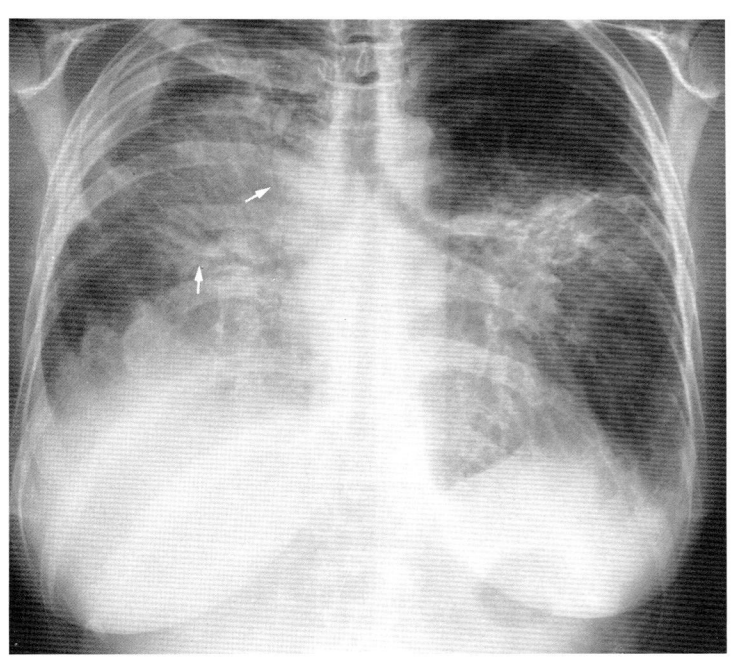

Fig. 5.**5a, b** **Bronchoalveolar cell carinoma.**
51-year-old patient with orthopnea. Confluent large opacities with air bronchogram. Left-sided apical loculated pleural effusion.

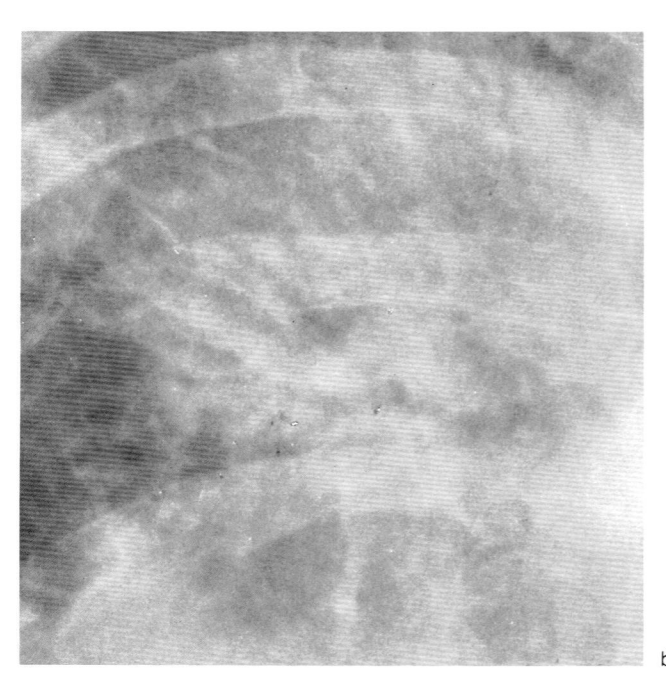

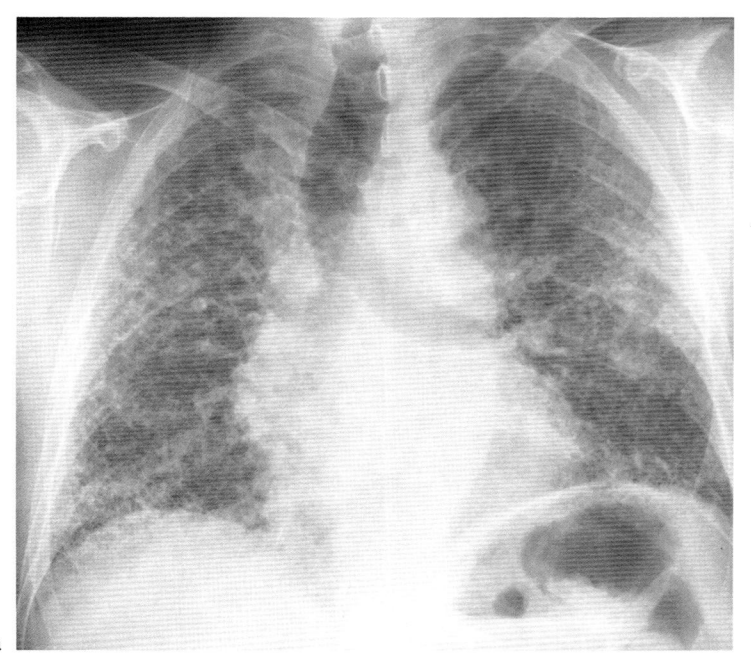

Fig. 5.**6a, b** **Disseminated bronchoalveolar cell carcinoma.**
58-year-old patient with massive sputum production of 1 L per day. Diffuse bilateral reticulonodular opacities.

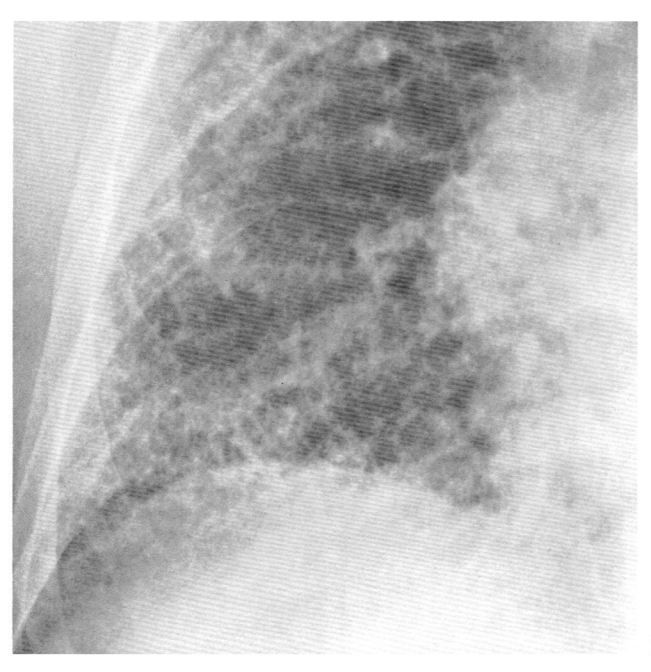

5. Neoplasms

Atelectasis and Lung Cancer

Total or partial atelectasis is the second most common radiographic finding in bronchogenic carcinoma. Usually an entire lobe is involved, producing displacement of the interlobar fissures and mediastinum, elevation of diaphragmatic leaflets, and approximation of ribs. Overpenetrated chest radiographs, conventional tomography, and CT can demonstrate the tumor mass and the bronchial stenosis. Occasionally, benign lesions can also lead to atelectasis of a lobe or an entire lung: Mucus plugs, foreign bodies, benign tumors, or inflammatory strictures have to be considered.

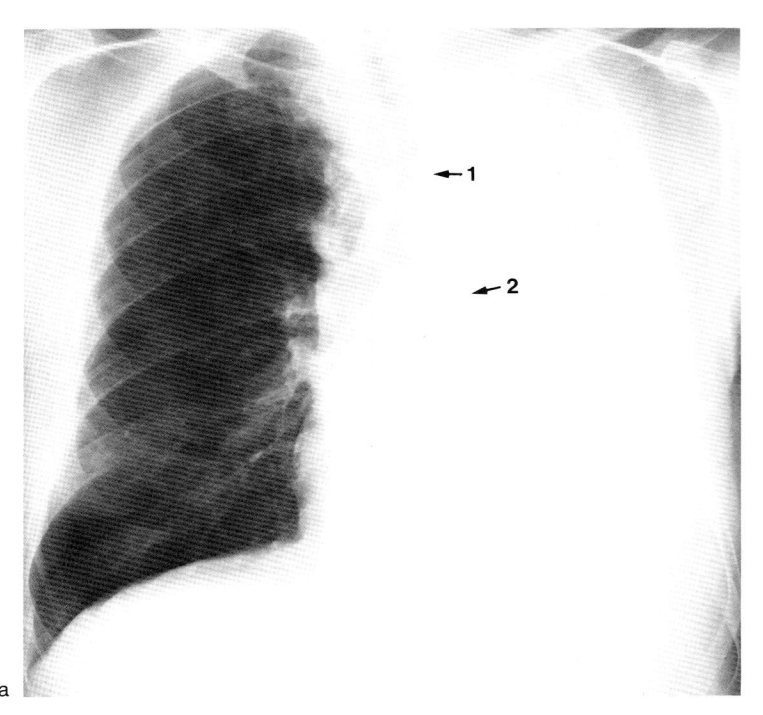

Fig. 5.7 a, b **Central bronchogenic carcinoma with complete atelectasis of entire left lung.**
58-year-old patient. Homogeneous opacification of left hemithorax. Tracheal shift to the left (1), cut-off, left mainstem bronchus, 1 cm distal to carina (2). Lateral projection shows only contour of right hemidiaphragm. Left pulmonary artery is obscured, and only right-sided posterior pleural line is visible (1).

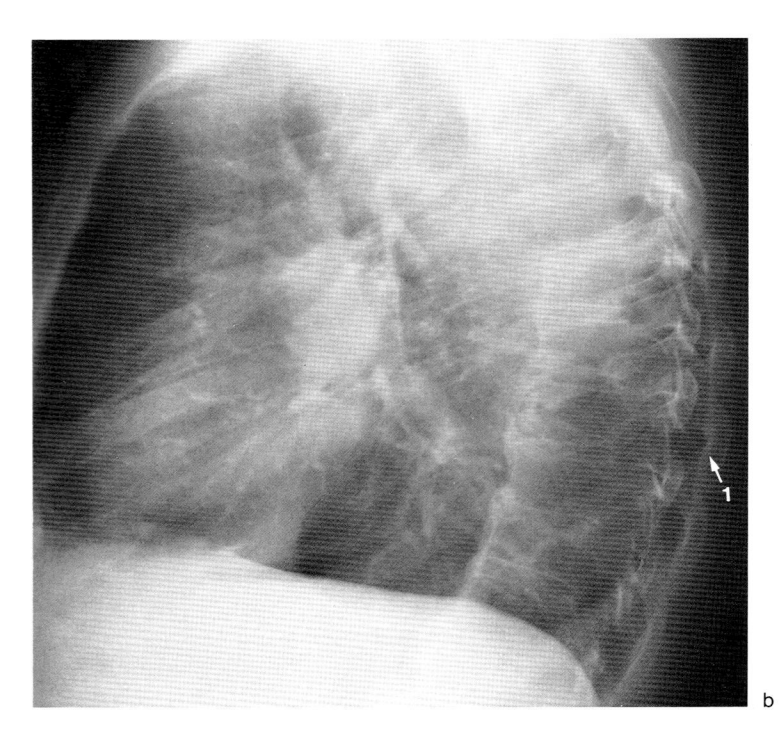

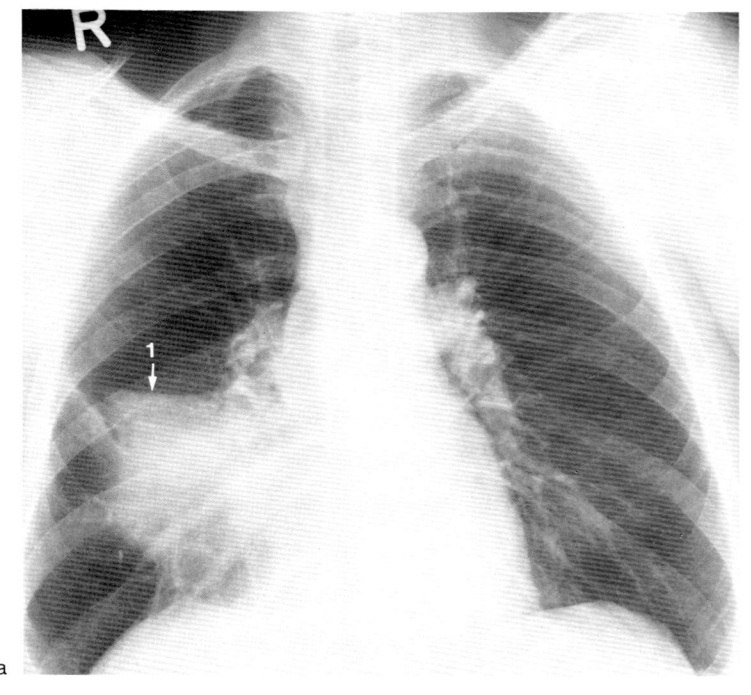

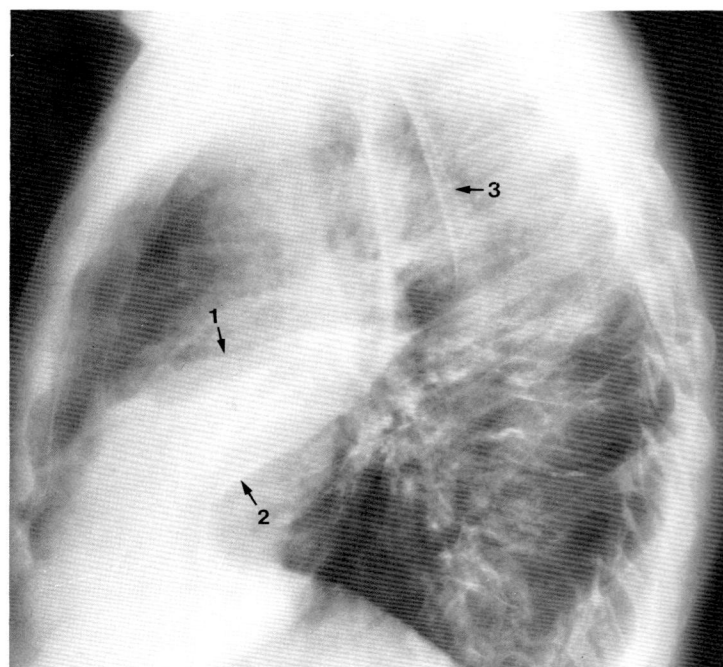

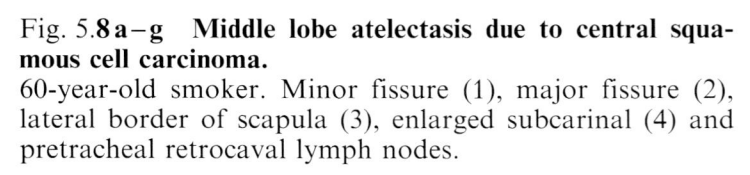

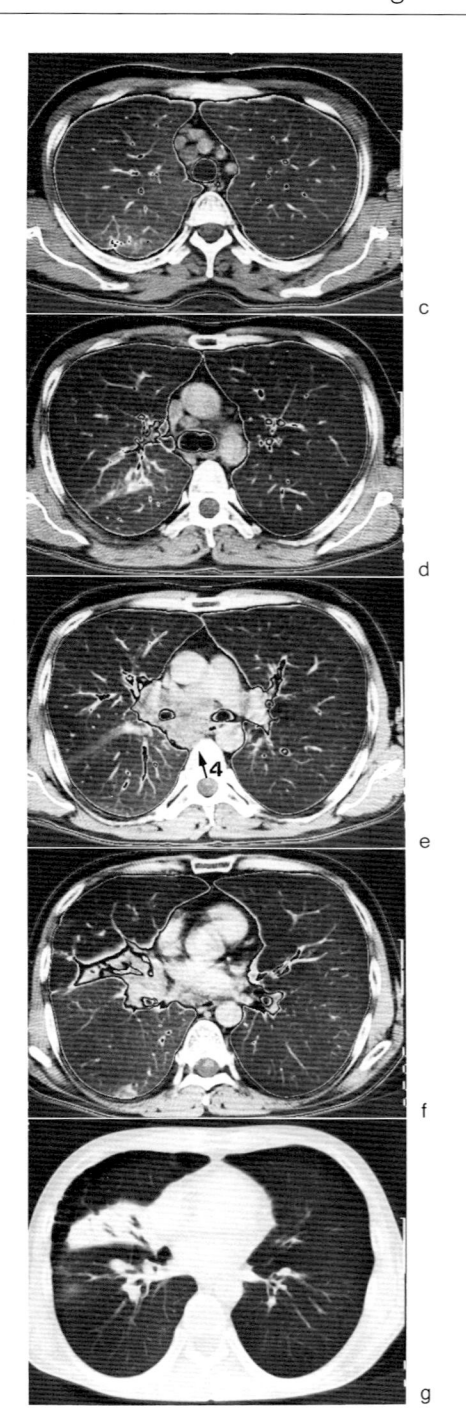

Fig. 5.8 a–g **Middle lobe atelectasis due to central squamous cell carcinoma.**
60-year-old smoker. Minor fissure (1), major fissure (2), lateral border of scapula (3), enlarged subcarinal (4) and pretracheal retrocaval lymph nodes.

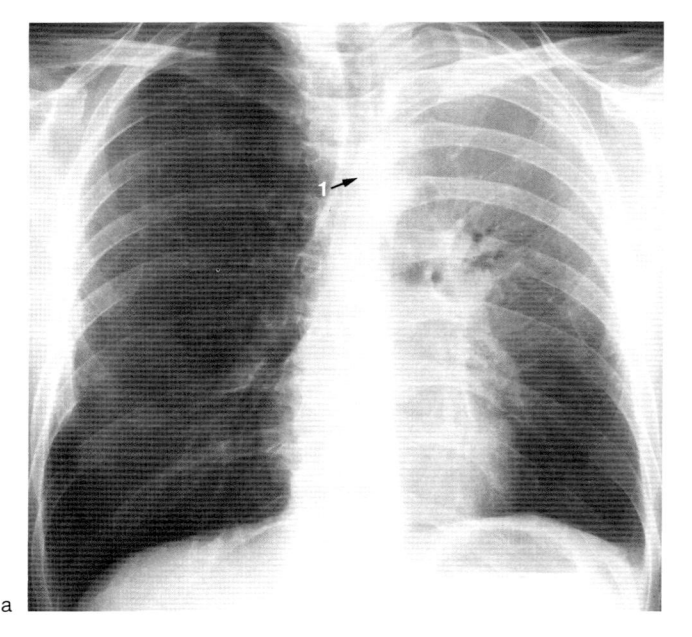

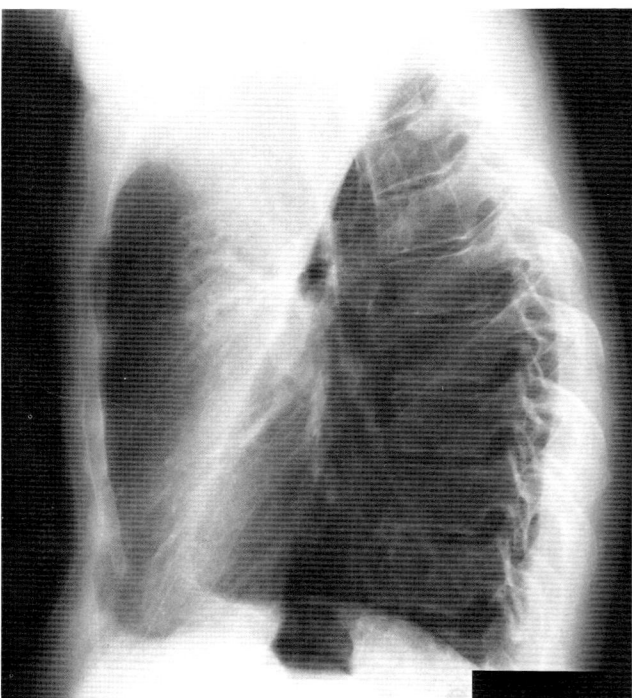

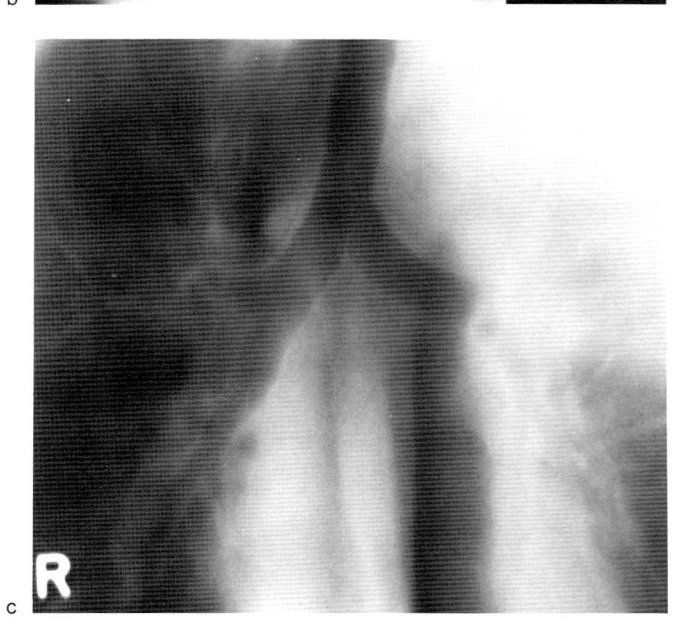

Fig. 5.9 a–c Left upper lobe atelectasis.
42-year-old smoker. Large cell carcinoma. Homogeneous opacification of collapsed left upper lobe. Leftward shift of trachea and anterior junction line (1). Conventional tomogram shows occlusion of left bronchus as well as azygos vein and azygoesophageal stripe.

Fig. 5.10 a–d Carcinoma left upper lobe bronchus.
48-year-old smoker. Incidental finding on routine chest radiograph. Partial atelectasis in anterior segment of left upper lobe with patchy opacification. Note primary tumor in region of left hilus (**d**) and the enlarged prevascular lymph node adjacent to ascending aorta (**b**).

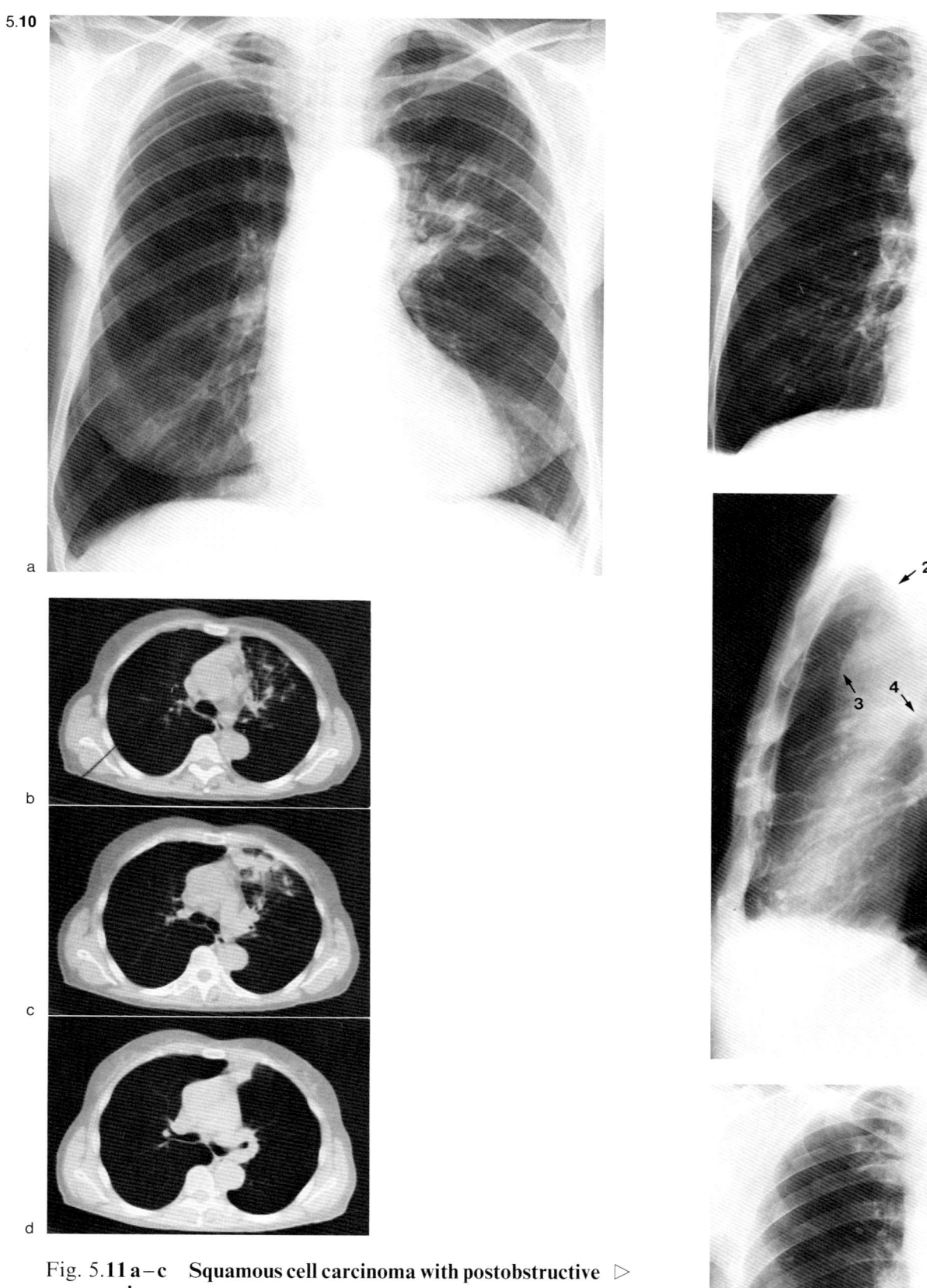

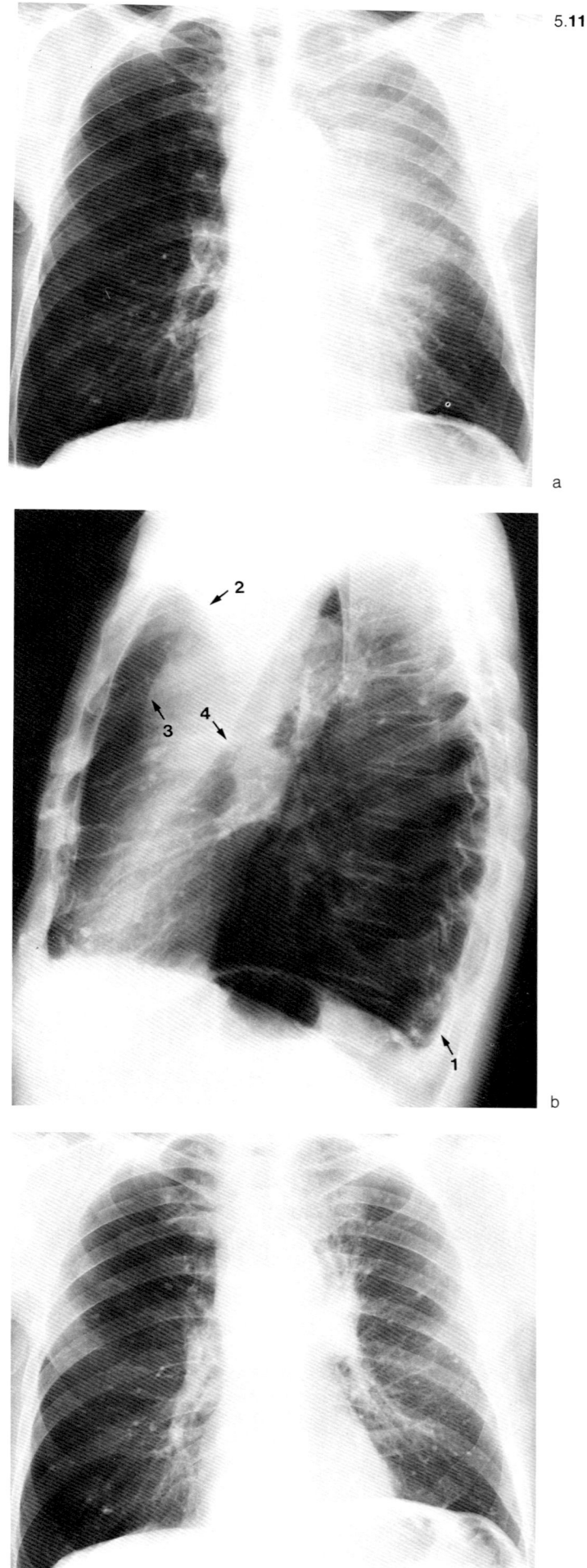

Fig. 5.11 a–c **Squamous cell carcinoma with postobstructive pneumonia.**
56-year-old smoker with previous history of varicella pneumonia.
Initial chest frontal and lateral radiograph (**a, b**) shows left upper lobe atelectasis with consolidation. Small, left, pleural effusion (1), contour of ascending aorta (3), anteriorly displaced major fissure (4), soft tissues, arm (2). After antibiotic therapy (**c**), consolidation clears, but loss of volume with elevation of left hemidiaphragm and left hilar mass persists.

136 5. Neoplasms

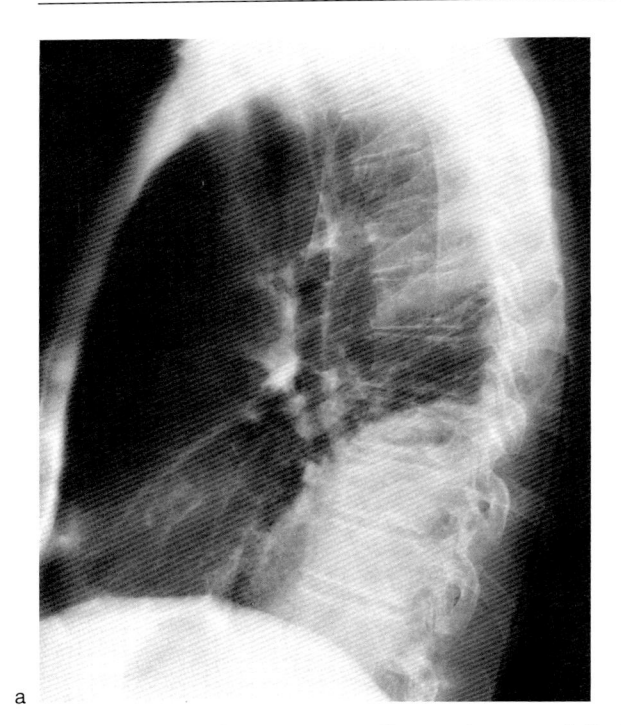

Fig. 5.**12 a, b Squamous cell carcinoma, left lower lobe bronchus.**

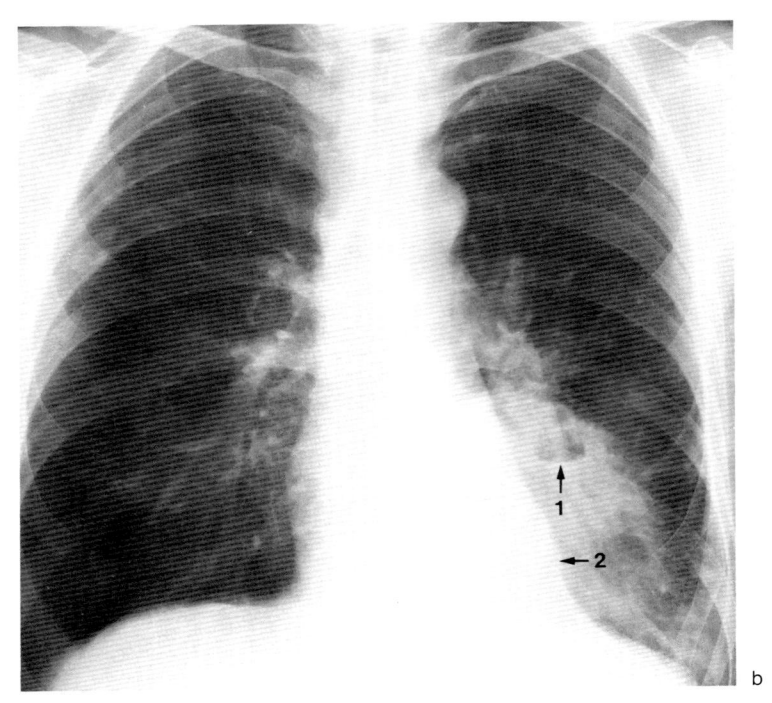

62-year-old smoker with hemoptysis. Chest frontal and lateral radiograph shows left lower lobe atelectasis with cavitation and fluid level (1). Left heart border preserved (2).

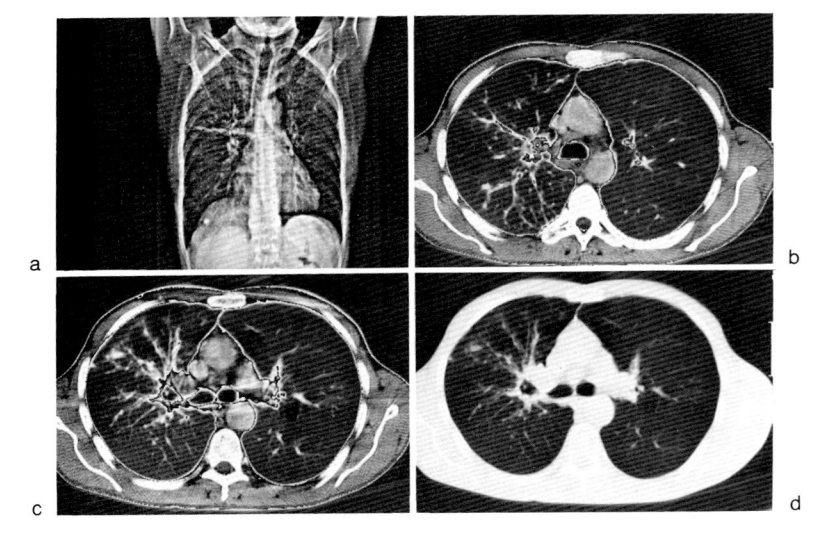

Fig. 5.**13 a–d Large cell carcinoma right upper lobe bronchus.**
52-year-old patient.
Subsegmental atelectasis of right upper lobe, anterior segment. Right hilar mass, with slightly enlarged right paratracheal and tracheobronchial lymph nodes.

Fig. 5.14a–j Bronchogenic carcinoma.
46-year-old smoker with a 30 pack-year history.
Left upper lobe atelectasis due to squamous cell carcinoma (**a, b**) with sparing of lingula; tumor extends bronchoscopically along the posterior wall of left main bronchus to carina. Note thickening of posterior wall of left main bronchus (**d**). After primary radiotherapy with 56 Gy (5600 rads), tumor has shrunk, and left upper lobe has reexpanded with only streaky residual opacities (**e, d**). Eventual tumor recurrence with left upper lobe atelectasis including lingula (**g, h**). No tumor recurrence in left main bronchus at bronchoscopy. Quantitative perfusion scan shows than only 38% of pulmonary blood flow supplies left lung. Delayed pneumonectomy (**j**). Patient free of disease 2 years after surgical procedure.

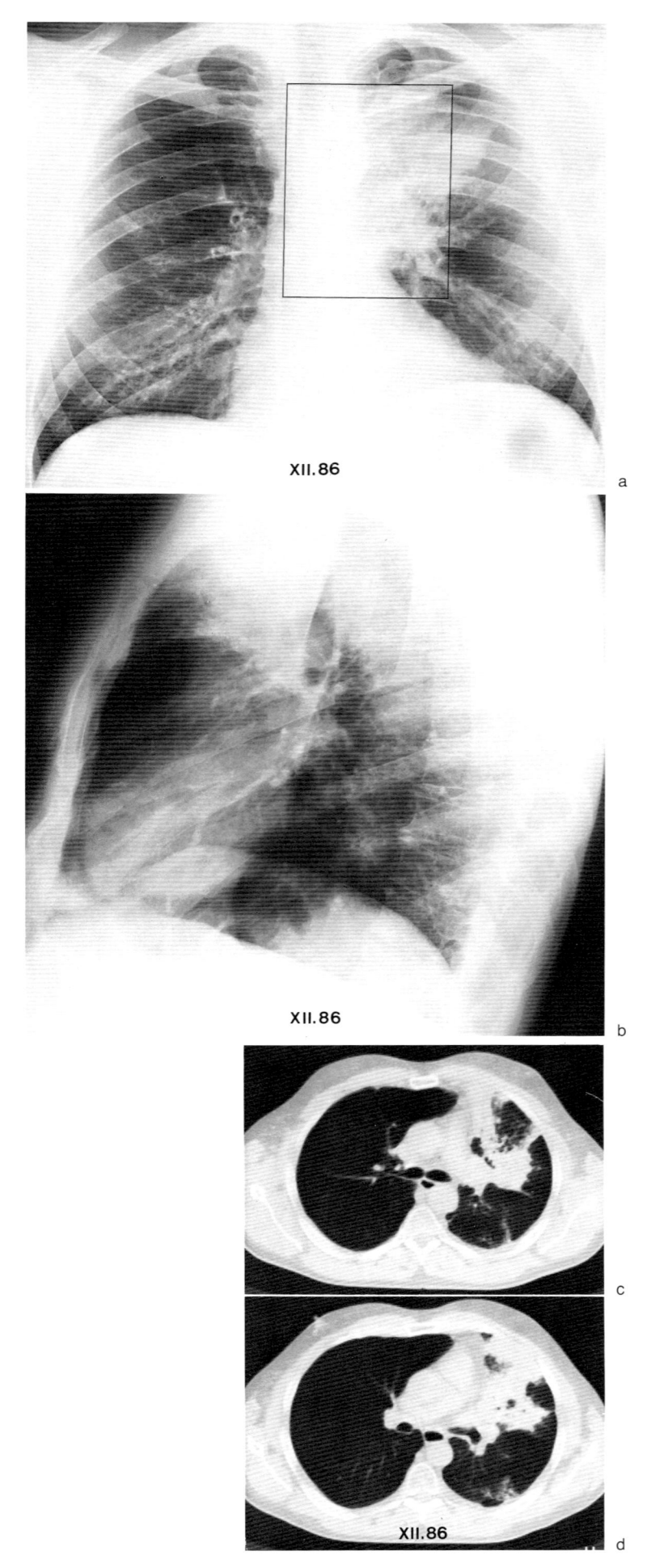

Fig. 5.14e–j ▷

138   5. Neoplasms

II.87

III.87

IX.87

IX.87

XII.87

Fig. 5.14e–j

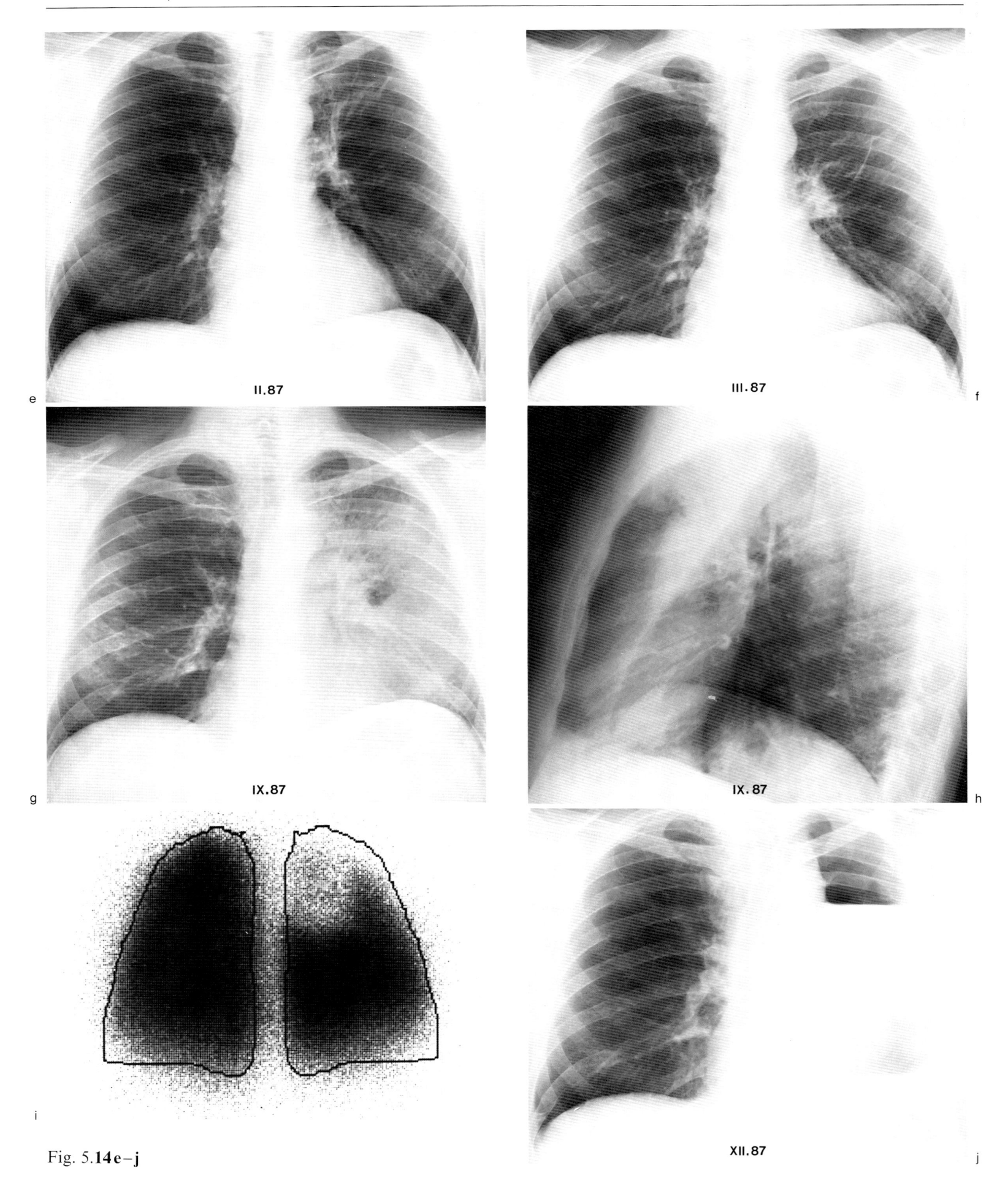

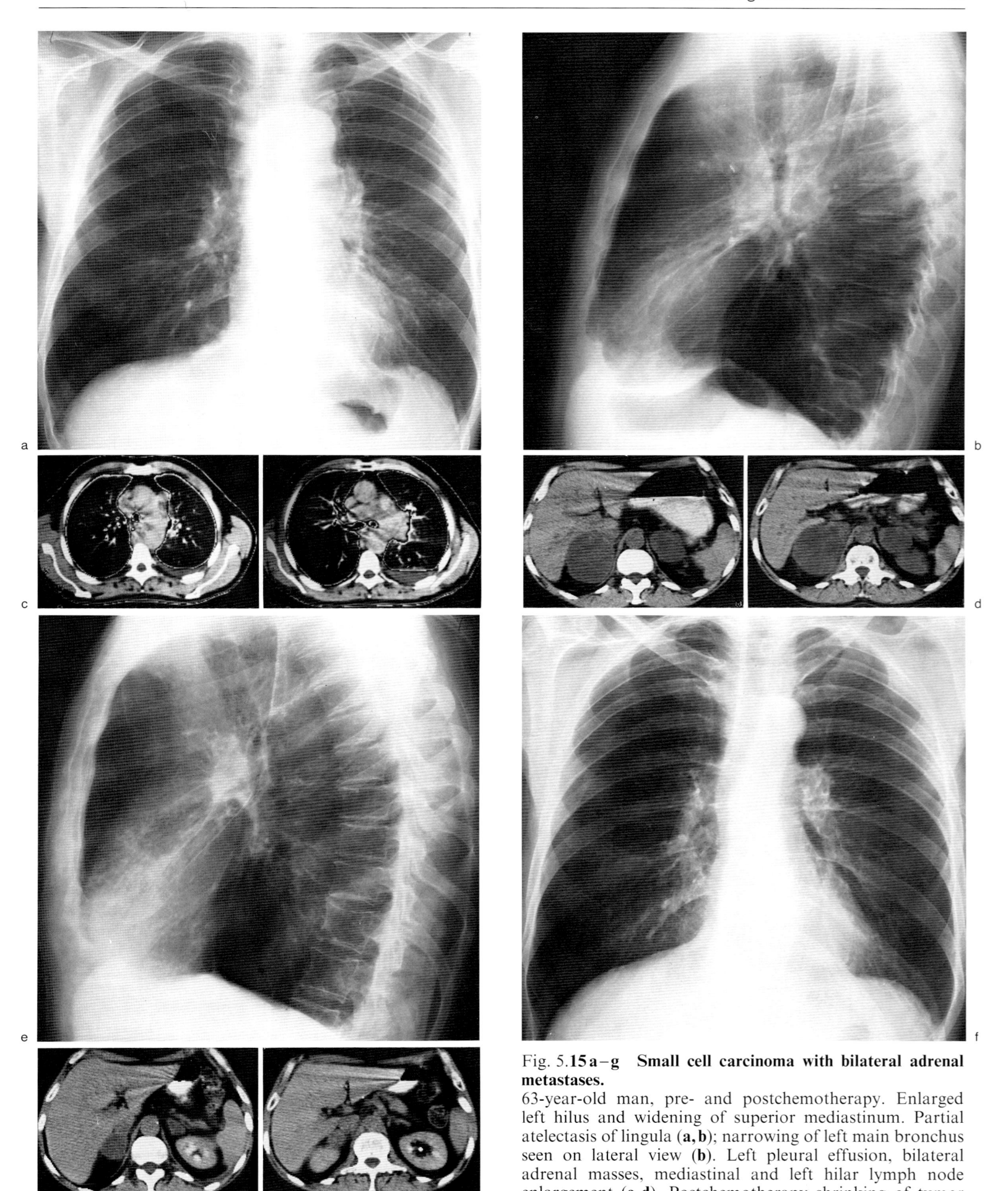

Fig. 5.**15 a−g Small cell carcinoma with bilateral adrenal metastases.**
63-year-old man, pre- and postchemotherapy. Enlarged left hilus and widening of superior mediastinum. Partial atelectasis of lingula (**a, b**); narrowing of left main bronchus seen on lateral view (**b**). Left pleural effusion, bilateral adrenal masses, mediastinal and left hilar lymph node enlargement (**c, d**). Postchemotherapy shrinking of tumor masses in the chest and adrenals (**e−g**).

140 5. Neoplasms

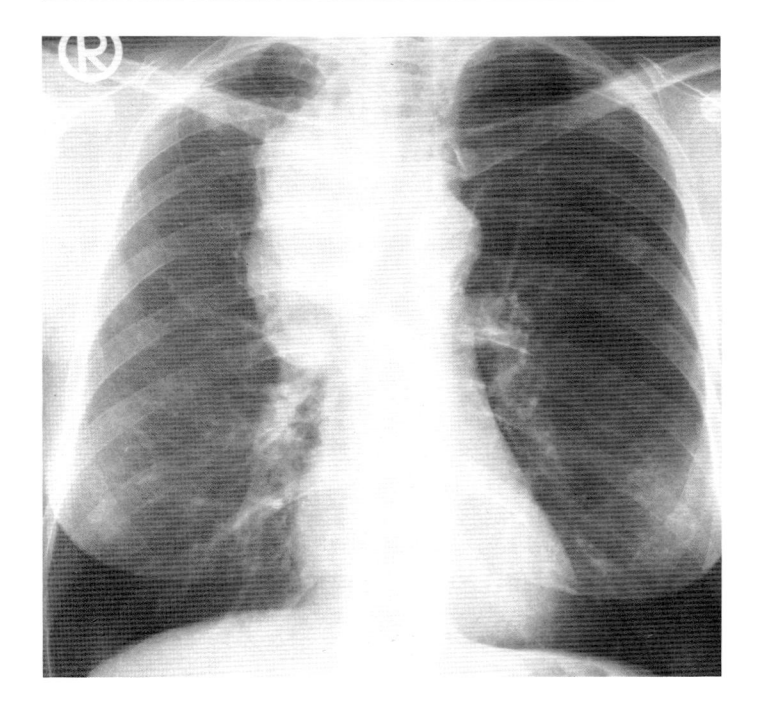

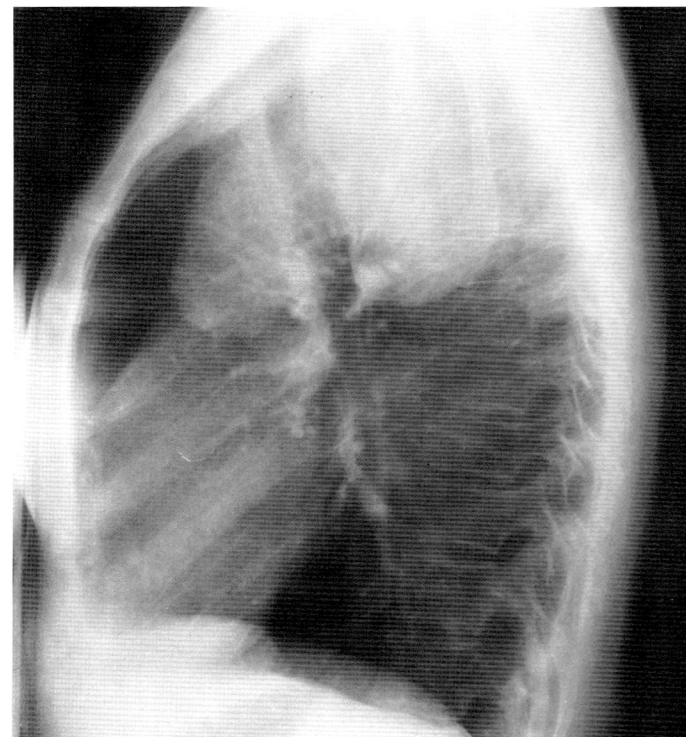

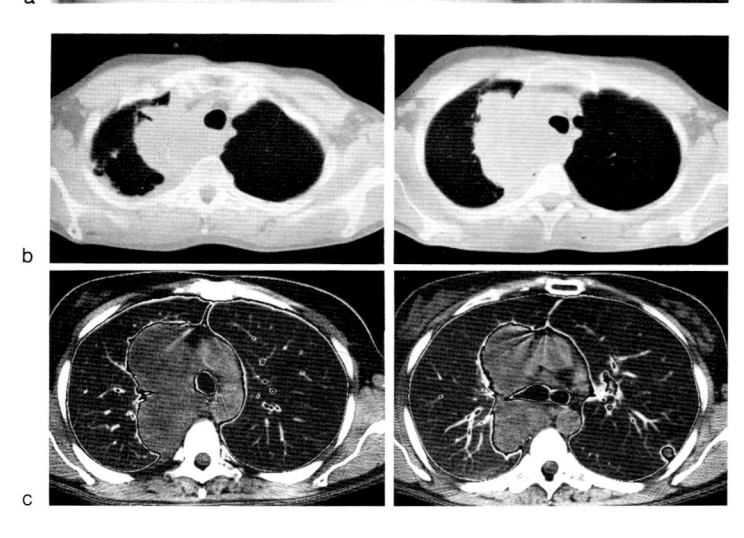

Fig. 5.16 a–c **Small cell carcinoma.**
43-year-old patient. Marked polycyclic widening of right paratracheal mediastinum. Tracheal deviation to the left. Left upper lobe solitary pulmonary nodule, probably represents a metastasis. CT demonstrates extent of tumor involvement with large paratracheal and retrotracheal component.

Central Bronchogenic Carcinoma, Hilar Mass

Some central bronchogenic carcinomas grow peribronchially before occluding the bronchial lumen; radiographically, they present as hilar masses before they lead to atelectasis. The tumor progressively enlarges in the suprahilar region then fills in the hilar angle and eventually obliterates the normal hilar structures. Strands of tumor extension can protrude from the hilar mass into the adjacent lung parenchyma. Enlarged lymph nodes can lead to similar hilar enlargement. CT can differentiate the tumor mass from enlarged hilar vessels.

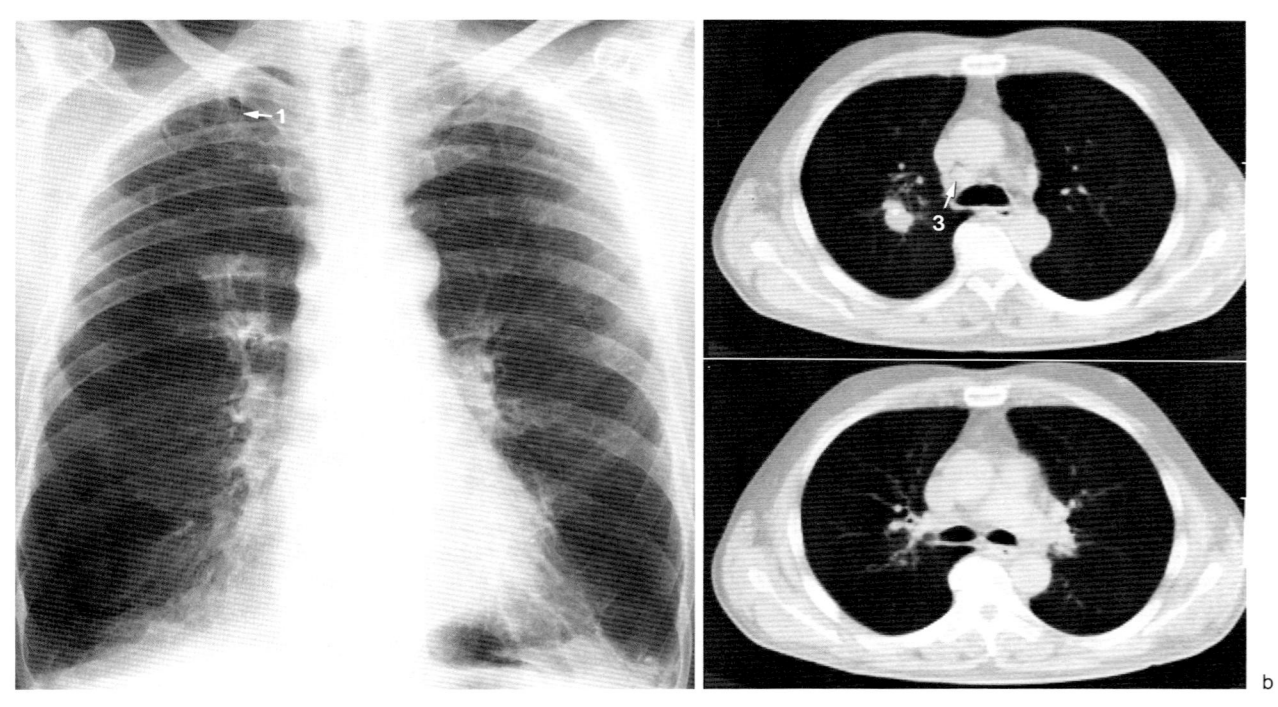

Fig. 5.17 a, b **Central small cell bronchogenic carcinoma.** 71-year-old patient with brain metastasis. Right lung suprahilar opacity, pretracheal retrocaval lymph node enlargement (3), emphysema with apical bullae (1).

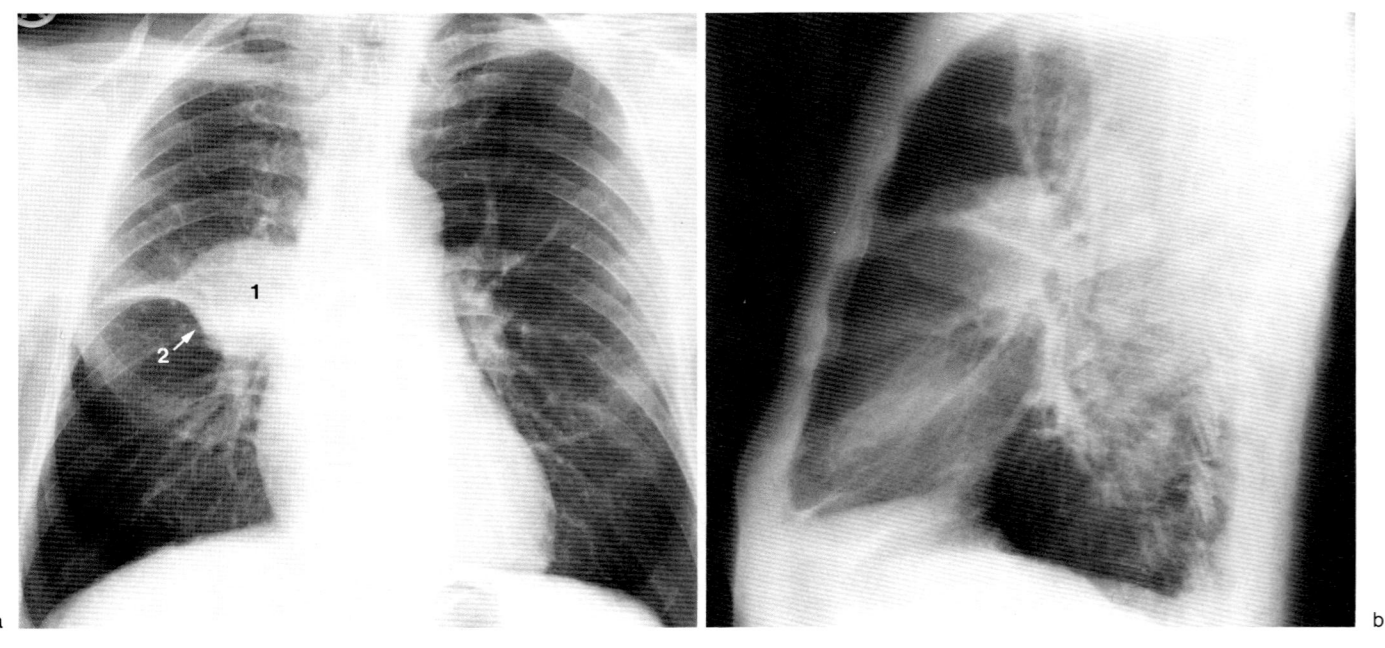

Fig. 5.18 a, b **Central bronchogenic carcinoma.** 66-year-old patient. Hilar mass (1) and partial atelectasis of anterior segment of right upper lobe, together forming a variant of Golden S-sign.

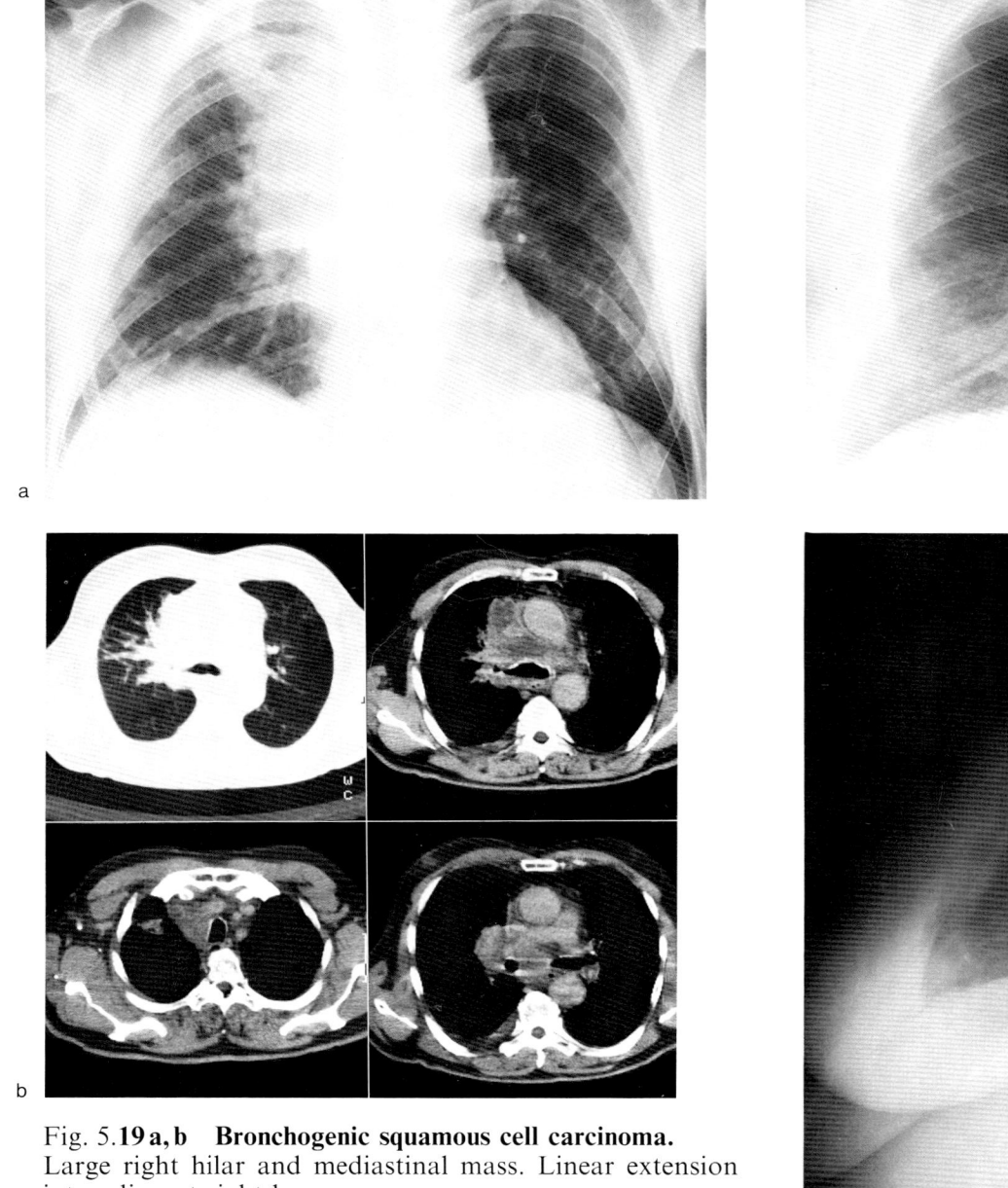

142   5. Neoplasms

Fig. 5.**19 a, b** **Bronchogenic squamous cell carcinoma.**
Large right hilar and mediastinal mass. Linear extension into adjacent right lung.

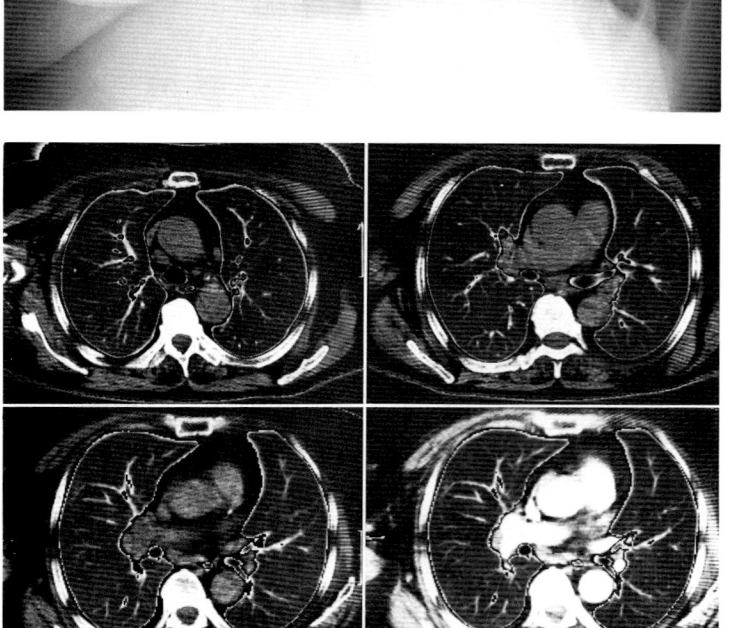

Fig. 5.**20 a–c** **Central squamous cell carcinoma.** ▷
66-year-old woman with pathological fracture of humeral neck. Right hilar angle is effaced with obvious lateral convexity. Right paratracheal mediastinum is widened.

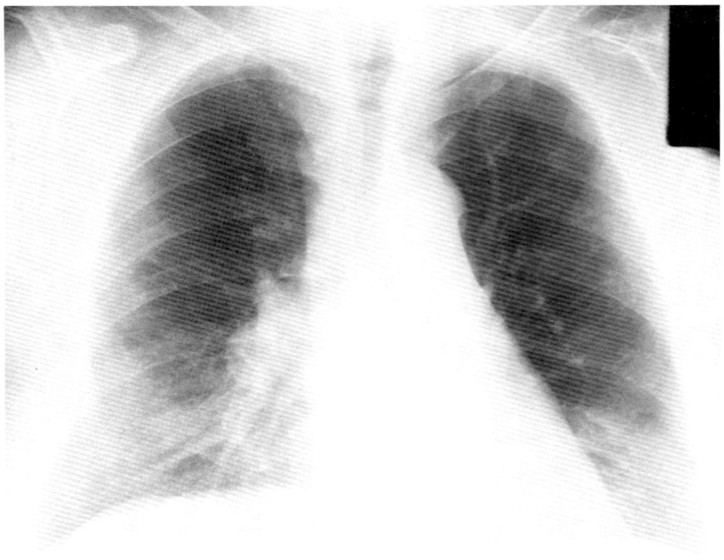

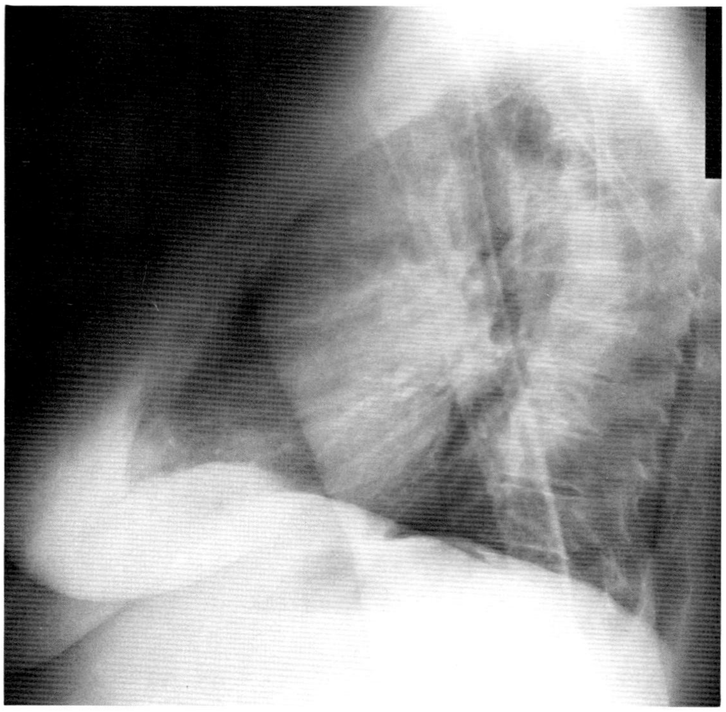

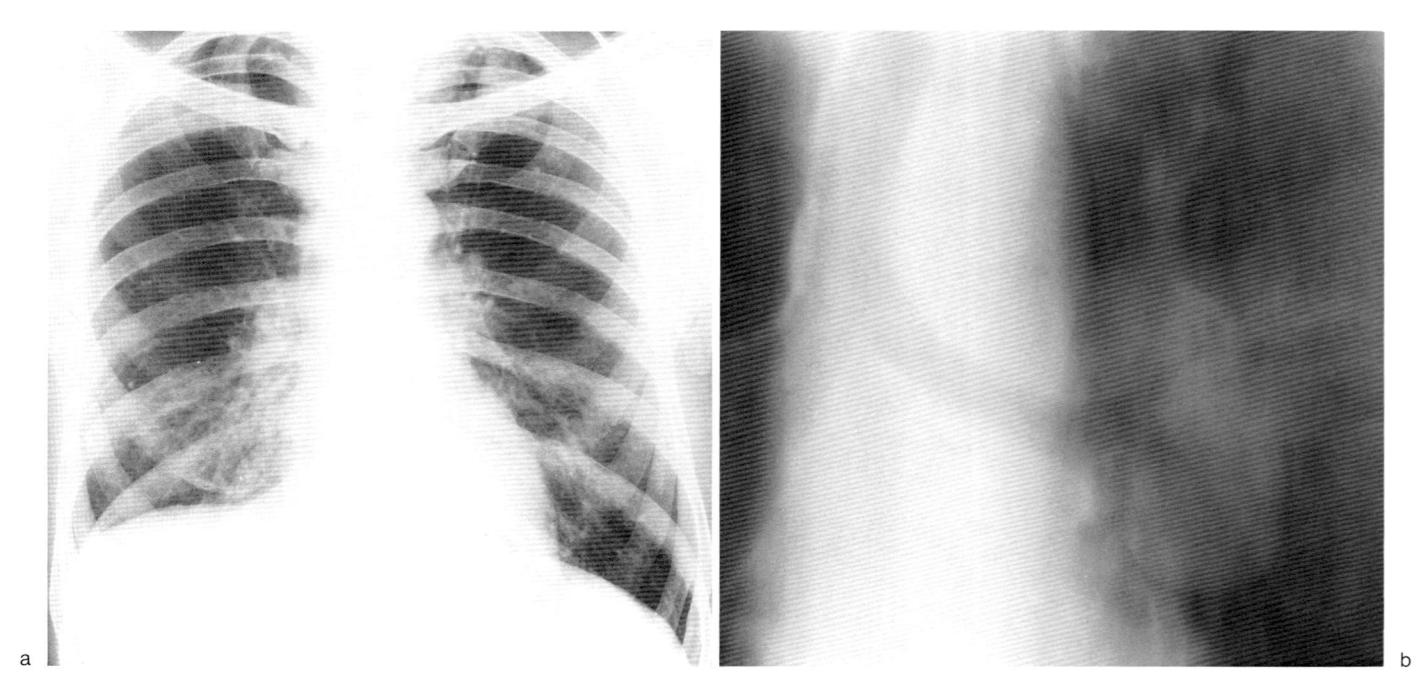

Fig. 5.**21 a, b Central squamous cell carcinoma**
Ill-defined, enlarged left hilum with slight narrowing of left upper lobe bronchus and undercutting of inferior left hilar contour, best seen on tomogram.

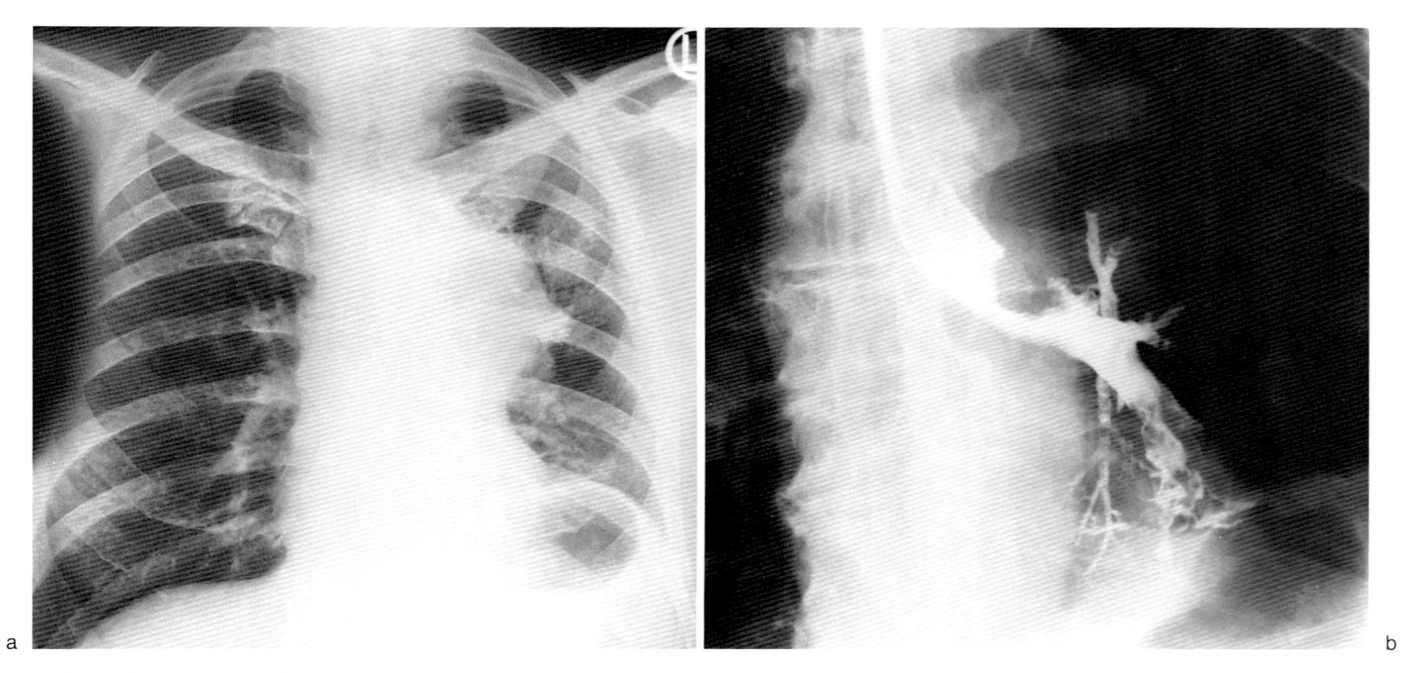

Fig. 5.**22 a, b Central bronchogenic adenocarcinoma.**
Large left hilar mass, obscuring aortic-pulmonic window. Postobstructive consolidation in left upper lobe. Elevation of left hemidiaphragm likely due to left phrenic nerve paralysis. Bronchogram confirms large intraluminal mass in left main bronchus with occlusion of left upper lobe bronchus.

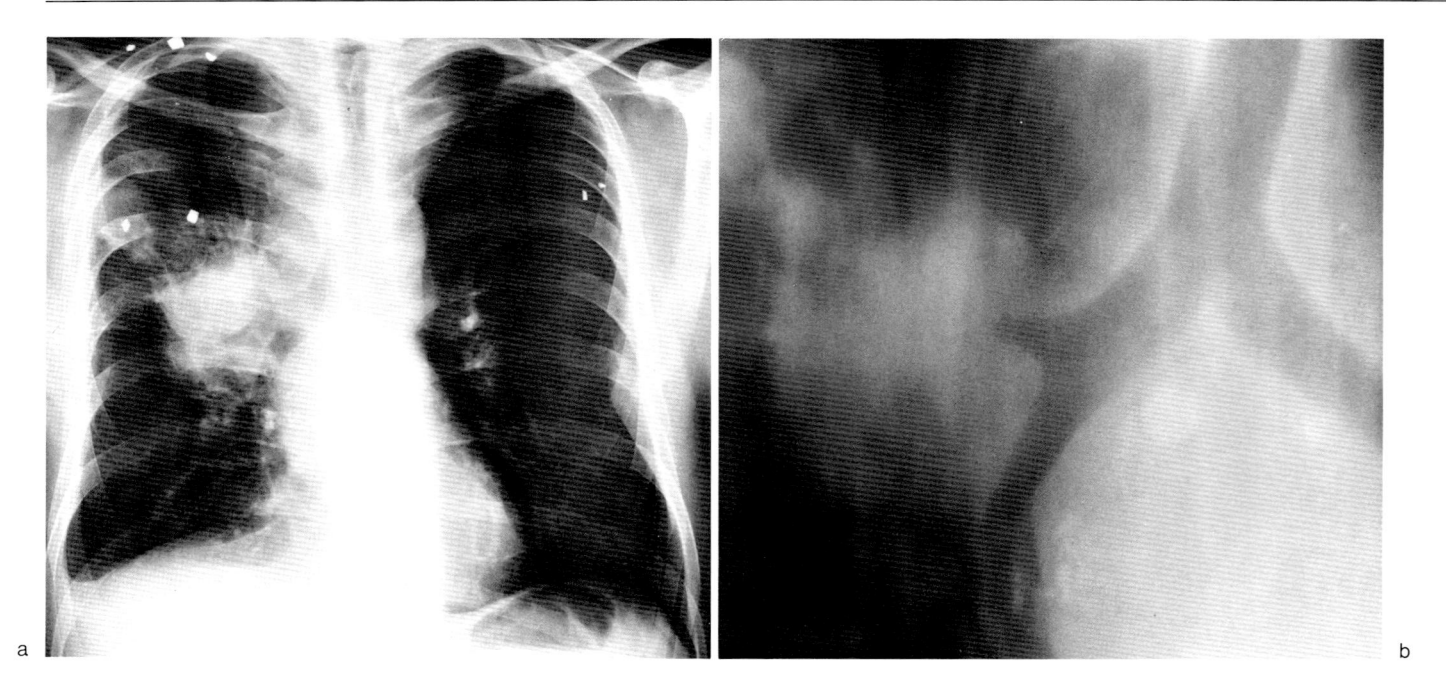

Fig. 5.**23 a, b   Central squamous cell carcinoma.**
Large right hilar mass occluding right upper lobe bronchus. Postobstructive retention of secretions in right upper lobe. Linear extension of tumor into surrounding parenchyma. Metallic fragments from old gunshot injury.

Superior Sulcus Tumor; Pancoast Syndrome

Pancoast, who was a radiologist, described in 1929 an apical bronchogenic carcinoma that originated from the region of the superior sulcus, formed by the subclavian vessels on the lung. The tumor infiltrates the chest wall, the brachial plexus, and the sympathetic trunk. Patients present with chest wall pain, weakness, and pain in the distribution of the ulnar nerve (C7–T1 roots) as well as Horner syndrome (meiosis, ptosis, enophthalmus, anhydrosis).

Radiologic features include apical mass, apical cap, and destruction of ribs or vertebral body. Rarely, benign inflammatory lesions like actinomycosis can mimic a superior sulcus tumor. Other malignant lesions like lymphoma, plasmacytoma, or even malignant mesothelioma can infrequently produce a Pancoast syndrome.

Fig. 5.24 **Pancoast tumor.**
67-year-old patient with biopsy-proven squamous cell carcinoma presents with excruciating shoulder pain, treated for 4 months for arthritis.
Near complete opacification of right upper lobe with destruction of several ribs. Several small cavities are visible within the tumor. Major fissure is visible, separating the tumor from noninvolved right lower lobe.

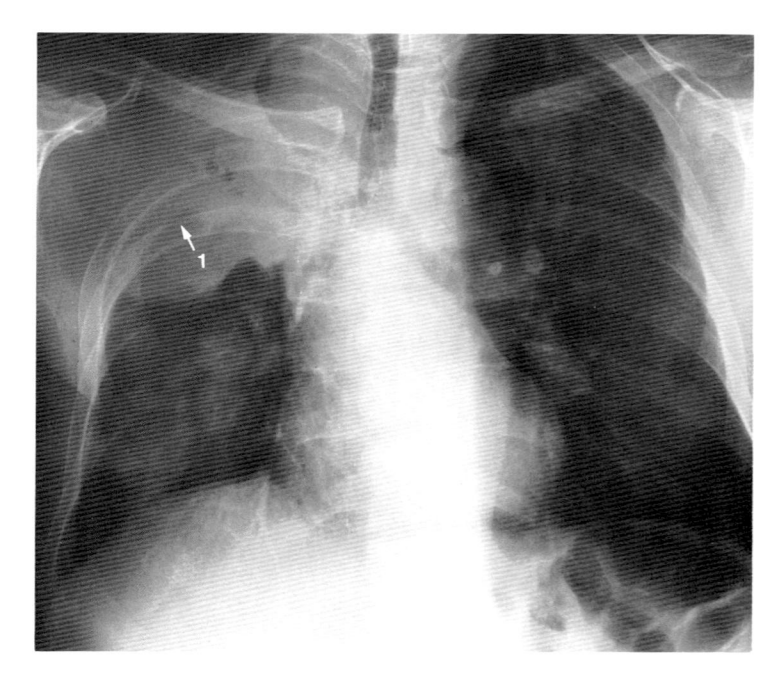

Fig. 5.25 **Pancoast tumor.**
MRI, coronal plane, spin-echo, T1-weighted scan. Large, right upper lobe mass invades the chest wall and the vertebral bodies, with extension into the spinal canal. Note invasion of scalene muscles on the right side of the lower neck.

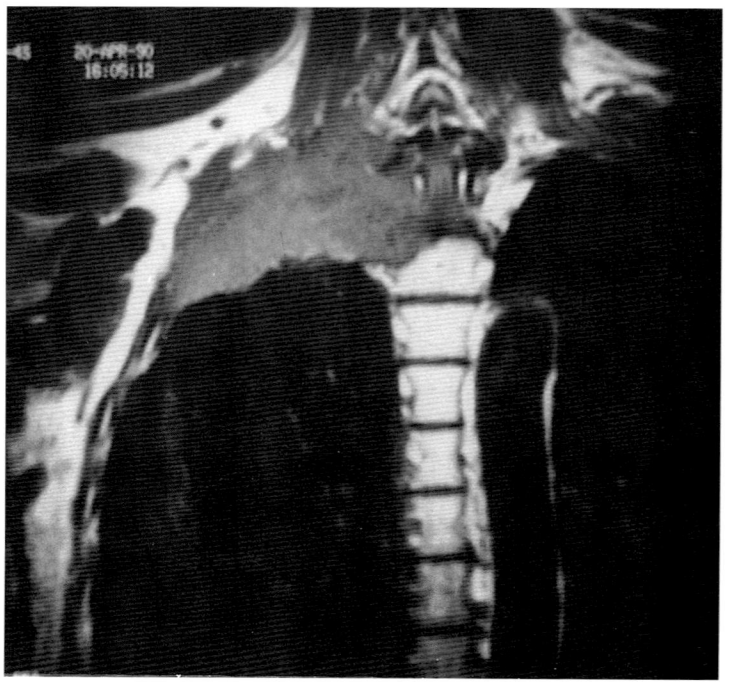

Fig. 5.**26 a–g Pancoast tumor.**
58-year-old patient with a 2-month history of right shoulder and arm pain and Horner syndrome. Biopsy proven squamous cell carcinoma. Right apical mass, abutting on posteromedial aspect of chest wall. Osteolytic destruction of third rib with transthoracic extension of tumor into paraspinal musculature (**d**).

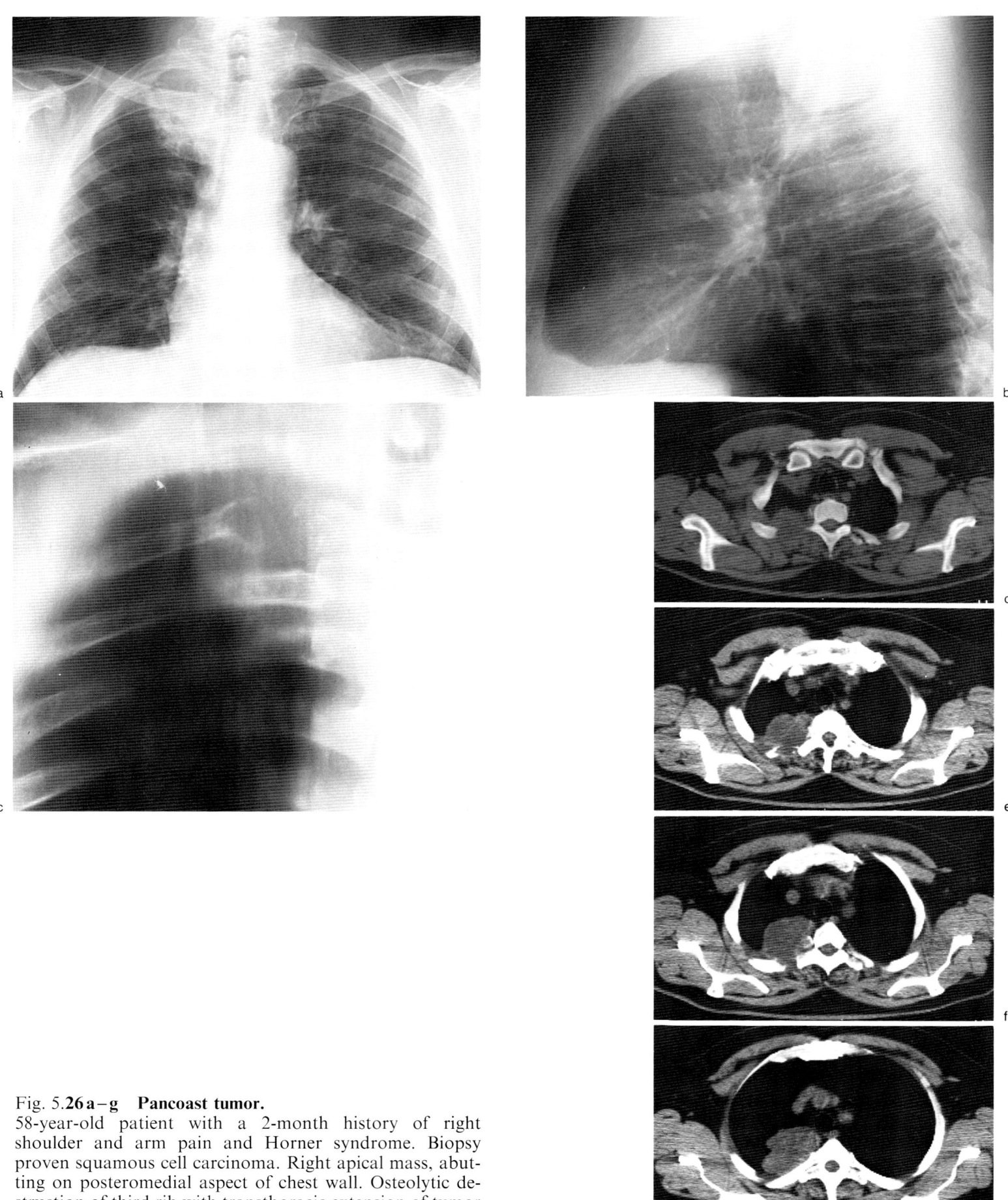

Superior Vena Cava Obstruction: Esophageal Invasion

Mediastinal or paramediastinal tumors, as well as enlarged metastatic lymph nodes, can compress or invade the superior vena cava and thus impair the venous return to the heart from the upper half of the body. Collateral circulation develops via the paraspinal venous plexus, internal thoracic veins, and intercostal veins; if the obstruction of the superior vena cava occurs distal to the junction with the azygos vein, then the latter participates, too, in diverting the blood to the inferior vena cava.

Clinical findings include swelling and venous congestion of the head, neck (Stokes collar), and arms. Venography or MRI can document the obstruction and the collateral circulation.

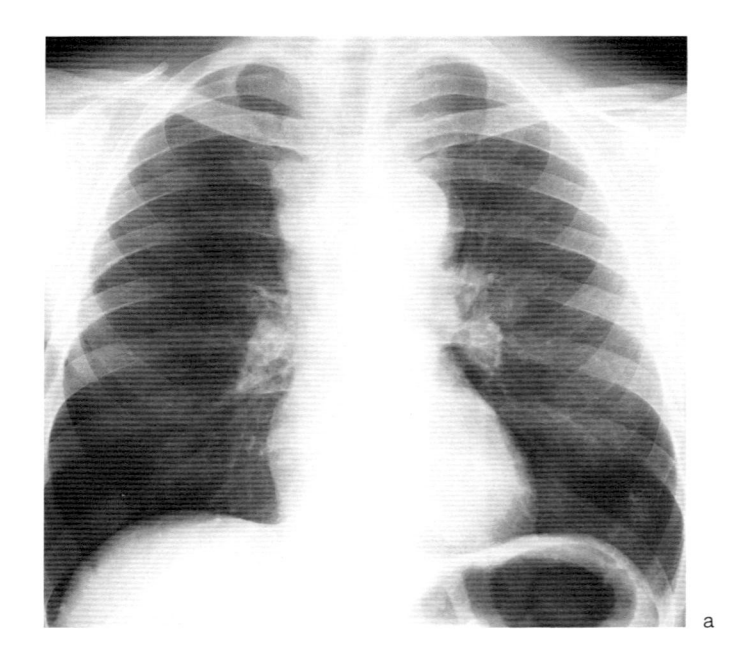

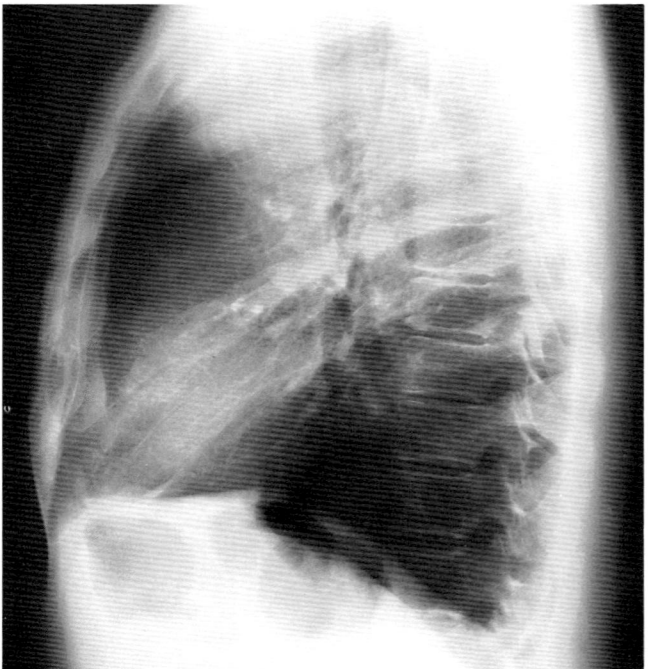

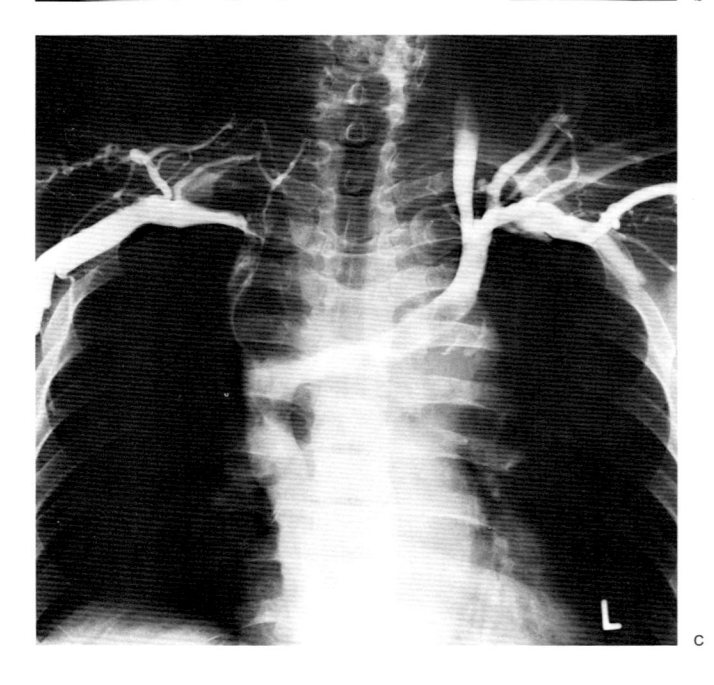

Fig. 5.27 a–c **Small cell bronchogenic carcinoma with mediastinal extension.**
66-year-old patient who has had eyelid edema for 2 weeks. Left hilar mass, superior mediastinal widening with thickening of right paratracheal mediastinum, and double contour of aortic arch. Obliteration of anterosuperior mediastinum as seen in lateral projection. Venogram shows occlusion of right jugular and subclavian veins as well as caudal displacement of left innominate vein.

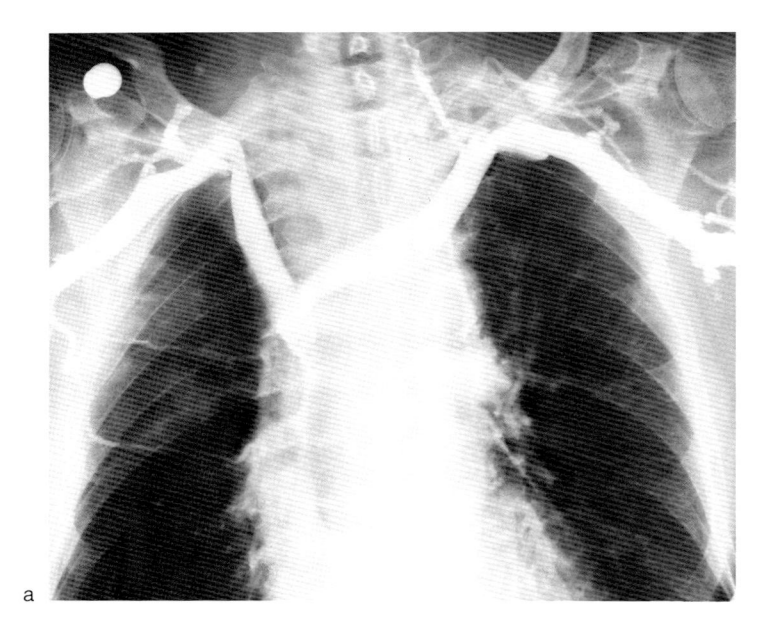

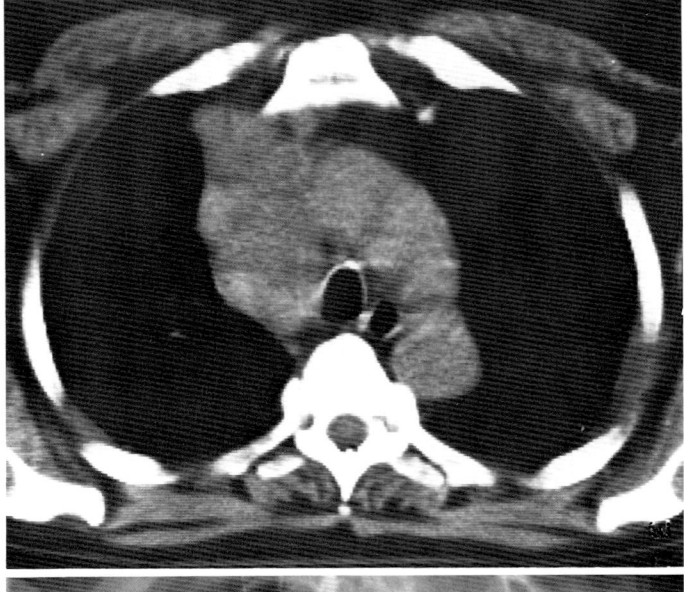

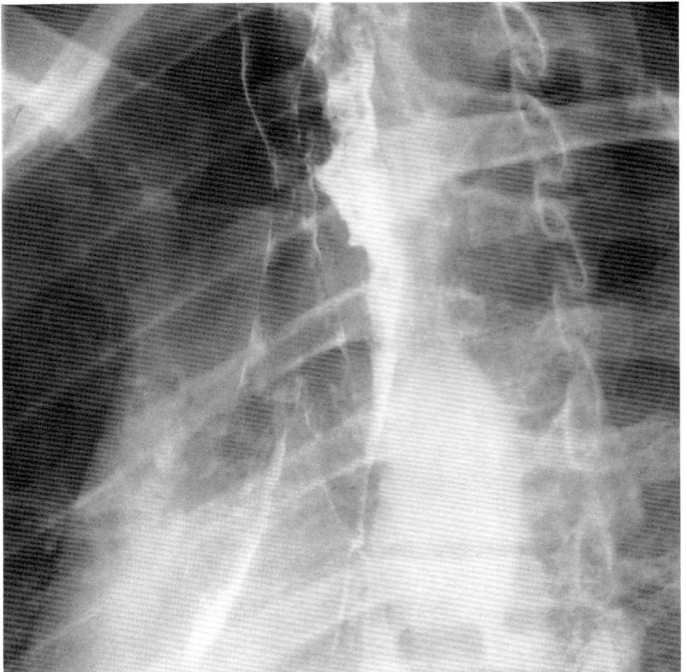

Fig. 5.28 a–c Central bronchogenic carcinoma with compression of superior vena cava and erosion into esophagus. Patient with dysphagia of 3 weeks' duration, episodic attacks of cough while eating, and swelling of head and neck. Extensive mediastinal lymph node enlargement (**b**) with obstruction of superior vena cava and collateral circulation over subclavian veins (**a**). Barium study shows tracheoesophageal fistula.

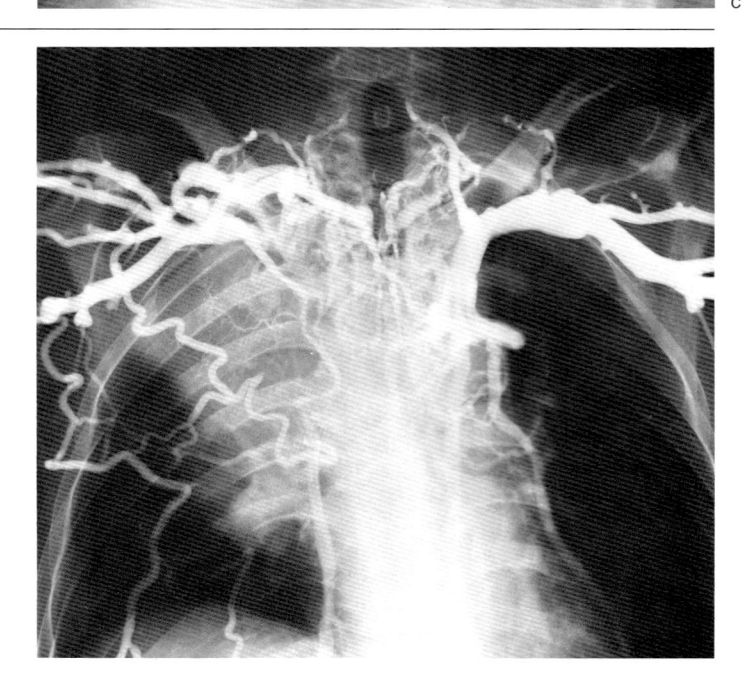

Fig. 5.29 Central bronchogenic carcinoma with right upper lobe atelectasis and compression of superior vena cava. Collateral circulation over hemiazygous, internal thoracic, and pectoral veins. Note complete occlusion of superior vena cava.

Malignant Lymphoma

Hodgkin and non-Hodgkin lyMphomas account for about 2% of all malignant tumors. The disease originates in the lymph nodes and can eventually involve the reticuloendothelial elements of parenchymal organs. Imaging modalities play an important role in staging lymphomas; the therapy and prognosis in Hodgkin's lymphoma are contingent on the stage at diagnosis. The histology result is more important than the stage in determining the therapy and prognosis for non-Hodgkin lymphoma. In the chest, enlarged mediastinal and hilar lymph nodes are seen initially. In stage IV disease, the lung parenchyma is also involved along bronchovascular bundles, as nodular disease, or as patchy consolidative disease.

References: 77, 103, 124.

Table 5.2 Ann Arbor staging of Hodgkin disease

Stage I	One lymph node group involved
Stage Ie	Transcapsular extralymphatic extension into lung
Stage II	Two or more lymph node groups on one side of diaphragm
Stage IIe	Transcapsular extralymphatic extension into lung
Stage III	Lymph node groups involved on both sides of diaphragm; spleen counts as lymph node group
Stage IIIe	Same as above with transcapsular extralymphatic extension
Stage IV	Involvement of parenchymal organs
A	No symptoms
B	Night sweats, more than 10% weight loss, fever

Table 5.3 Histologic classification of Hodgkin lymphoma (Rye classification)

	Prevalence
1. Lymphocyte predominance	15%
2. Nodular-sclerosing	40%
3. Mixed cellularity	30%
4. Lymphocyte depletion	15%

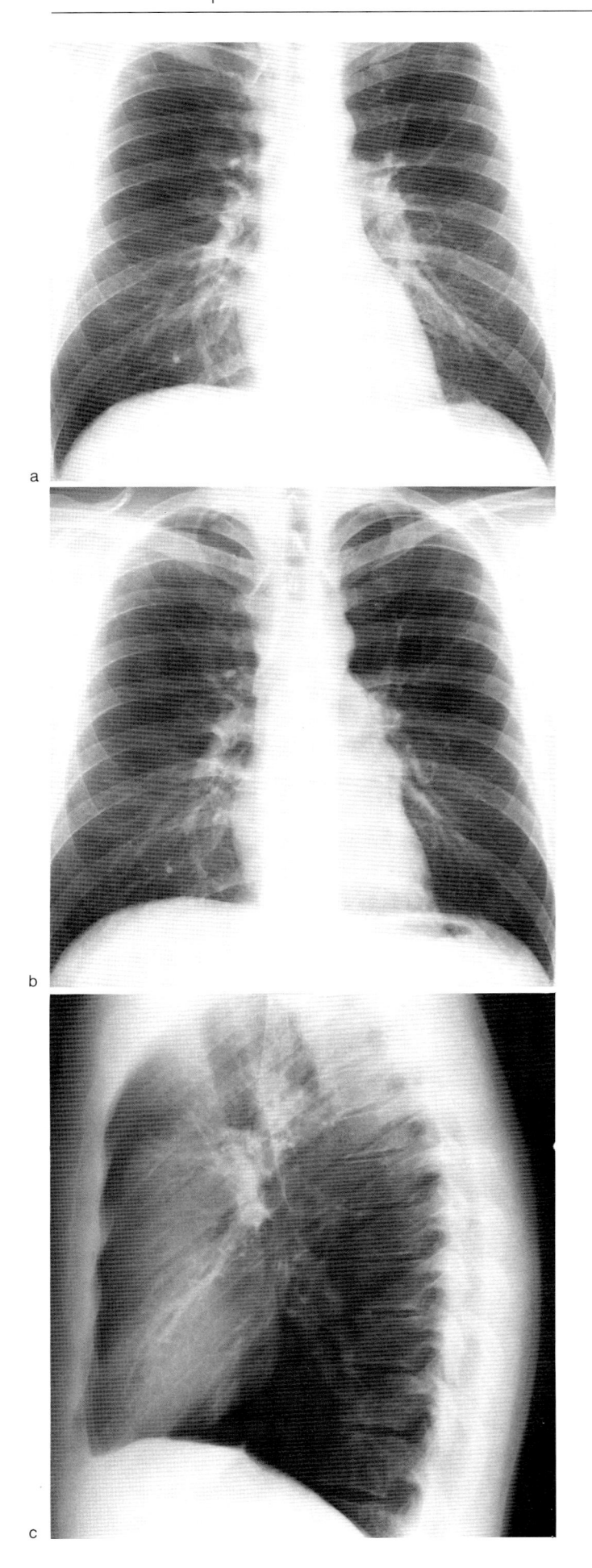

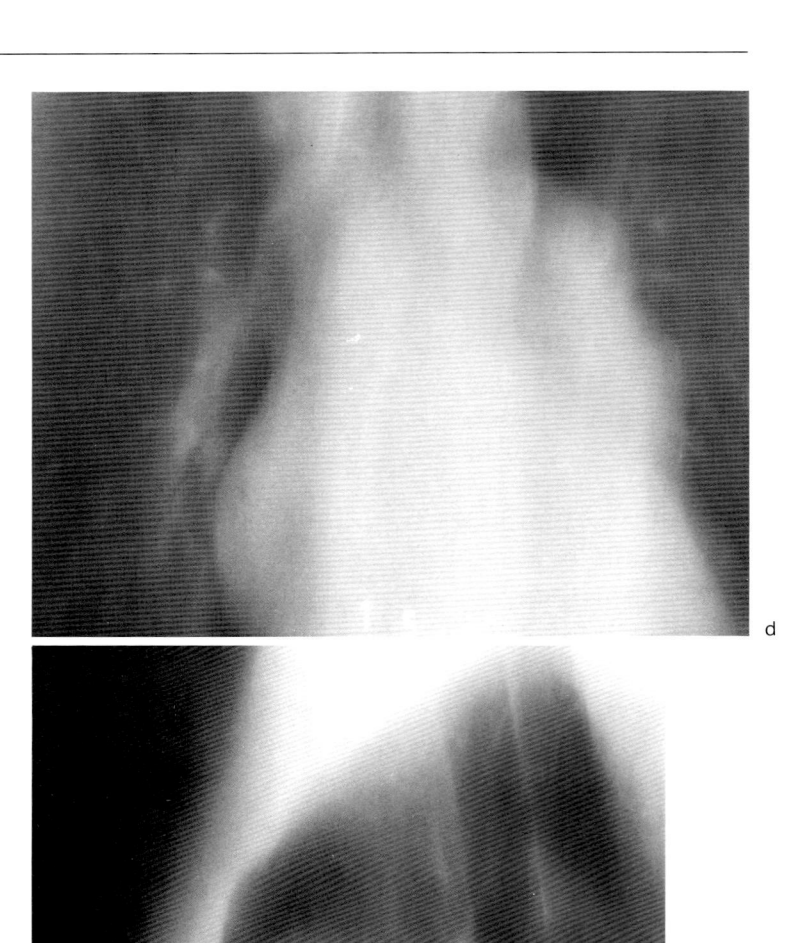

Fig. 5.30 a–e Hodgkin disease.
26-year-old, asymptomatic patient. Initial film (**a**) prior to current routine chest radiograph (**b**) is normal. Now an anterior mediastinal mass is visible, superimposed on left hilus, with polycyclic left lateral contour.

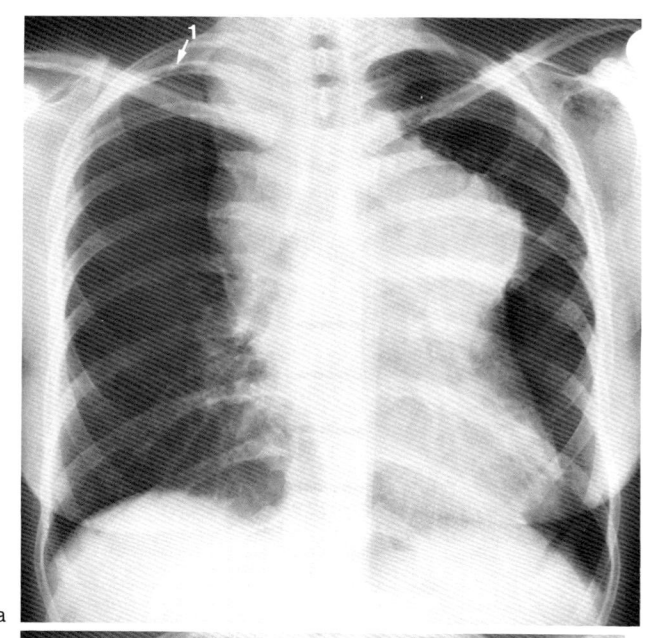

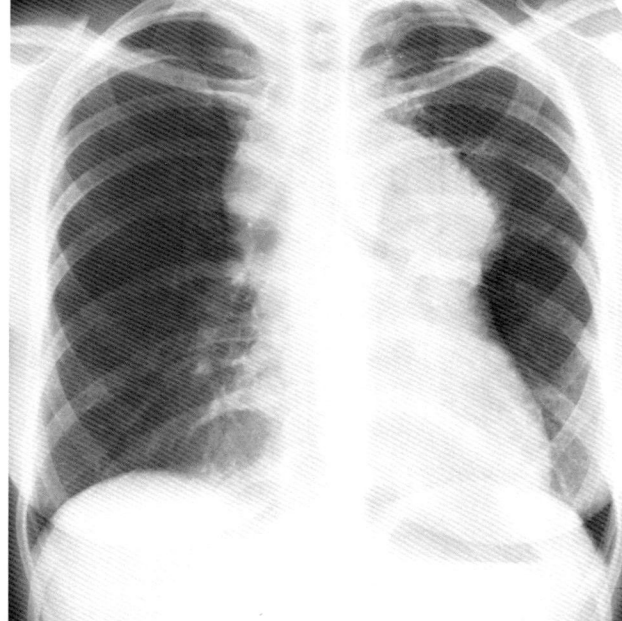

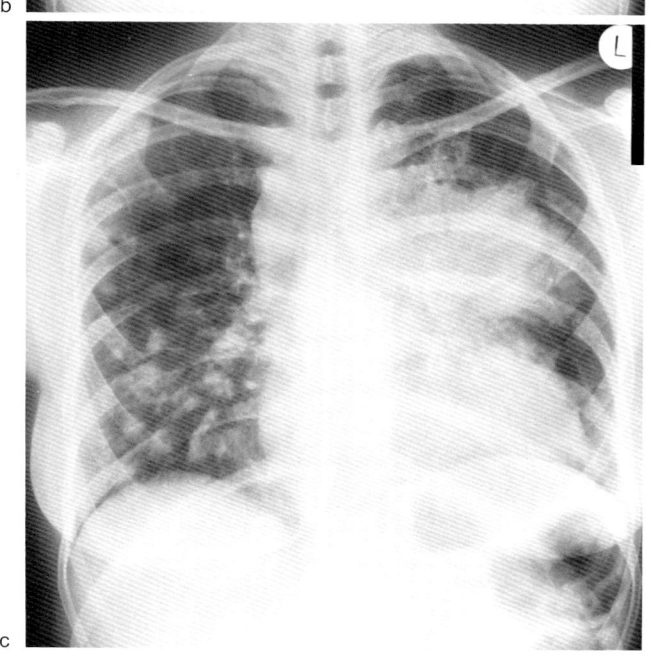

Fig. 5.**31 a–d Hodgkin disease.**
32-year-old patient. Biopsy of axillary lymph nodes yields nodular-sclerosing Hodgkin disease. Downhill course leading to death within 1 year. Initial chest film (**a**) shows massive anterior mediastinal, aortic-pulmonic window, right paratracheal, and right paracardiac lymph node enlargement. Note obscuration of right heart border. Right apical cap (1). After chemotherapy, slight regression of lymph node masses. Follow-up films (**c, d**) show progressive involvement of lung parenchyma with air bronchogram (2). Left pleural effusion. Stomach gas bubble slightly impinged upon, probably by enlarged spleen (3).

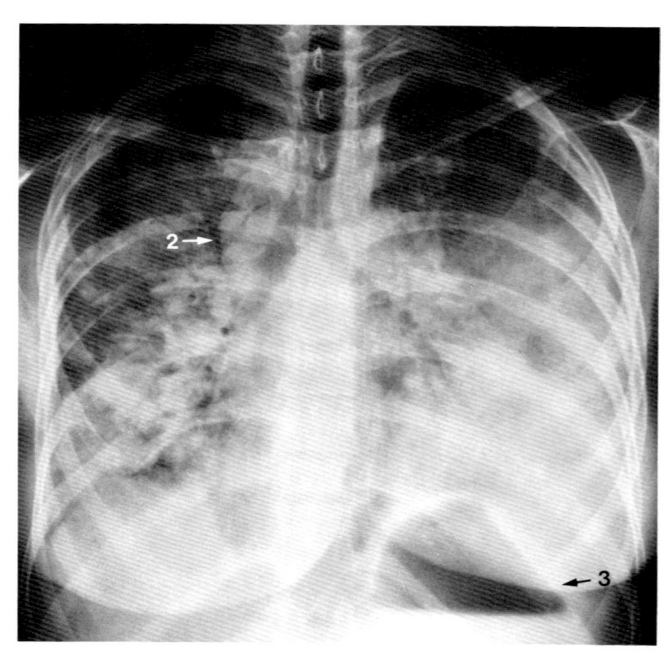

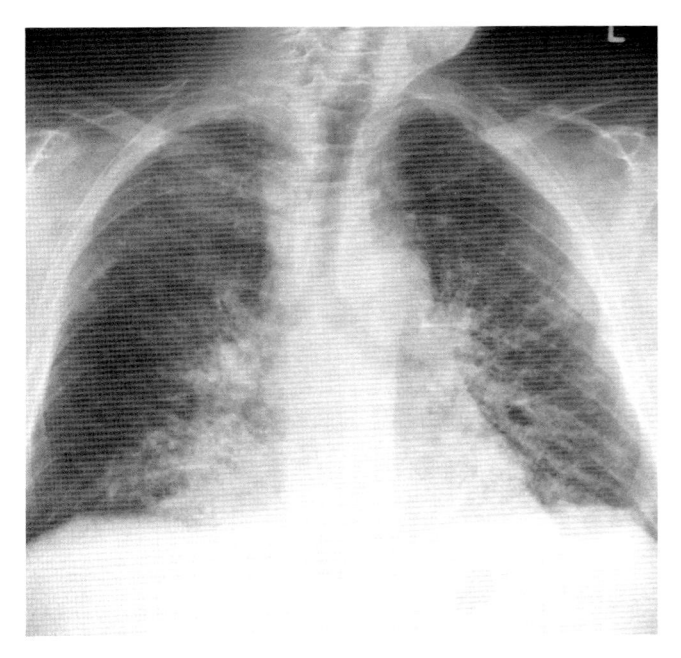

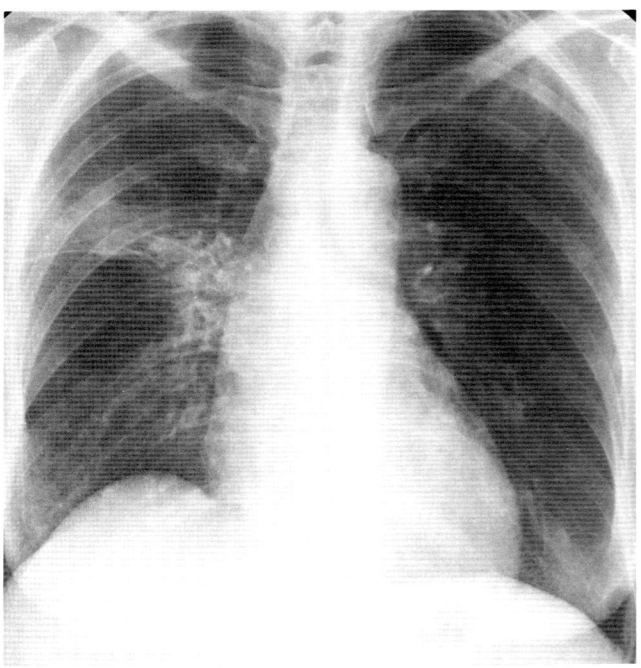

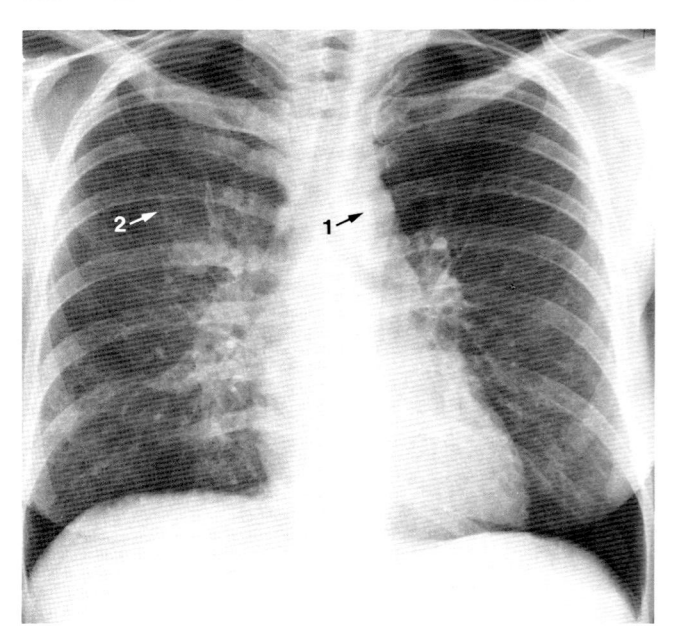

Fig. 5.32 Hodgkin disease.
60-year-old patient complaining of shortness of breath. Multiple linear opacities radiating from hilus along bronchovascular bundles.

Fig. 5.33 Hodgkin disease with lung involvement.
58-year-old patient with recurrence outside the radiation portal, 3 years after initial therapy. Nodular opacity in left upper lobe, in infraclavicular location. Consolidation of anterior segment of right upper lobe with partial atelectasis and slight cranial retraction of minor fissure.

Fig. 5.34 Hodgkin disease.
37-year-old patient with cough for 2 months. Ill-defined, right suprahilar nodule with linear extension into surrounding lung (2). Left paratracheal lymph node enlargement (1).

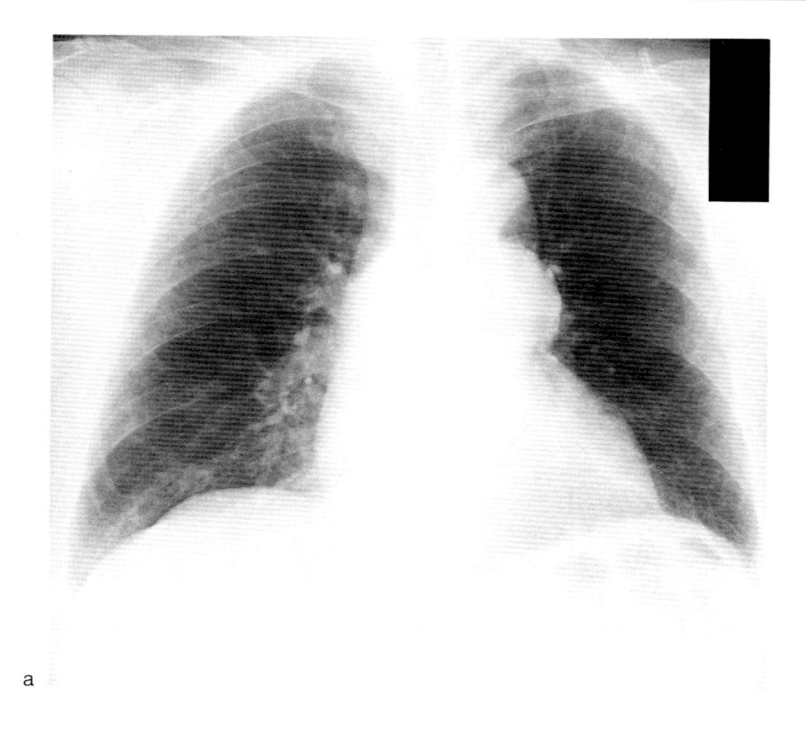

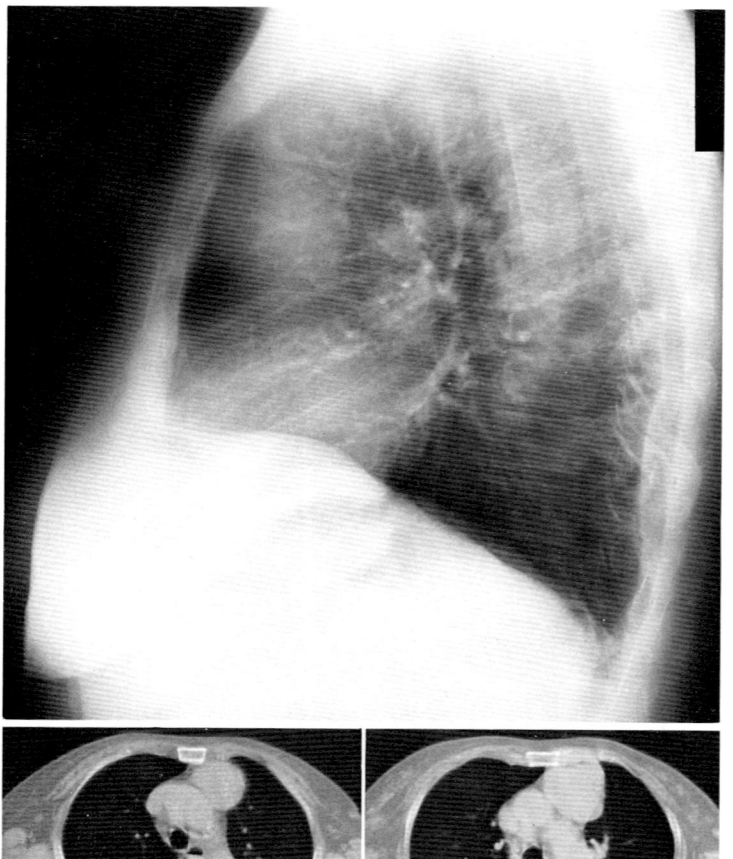

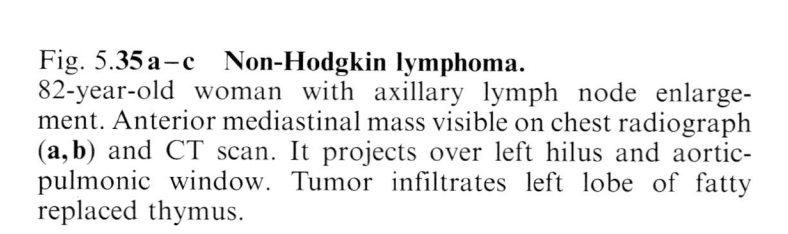

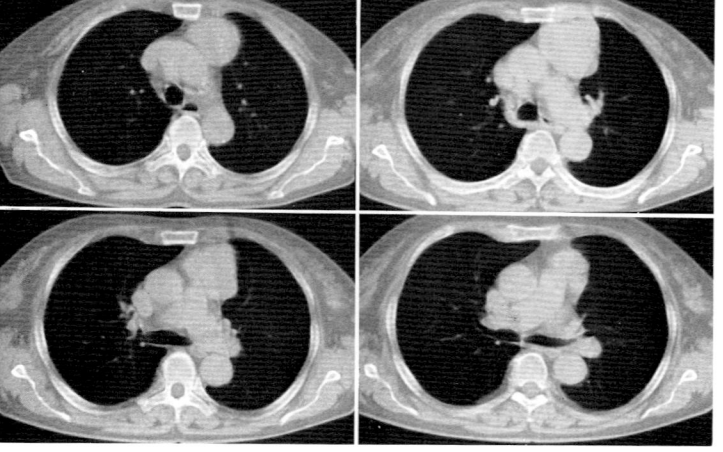

Fig. 5.35 a–c **Non-Hodgkin lymphoma.**
82-year-old woman with axillary lymph node enlargement. Anterior mediastinal mass visible on chest radiograph (**a, b**) and CT scan. It projects over left hilus and aortic-pulmonic window. Tumor infiltrates left lobe of fatty replaced thymus.

5. Neoplasms

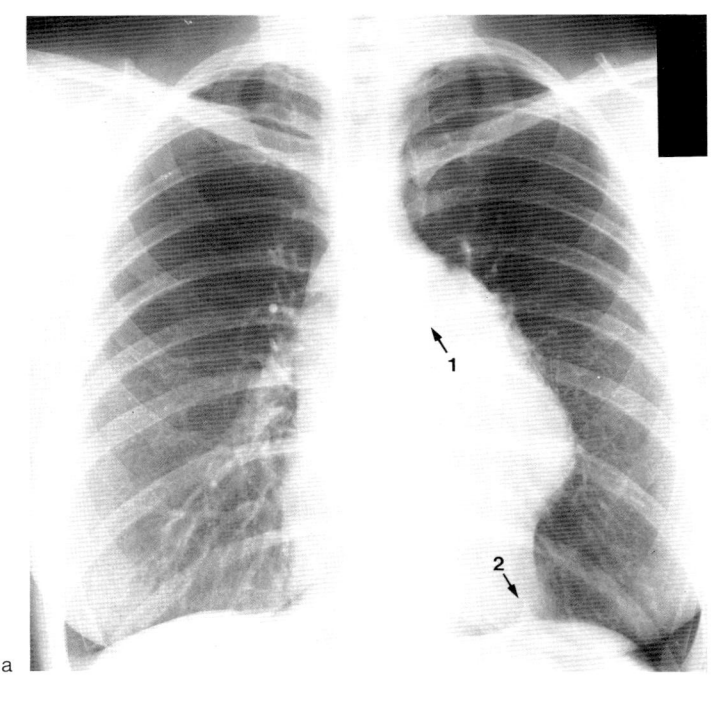

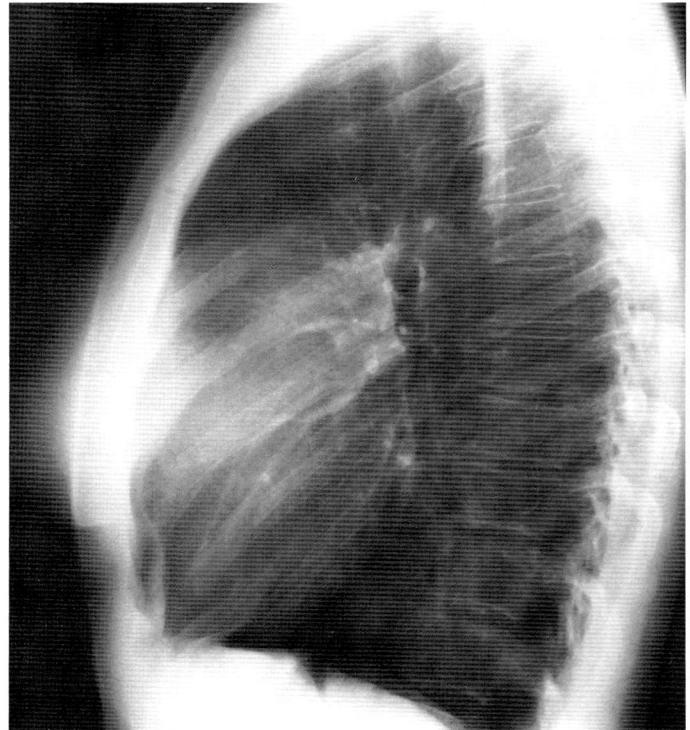

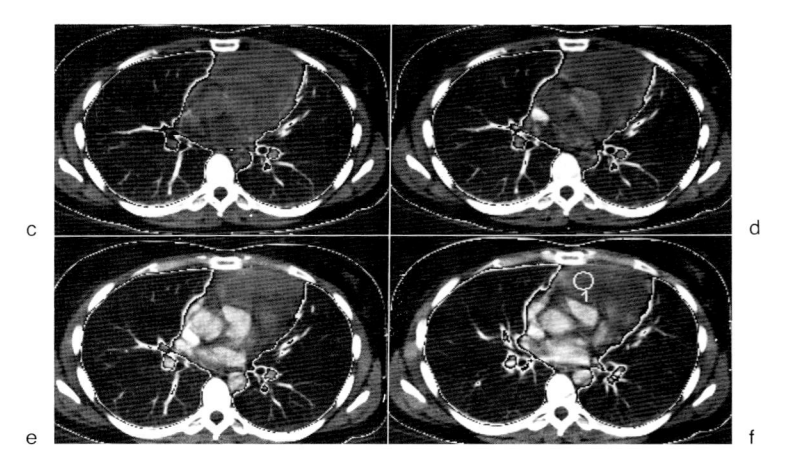

Fig. 5.36 a–f Non-Hodgkin lymphoma.
37-year-old patient with lymphoblastic lymphoma. Large anterior mediastinal mass with obliteration of aortic arch contour (1). Mediastinal mass ends at level of clavicles, which indicates its anterior location. Marked regression of tumor after three cycles of chemotherapy.

Fig. 5.37 a–d T-cell lymphoma.
23-year-old woman with weight loss over 3 months. Polycyclic widening of superior mediastinum. Obscuration of aortic arch (1). Mediastinal mass fades above level of clavicles, since it is located anteriorly and is not outlined by lung above that level (**a**). The anterior position of the mass is confirmed on the lateral view (**b**). After three cycles of chemotherapy, the mass has nearly completely resolved (**c, d**).

Fig. 5.38 a, b Non-Hodgkin lymphoblastic lymphoma.
17-year-old patient. Massive superior mediastinal widening. Obscuration of aortic arch (1). Marked regression of tumor after radiation and chemotherapy. Anterior junction line (2).

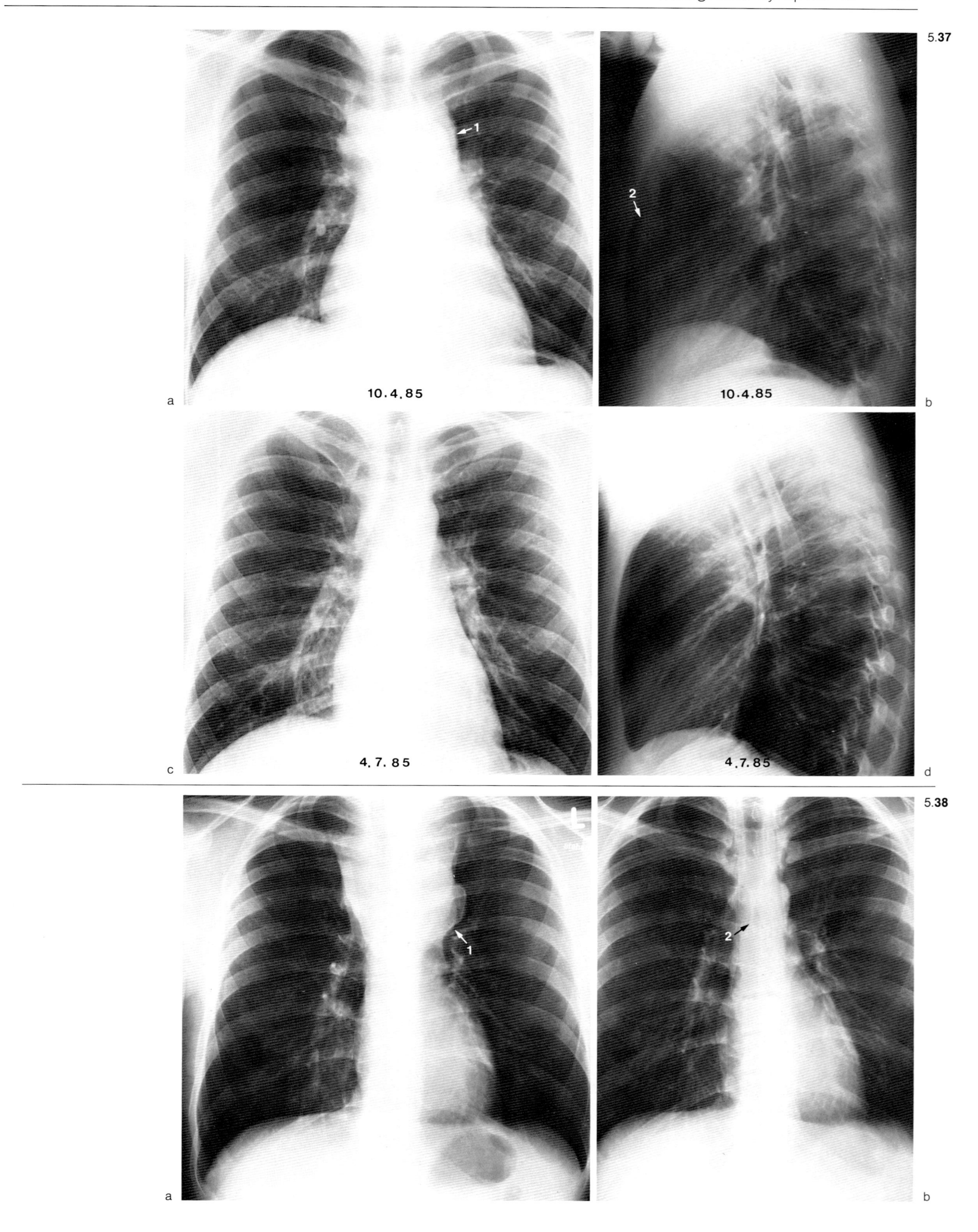

Malignant Lymphoma 155

5.37

a 10.4.85
b 10.4.85
c 4.7.85
d 4.7.85

5.38

a
b

156 5. Neoplasms

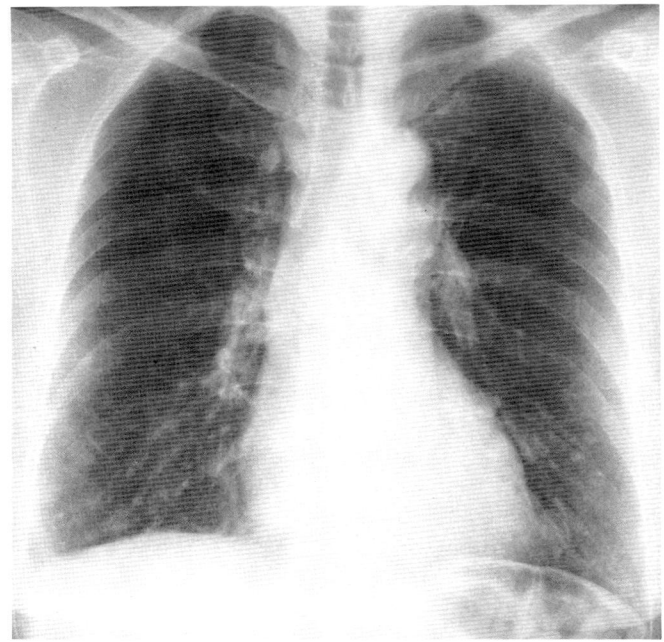

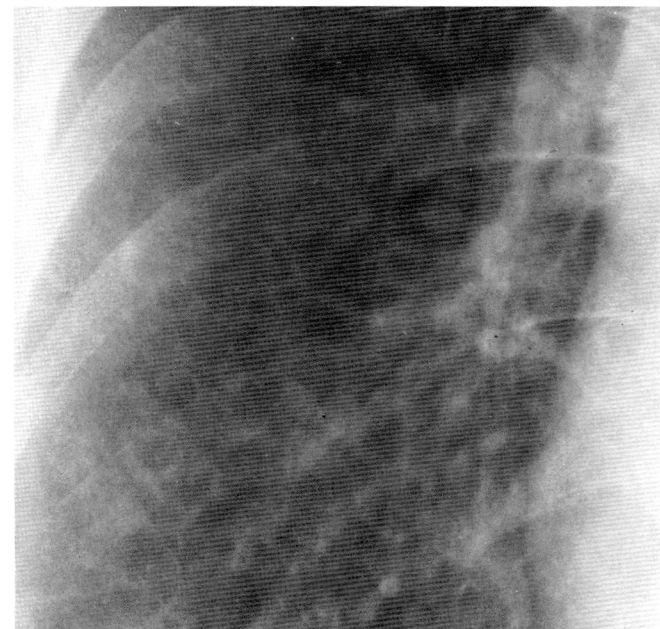

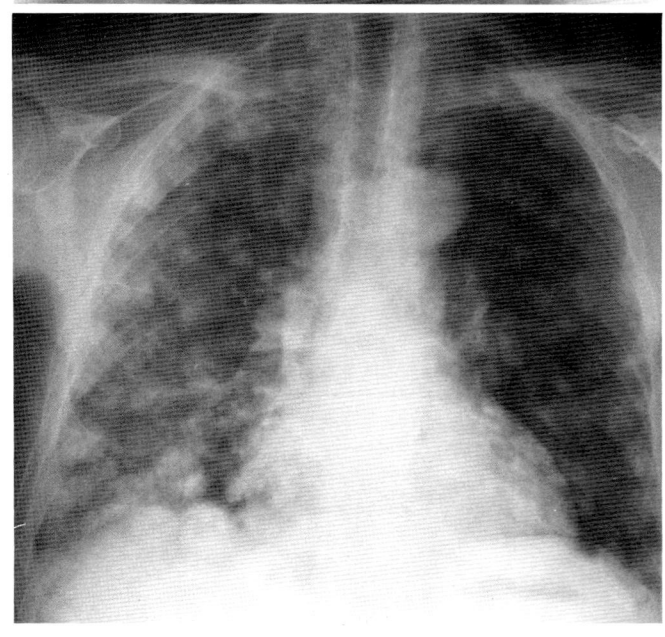

Metastatic Disease

In Western industrialized countries, 20–25% of people will develop a tumor during their lifetime, and of those, 20–30% will metastasize to the lung. They can form nodular lesions, lymphangitic carcinomatosis, pneumonia-like lesions, and rarely embolic carcinomatosis with pulmonary arterial hypertension.

Nodular Metastasis

Tumor cells reach the lung capillaries via the systemic venous circulation. The generalizing site can be in the systemic circulation and then reach the pulmonary capillary bed first or else the tumor can be located in the portal venous bed; in the latter case, lung metastases occur subsequent to liver metastasis. A solitary metastasis cannot be differentiated from other solitary pulmonary nodules without a biopsy. Only 4% of solitary pulmonary nodules turn out to represent a metastasis from an unknown primary. Multiple pulmonary nodules have an 80% chance of representing a metastasis from an unknown primary tumor.

Fig. 5.**39 a–c** **Multiple, small, nodular metastases.**
55-year-old woman 9 months after thyroidectomy for anaplastic thyroid carcinoma.
Initial chest radiograph reveals multiple, bilateral nodules 1–1.5 cm in diameter primarily distributed in the lower lung zones (**a, b**). One year later (**c**), the metastases have increased in size to 2–4 cm in diameter and now involve all lung zones.

Fig. 5.40 a–c **Metastatic choriocarcinoma.**
25-year-old patient with testicular choriocarcinoma who had undergone, orchiectomy, retroperitoneal lymph node dissection, and chemotherapy. Initial chest film shows an anterior mediastinal mass. Several months later, multiple, rapidly growing, pulmonary masses have developed.

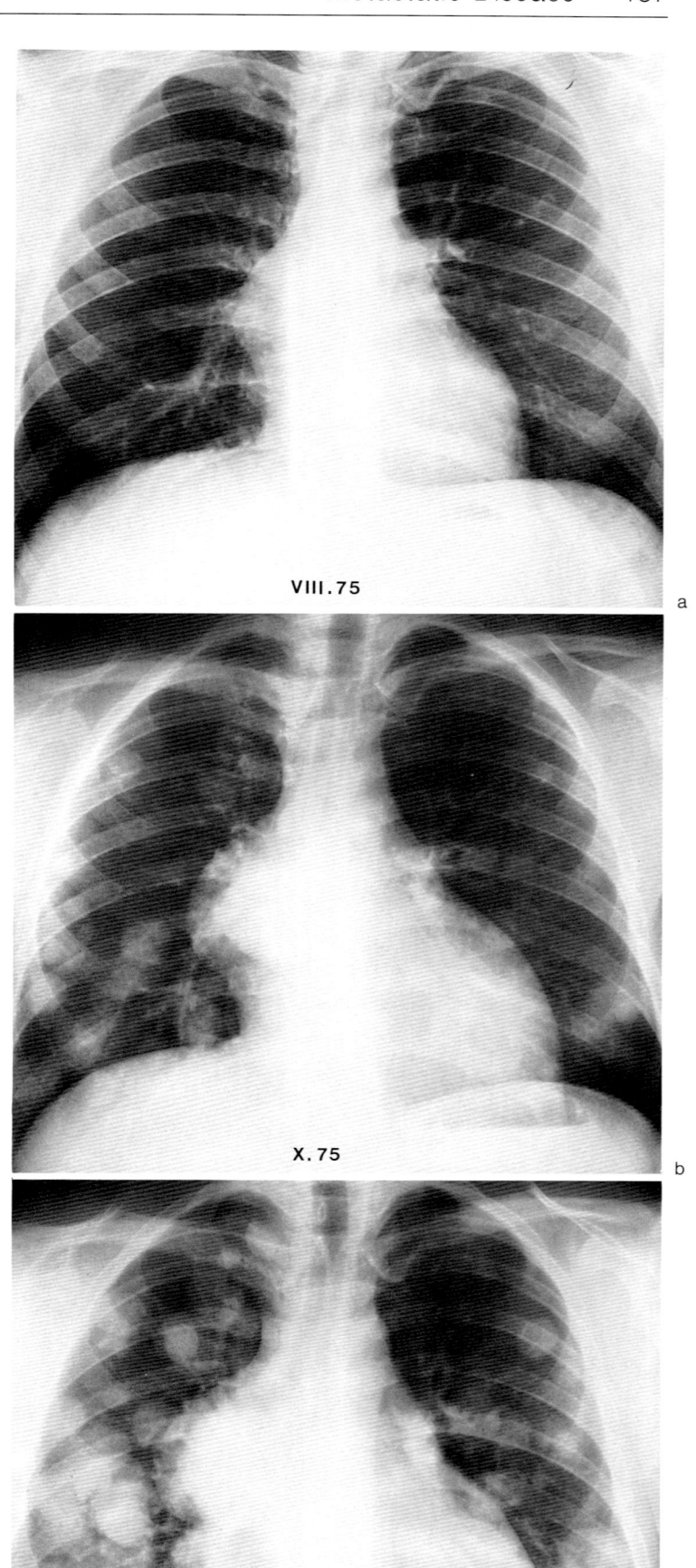

158   5. Neoplasms

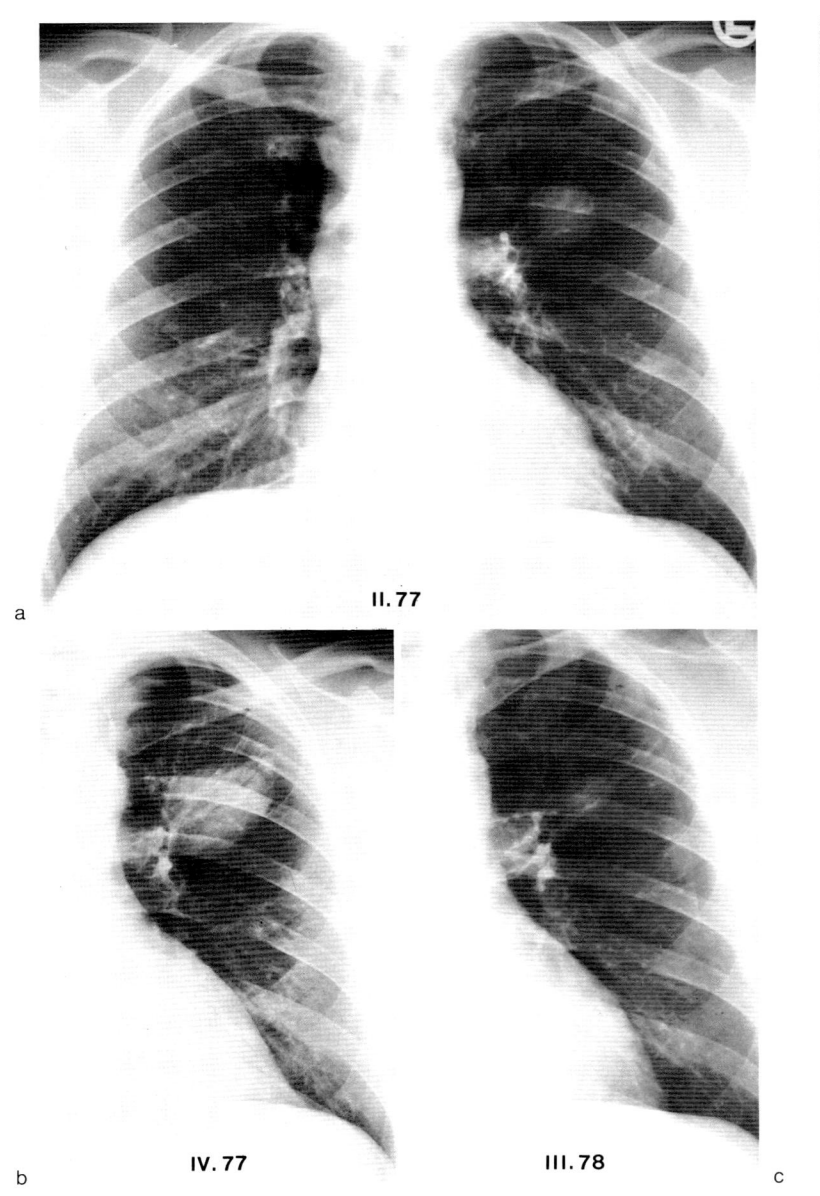

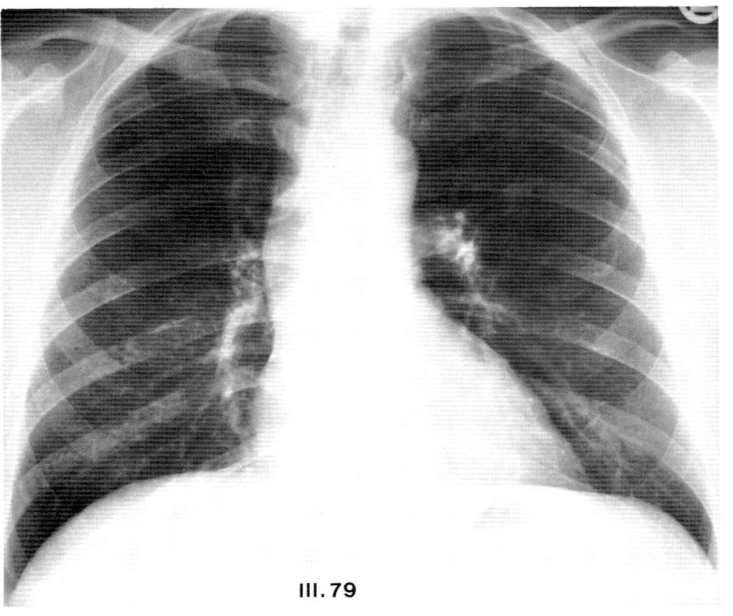

a   II.77

b   IV.77

c   III.78

d   III.79

Fig. 5.**41 a–d   Solitary pulmonary metastasis.**
43-year-old patient with renal cell carcinoma. Pulmonary lesion discovered 1 month before nephrectomy. Over the course of 2 years, the lesion disappears, without further adjuvant therapy.

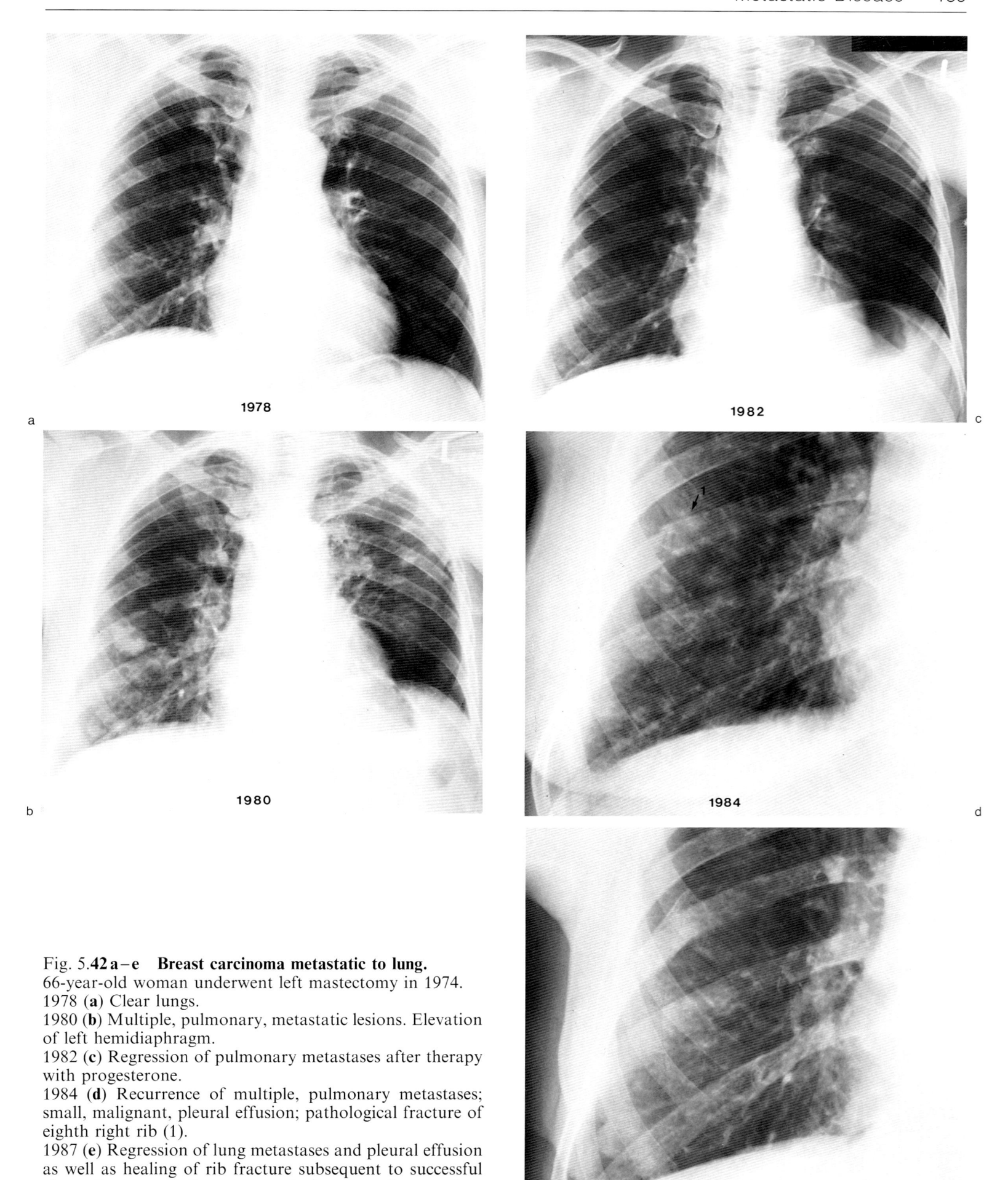

Fig. 5.42 a–e Breast carcinoma metastatic to lung.
66-year-old woman underwent left mastectomy in 1974.
1978 (**a**) Clear lungs.
1980 (**b**) Multiple, pulmonary, metastatic lesions. Elevation of left hemidiaphragm.
1982 (**c**) Regression of pulmonary metastases after therapy with progesterone.
1984 (**d**) Recurrence of multiple, pulmonary metastases; small, malignant, pleural effusion; pathological fracture of eighth right rib (1).
1987 (**e**) Regression of lung metastases and pleural effusion as well as healing of rib fracture subsequent to successful chemotherapy. Patient succumbed eventually to liver metastases.

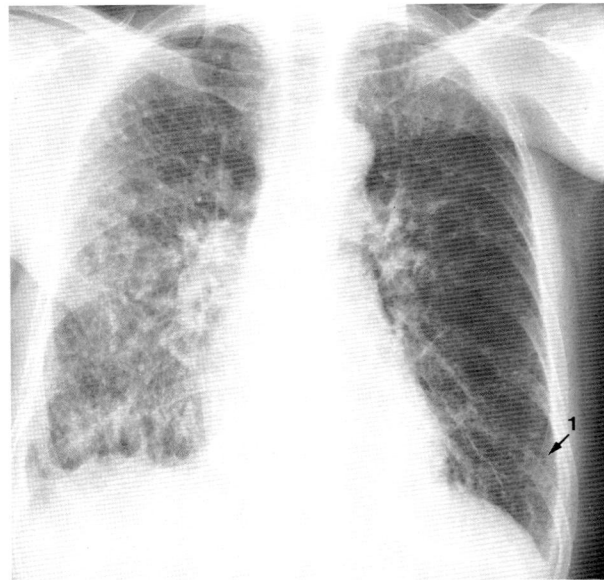

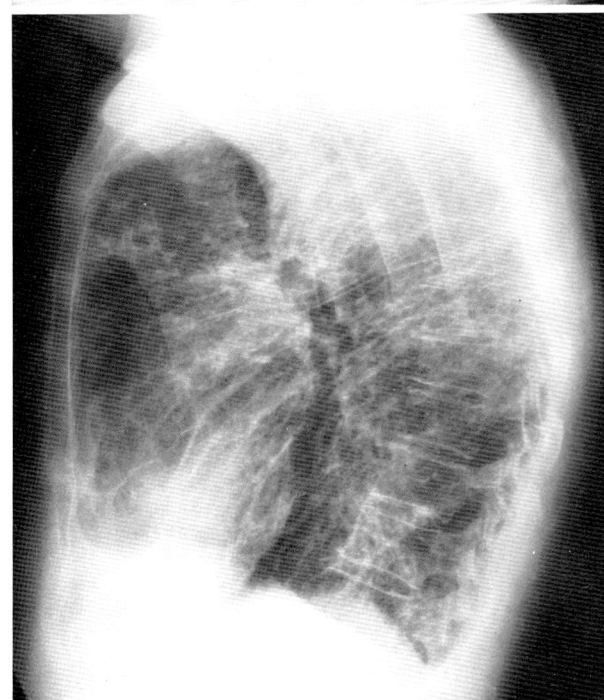

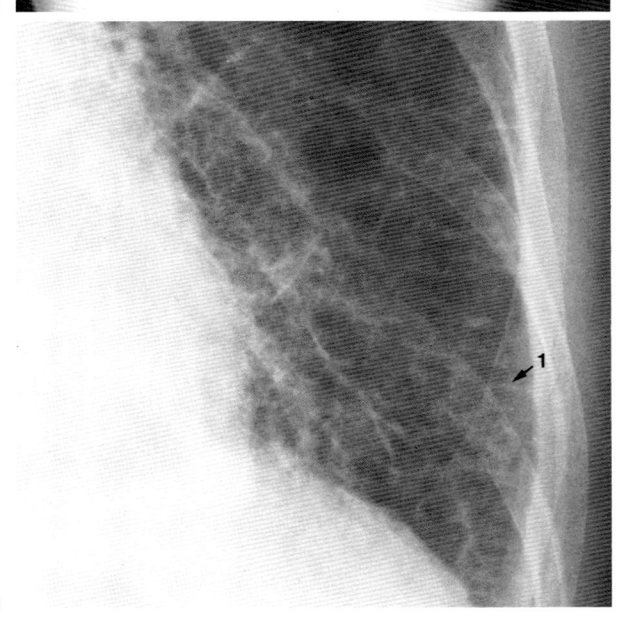

Lymphangitic Carcinomatosis

This form of metastatic disease occurs due to hematogenous micrometastases to the lung with subsequent centripetal growth towards the hilus in 75% of cases. In 25% of cases, centrifugal growth of the tumor occurs from enlarged hilar or mediastinal lymph nodes into the periphery. The majority of afflicted patients have an adenocarcinoma (80%). In 50% of patients, symptoms, like dyspnea, appear before definite plain film radiologic findings become visible. Carcinoma of the pancreas, colon, stomach, cervix, endometrium, ovary, prostate, and thyroid is likely to produce bilateral lung disease. Lung and breast primary tumors can lead to asymmetric or unilateral lung disease.

Reactive fibrosis, drop in compliance of the lung, and ventilation-perfusion mismatch explain the severe dyspnea. The median survival of such patients is 5 months. Radiologically reticular and reticulonodular opacities and Kerley B lines predominate. An accompanying malignant pleural effusion can frequently be present. High-resolution CT can detect the disease earlier than plain films. Polygones, thickened interlobular septa, thick nodular bronchovascular bundles ("string of beads"), and central dots in the center of secondary pulmonary lobules are characteristic.

Fig. 5.**43a-c** **Lymphangitic carcinomatosis.**
63-year-old patient with severe dyspnea, years after bilateral mastectomies. Diffuse, bilateral, linear and reticular markings. Kerley B lines (1).

Fig. 5.**44a-d** **Lymphangitic carcinomatosis with malignant pleural effusion.**
52-year-old patient treated for breast carcinoma a year prior to current admission for severe dyspnea. Chest film shows confluent, diffuse, linear and reticular opacities as well as right pleural effusion. Slight improvement (c) after chemotherapy with subsequent rapid deterioration (b,d). Right effusion extends into major fissure (d) (1).

Fig. 5.**45a, b**
Nodular metastases and atelectasis due to lymphatic spread of tumor in the bronchial wall and subsequent occlusion of its lumen. Autopsy proof.

Metastatic Disease 161

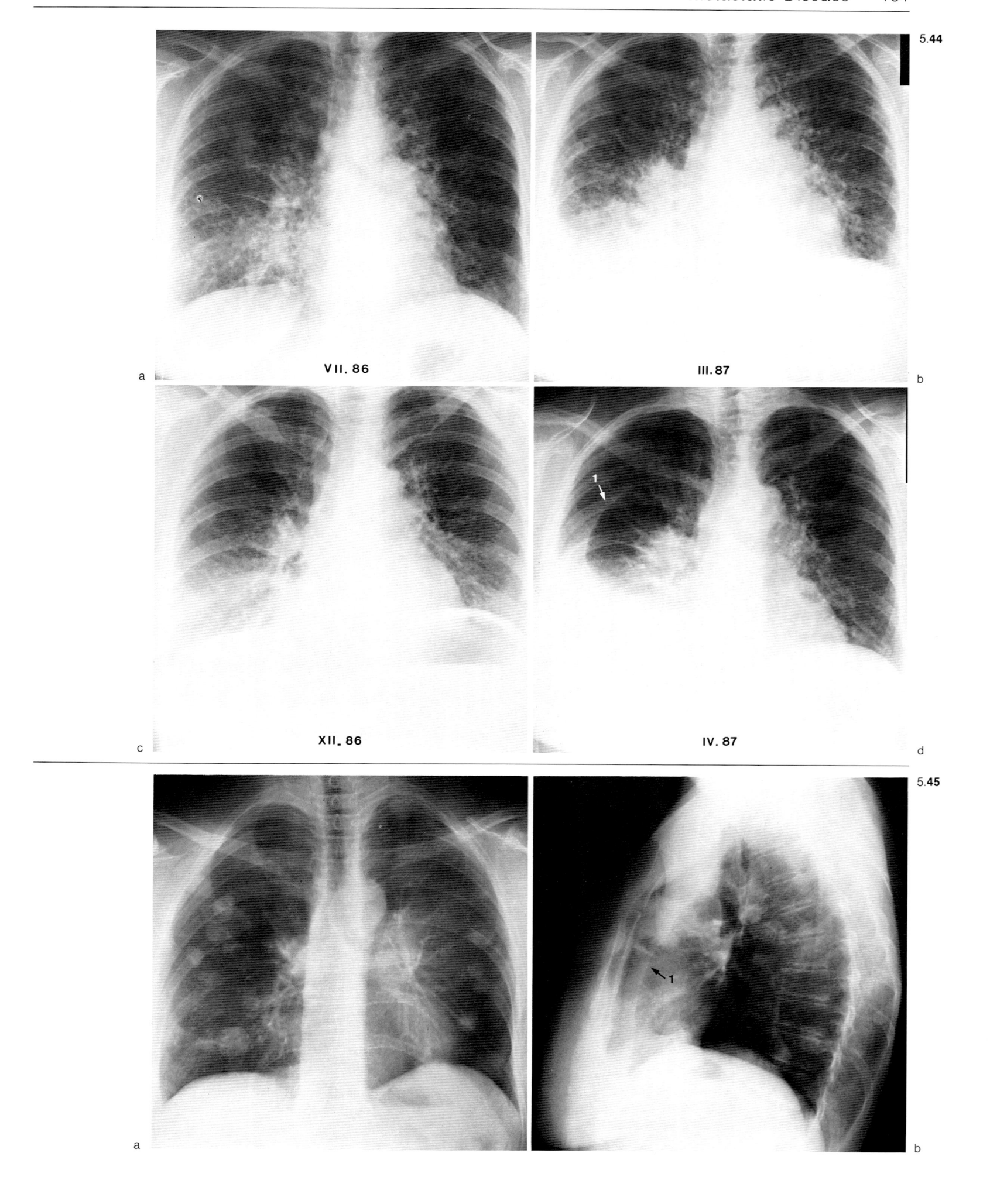

5.44

a   VII. 86

b   III. 87

c   XII. 86

d   IV. 87

5.45

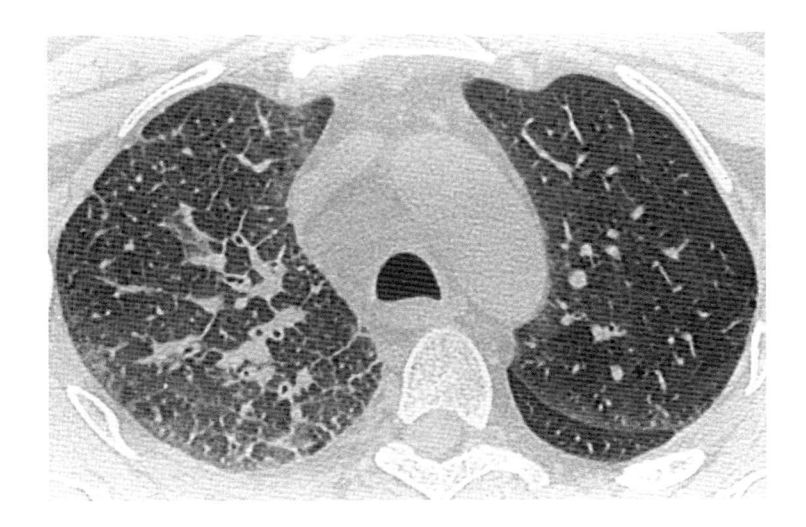

Fig. 5.46 Patient with bronchogenic carcinoma and right-sided unilateral lymphangitic carcinomatosis. High-resolution CT scan shows thickening of interlobular septa, thickening of bronchovascular bundles, and ground glass opacities. Note enlarged pretracheal-retrocaval lymph node.

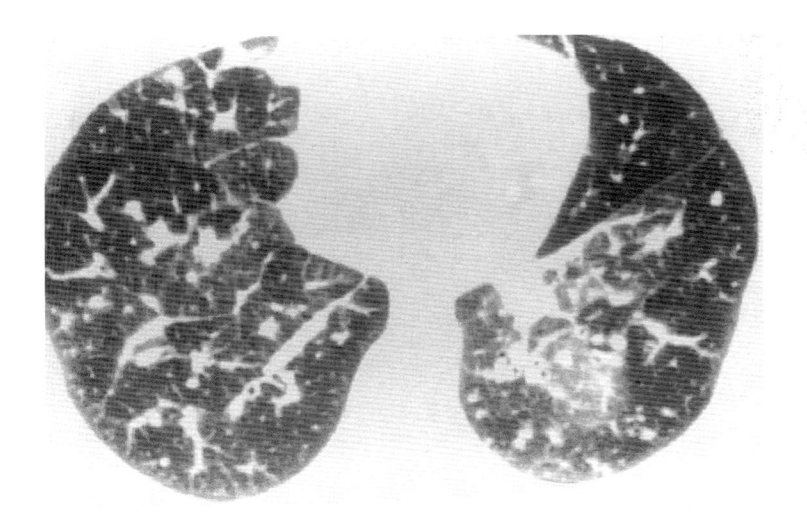

Fig. 5.47 **Lymphangitic carcinomatosis from carcinoma of the cervix.**
42-year-old woman with dyspnea. High resolution CT scan displays thickening of bronchovascular bundles, bronchial walls, interlobular septa and interlobar fissures. Ground glass opacities are visible in the left lower lobe.

Multiple pulmonary metastases can be resected under special circumstances. In most cases, the metastases can be only temporarily influenced by chemotherapy. Rarely, pulmonary metastases from renal cell carcinoma can regress after resection of the primary tumor.

Unusual Intrathoracic Tumors and Related Conditions

Benign tumors account for only 2–4% of all intrathoracic neoplasms. Accurate diagnosis necessitates a biopsy. A typical pattern of popcorn calcification or fat content on CT scan make a hamartoma likely and a biopsy unnecessary. Benign tumors have a doubling time longer than 2 years and a smooth sharp contour. Frequently, they are solitary.

Multiple benign lung tumors can be hamartomas (Cowden syndrome), squamous cell papillomas, and multiple leiomyomas (so-called benign metastasizing leiomyoma of the uterus).

Fig. 5.48 a–c **Chondroma, autopsy proven.**
66-year-old patient. Solitary pulmonary nodule projecting over the seventh anterior right rib. CT scan demonstrates central calcifications.

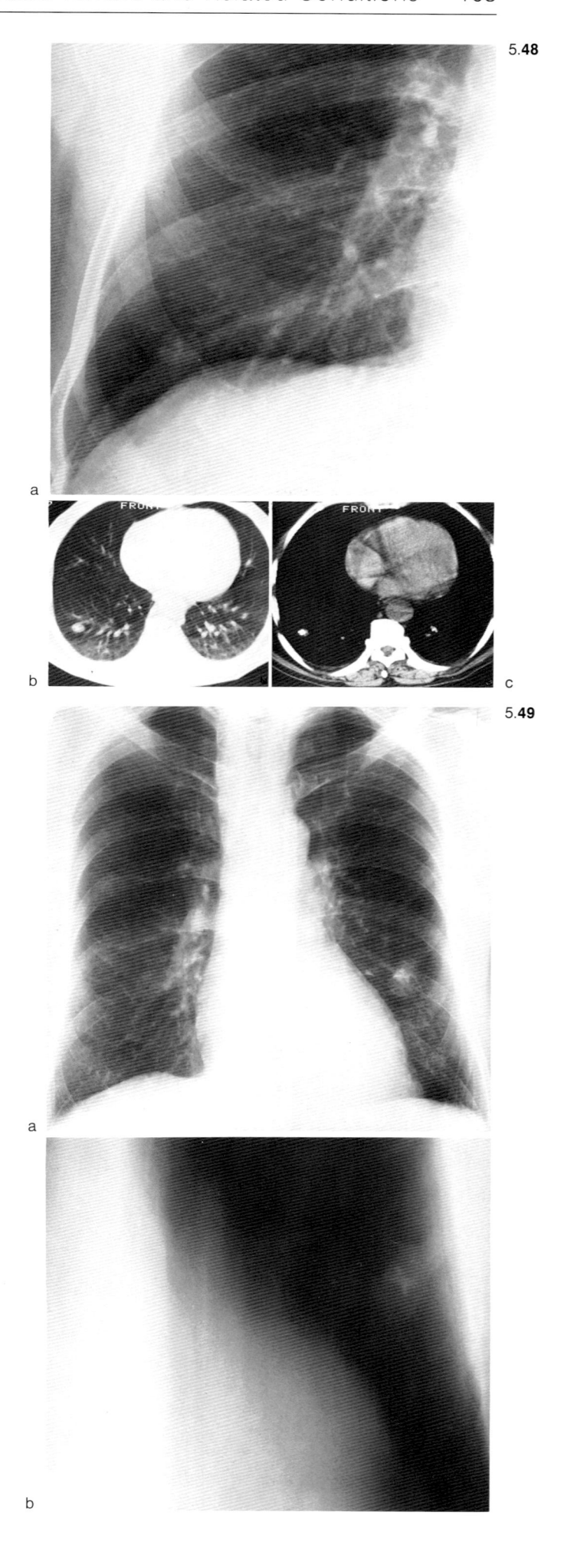

Fig. 5.49 a, b **Hamartoma, autopsy proven.**
Solitary pulmonary nodule with popcorn calcification, stable for 2 years.

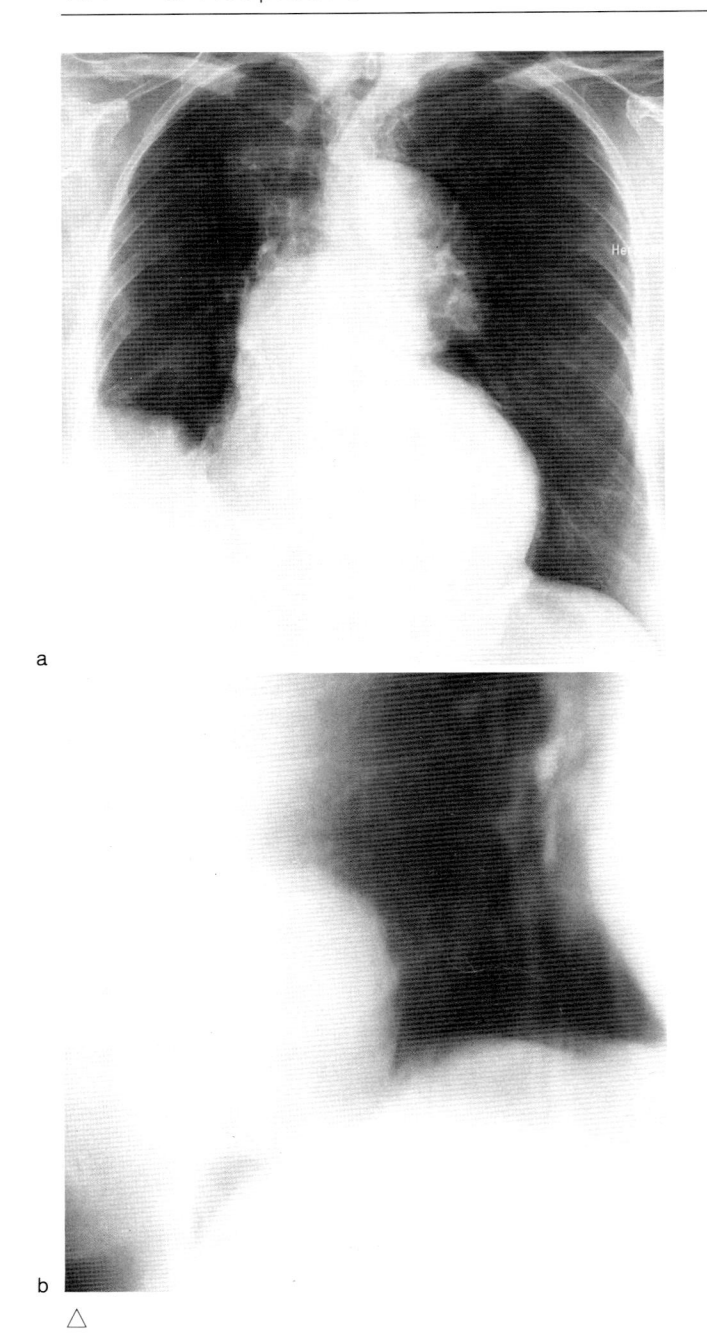

Fig. 5.50 a, b Neurinoma, surgically verified.
76-year-old patient. Large (6 cm in diameter), smoothly marginated, right lower lobe mass.

Fig. 5.51 a–c Bronchial carcinoid in bronchus intermedius.
32-year-old patient with recurrent pneumonias. Biopsy-proven nodular mass projects over bronchus intermedius (**a**). Linear tomogram displays abnormality better (**b**). Expiratory film demonstrates marked air-trapping on the right side with contralateral mediastinal shift.

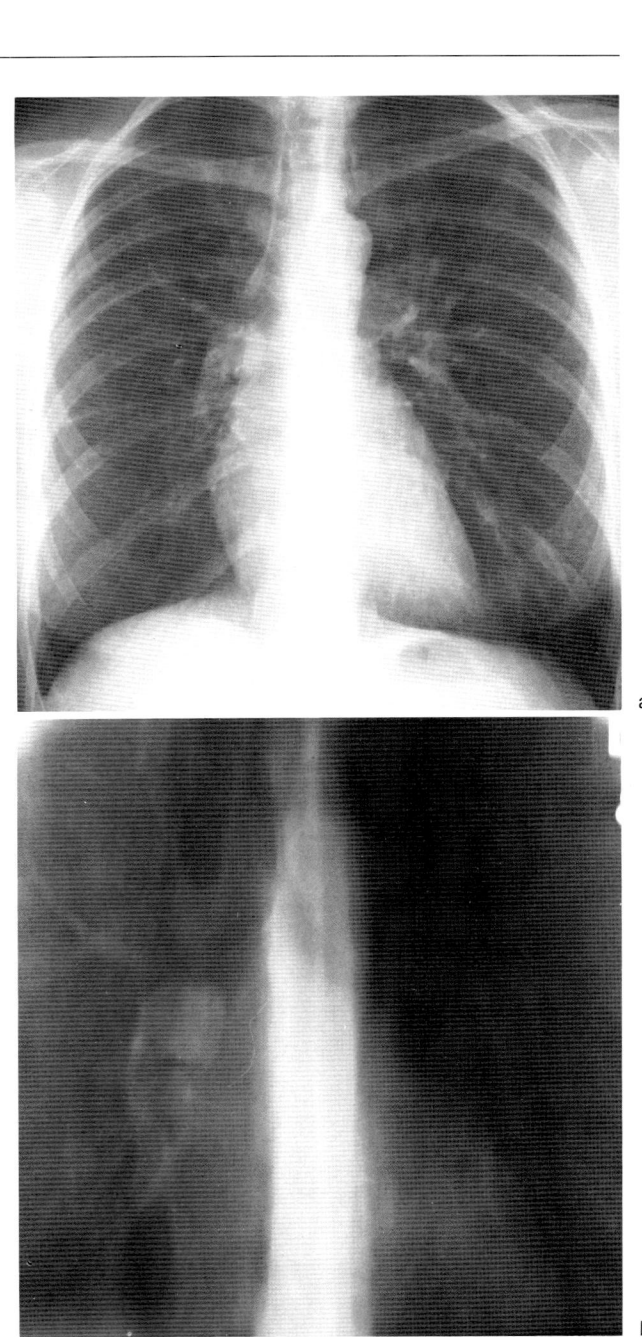

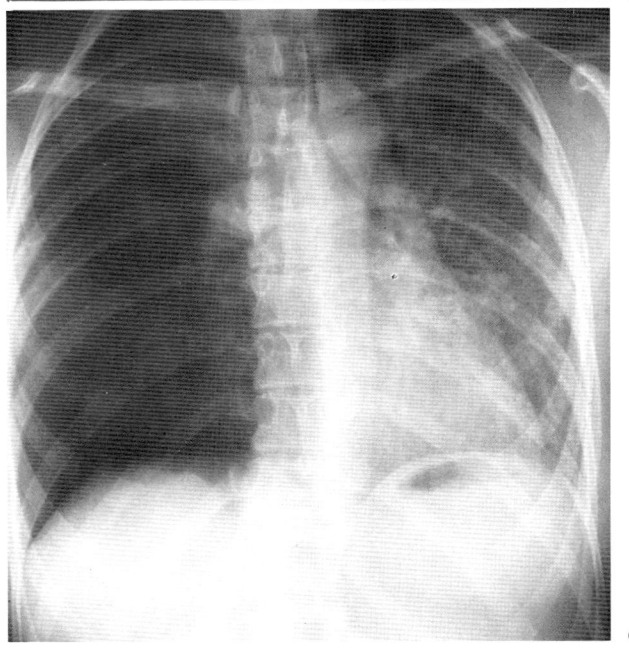

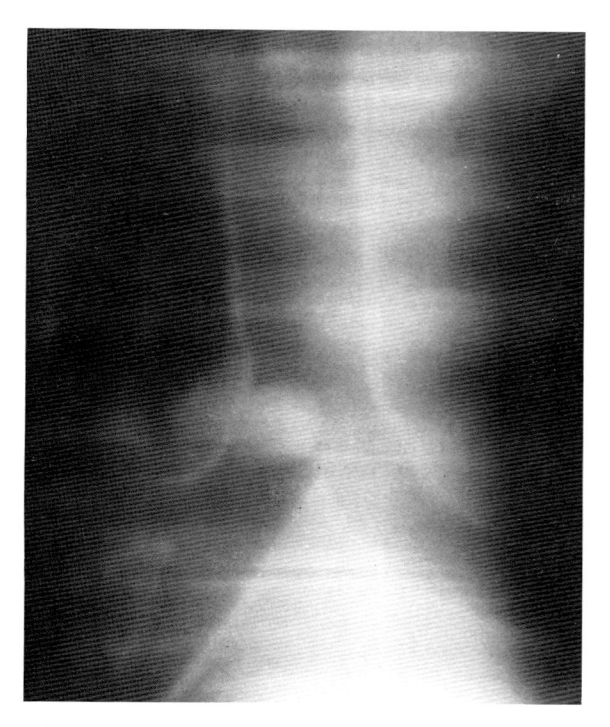

Fig. 5.**52** **Fibroma.**
Patient with stridor of several years' duration. Nodular mass within air column of distal trachea and right mainstem bronchus.

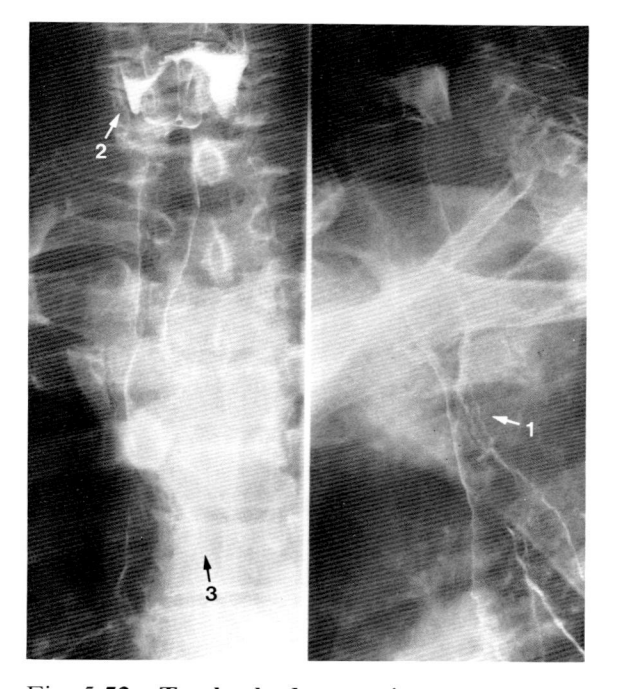

Fig. 5.**53** **Tracheal adenocarcinoma.**
Irregular tracheal narrowing, 4 cm proximal to bifurcation (1); piriform sinus (2), carina (3).

Fig. 5.**54a–c** **Tracheal papillomatosis.**
9-year-old child with dyspnea and stridor. Irregular filling defects in tracheal air column (1), intrapulmonary nodules, azygoesophageal stripe (2), descending aorta (3).

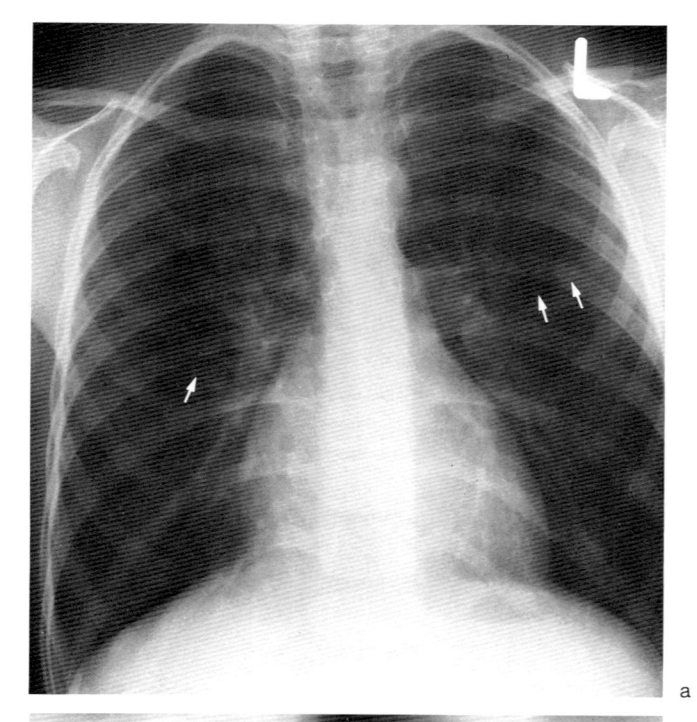

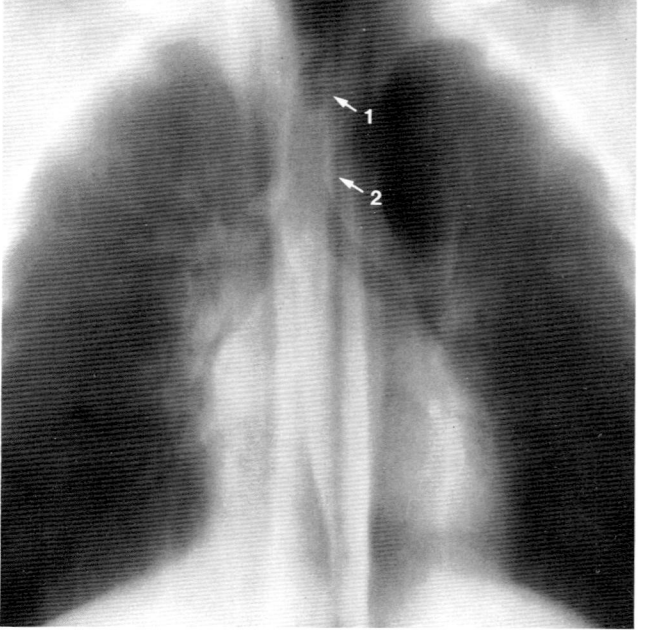

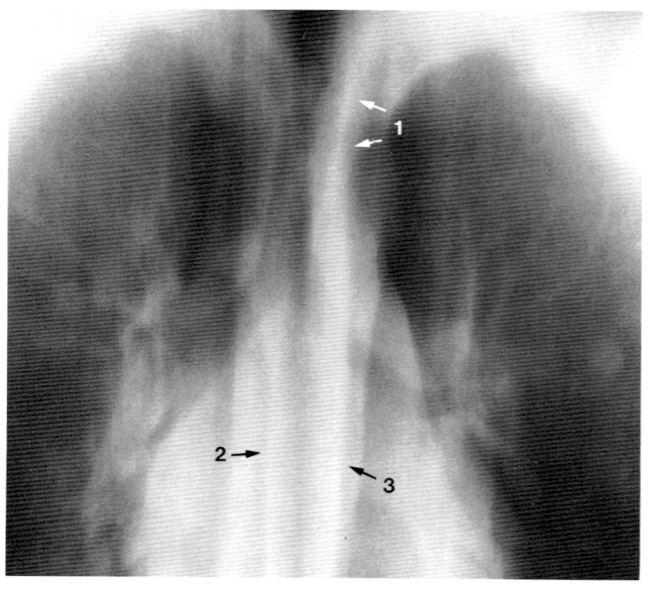

6. Vascular Disease

Pulmonary Vascular Congestion

Pulmonary vascular engorgement is a frequent occurrence and is due to either left ventricular failure or mitral valve stenosis. Left ventricular failure is reported to affect 1% of the population with an annual incidence of approximately 3 per 1000. The prognosis of congestive heart failure is poor: Annual mortality is in excess of 50%. The pulmonary venous hypertension leads to subliminal interstitial edema, decrease in basilar lung compliance, and reactive basilar vasoconstriction and results in cranial redistribution of the pulmonary vascular flow.

Radiographic signs of left ventricular failure include:

- Dilatation of central pulmonary vessels and peripheral plethora. Comparison with previous films allows the detection of subtle changes.
- Interstitial pulmonary edema with poor definition of peripheral pulmonary vessels, peribronchial cuffing, thickening of interlobar fissures, Kerley lines representing thickened interlobular septa, and perihilar haze.
- Alveolar pulmonary edema with confluent opacification due to fluid-filled acini in a perihilar and dependent location.
- Cardiomegaly
- Pleural effusions

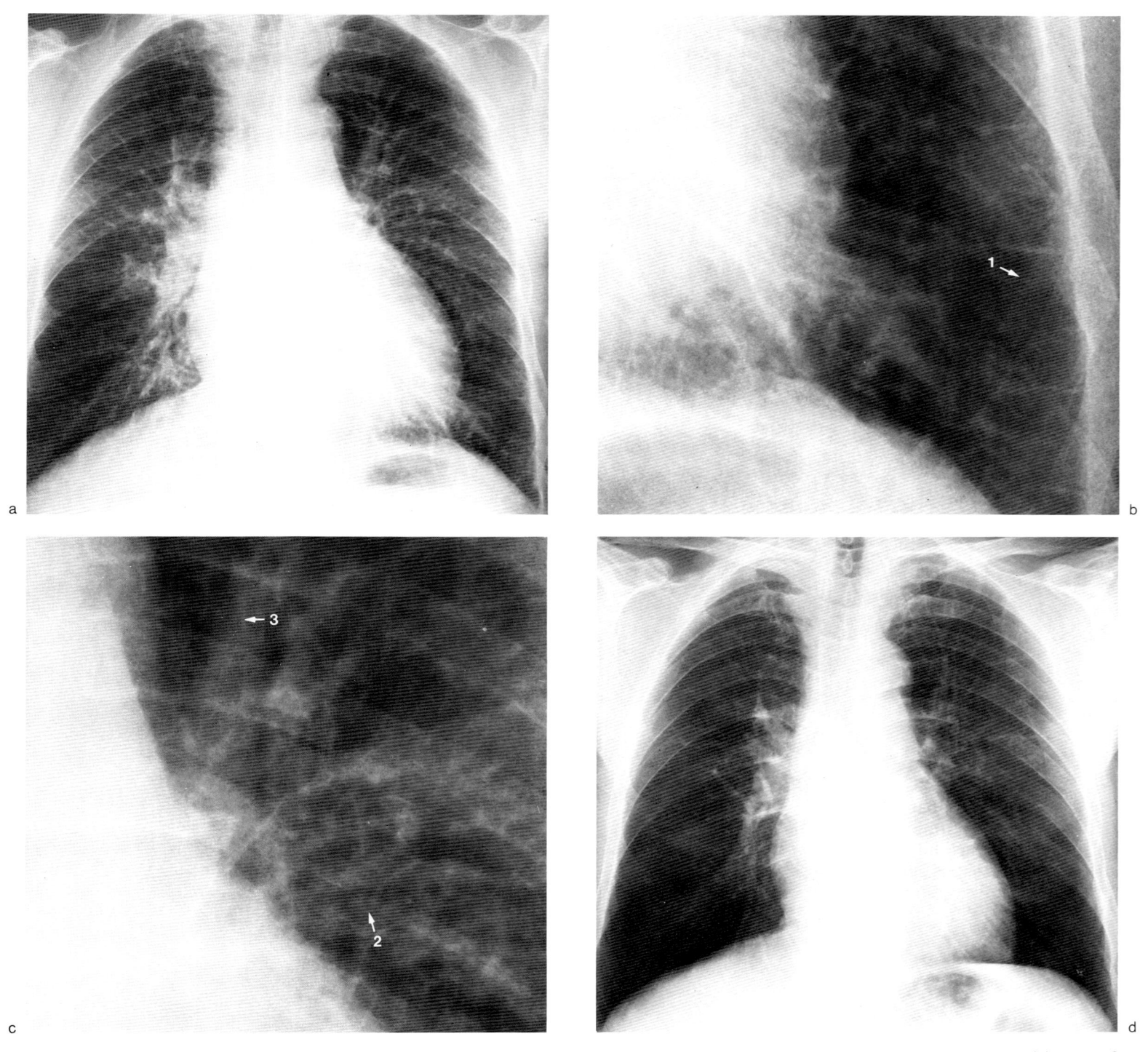

Fig. 6.1 a–d Left ventricular failure with marked interstitial edema.
Enlarged cardiac silhouette, Kerley B (1) and A lines (2). Dilated upper lobe pulmonary vessels (3) as evidence of cephalization of pulmonary vascular flow. Follow-up 2 weeks later (**d**) reveals clearing of failure.

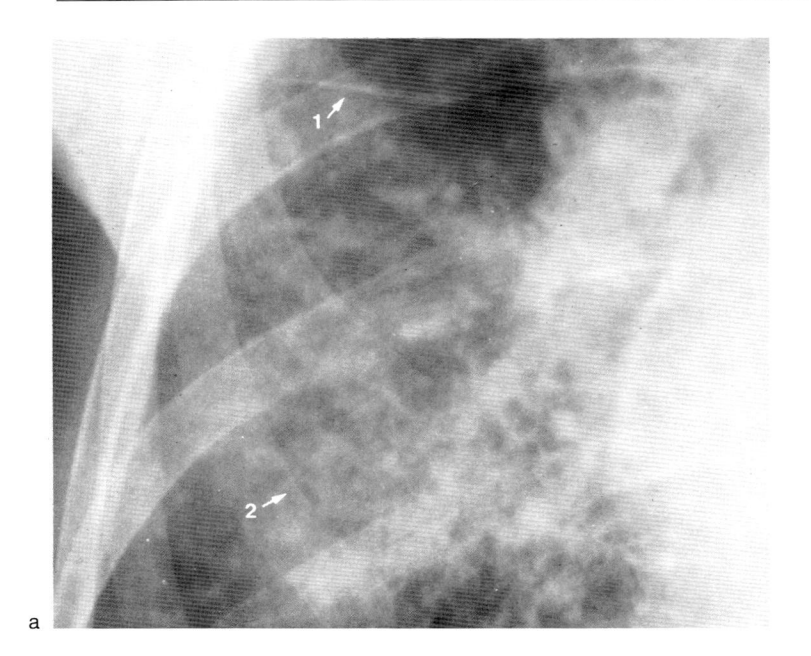

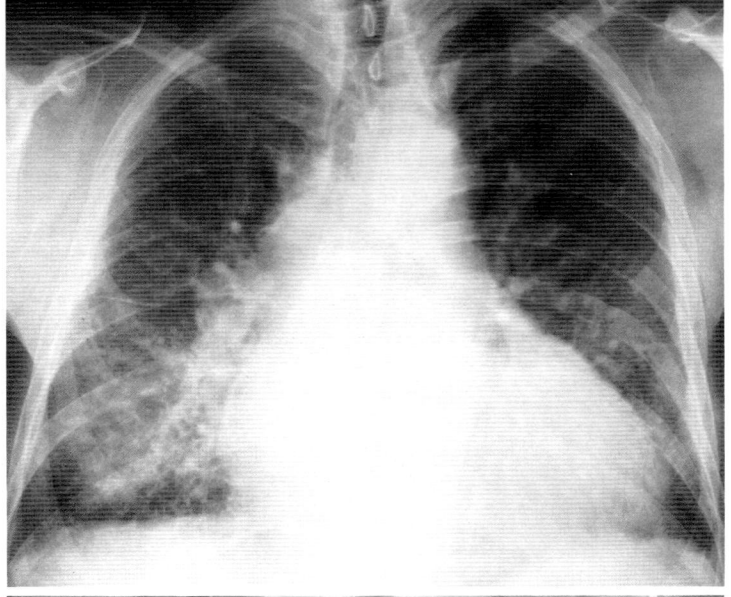

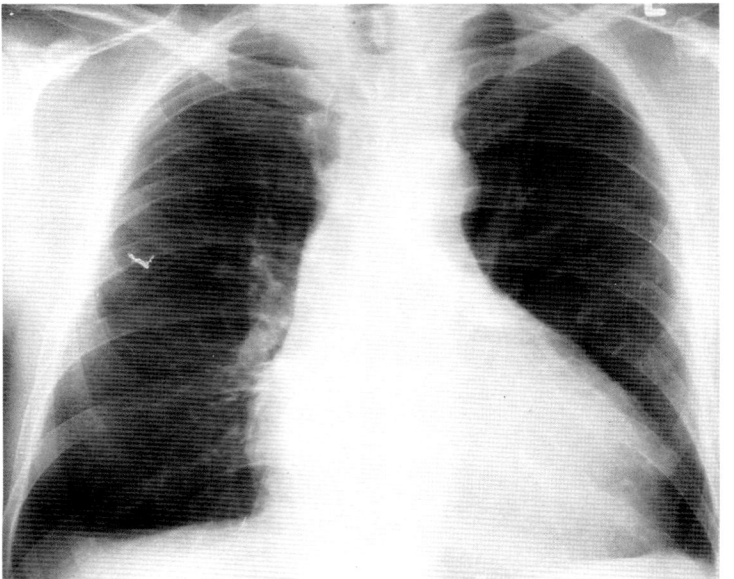

Fig. 6.2 a–c **Pulmonary edema.**
Left ventricular failure due to alcoholic cardiomyopathy; enlarged, ill-defined hilar structures. Clearing of pulmonary edema but persistent cardiomegaly.

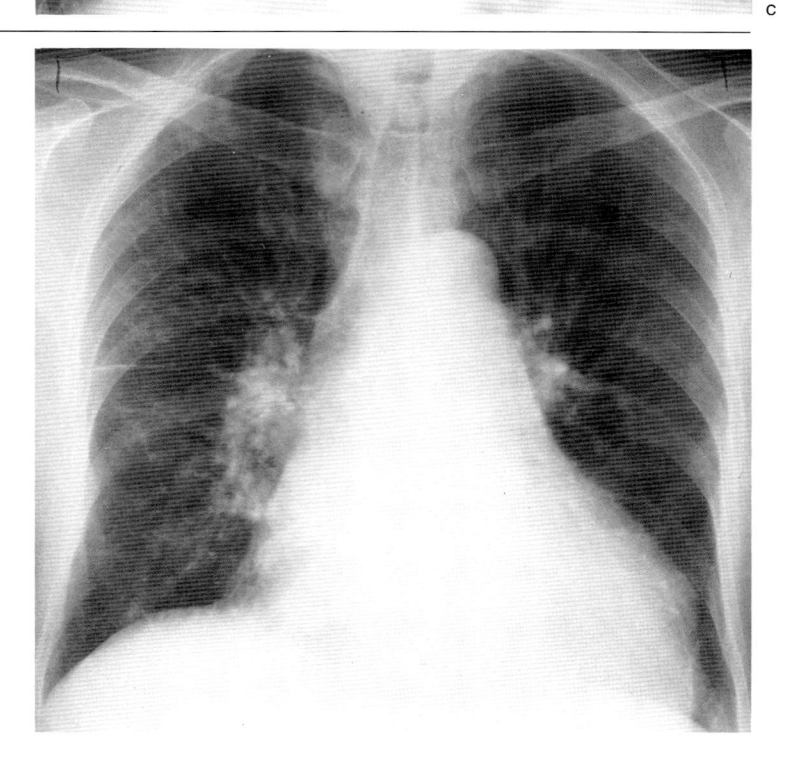

Fig. 6.3 **Left ventricular failure.**
Cephalization of pulmonary vascular flow, cardiomegaly, dilated central pulmonary vessels, thickened minor fissure.

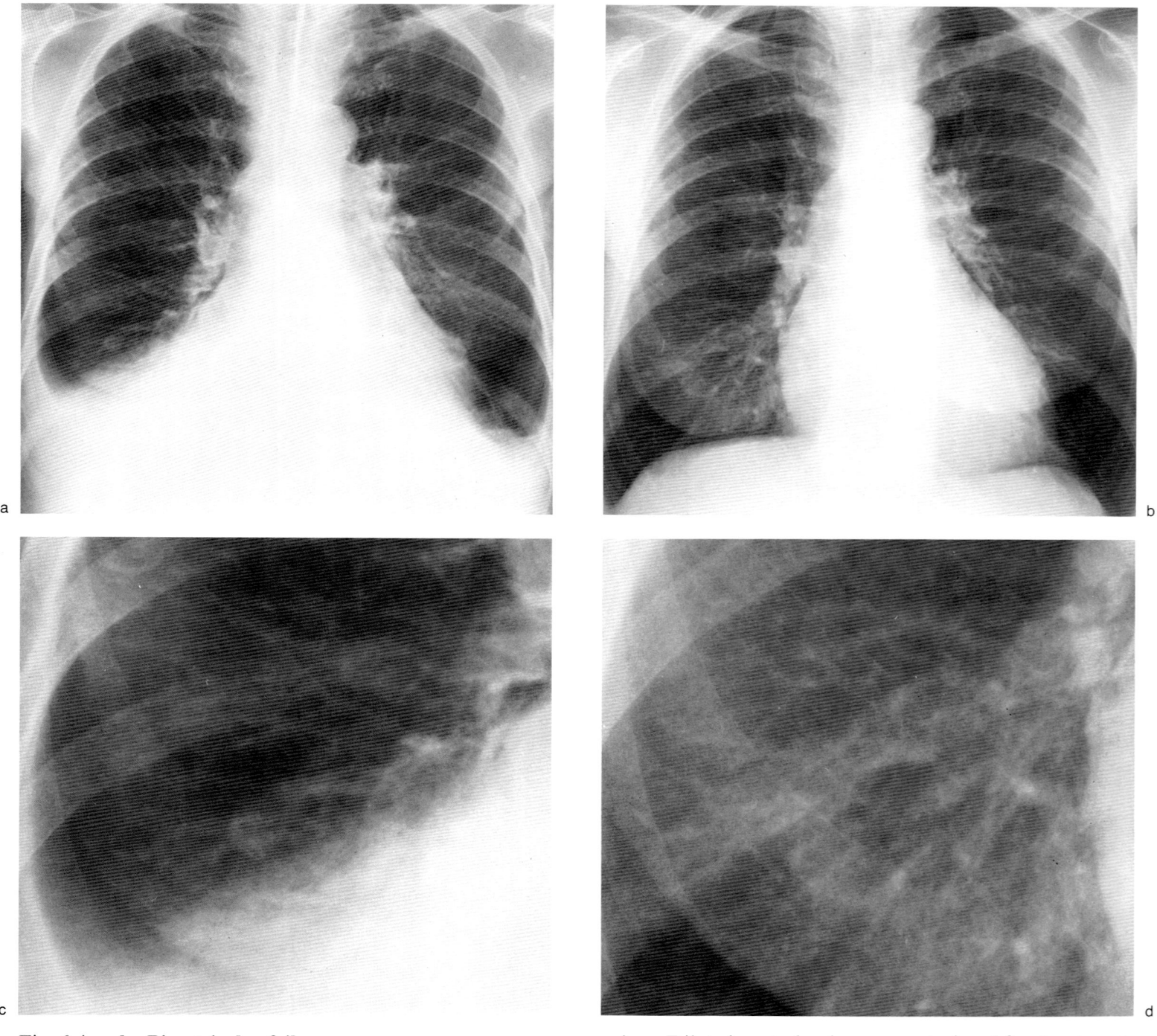

Fig. 6.4 a–d **Biventricular failure.**
60-year-old patient with orthopnea, paroxysmal nocturnal dyspnea, and ankle edema.
Bilateral pleural effusions, right greater than left, obscuring the diaphragm, the costophrenic and the cardiophrenic sulcus. Dilated central pulmonary arteries. After treatment, clearing of pleural effusions, increased lung volumes, decreased pulmonary vascular engorgement.

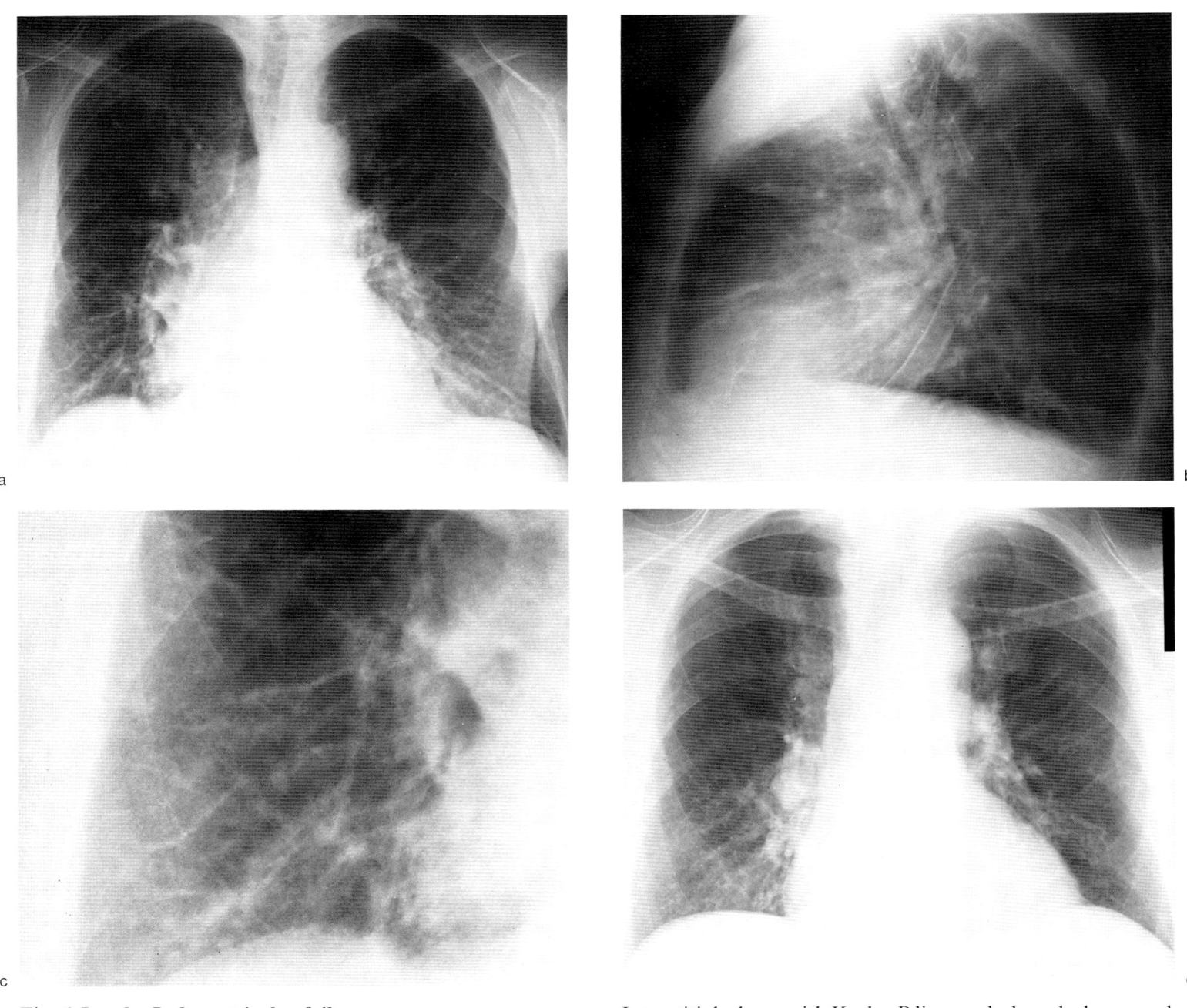

Fig. 6.5 a–d Left ventricular failure.
80-year-old patient with orthopnea.

Interstitial edema with Kerley B lines, subpleural edema, and thickening of major fissures. Marked improvement after 3 weeks of intense therapy (**d**) with digitalis and diuretics.

Pulmonary Edema

Pulmonary venous hypertension due to increased left ventricular filling pressures leads to pulmonary vascular engorgement and transudation of fluid into the interstitium of the pulmonary parenchyma. This usually happens when the end diastolic left ventricular pressure exceeds 20–25 mmHg. Further pressure increase to 30 mmHg results in failure of tight junctions of alveolar epithelial cover with subsequent alveolar flooding and alveolar edema. Kerley lines and a gravitational perihilar and basilar distribution of pulmonary edema are characteristic for left ventricular failure, overhydration, or even renal failure.

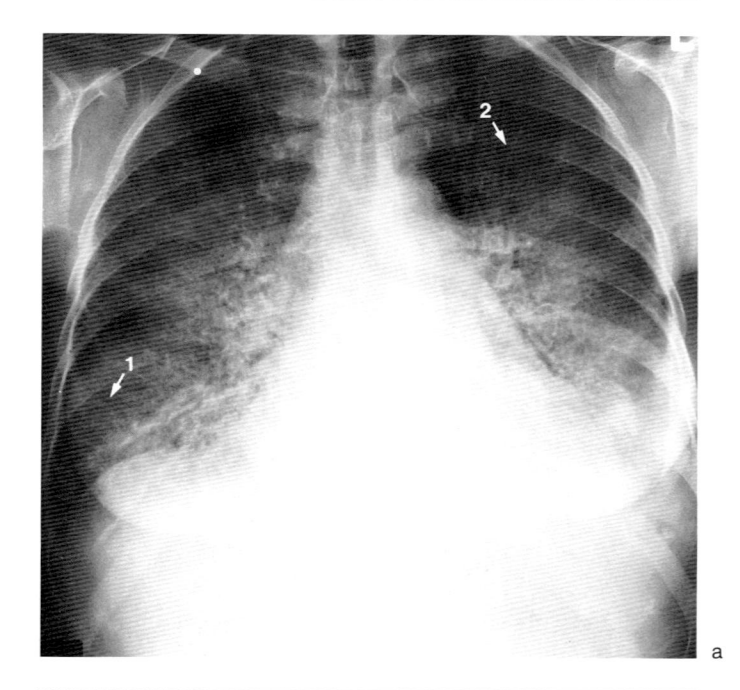

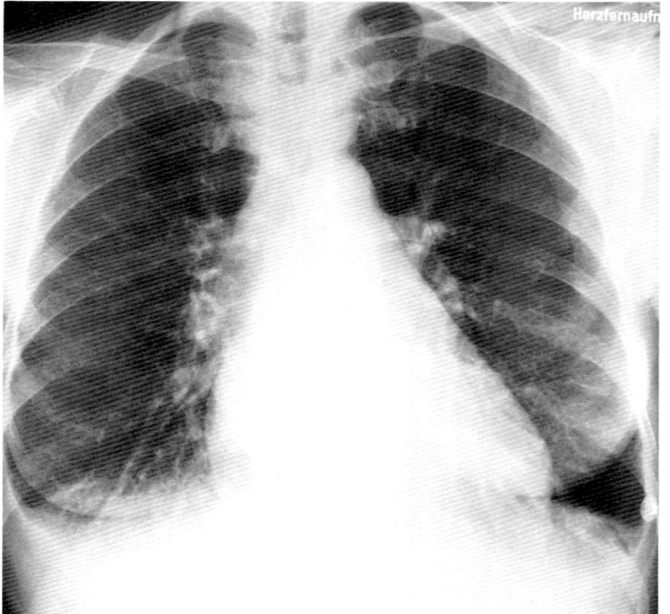

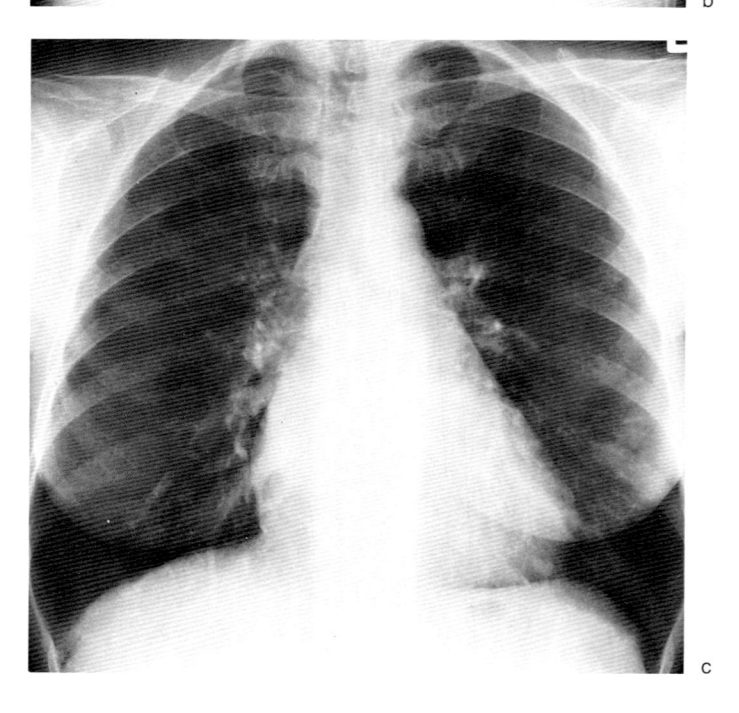

Fig. 6.6 a–c **Pulmonary edema due to left ventricular failure.**
64-year-old patient with dyspnea, nocturia, and pedal edema. Alveolar and interstitial edema combined. Perihilar opacification, pleural effusions, Kerley B (1) and A (2) lines. Improved after therapy with diuretics for 10 days (**c**).

6. Vascular Disease

Fig. 6.**7a,b** **Asymmetric pulmonary edema.**
63-year-old patient with acute myocardial infarction, preferentially lying on his left side. Poor definition of both hilar regions, right pleural effusion (1), major fissure (3). Two weeks later, significantly improved (**b**).

Fig. 6.**8a,b** **"Batwing" pulmonary edema.**
70-year-old patient with severe congestive heart failure. Two weeks later, markedly improved (**b**).

Fig. 6.**9a,b** **Interstitial pulmonary edema; renal failure.**
25-year-old patient with acute glomerulonephritis. Enlarged cardiac silhouette, interstitial pulmonary edema, left pleural effusion. Previous film (**b**) taken 6 weeks earlier is normal.

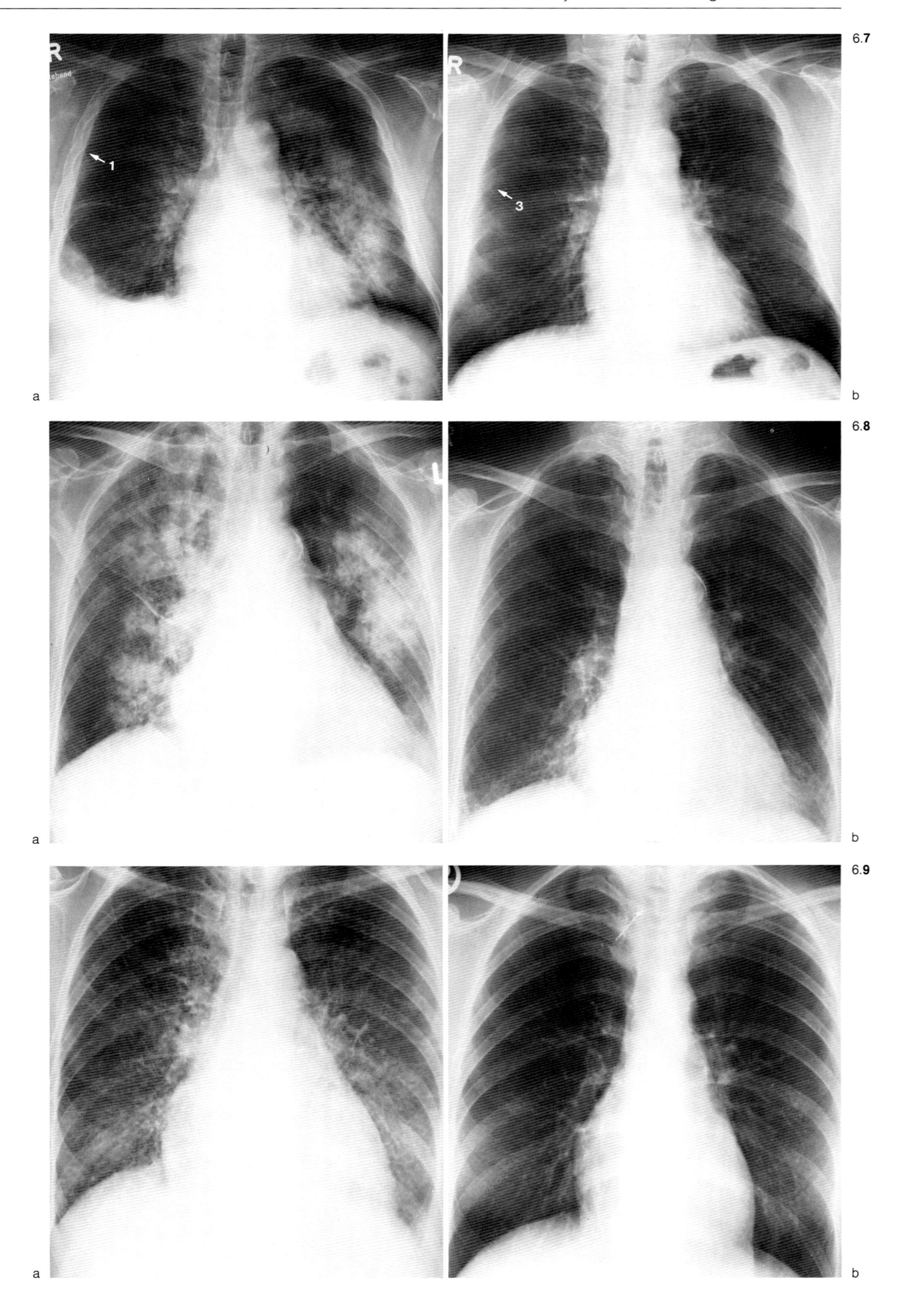

Pulmonary Vascular Congestion 175

6.7

6.8

6.9

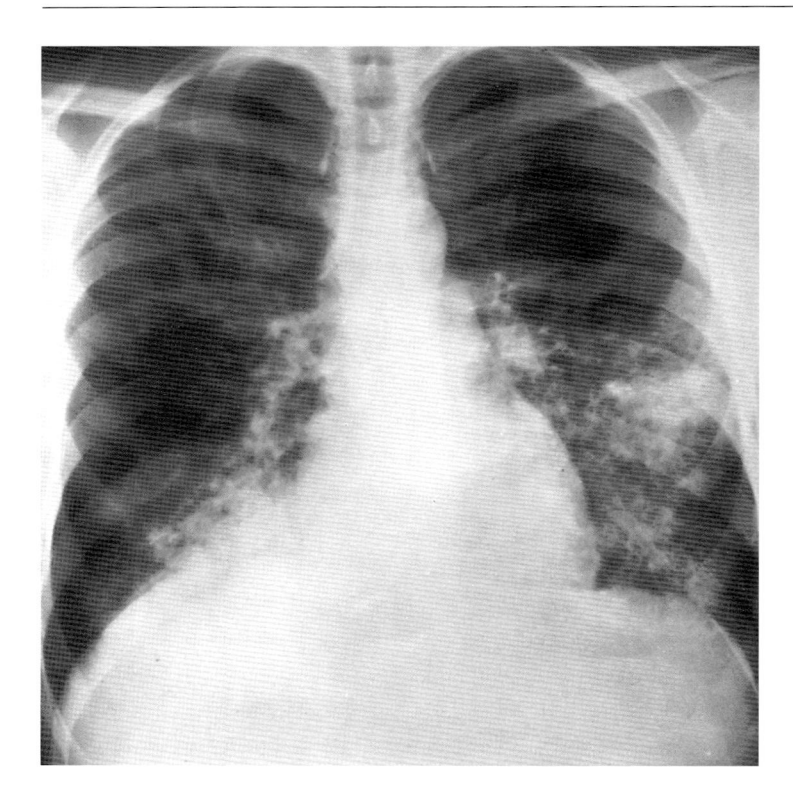

Fig. 6.10 Mountain climber with high altitude pulmonary edema. Chest radiograph shows bilateral extensive patchy consolidation.

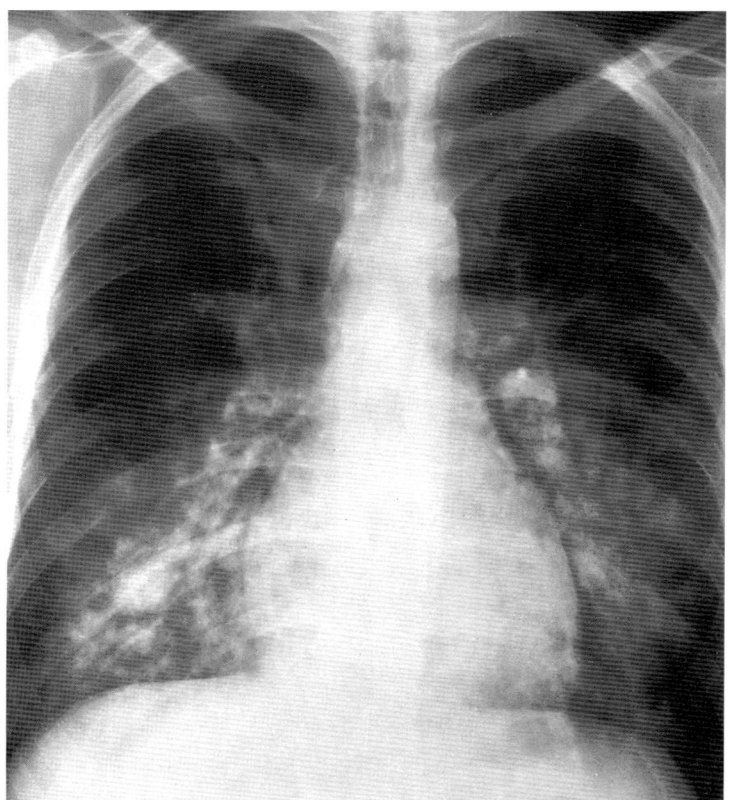

Fig. 6.11 Mountain climber with high altitude pulmonary edema. Chest radiograph shows bilateral perihilar and lower lobe consolidation with dilated central pulmonary arteries due to hypoxic vasoconstriction and pulmonary arterial hypertension. Normal cardiac size.

Chronic Pulmonary Venous Hypertension – Mitral Stenosis

Mitral stenosis is the most common cause of chronic pulmonary vascular congestion. It leads to hemosiderosis and pulmonary fibrosis. Radiographic features include reticulonodular and micronodular changes as well as irreversible Kerley lines, indicative of thickening of the interlobular septa. Microhemorrhages induce the formation of small granulomatous nodules which account for the miliary pattern visible in hemosiderosis. Rarely, true ossifications can form in the interstitium. Similar to the situation in acute left ventricular failure, the central pulmonary vessels and the main pulmonary artery segment are dilated. Cephalization of the pulmonary vascular flow is visible towards the upper lung zones. Radiographic findings in mitral stenosis are characterized by dilatation of the left atrium and right ventricle, widening of the tracheal angle of bifurcation, obscuration of the upper retrocardiac space, and double contour in the region of the right atrium.

The contact surface of the right ventricle with the sternum exceeds a third of the sternal length. Straightening of the left heart border occurs due to enlargement of the main pulmonary artery, the left atrial appendage, and the pulmonary outflow tract, and is also due to levorotation of the heart.

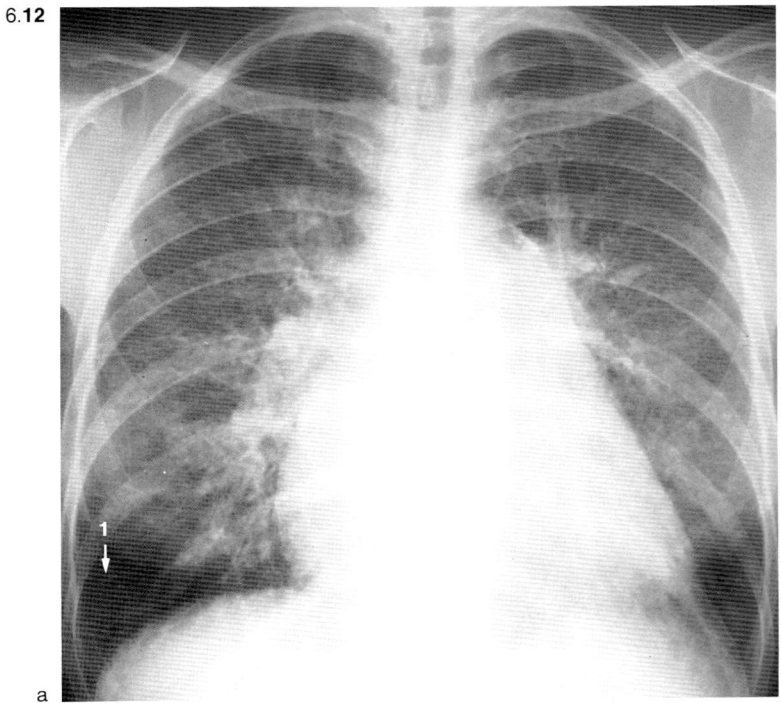

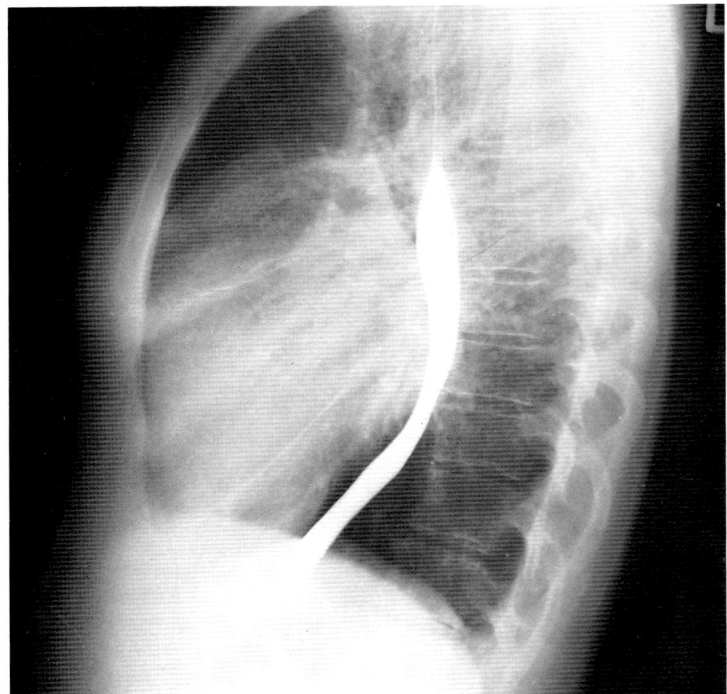

Fig. 6.12 a–e Mitral stenosis with chronic pulmonary vascular engorgement.
55-year-old patient with a 20-year history of known mitral valve disease. Cardiomegaly with mitral configuration: straightening of left heart border, dilated main pulmonary artery segment and left atrial appendage, double contour of right atrium, dilated central pulmonary vessels, narrowing of retrocardiac space, increased contact surface of right ventricle with the sternum. After conservative therapy (d, e), the cardiac silhouette has decreased in size, the pulmonary vascular engorgement has diminished, and the pulmonary edema has cleared. Miliary nodular pattern persists due to hemosiderosis.

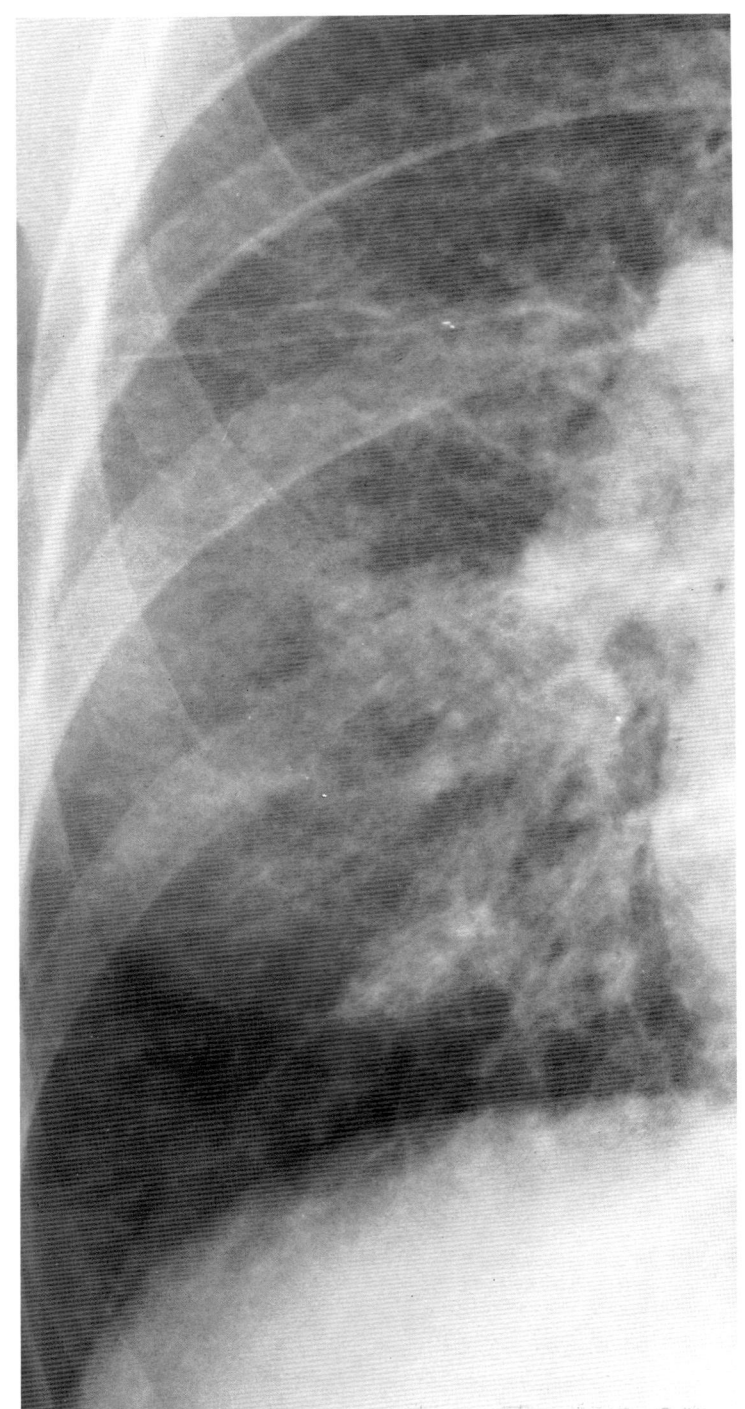

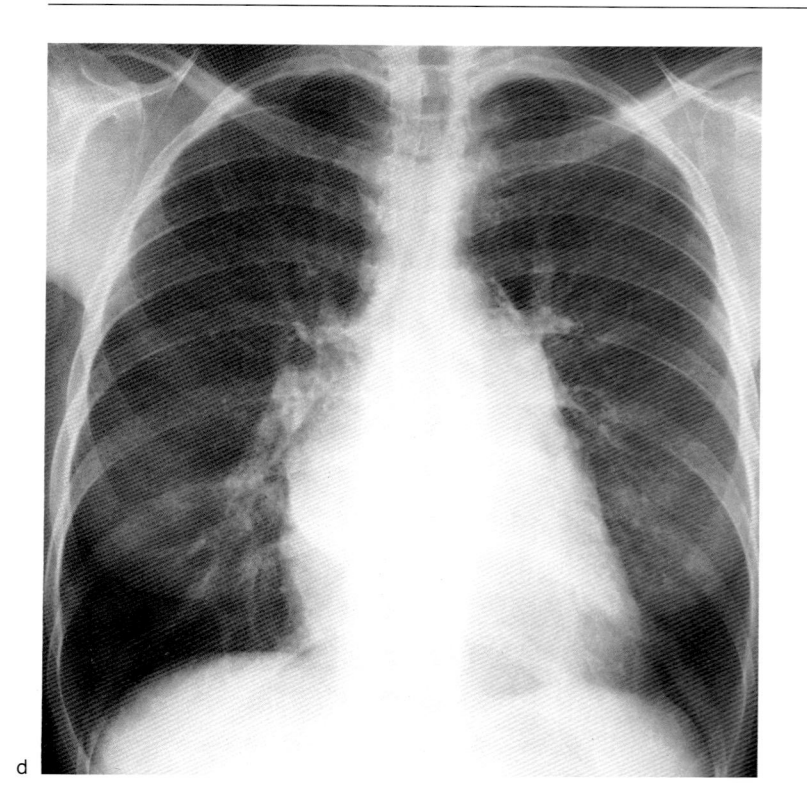

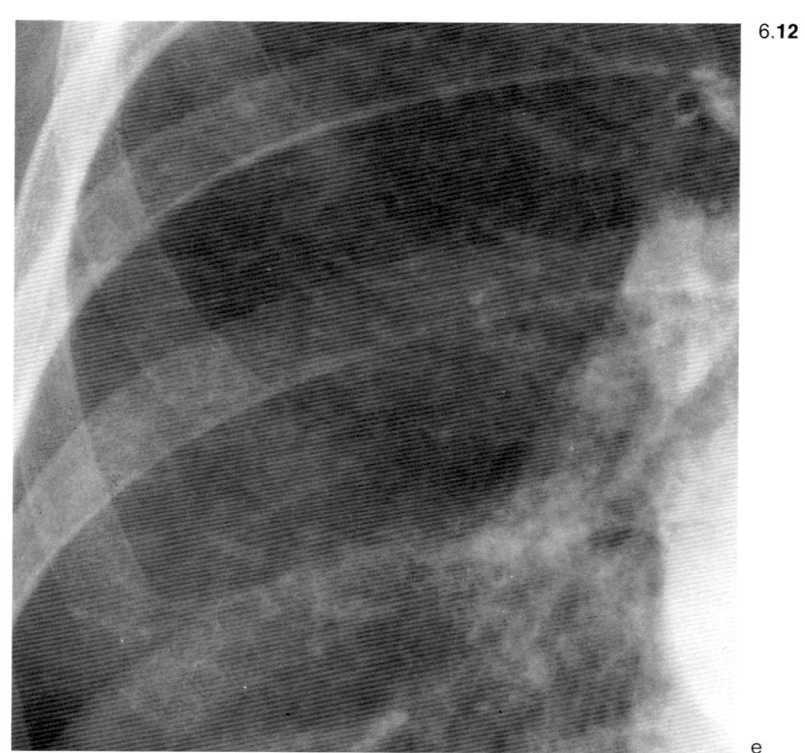

Pulmonary Vascular Congestion 179

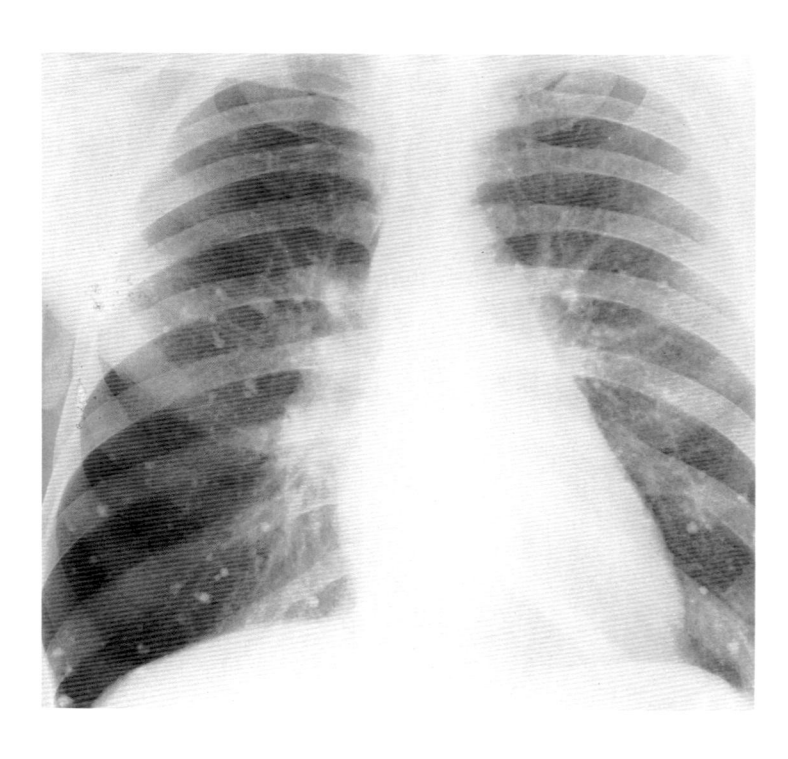

Fig. 6.13 Pulmonary ossification; chronic mitral valve disease.
40-year-old woman with a 20-year history of mitral stenosis. Straightening of left heart border, convex main pulmonary artery segment, nodular ossifications in both lower lung zones.

Pulmonary Embolism

Pulmonary emboli impede the perfusion of the subtending lung parenchyma. Bronchial arteries supply the necessary oxygen and nutrients; thus, true infarction and necrosis of lung parenchyma occur in about 10% of cases. The most common radiographic finding is a normal chest (42%). Subsegmental atelectases, low lung volumes, small pleural effusions, regional oligemia, evidence of pulmonary arterial hypertension, ipsilateral hilar enlargement due to a large saddle embolus, contralateral pulmonary edema, and focal consolidation due to hemorrhage without necrosis are just a few of the signs of pulmonary embolism. A wedge-shaped area of consolidation in subpleural location, also called the Hampton hump, is suggestive of an infarct. It is composed of multiple, confluent, hemorrhagic secondary lobules.

Ventilation perfusion scanning demonstrates multiple subsegmental, segmental, or lobar perfusion defects with preserved ventilation (mismatch). Angiography shows either an abrupt arterial cut-off or the actual emboli as filling defects in the column of contrast.

References: 61, 90, 158.

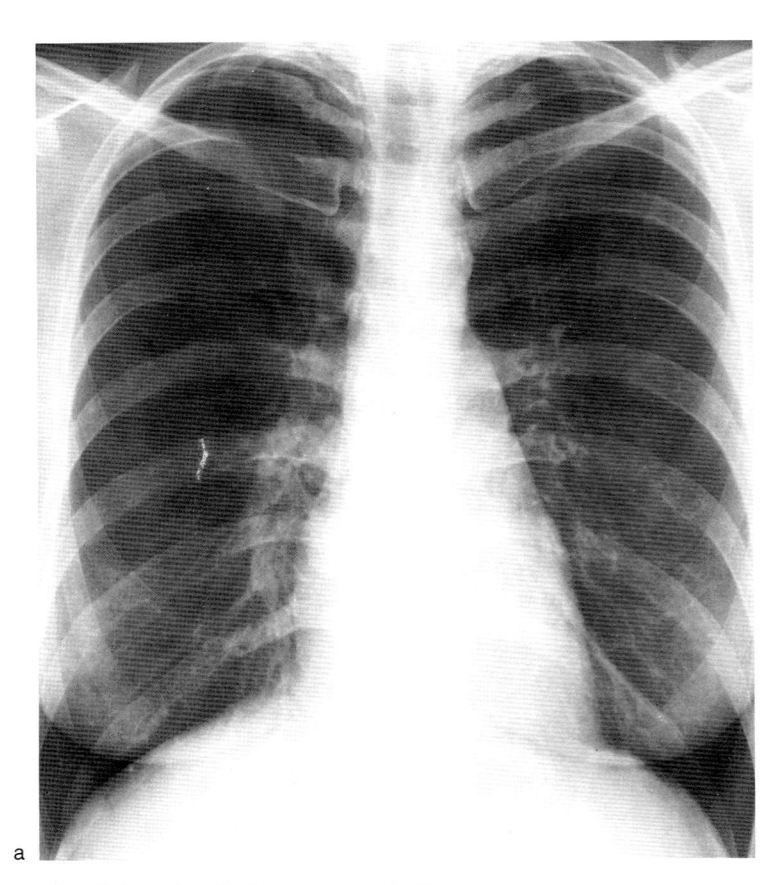

Fig. 6.14a, b **Pulmonary embolism.**
27-year-old patient who experienced dyspnea after gynecologic surgery. Normal chest radiograph except for subtle oligemia in right upper lobe (Westermark sign). Ventilation-perfusion scan demonstrates multiple, wedge-shaped perfusion defects.

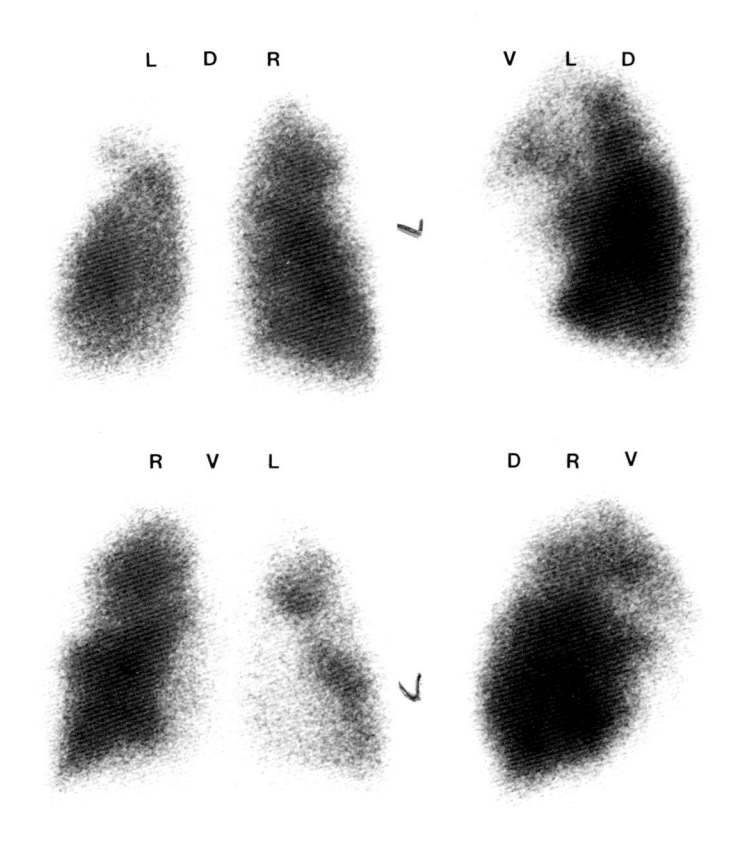

Pulmonary Embolism

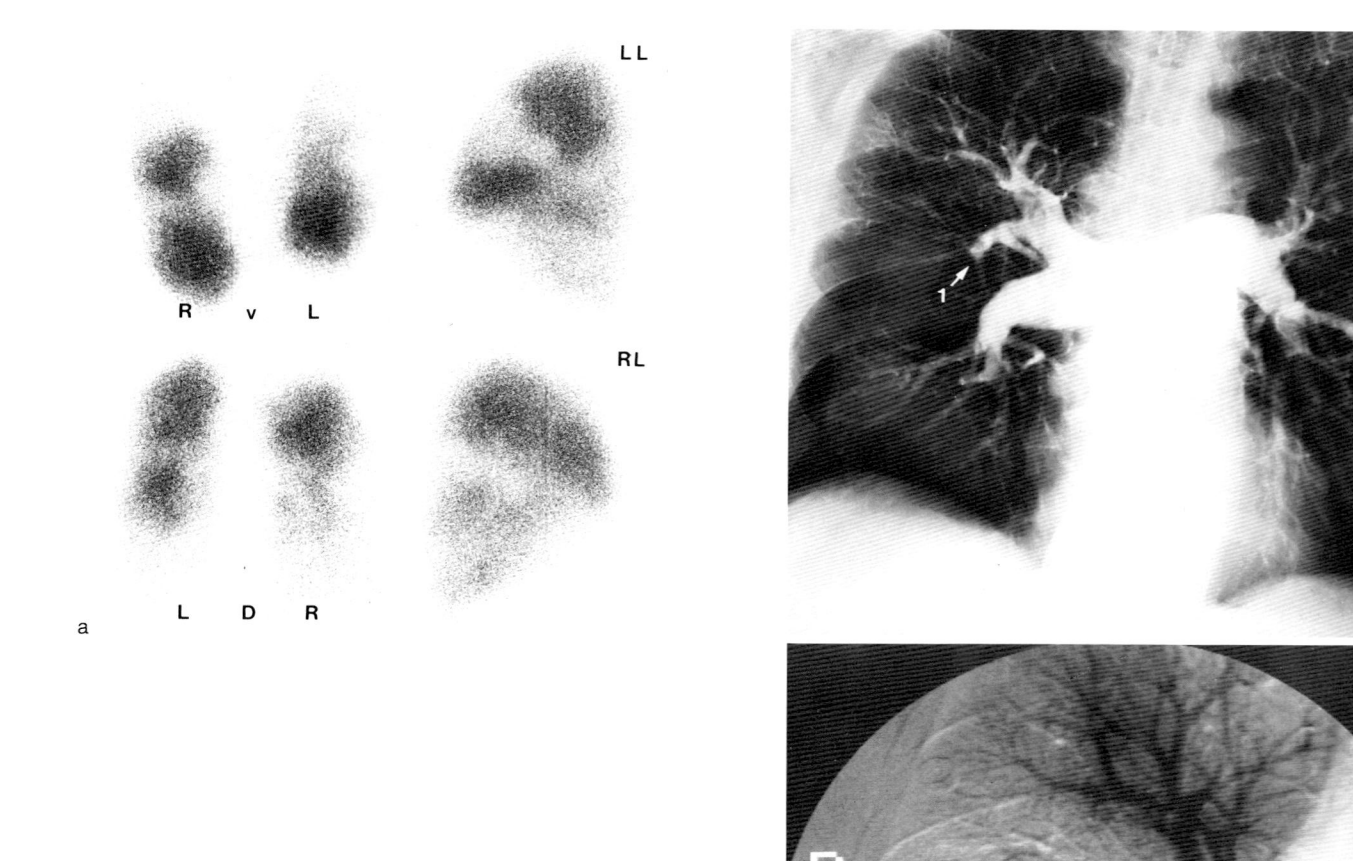

Fig. 6.15 a–c **Pulmonary embolism.**
76-year-old patient with known pancreatic carcinoma. Multiple, wedge-shaped perfusion defects seen on ventilation-perfusion scan. Pulmonary angiogram demonstrates abrupt cut-off of both anterior segmental pulmonary arterial branches (1 right, 2 left).

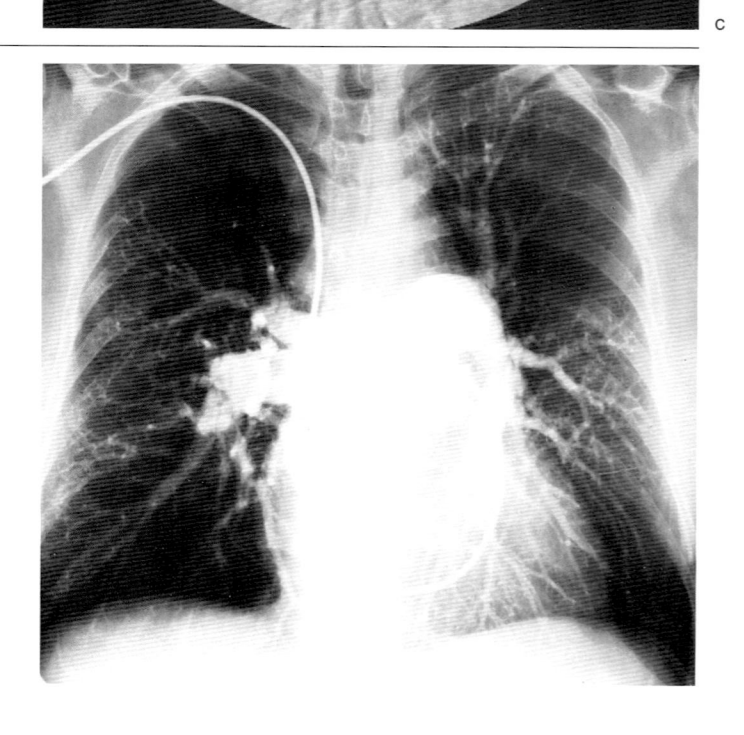

Fig. 6.16 **Pulmonary embolism.**
48-year-old patient, 5 days after orthopedic surgical procedure on knee joint. Pulmonary angiogram shows occlusion of right upper lobe pulmonary artery.

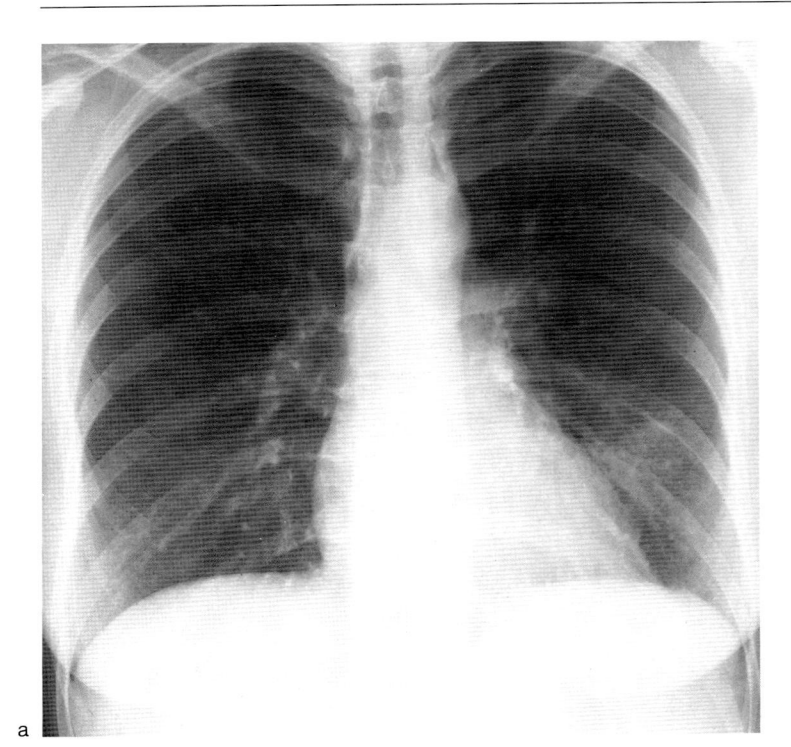

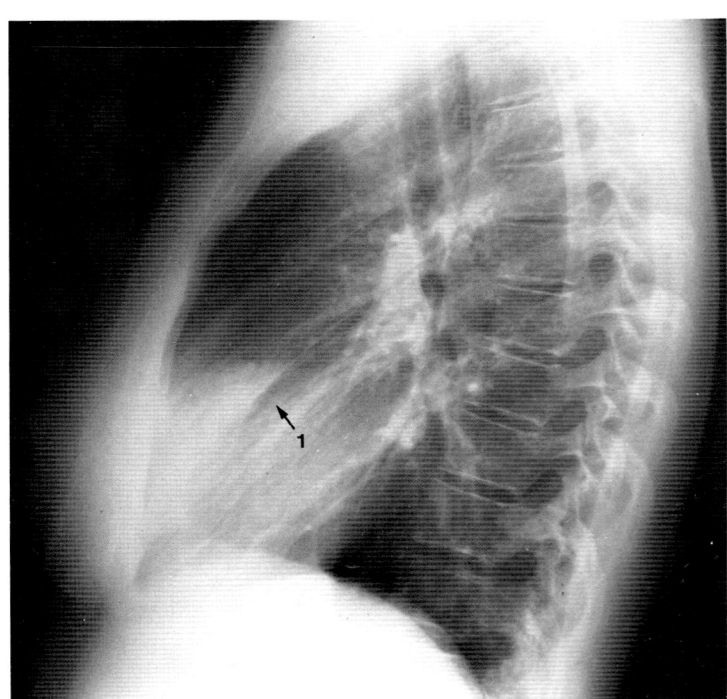

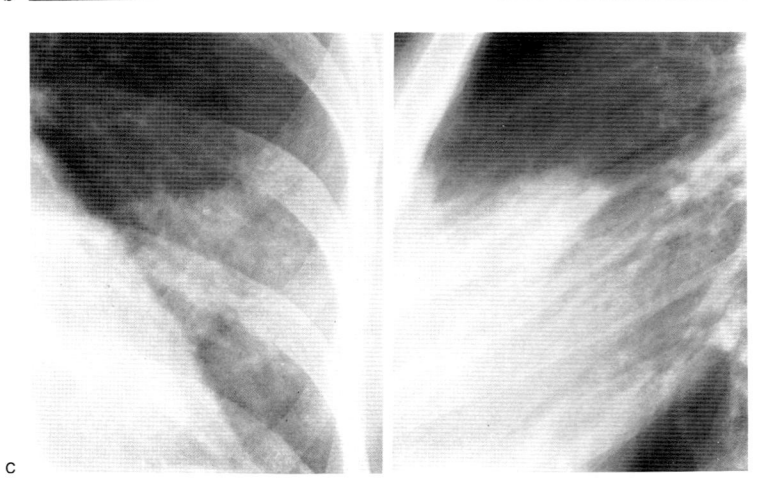

Fig. 6.17 a–c **Pulmonary infarct.**
27-year-old patient on oral contraceptives with chest pain, hemoptysis. Wedge-shaped opacity in superior segment of lingula.

Fig. 6.18 a–c **Pulmonary infarct.**
74-year-old patient with chronic left ventricular failure and acute episode of chest pain. Right basilar consolidation with discoid atelectasis. Perfusion scan shows right basilar perfusion defects. After a week, area of consolidation has diminished concentrically from the periphery (melting iceberg sign of Woesner).

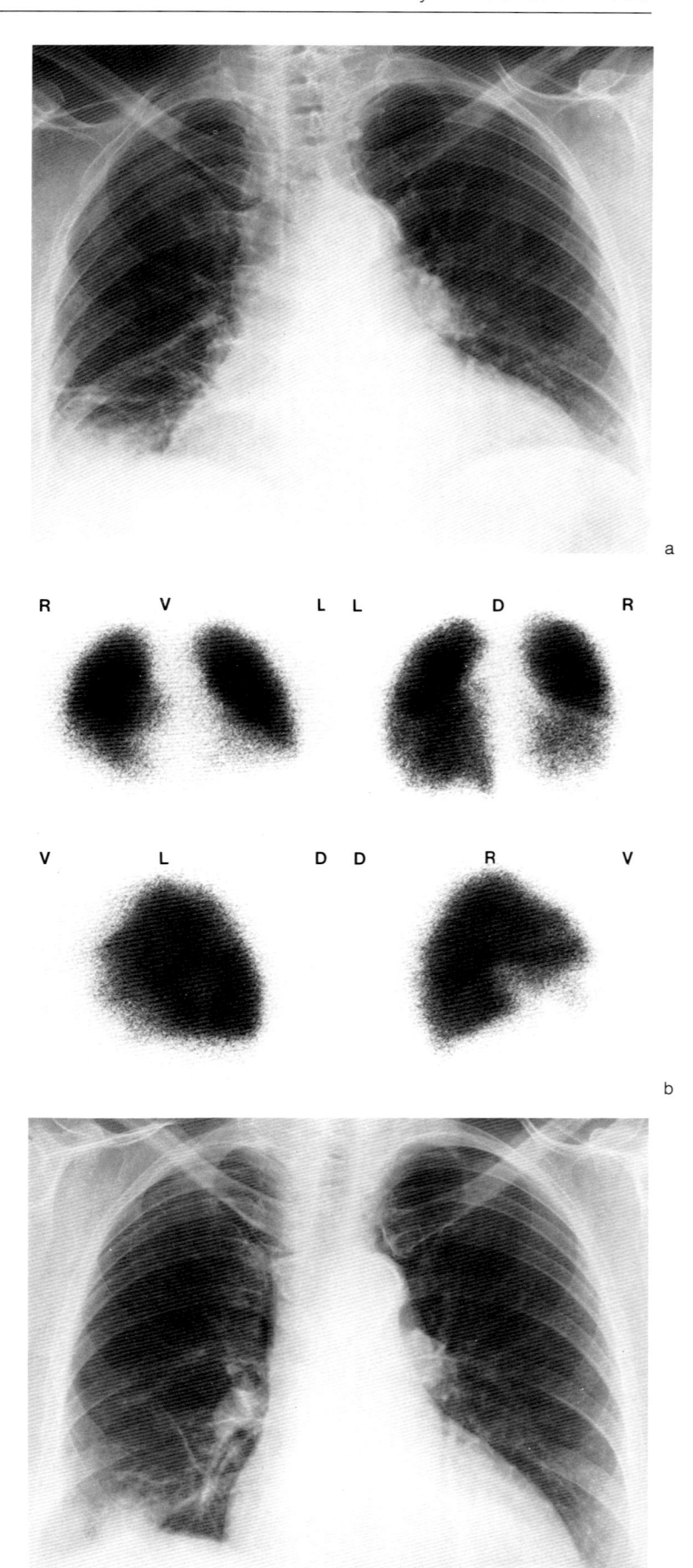

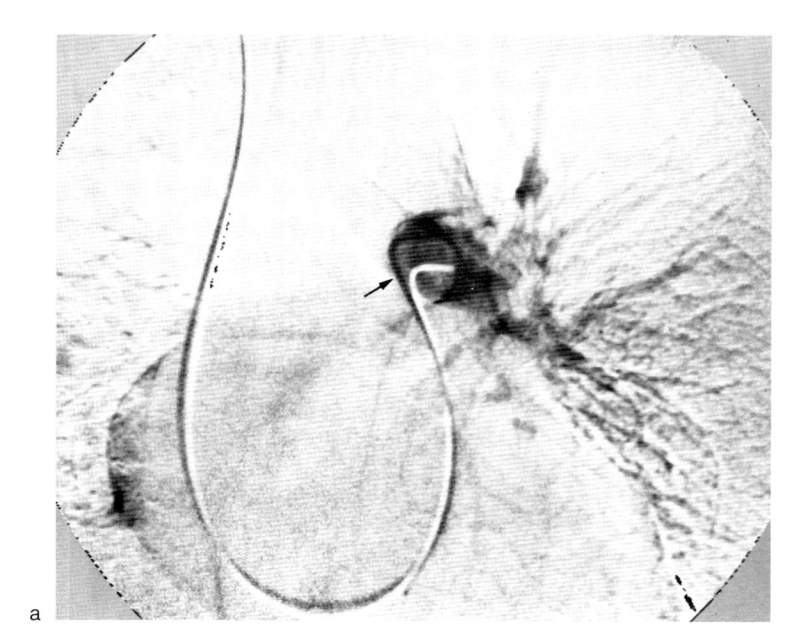

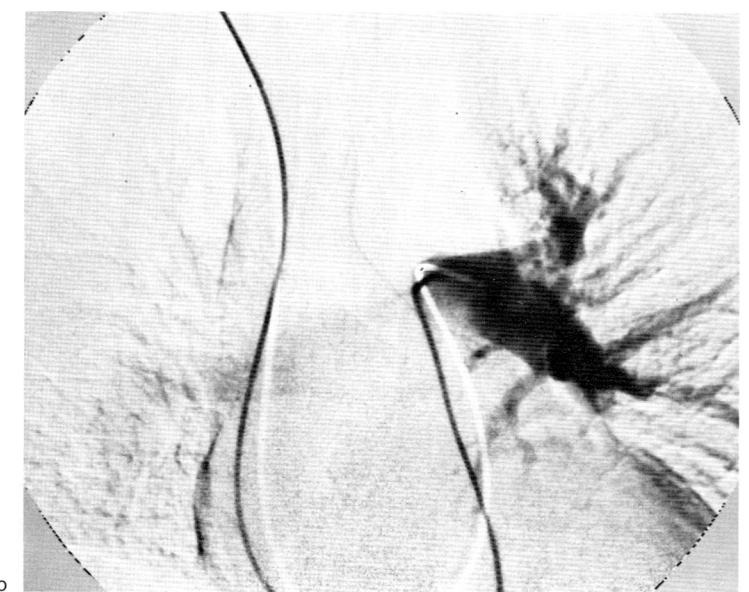

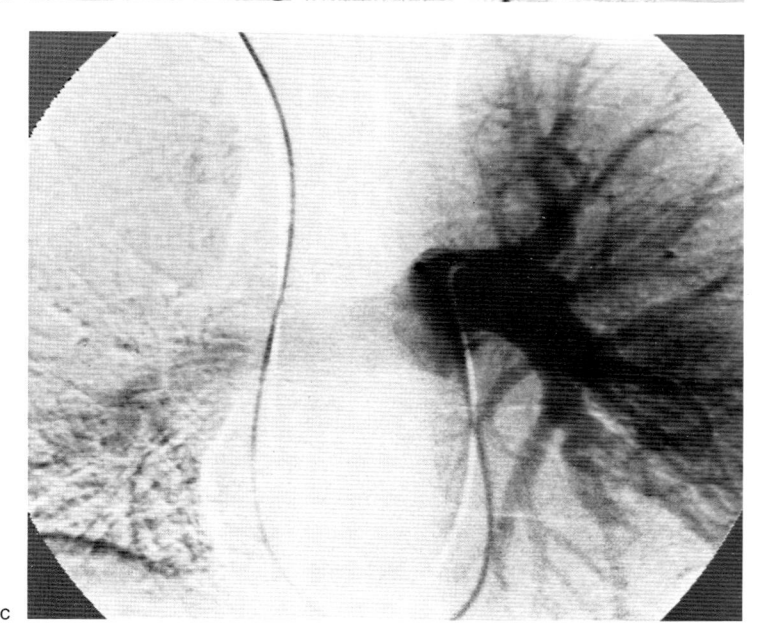

Fig. 6.19 a–c Transcatheter fibrinolytic therapy of pulmonary embolus.
Catheter impinges on thromboembolus and cannot be advanced further into pulmonary artery. Follow-up at 24 h (**b**) and 48 h (**c**) after streptokinase infusion. Recanalization of upper lobe and then lower lobe artery.

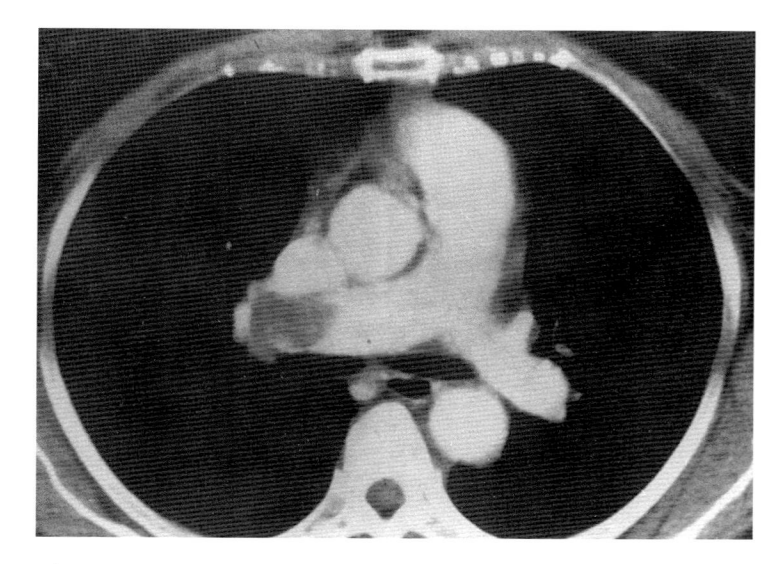

Fig. 6.20 **Pulmonary embolus in right pulmonary artery.** Contrast-enhanced CT scan reveals a low-attenuation filling defect in distal intrapericardiac segment of right pulmonary artery.

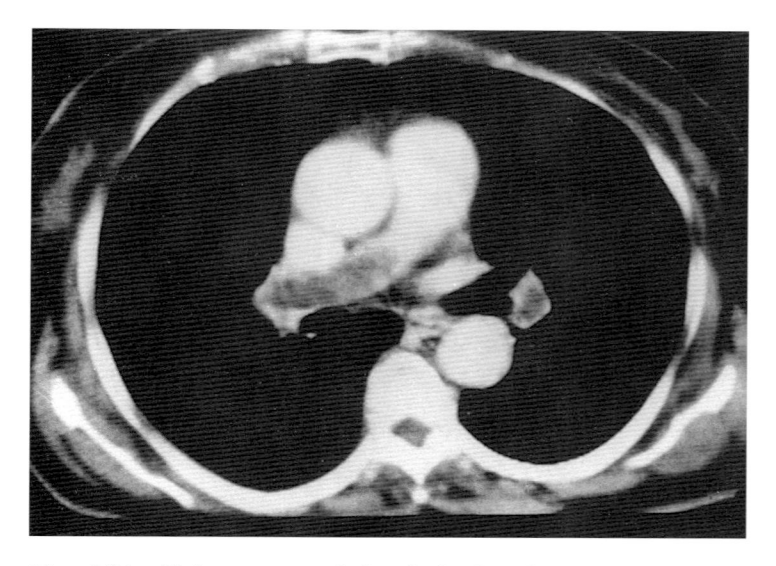

Fig. 6.21 **Pulmonary embolus in both pulmonary arteries.** Contrast-enhanced CT scan shows low-attenuation filling defects in right intrapericardiac pulmonary artery and left lower lobe pulmonary artery.

Discoid Atelectasis

Discoid atelectasis, also called plate-like or subsegmental atelectasis, is a frequent finding and indicates a local disturbance in aeration. They tend to form in the vicinity of linear lung scars and accessory fissures. Theoretically, collateral ventilation through the pores of Kohn should avert the formation of subsegmental atelectasis. A bland alveolitis with a lack of surfactant and temporary occlusion of the collateral pathways in tandem with obstruction of a small bronchus has to be postulated. Radiologic features include bands of opacity 1–3 mm in thickness and 4–10 cm in length, always abutting the pleura. They occur preferentially in the lower lobes. Oblique discoid atelectasis usually abuts the major fissure.

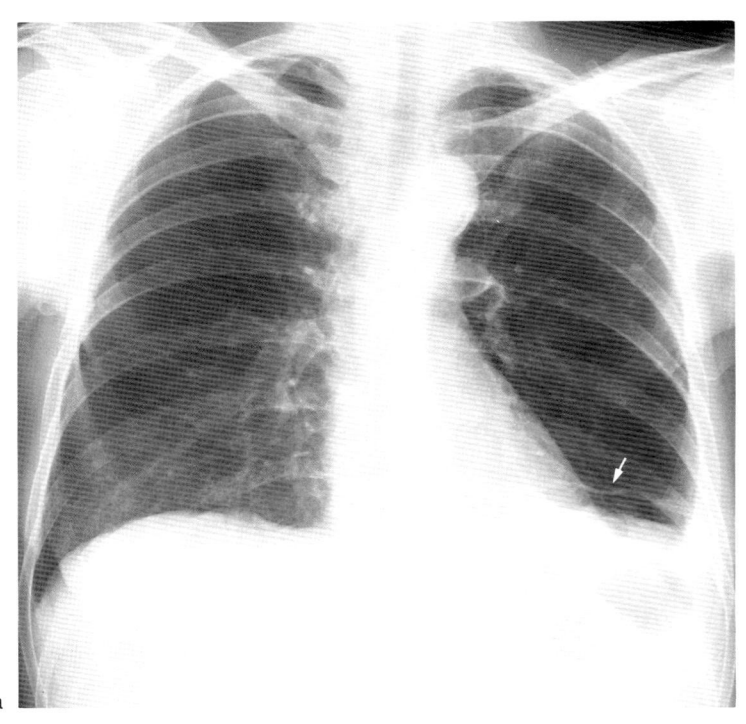

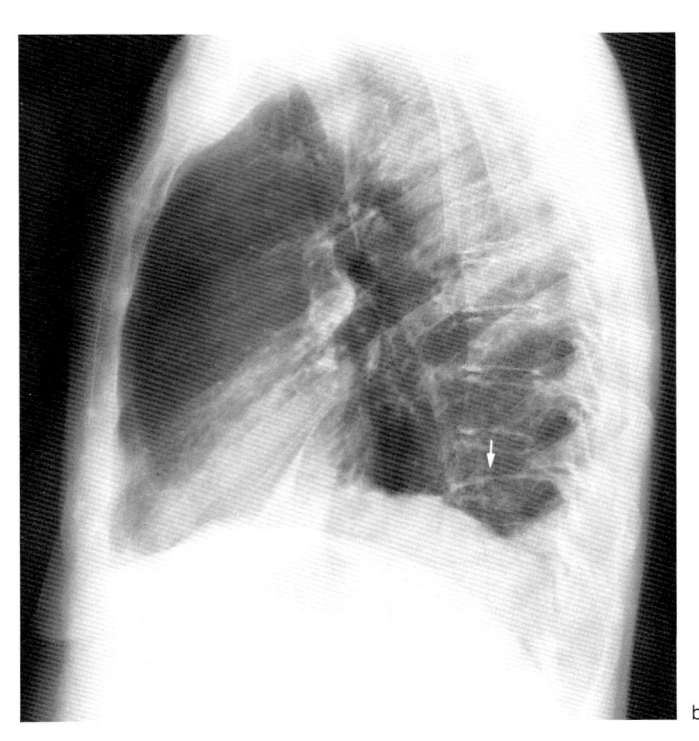

Fig. 6.**22 a, b   Discoid atelectasis.**
58-year-old patient with acute pancreatitis. Left pleural effusion. Slight elevation of left hemidiaphragm. Left basilar discoid atelectasis.

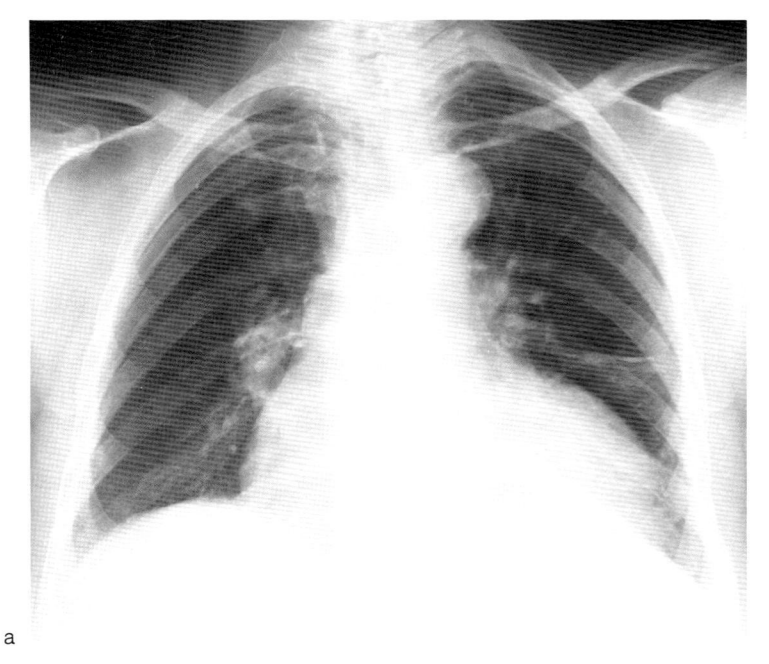

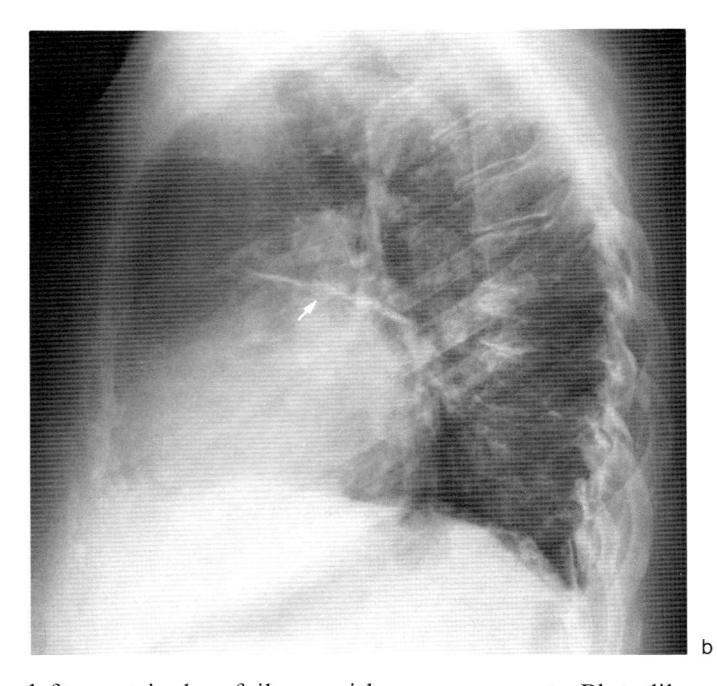

Fig. 6.**23 a, b   Discoid atelectasis.**
Chronic left ventricular failure with cardiomegaly and left ventricular failure with engorgement. Plate-like atelectasis in left lung.

7. Trauma

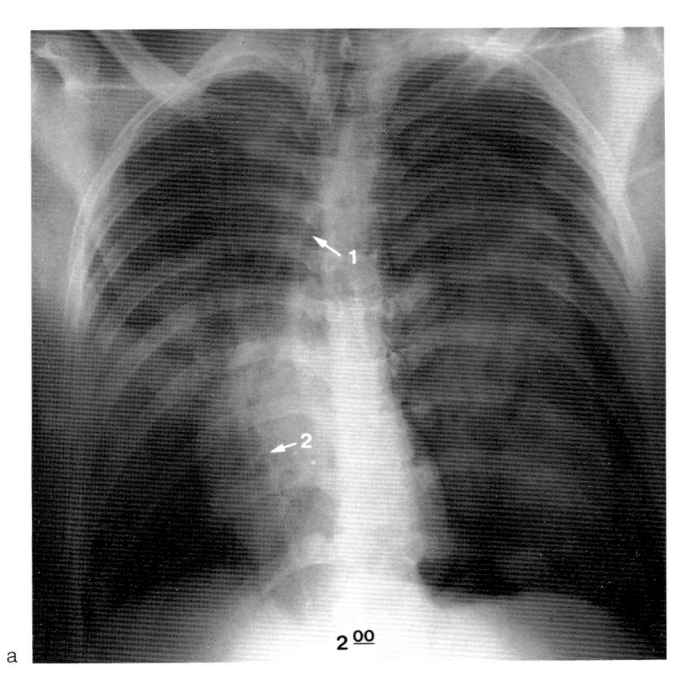

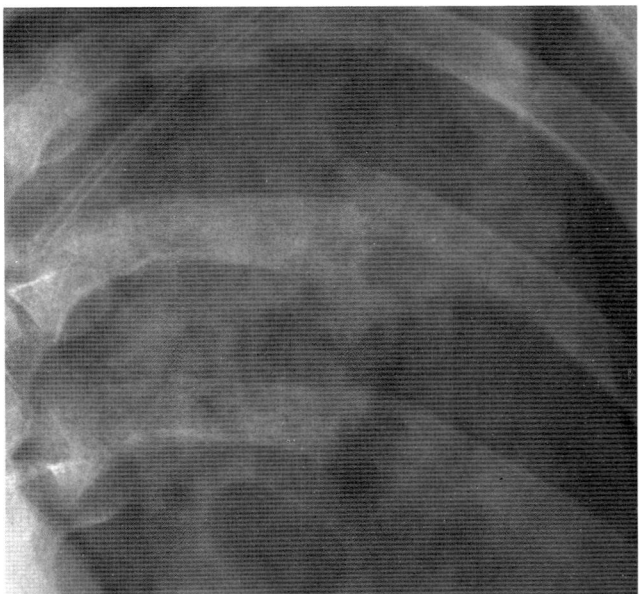

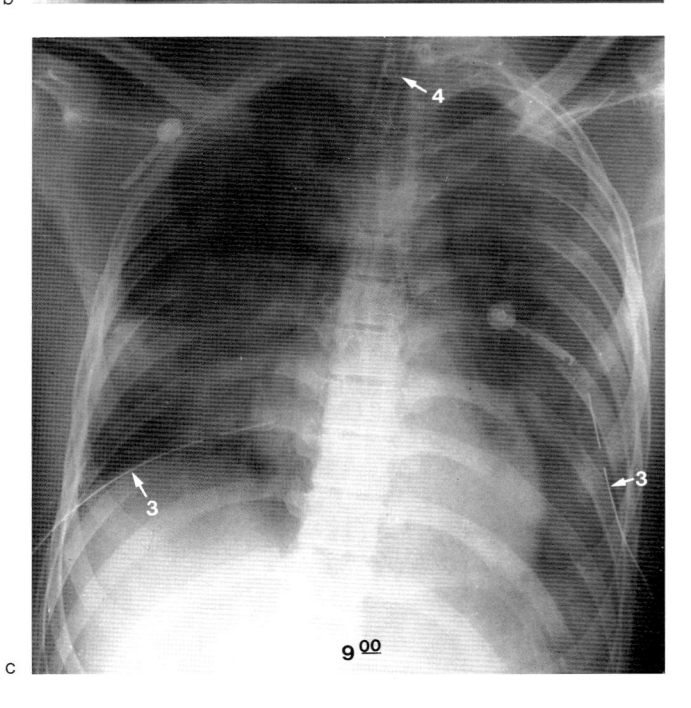

Traumatic Pneumothorax

Pneumothorax can be classified as closed simple, closed tension, or open. Blunt or penetrating trauma can lead to pneumothorax. Fractured ribs puncture the visceral pleura in two-thirds of cases, pulmonary laceration due to effects of inertial mechanisms, spallation, or implosion induce a pneumothorax in one-third.

Stab wounds are more likely to induce a pneumothorax than bullet wounds because the projectiles seal the pleura due to coagulation from the heat. Tension pneumothorax forms due to a check-valve mechanism that allows air to enter the pleural space in inspiration, yet traps it in expiration. The supra-atmospheric pressure build-up occurs in expiration and shifts the mediastinum to the contralateral side. Compression of the normal lung can lead to respiratory failure. The venous return to the heart is not impaired in inspiration, since a markedly negative inspiratory pressure helps avoid venous congestion. A tension pneumothorax not influenced by chest tube suction should bring the possibili4y of tracheobronchial rupture to mind.

Fig. 7.1 a–c **Tension pneumothorax with acute respiratory failure.**
18-year-old patient after a motor vehicle accident. Multiple left-sided rib fractures. Mediastinal shift to the right, anterior junction line (1), increased permeability pulmonary edema, air bronchogram (2), thoracostomy tubes (3), endotracheal tube (4).

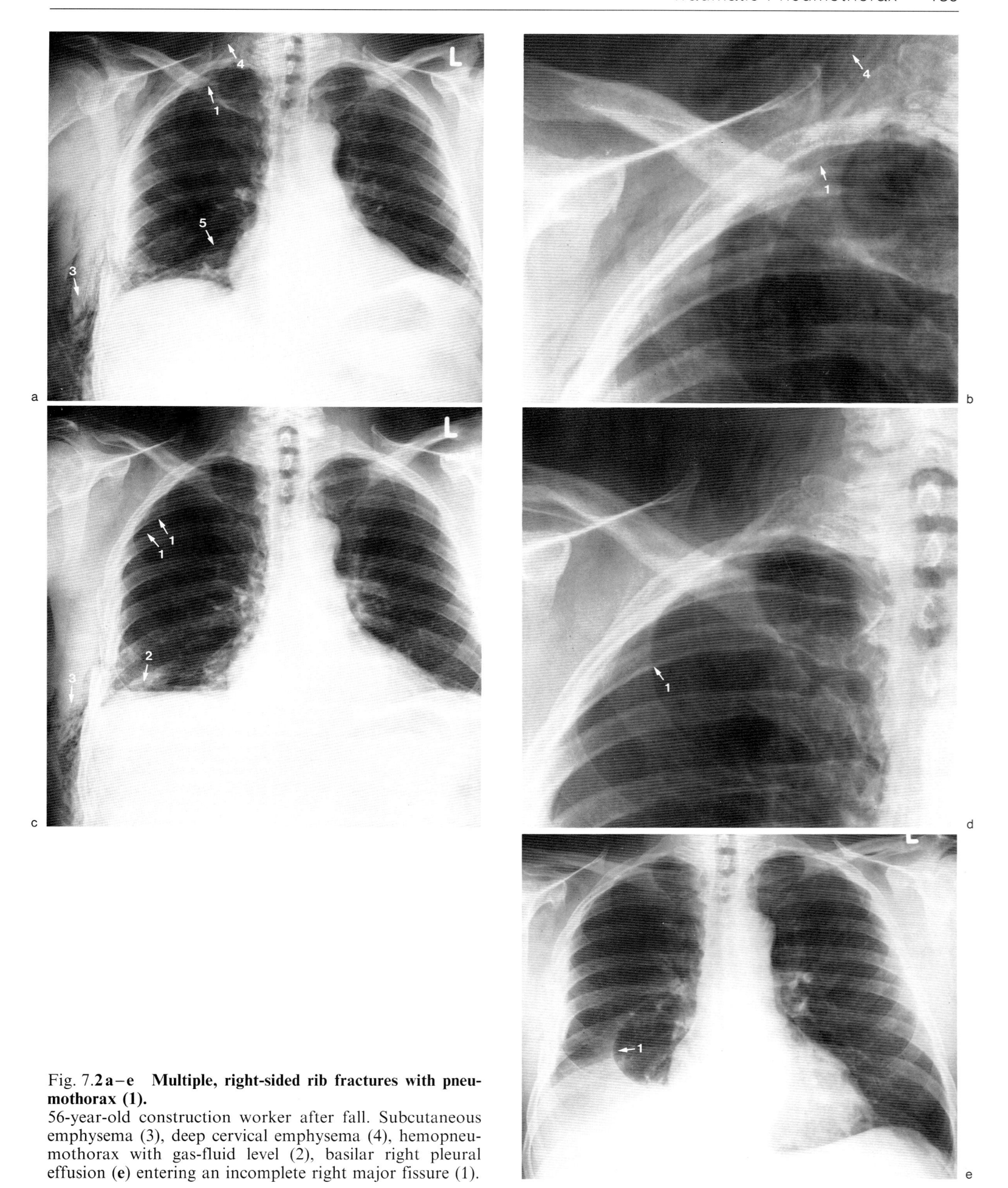

Fig. 7.2 a–e Multiple, right-sided rib fractures with pneumothorax (1).
56-year-old construction worker after fall. Subcutaneous emphysema (3), deep cervical emphysema (4), hemopneumothorax with gas-fluid level (2), basilar right pleural effusion (e) entering an incomplete right major fissure (1).

190   6. Vascular Disease

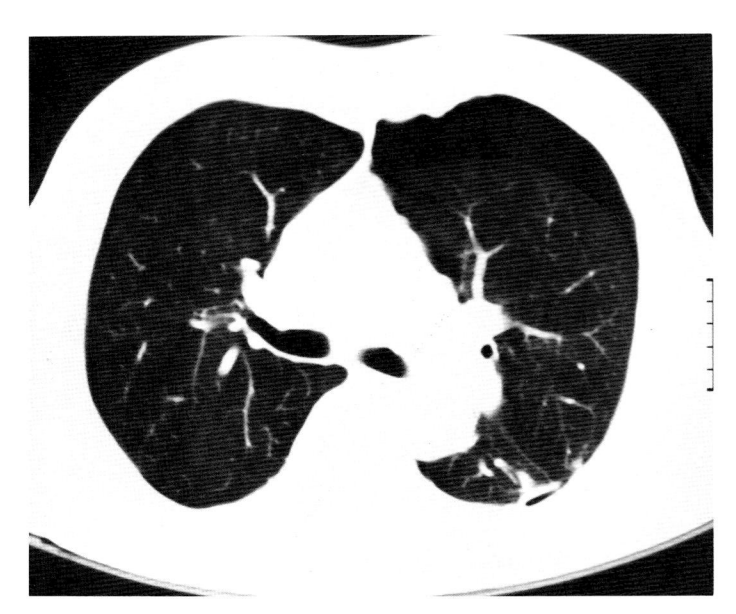

Fig. 7.3 **Posttraumatic left pneumothorax in supine patient.**
Free pleural air accumulates anteriorly.

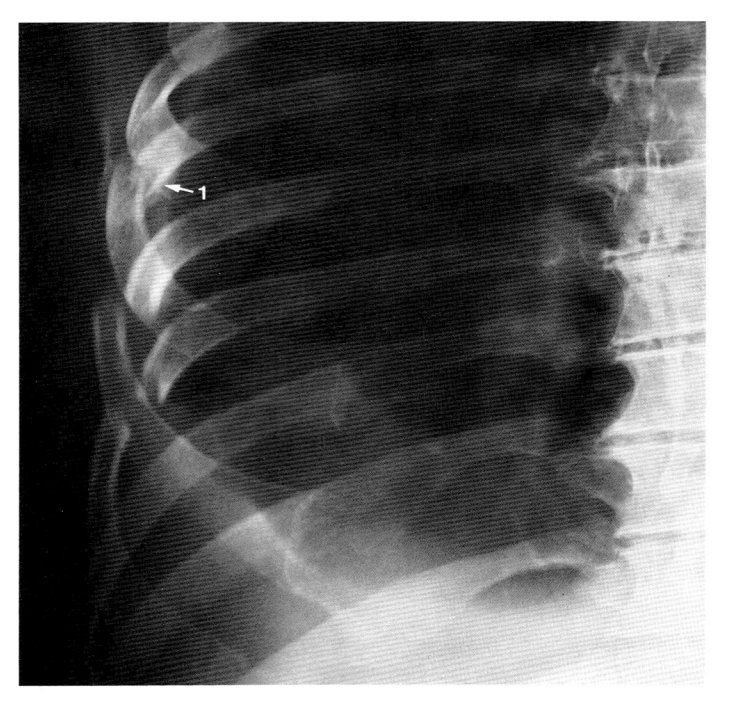

Fig. 7.4 **Displaced rib fractures with pleural hematoma (1).**

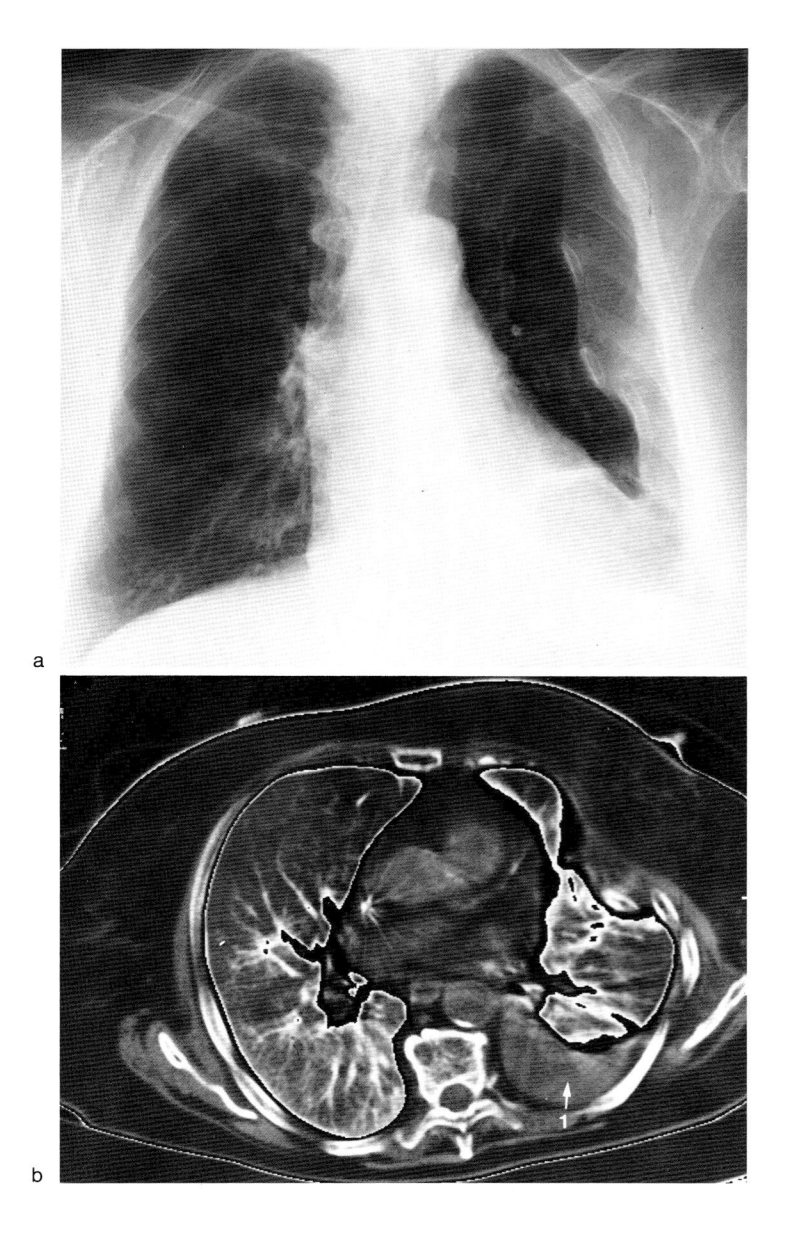

Fig. 7.5 a, b **Flail chest.**
Multiple segmental rib fractures with inward curving of chest wall. Hemothorax (1).

Pneumomediastinum

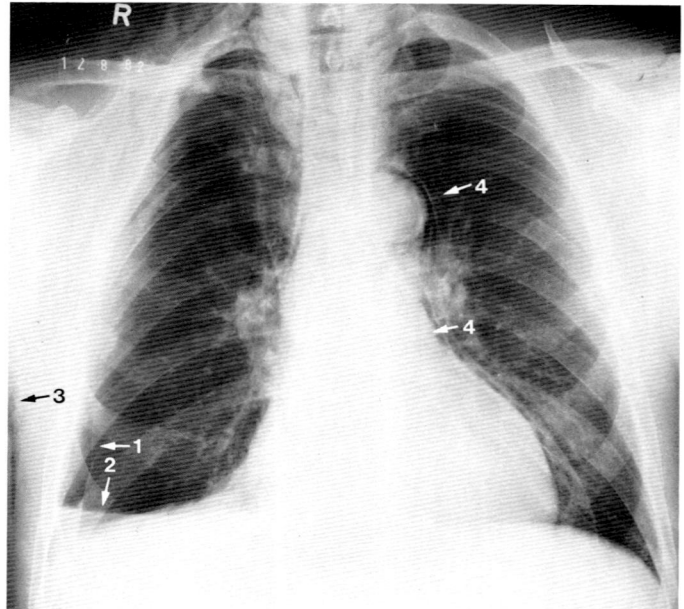

Fig. 7.6 54-year-old coal worker. Multiple, right-sided rib fractures, hemopneumothorax (1) with gas-fluid level (2), subcutaneous emphysema (3), pneumomediastinum (4).

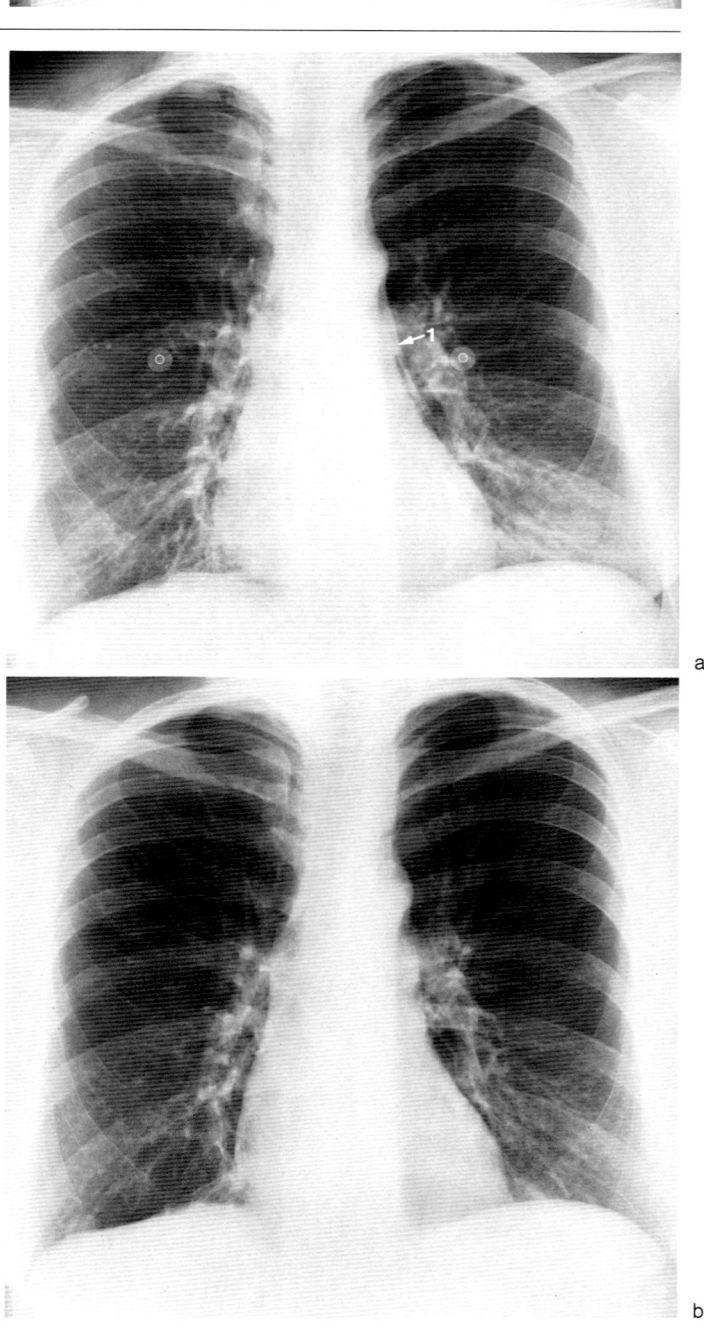

Fig. 7.7 a, b **Pneumomediastinum (1).**
36-year-old patient after steering wheel injury. Separation of mediastinal pleura by interstitial air (**a**). One week later, pneumomediastinum resolved (**b**).

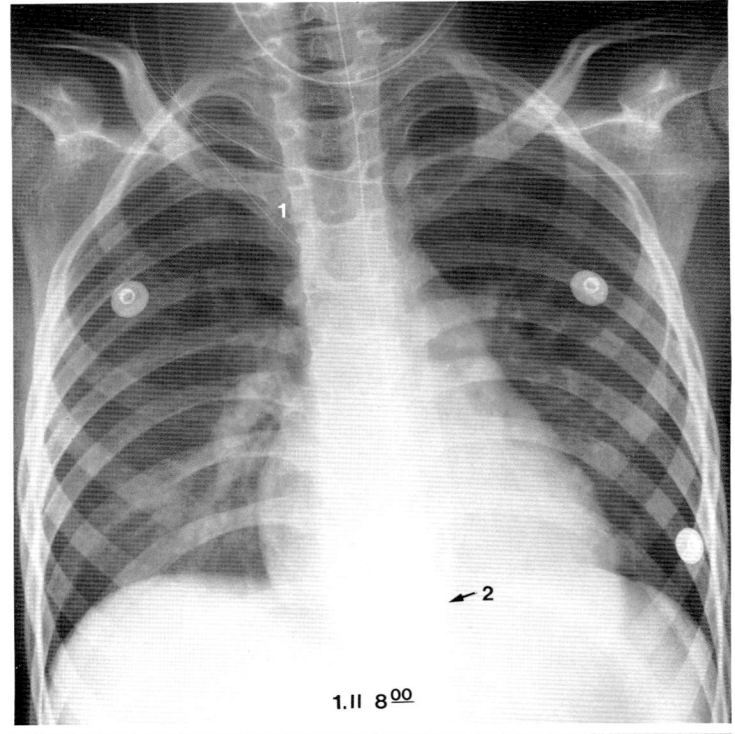

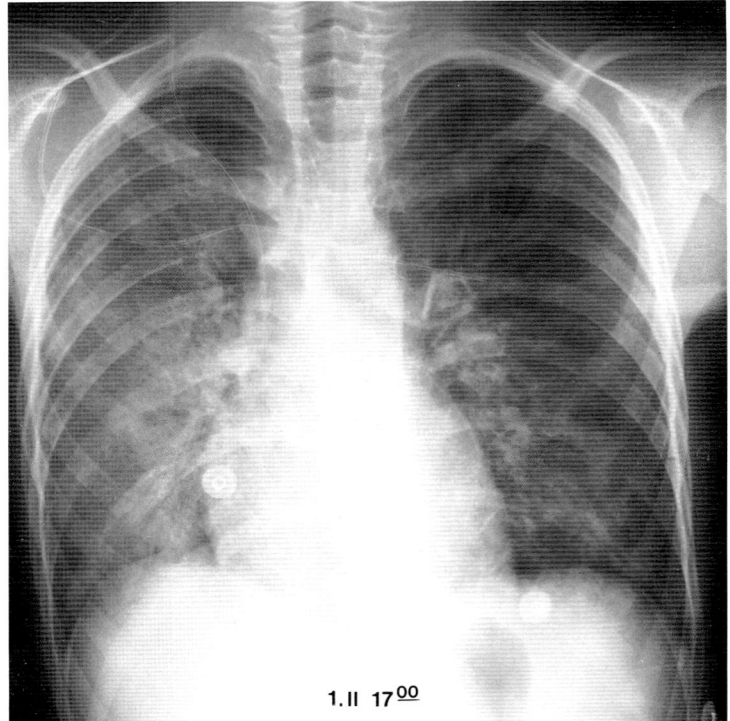

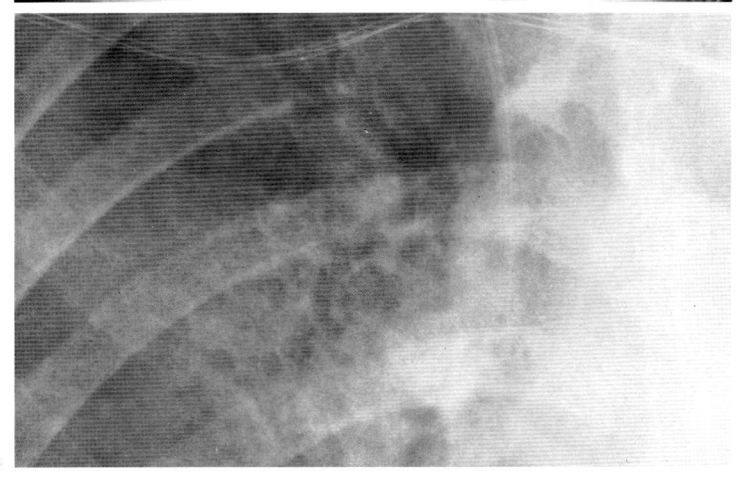

Adult Respiratory Distress Syndrome (ARDS)

ARDS or shock lung is a life-threatening disease with a 50–70% mortality. It represents a monotonous reaction of the lung to a wide array of noxious events, including hypovolemic shock, sepsis, aspiration, fat embolism syndrome, blood transfusions, and massive contusion.

Increased permeability pulmonary edema results from the interaction of leukocytes with the alveolocapillary membrane. Pathologically, the exudative phase lasts for 7–10 days and is followed by the proliferative phase, which eventually can lead to end-stage lung with intra-alveolar and interstitial fibrosis.

Radiologically, in the first 12–48 h, the lungs are clear and have low volumes. Only rarely are interstitial changes visible. Patchy, peripheral opacities appear, tend to become confluent, and exhibit air bronchograms. Ground glass opacification and microcystic changes follow, particularly in mechanically ventilated patients. Clinically, these patients are hypoxemic, have low pulmonary compliance, and require intubation and mechanical ventilation.

References: 60, 63, 86, 108, 130.

Fig. 7.8 a–h **Posttraumatic ARDS.**
11-year-old patient after car accident. Fracture of tibia and fibula. Three hours after the accident, ground glass opacification of both lung bases is present. Jugular venous catheter (1), nasogastric tube (2). Twelve hours after the accident, increased asymmetric opacification with involvement of entire lung. Air bronchogram (1) visible. After intubation, slight change in the pattern of consolidation (d–f). After extubation, 1 week after the accident, development of bibasilar pneumonia. Three weeks later (h), patient is asymptomatic and is discharged on crutches.

Adult Respiratory Distress Syndrome (ARDS) 193

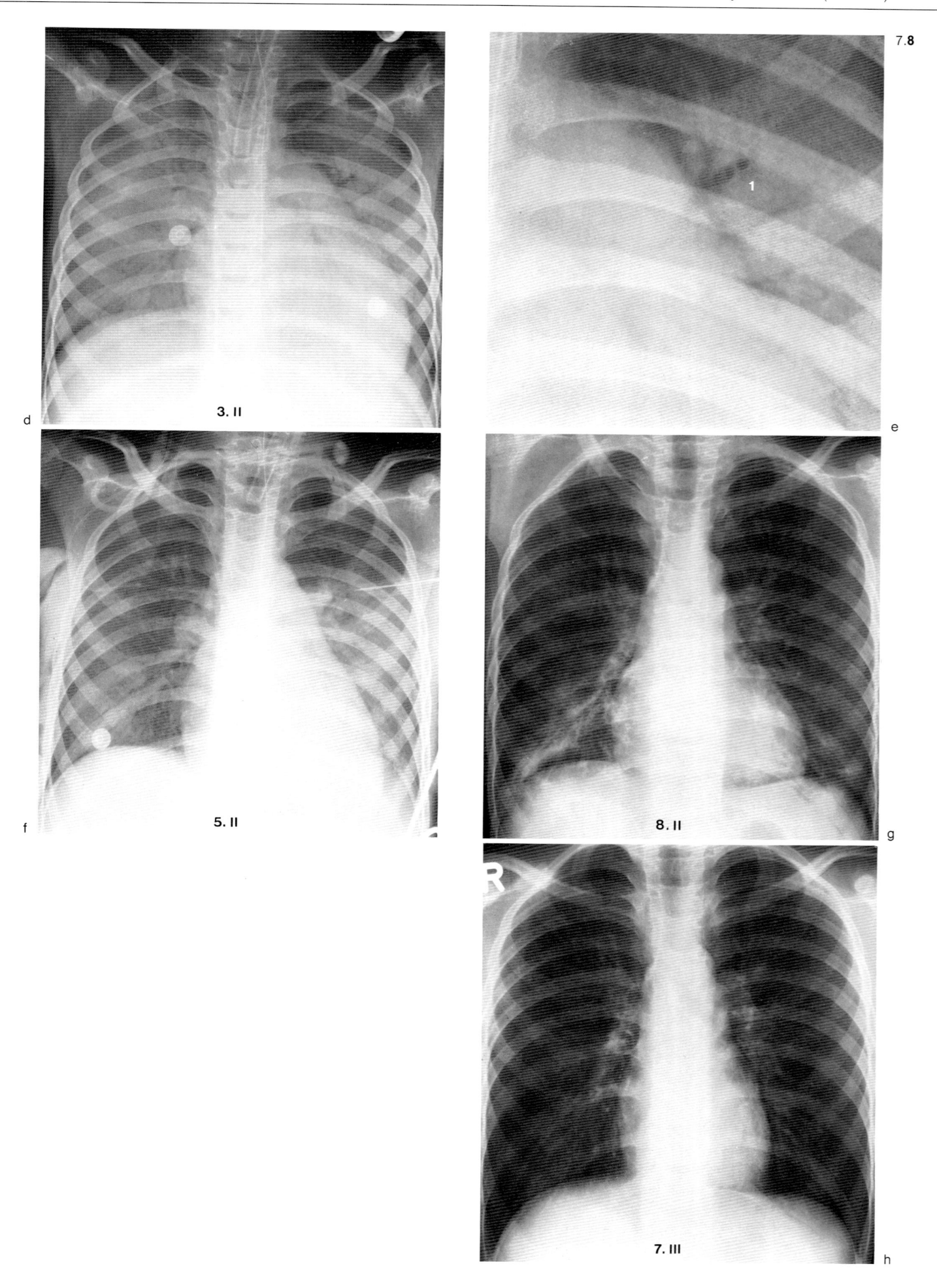

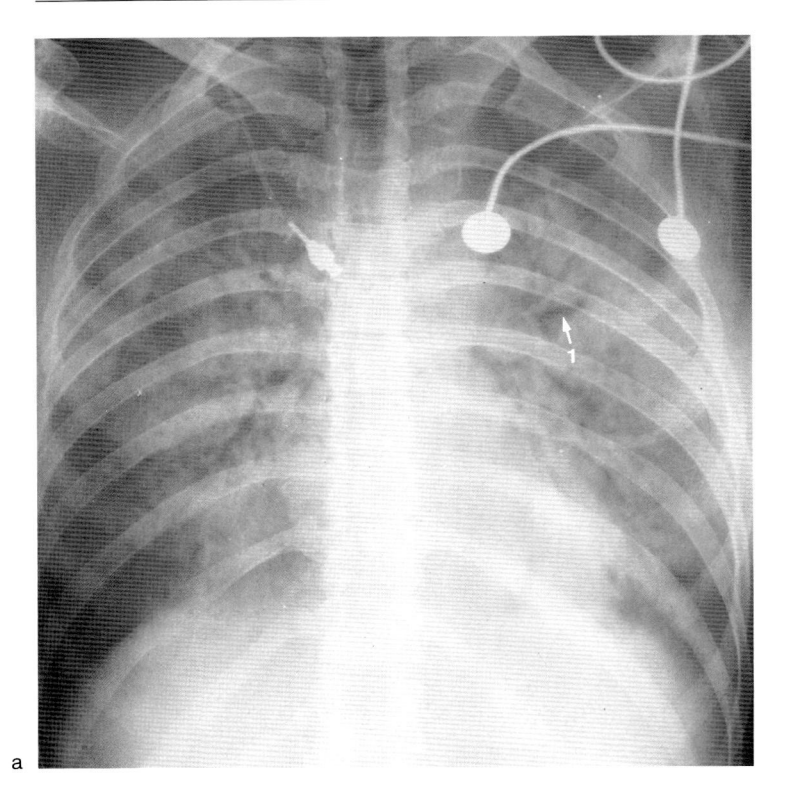

Fig. 7.9 a, b **Staphylococcal sepsis with fatal ARDS due to pyelonephritis.**
Confluent opacification of both lungs. Air bronchogram visible (1).

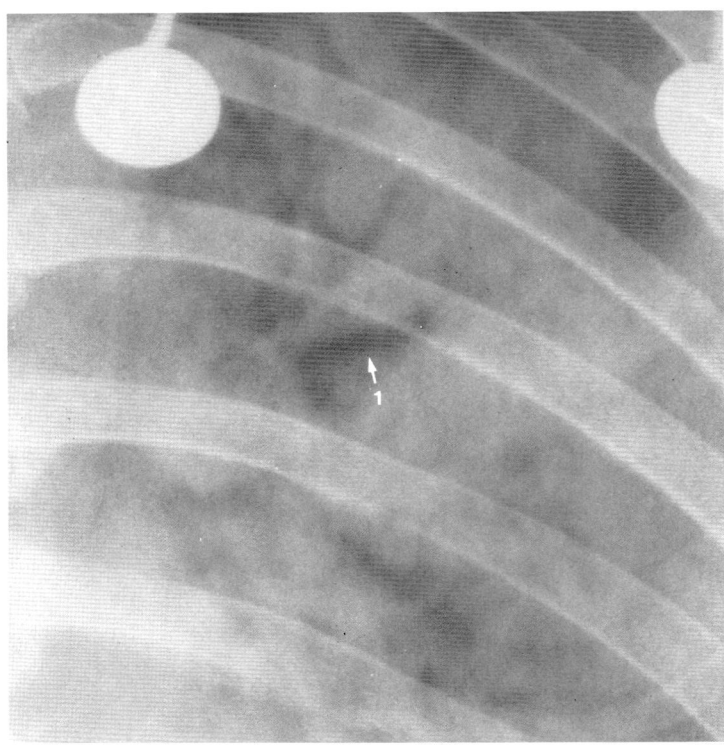

Adult Respiratory Distress Syndrome (ARDS) 195

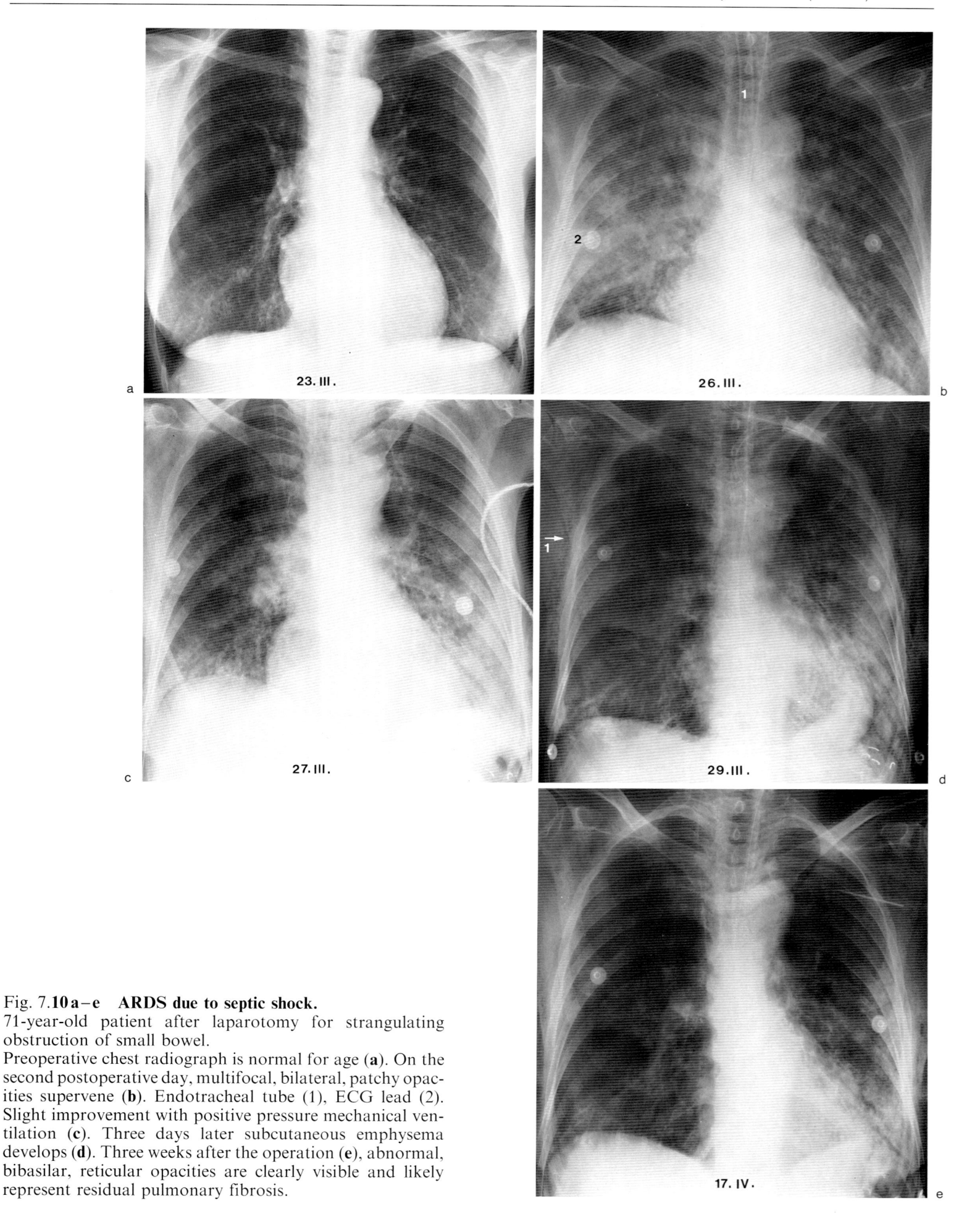

Fig. 7.10 a–e **ARDS due to septic shock.**
71-year-old patient after laparotomy for strangulating obstruction of small bowel.
Preoperative chest radiograph is normal for age (**a**). On the second postoperative day, multifocal, bilateral, patchy opacities supervene (**b**). Endotracheal tube (1), ECG lead (2). Slight improvement with positive pressure mechanical ventilation (**c**). Three days later subcutaneous emphysema develops (**d**). Three weeks after the operation (**e**), abnormal, bibasilar, reticular opacities are clearly visible and likely represent residual pulmonary fibrosis.

Pulmonary Contusion, Traumatic Pneumatocele

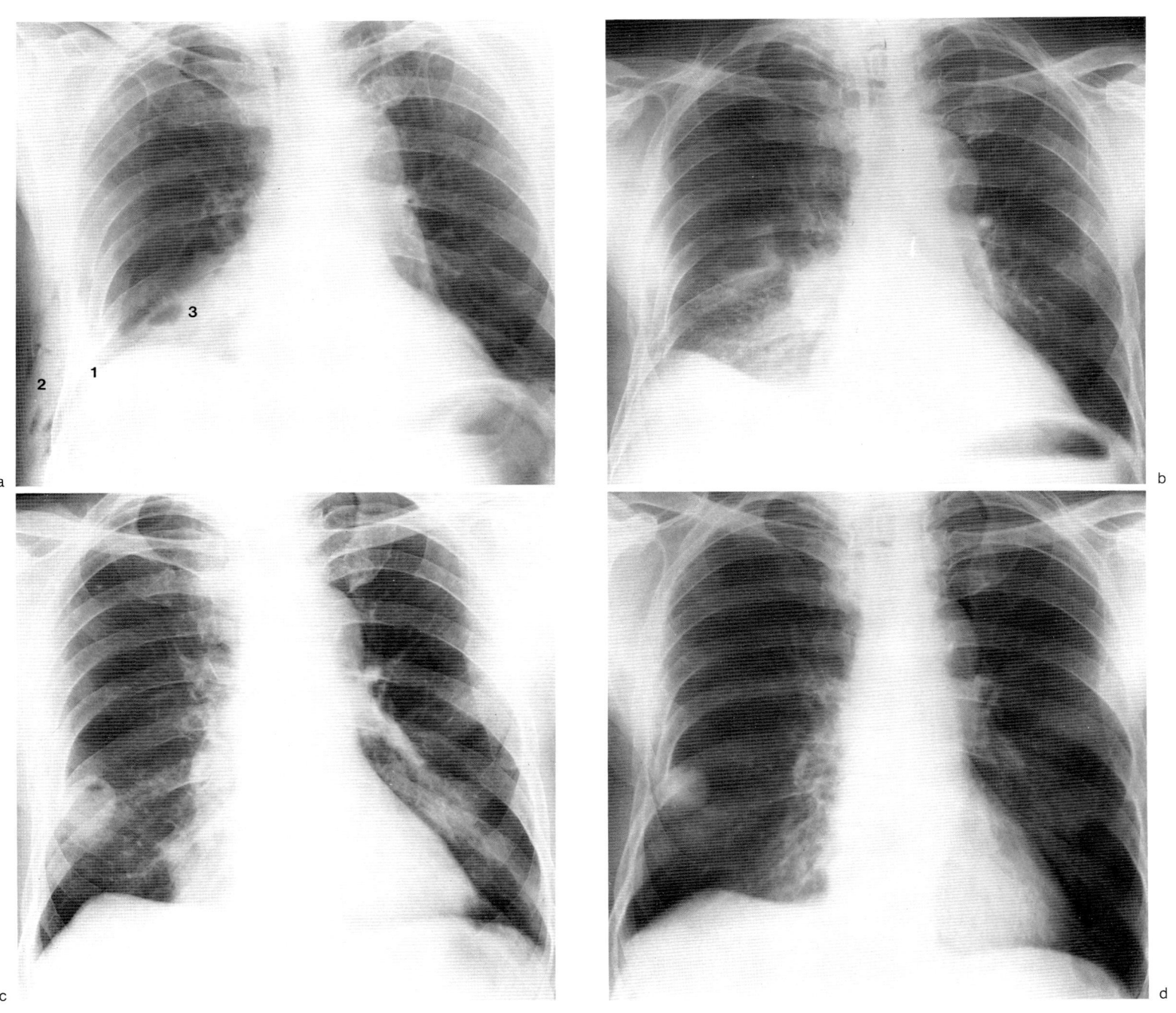

Fig. 7.**11 a–d** Multiple rib fractures in a 71-year-old patient after car accident led to traumatic pneumatocele. Blunted right costophrenic sulcus (1) due to hemothorax. Subcutaneous emphysema (2). Consolidated right lower lobe with cystic lucency within it. Progressive reexpansion and clearing of right lower lobe with formation of an intrapulmonary hematoma, due to accumulation of blood in the lacerated lung.

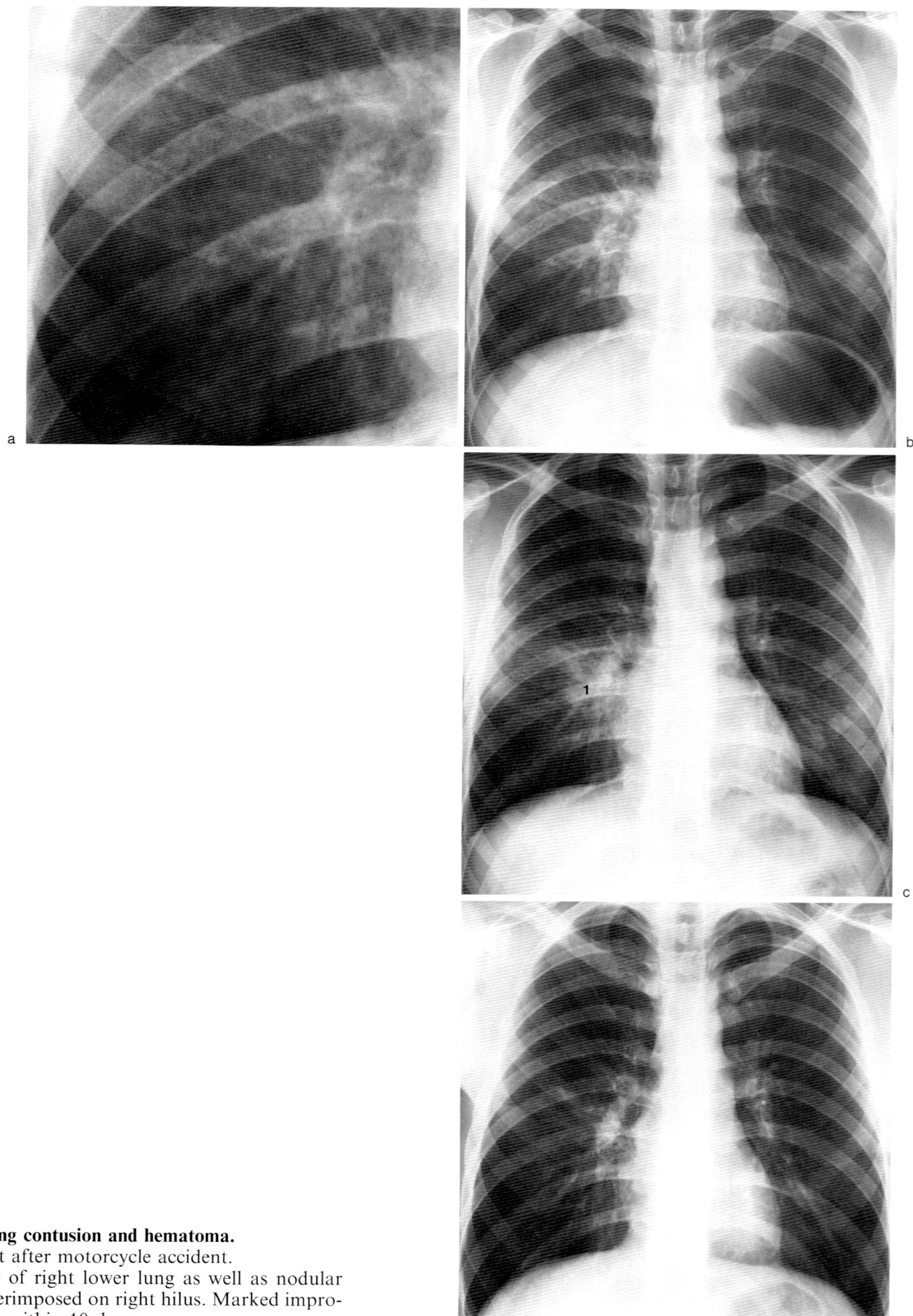

Fig. 7.**12 a–d Lung contusion and hematoma.**
18-year-old patient after motorcycle accident.
Ill-defined opacity of right lower lung as well as nodular hematoma (1) superimposed on right hilus. Marked improvement of findings within 10 days.

Lines, Tubes and Their Complications

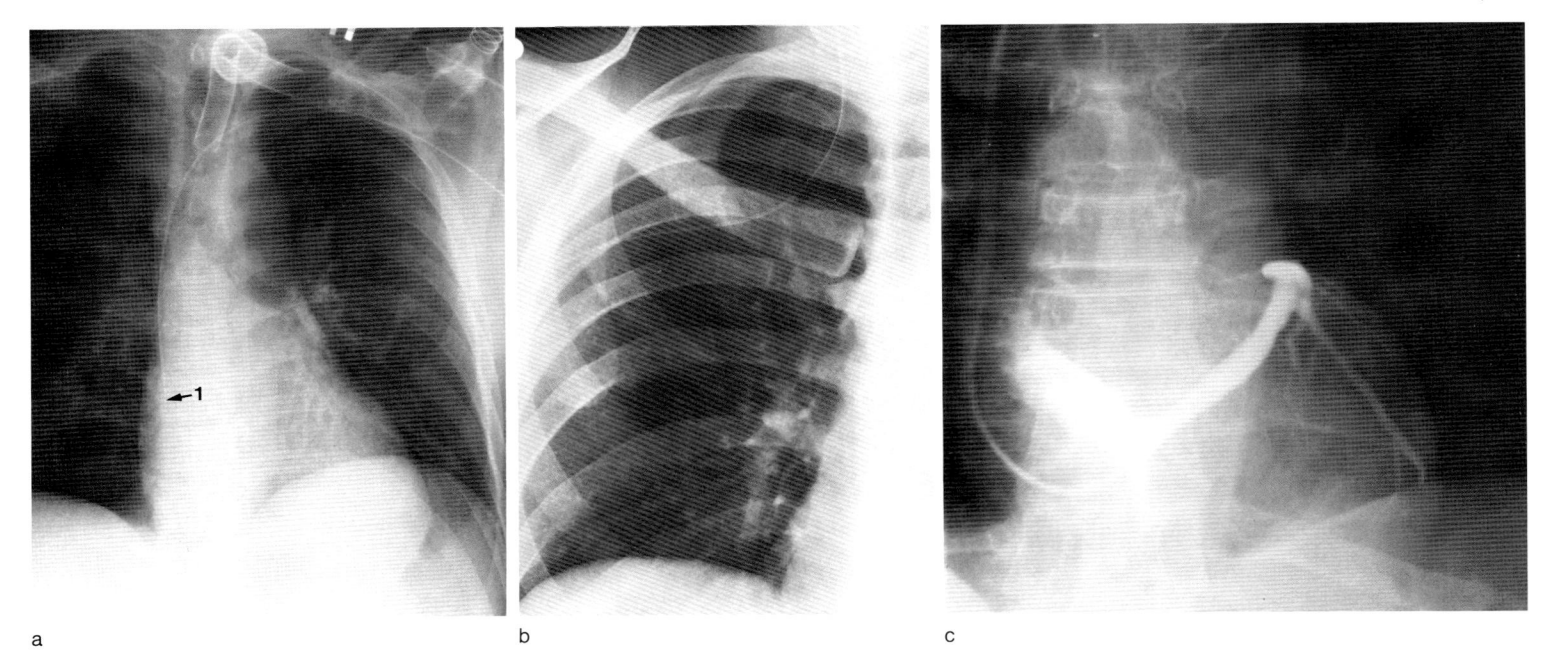

Fig. 7.**13a** Subclavian line in right atrium. **b** Subclavian line in internal jugular vein. **c** Central line enters coronary sinus.

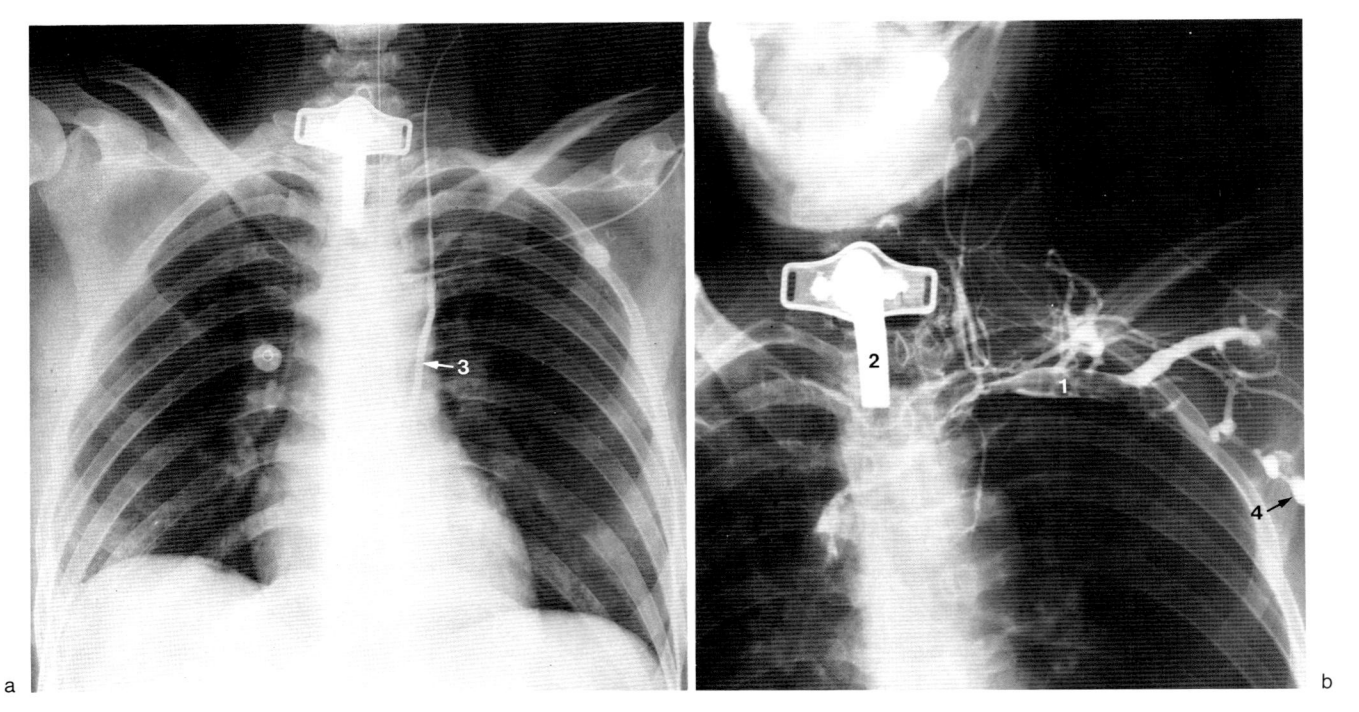

Fig. 7.**14a,b** Left jugular line in internal mammary vein in patient with 5-month-old thrombosis of left subclavian vein. Filling defect (1), tracheostomy tube (2), internal mammary vein (3), venous valves (4).

Fig. 7.**15** Pneumothorax after insertion of central venous line.

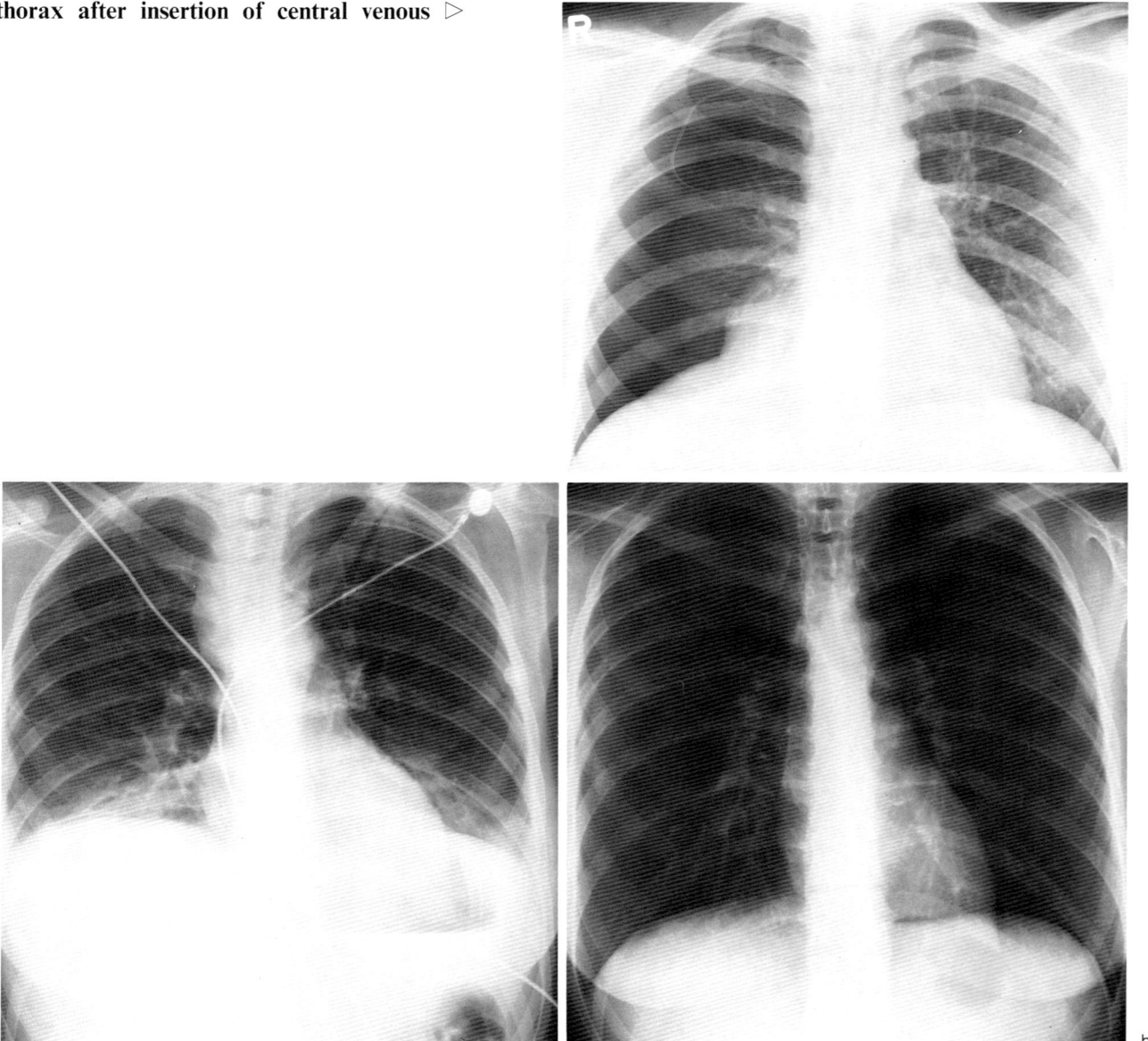

Fig. 7.**16 a, b** **Mediastinal hematoma as a sequel of right subclavian puncture.** Small pneumoperitoneum under right hemidiaphragm due to laparotomy (**a**). Two months later (**b**), normal chest.

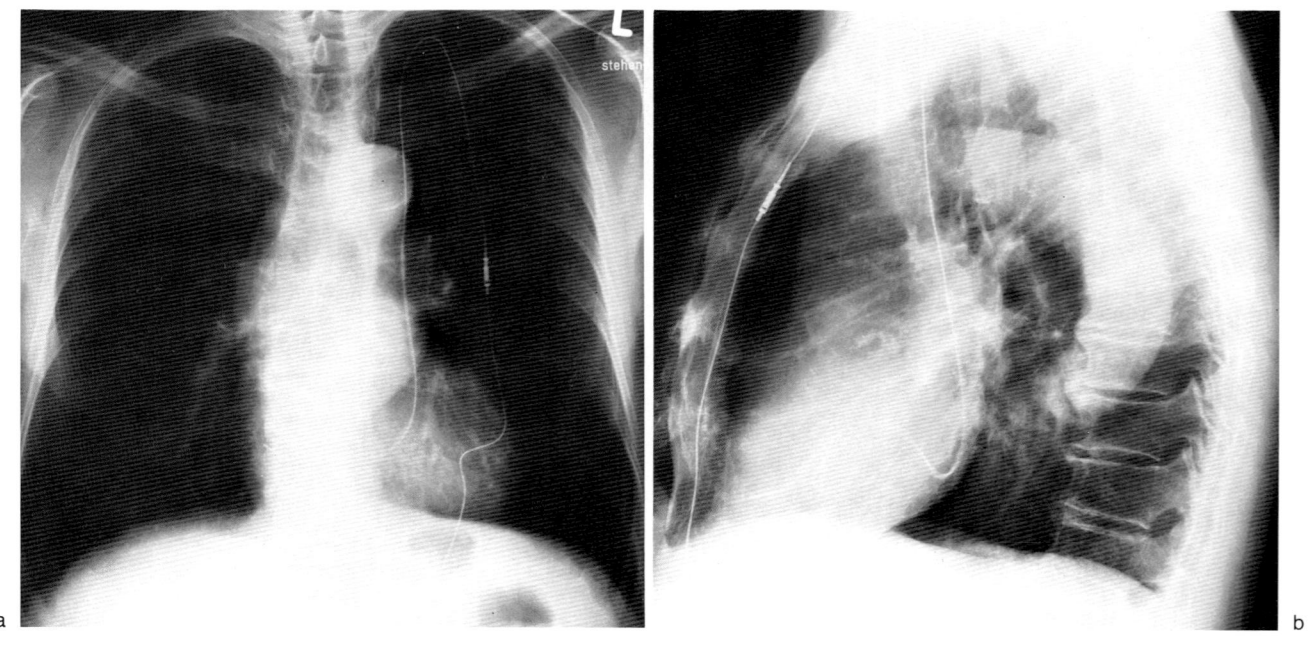

Fig. 7.**17 a, b** Left jugular line inserted into left persistent superior vena cava. Line enters right atrium through coronary sinus.

Postoperative Chest

Fig. 7.18 a–c Right hydrothorax after pneumonectomy.

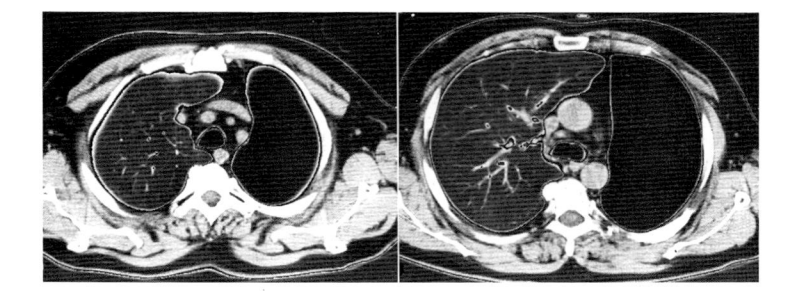

Fig. 7.19 Status after left pneumonectomy with vacant left hemithorax.

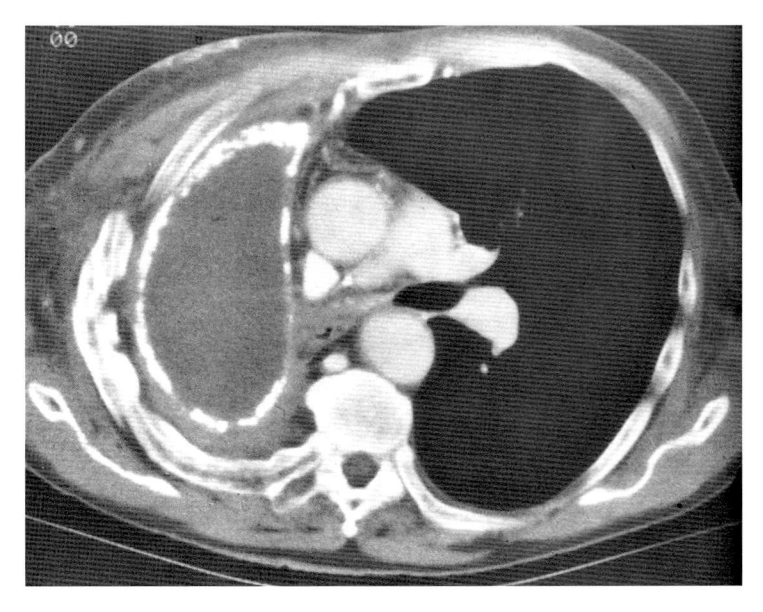

Fig. 7.20 **Status after remote right pneumonectomy for bronchogenic carcinoma.**
No tumor recurrence. Residual fluid in vacant hemithorax with shell-like calcification of parietal pleura and areolar tissue between calcification and ribs.

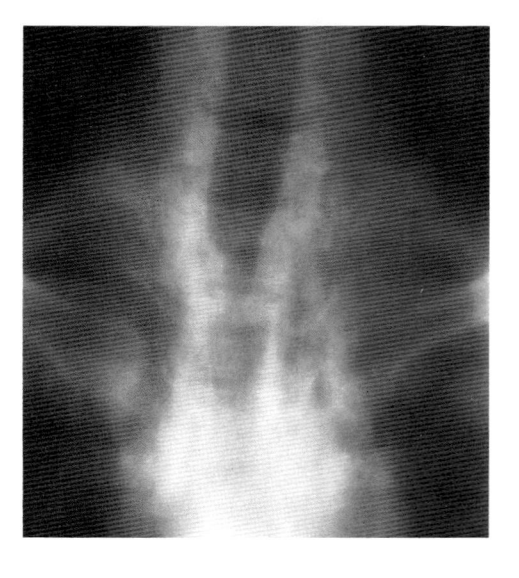

Fig. 7.21 Tracheal stenosis after tracheostomy.

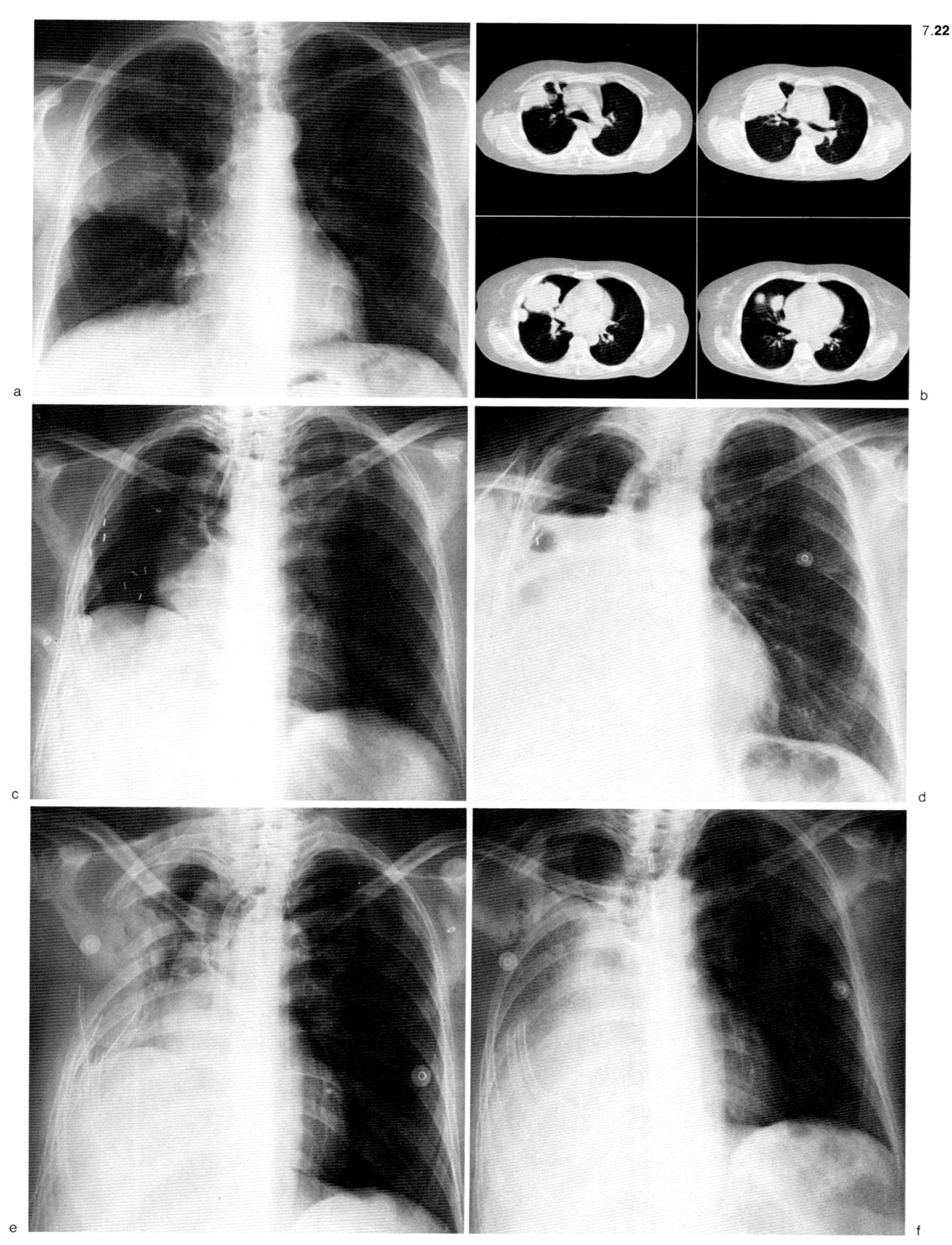

Fig. 7.22 a–f **Right-sided pneumonectomy for resection of primary pulmonary leiomyosarcoma.**
61-year-old patient presents with chest pain. Tumor diagnosed by percutaneous needle aspiration biopsy. Homogeneous, polycyclic, right upper lobe mass (**a, b**). Right pneumonectomy performed (**c**), surgical clips, elevation of right hemidiaphragm, rightward mediastinal shift, endotracheal tube. One week later, hydropneumothorax (**d**). Chest wall resection performed 2 weeks later because of microscopic chest wall invasion (**e**). Discharge film (**f**).

202   7. Trauma

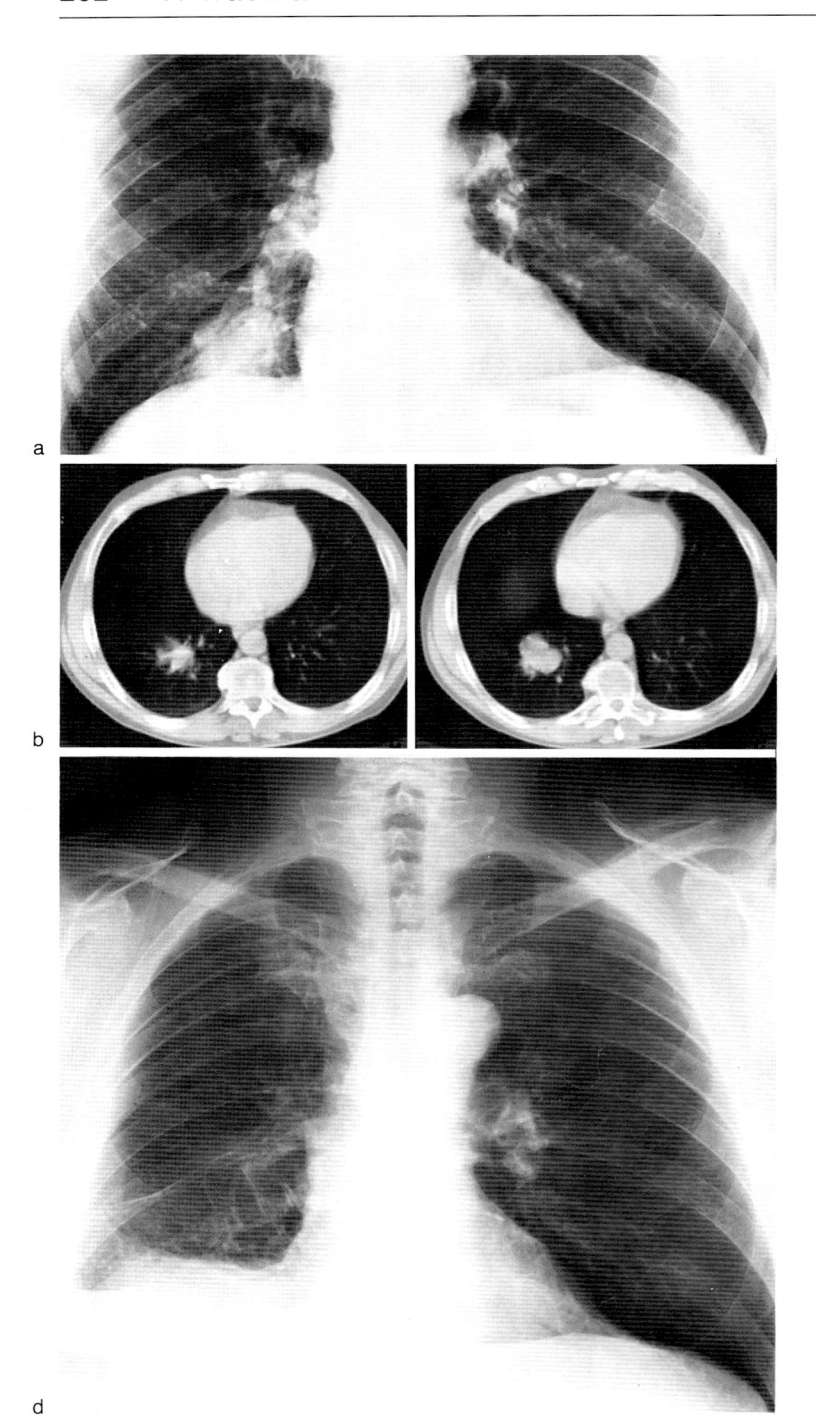

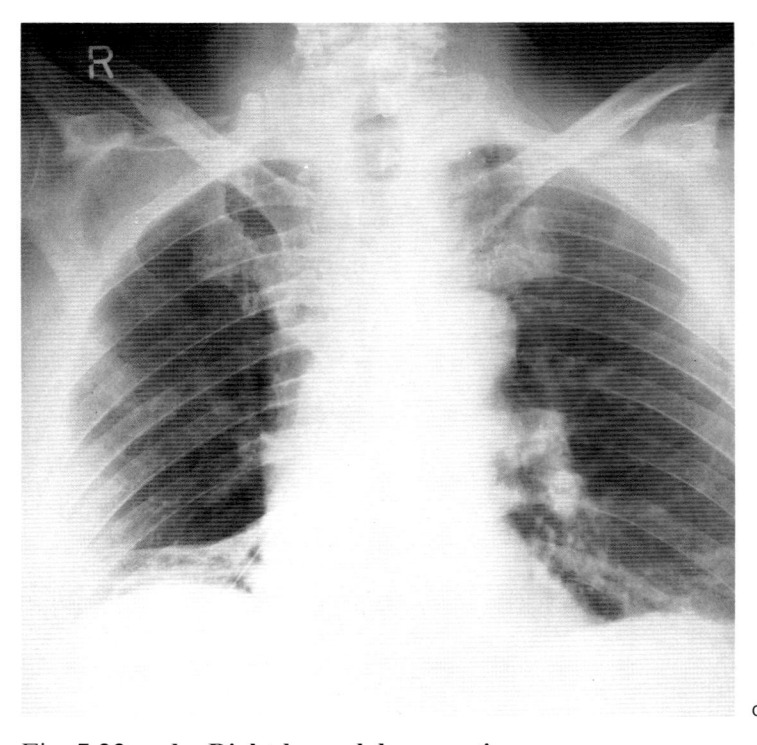

Fig. 7.23 a–d **Right lower lobe resection.**
59-year-old patient with squamous cell carcinoma of right lower lobe. Transient right middle lobe atelectasis. Right lower lobe tumor (**a, b**). Postoperative right middle lobe atelectasis (**c**). Delayed postoperative films show re-expansion of right middle lobe and right basilar pleural scarring. Right interlobular pulmonary artery is absent. Compensatory dilatation of left pulmonary artery.

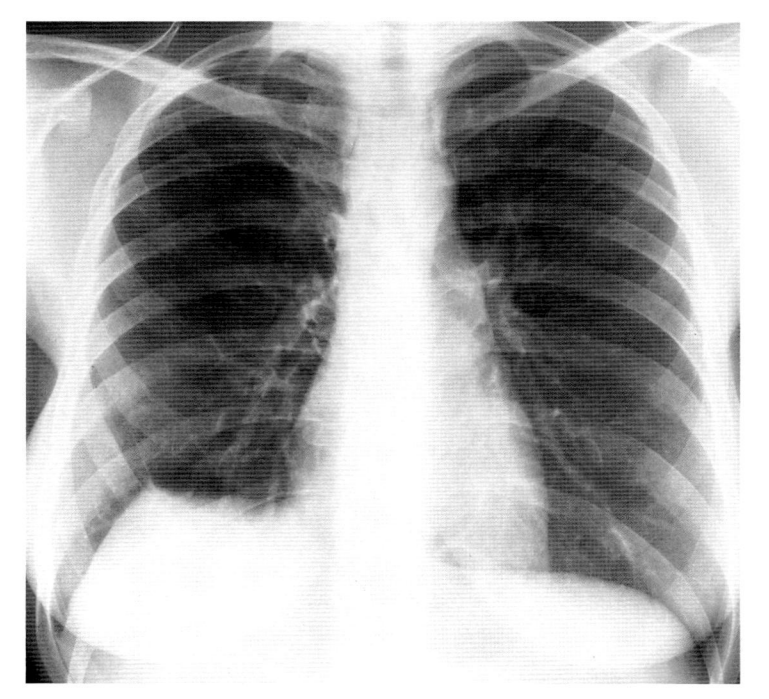

Fig. 7.**24** **Remote right upper lobe lobectomy.**
Right pulmonary artery elevated, right lung smaller and more lucent than left side. Right hemidiaphragm elevated with slight tenting of pleura ("juxtaphrenic peak"), typical of loss of volume in upper lobe region.

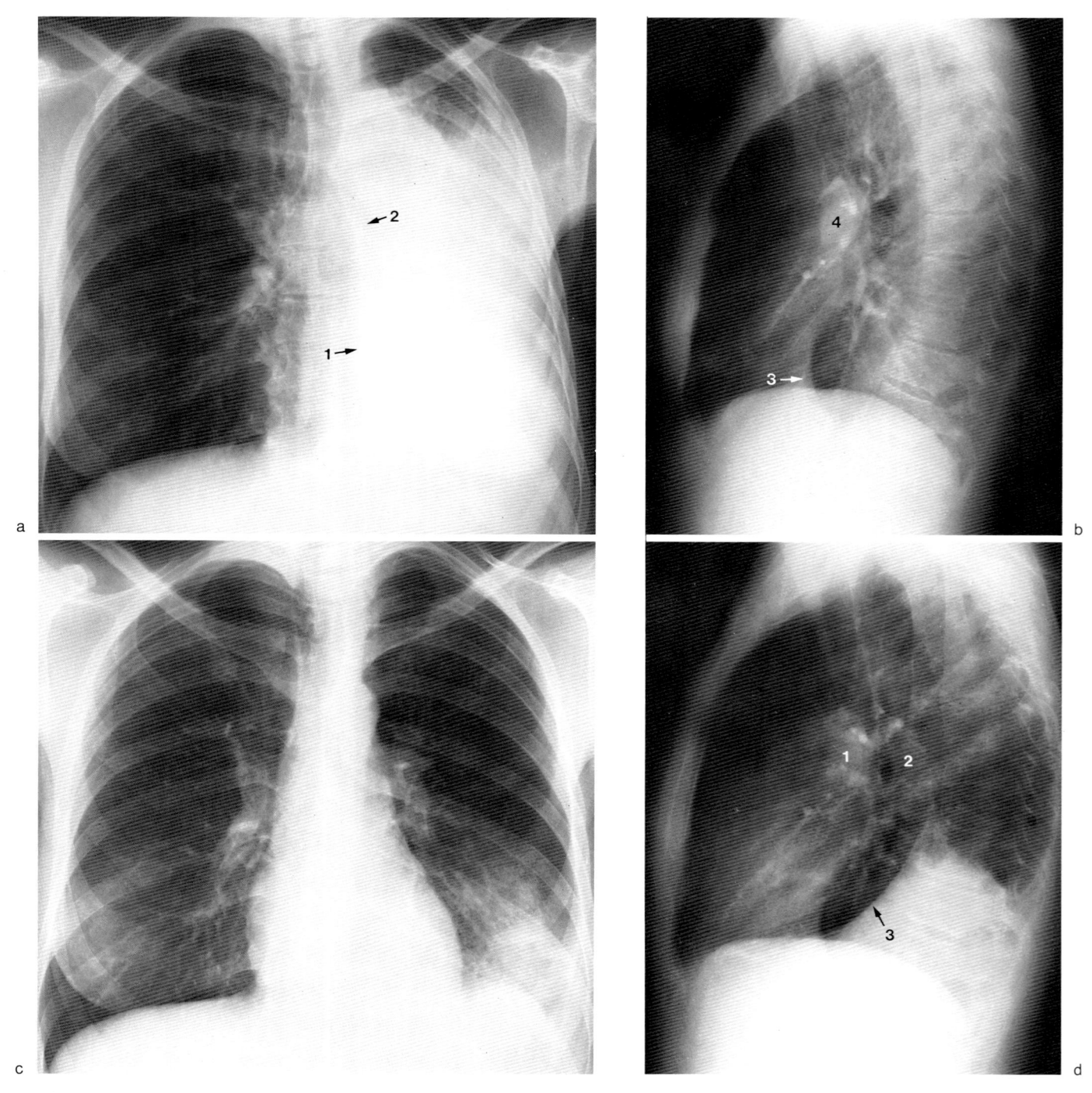

Fig. 7.25 a–d **Near complete atelectasis of left lung with sparing of apical region of left upper lobe.**
41-year-old patient with mucous plugs after cholecystectomy. Opacification of most of the left hemithorax with cardiomediastinal shift to the left (**a**) Azygoesophageal stripe (1), anterior junction line (2), inferior vena cava (3), right pulmonary artery (4). Note absence of left pulmonary artery visualization on lateral view (**b**). Atelectasis of anterobasal and posterobasal segments of left lower lobe (**c,d**). Right pulmonary artery (1), left pulmonary artery (2), major fissure (3).

8. Congenital Malformations

Bronchogenic Cysts

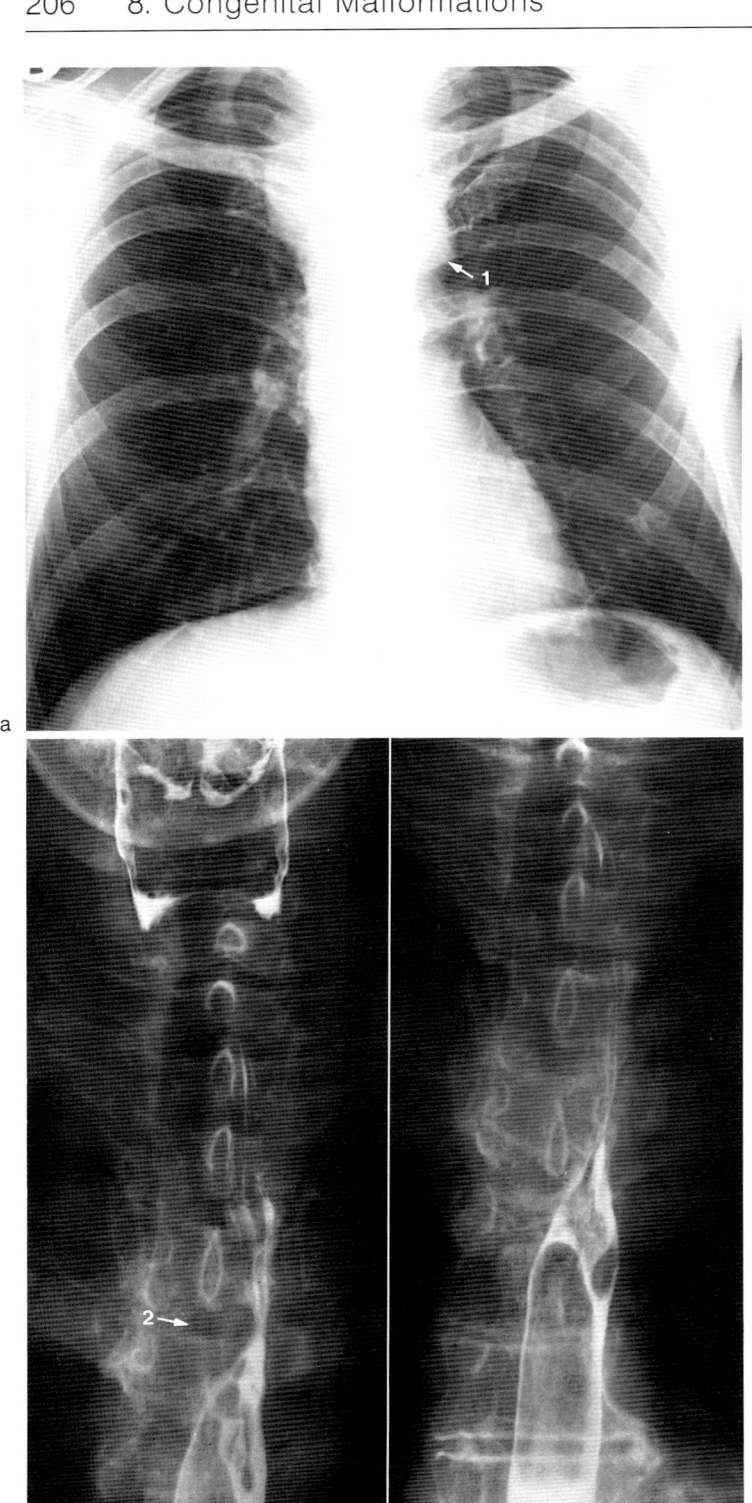

Bronchogenic cysts are filled with mucus, and their inner surface is covered by respiratory ciliated epithelium. They represent the most common bronchial malformation and originate from rudimentary bronchial buds. The majority occur in the mediastinum, particularly in a subcarinal and paratracheal location as well as in the lung parenchyma. Radiologic features include a homogeneous, sharply marginated, intrapulmonary mass with occasional wall calcification. These lesions contain gas or gas-fluid levels only if a communication with the rest of the bronchial tree is established, usually after an infection.

References: 129, 164.

Fig. 8.1 a–c **Mediastinal bronchogenic cyst.**
Patient complains of dysphagia. Superior mediastinal widening. Aortic arch (1) partially obliterated. Mass effect on right lateral aspect of esophagus (2). CT proves cystic nature of pretracheal, retrocaval mass.

Fig. 8.2 a, b **Mediastinal bronchogenic cyst, autopsy proven.**
Retrotracheal mass with circular calcification (1).

Fig. 8.3 a, b **Communicating intrapulmonary bronchogenic cyst.**
Large, thin-walled cavity in right lower lobe.

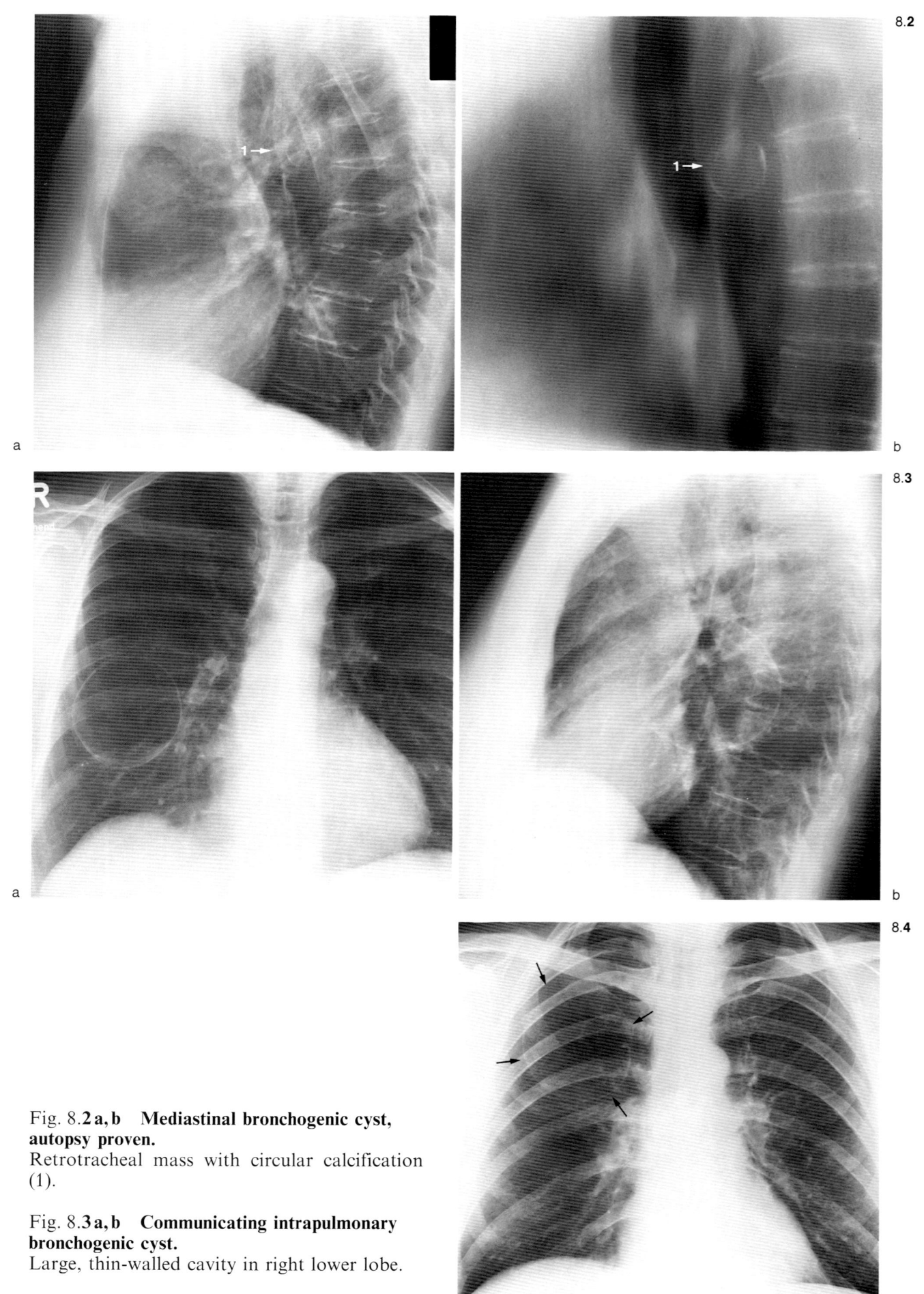

Fig. 8.4 **Communicating bronchogenic cyst.**
Thin-walled cavity in right upper lobe.

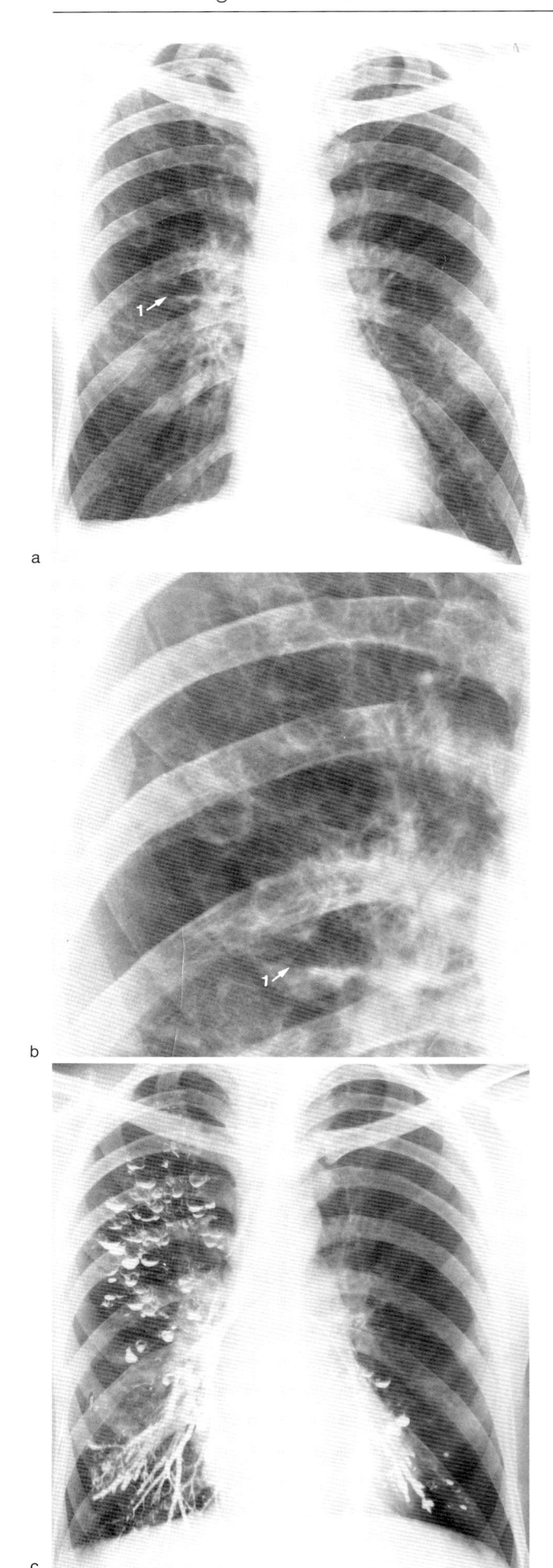

Cystic-Adenomatoid Malformation

Cystic-adenomatoid malformation (CAM) represents a hamartomatous transformation of the lung. Multiple cysts replace the lung parenchyma. Type I is composed of one or several large cysts, type II is formed by multiple smaller cysts, and type III is macroscopically solid but is composed of microscopic cysts.

Usually an entire lobe, frequently the left upper lobe, is involved. At birth, the mass can be lucent or opaque, can compress the remaining normal lung, and can at first glance mimic a diaphragmatic hernia. It can lead to acute respiratory failure.

In rare instances, CAM can be recognized later in life, even in adulthood. The differential diagnosis in adults includes cystic bronchiectasis, emphysematous bullae, infected bronchogenic cysts, or intralobar sequestrations.

◁ Fig. 8.**5 a–c Cystic bronchiectasis mimics CAM.**
Multiple ring shadows throughout right upper lobe. Gas-fluid levels are visible (1). Bronchography demonstrates right upper lobe and left lower lobe bronchiectasis.

Fig. 8.**6 a–c Cystic bronchectasis.**
Small, hyperlucent left lung. Coned-down view and tomogram show multiple cystic spaces.

Fig. 8.**7 a–c Multiple bronchogenic cysts.**
Recurrent bronchitis, with surgical proof. Multiple ring shadows in right lower lobe with fluid levels in right paracardiac location.

Cystic-Adenomatoid Malformation 209

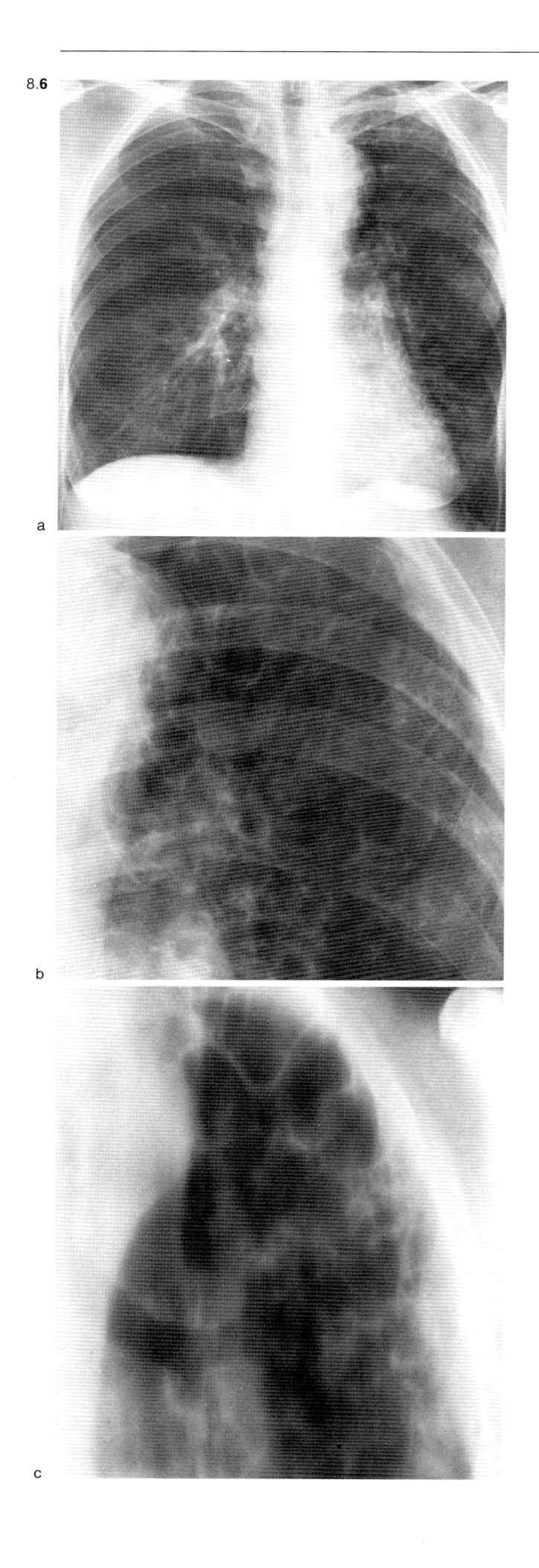

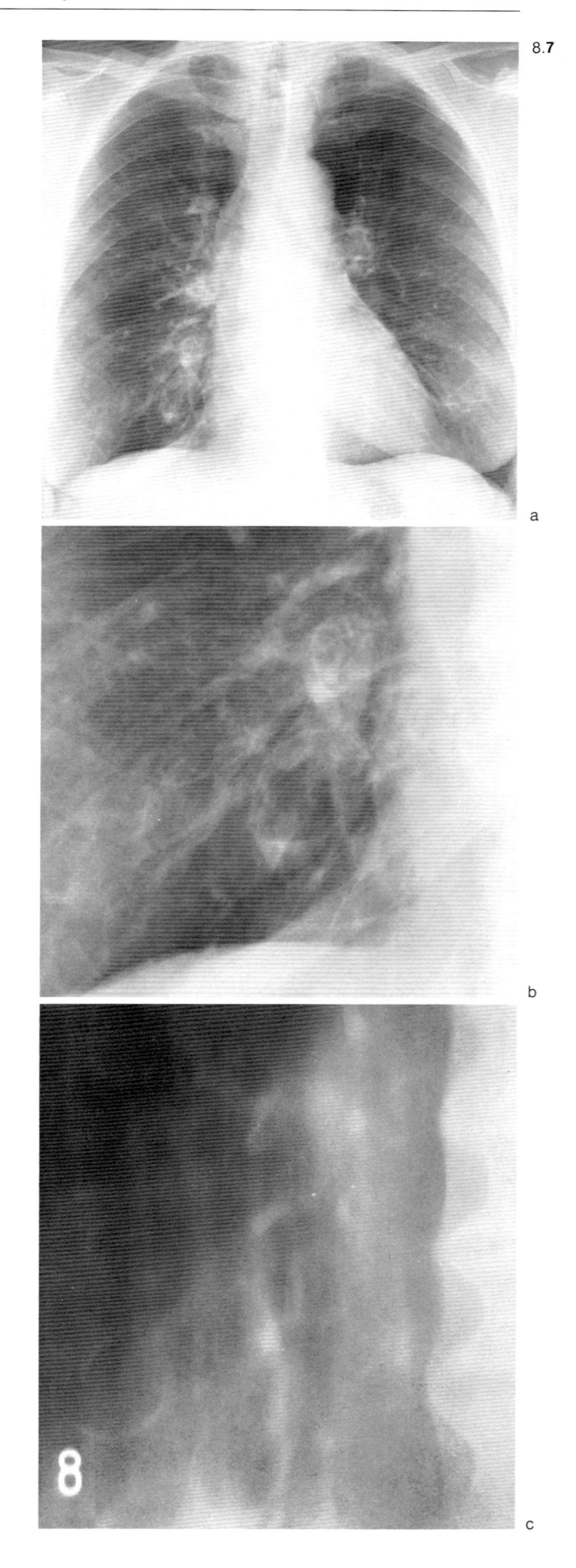

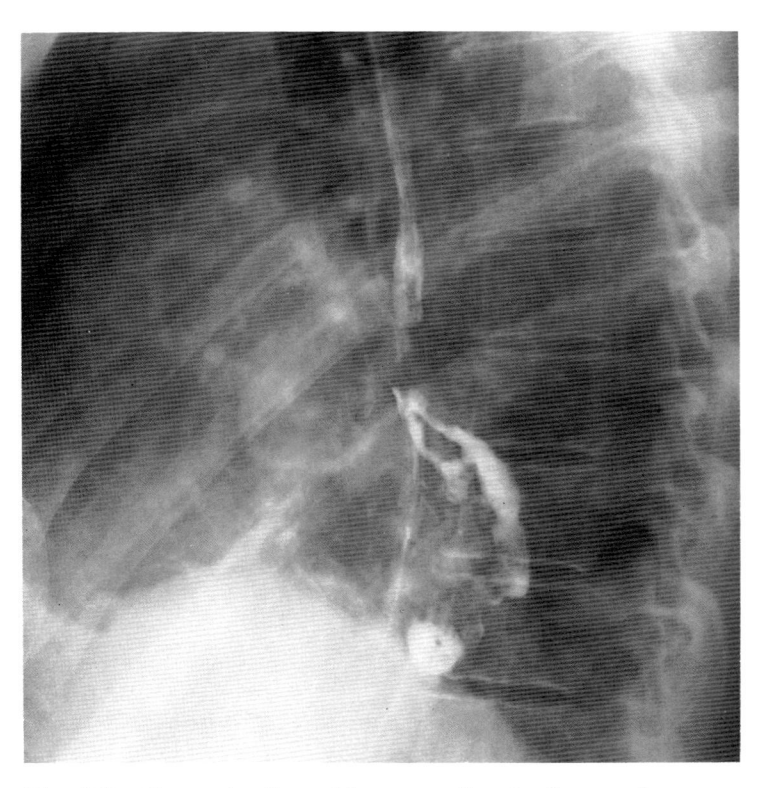

Fig. 8.8 **Sequestration with connection to the esophagus.** 48-year-old patient with recurrent pneumonias over many years. Barium esophagram demonstrates a connection between the esophageal lumen and the posterobasal region of the left lower lobe.

Pulmonary Sequestration

Sequestrations result from a malformed accessory lung bud that does not connect with the tracheobronchial tree. They originate from the foregut and can connect with the esophagus or the stomach.

Extralobar sequestrations have their own pleural cover and a systemic arterial supply, and their venous drainage proceeds to the right atrium. They are associated with other congenital anomalies and become symptomatic in the first year of life.

Intralobar sequestrations do not have a separate pleural cover but do have a systemic arterial supply, while their venous drainage is to the left atrium. They can become infected and then communicate with the bronchial tree. Intralobar sequestrations are discovered later in life.

The majority are congenital, though some could be acquired, and represent a chronic pneumonia with abscess formation and parasitization of bronchial and other systemic arteries. The radiological features include homogeneous, sharply marginated, lower lobe masses, in juxtaposition to the diaphragm, more frequently on the left than on the right side. If the mucus-filled sequestration becomes infected and perforates into an adjacent bronchus, then gas-fluid levels or cavities can become visible. Angiographic examinations are most important in elucidating the nature of such masses or cavities. Usually, a large splanchnic branch off the thoracic or abdominal aorta supplies the sequestration.

References 73, 82, 154.

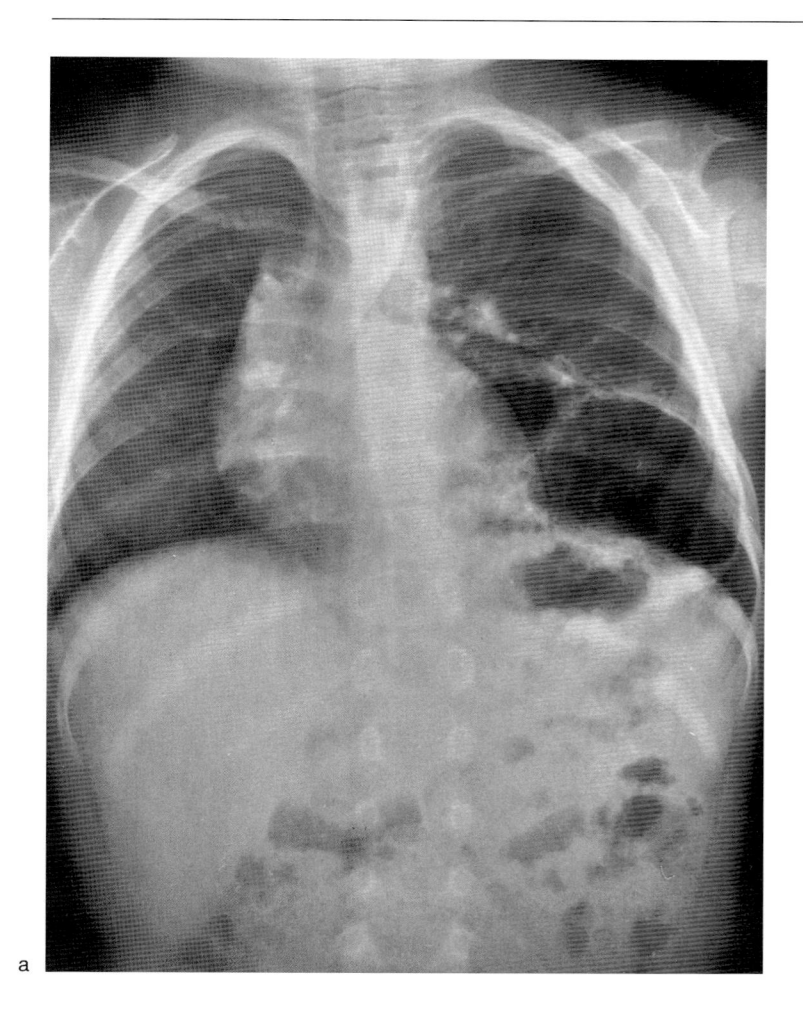

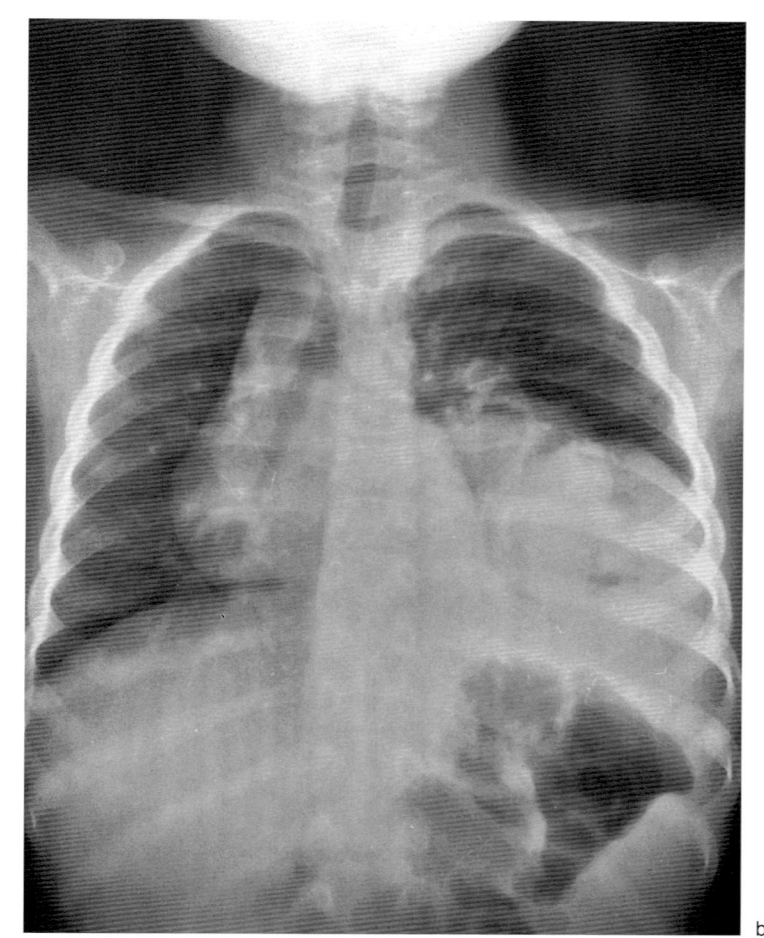

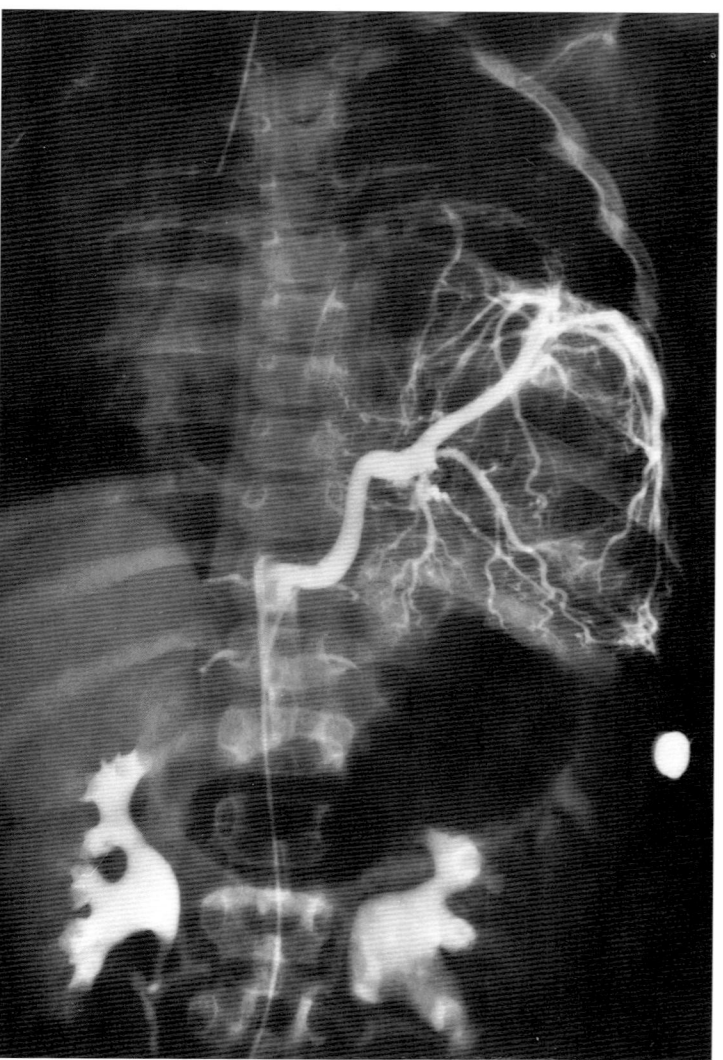

Fig. 8.**9 a–c Child with intralobar sequestration.**
Initial chest film shows multicystic left lower lobe mass displacing cardiac silhouette to the right (**a**). **b** Four months later, pneumonic consolidation opacifies the mass in the left lower lobe. **c** Aortogram demonstrates splanchnic systemic vessels supplying the left lower lobe mass.

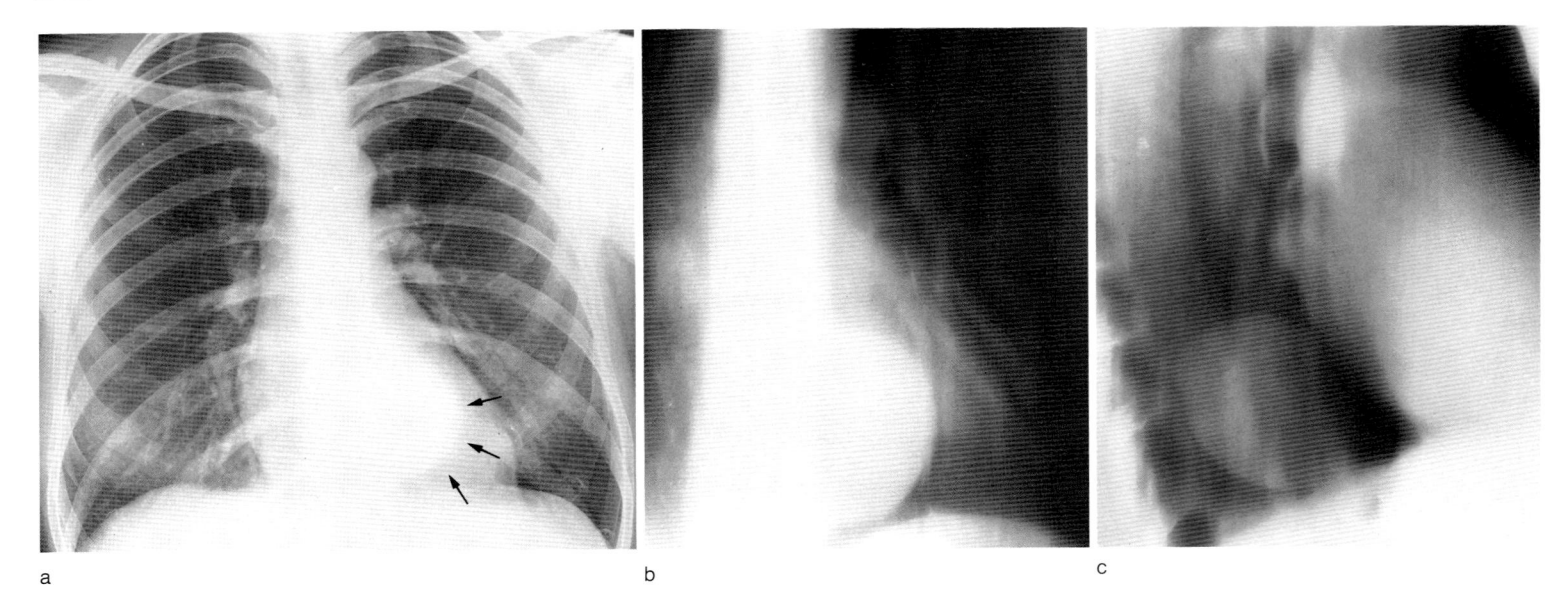

Fig. 8.10 a–c   Extralobar sequestration, surgically proven.
Large, left, lower lobe, paraspinal mass suspicious of tumor.

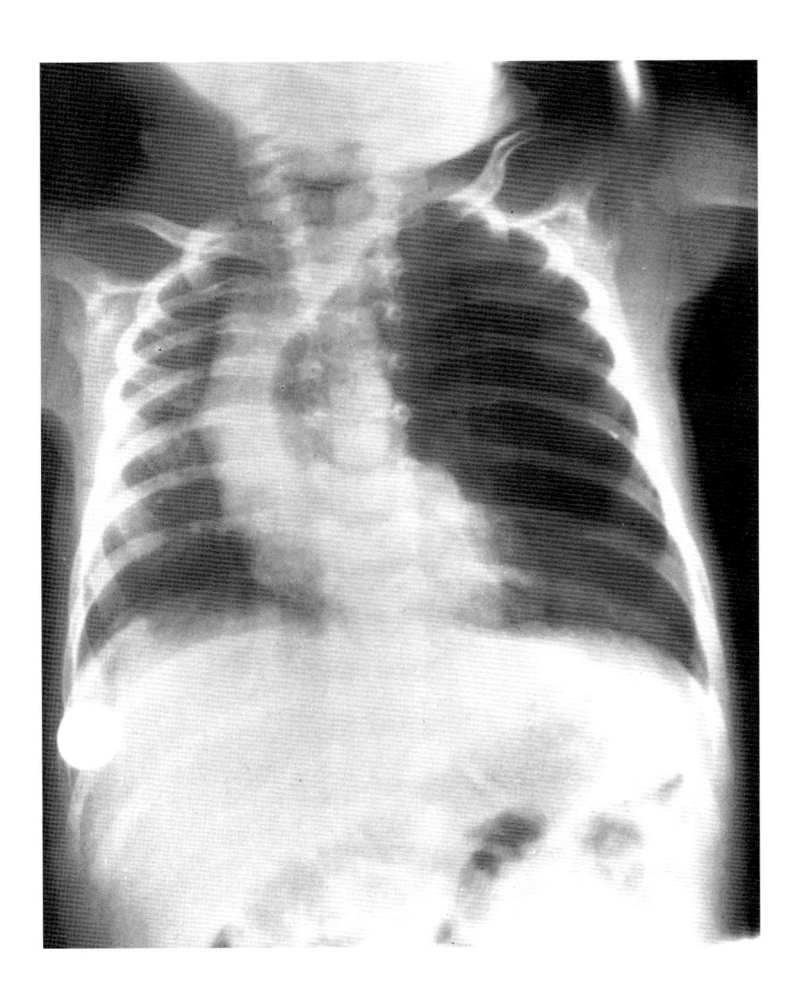

Fig. 8.11   Congenital lobar emphysema in a newborn.
Marked hyperexpansion of left upper lobe with herniation of lung to the right and accompanying cardiomediastinal shift.

Pulmonary Sequestration 213

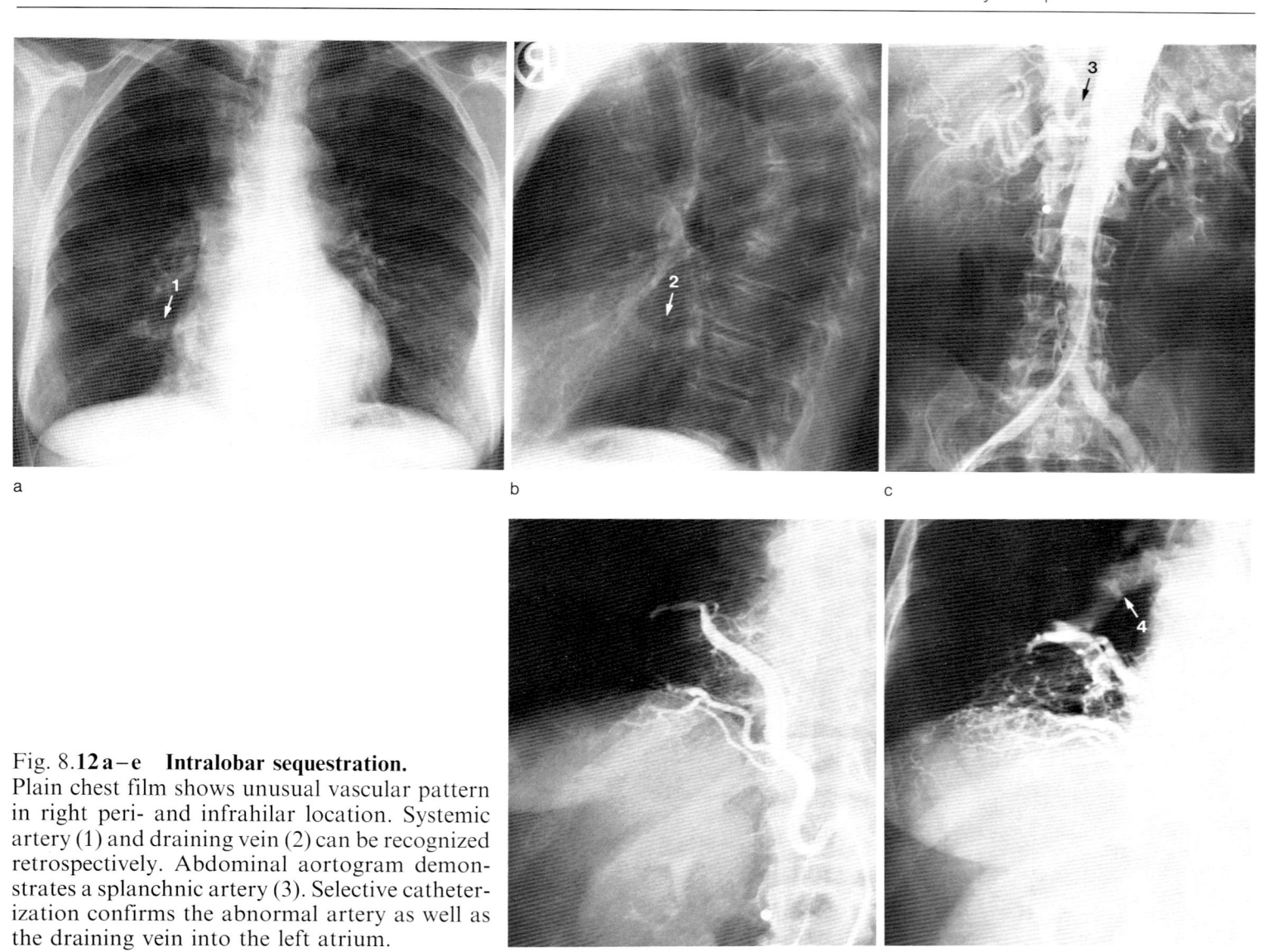

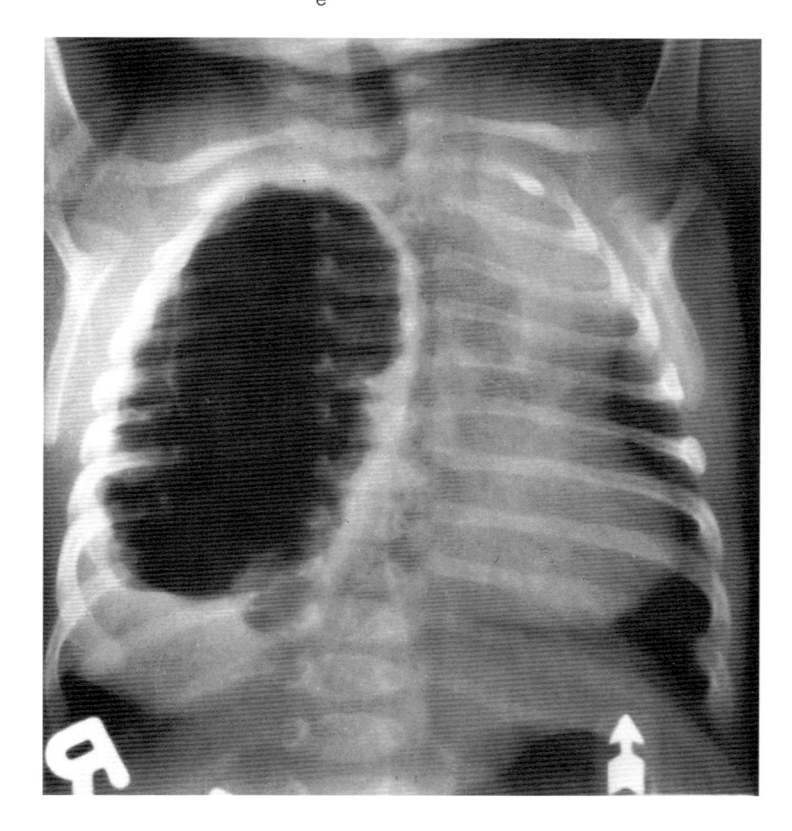

Fig. 8.12 a–e **Intralobar sequestration.**
Plain chest film shows unusual vascular pattern in right peri- and infrahilar location. Systemic artery (1) and draining vein (2) can be recognized retrospectively. Abdominal aortogram demonstrates a splanchnic artery (3). Selective catheterization confirms the abnormal artery as well as the draining vein into the left atrium.

Fig. 8.13 **Cystic adenomatoid malformation in an infant.**
Large, gas-filled, cystic structure replaces the right upper lobe. Cardiomediastinal shift to the left side is present.

Vascular Malformations of the Lung

The most common anomaly in this group is the arteriovenous malformation of the lung. It is associated with Weber–Rendu–Osler disease in 50% of cases. In 30% of patients, multiple arteriovenous malformations can be found at angiography. Over 50% of patients are asymptomatic, yet others have hemoptysis, dyspnea, cyanosis, paradoxical embolism with strokes brain abscesses, finger clubbing, or polycythemia. These arteriovenous malformations are usually located in the periphery of the lower lobes. CT scanning and pulmonary angiography are important to identify the size, location, and number of the arteriovenous malformations as well as the number and course of supplying and draining vessels.

Abnormal venous return can lead to aberrant drainage of the pulmonary veins into the superior or inferior vena cava; this anomaly results in a left to right shunt. The hypogenetic lung syndrome consists of a hypoplastic right lung and a large draining vein, the so-called scimitar, which enters the inferior vena cava, right atrium, or portal vein. The appearance of the draining vein is characteristic.

References: 14, 28, 58, 75, 95.

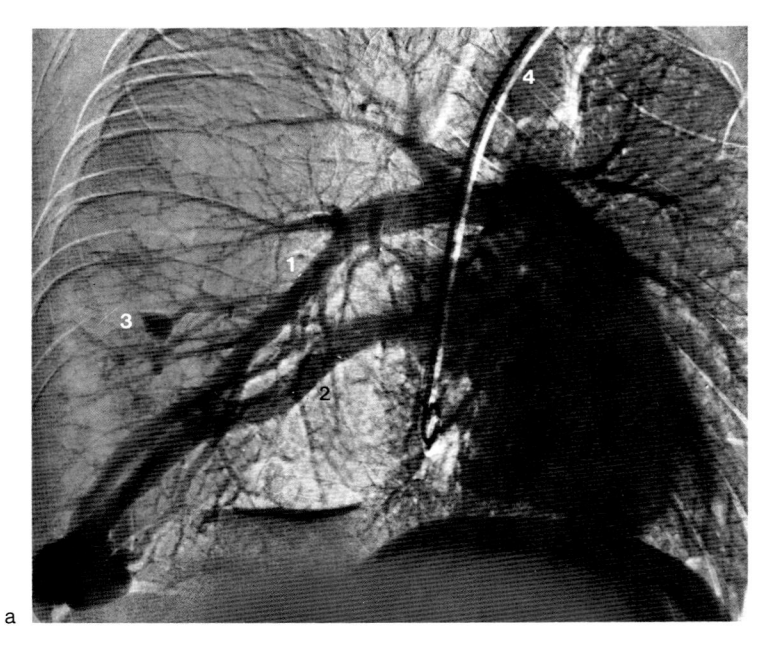

Fig. 8.**14a,b Arteriovenous malformation in right lower lobe.**
Patient with an episode of hemoptysis. Chest film demonstrates a peripheral, solitary, pulmonary nodule with questionable supplying vessel. Pulmonary angiogram shows feeding artery (1), draining vein (2), additional smaller malformations (3). Pigtail catheter in right atrium (4).

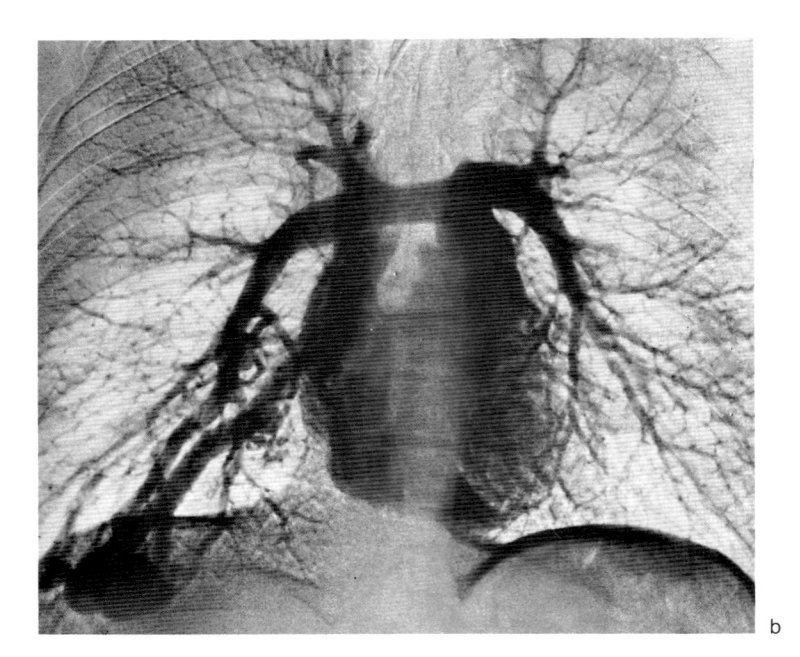

Fig. 8.**15 a–c Scimitar syndrome.**
Scimitar-shaped tubular opacity courses in right paracardiac location (1) and enters into inferior vena cava. Catheterization yielded a left to right shunt of 25%.

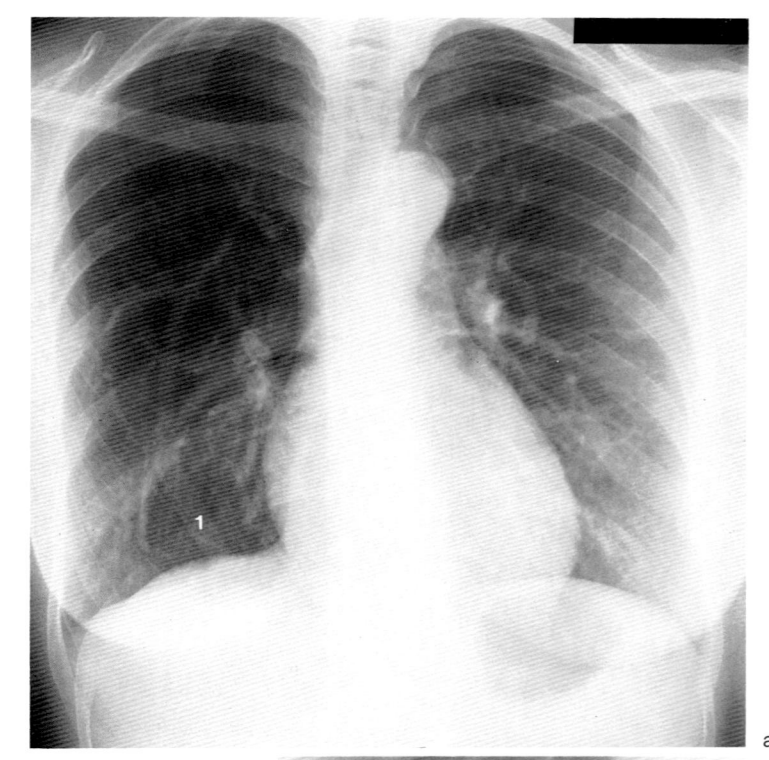

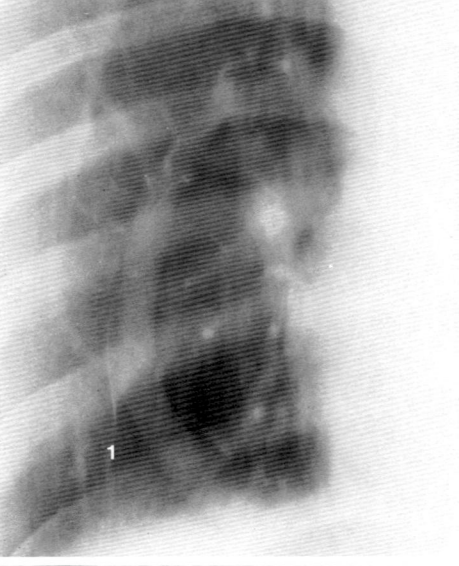

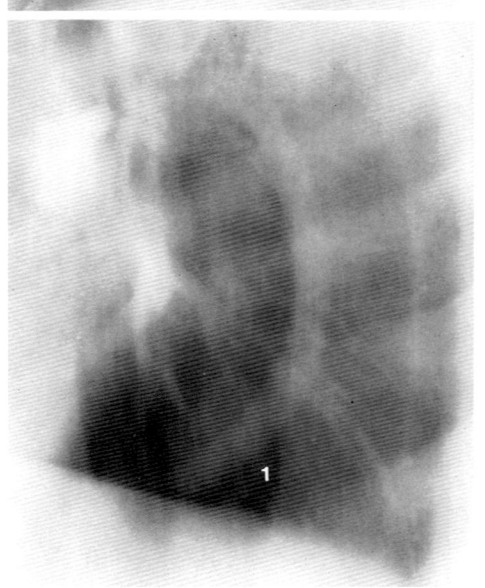

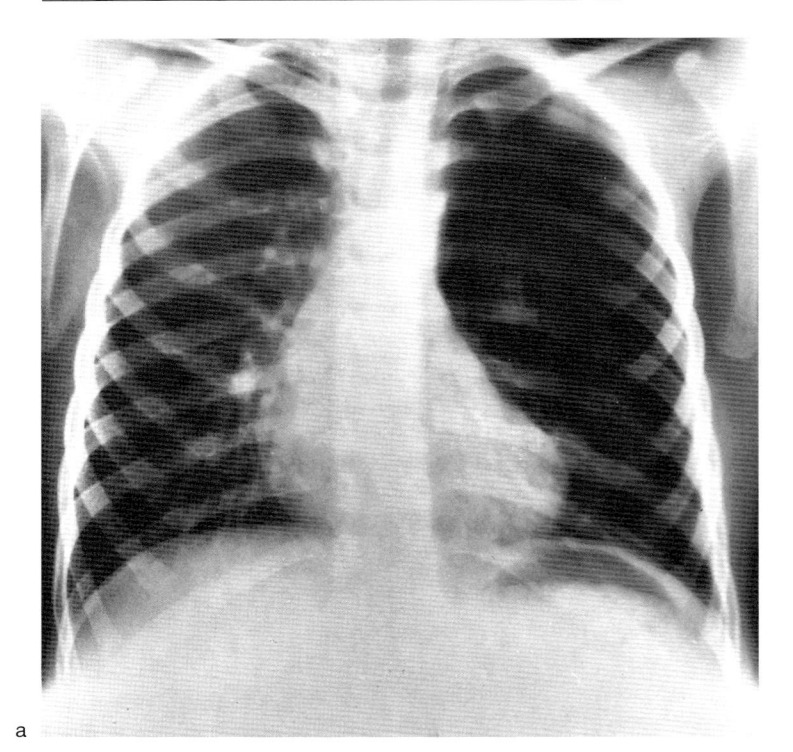

Fig. 8.16a, b   Congenital bronchial atresia to the left upper lobe.
Chest radiograph shows a hyperexpanded left upper lobe and a rounded left parahilar nodule. **a** Hyperexpansion is due to collateral ventilation from lingula and left lower lobe. Parahilar nodule represents a mucoid impaction distal to focal atresia of left upper lobe bronchus. **b** Bronchogram confirms absent left upper lobe bronchus and caudad displacement of lingular and left lower lobe bronchi.

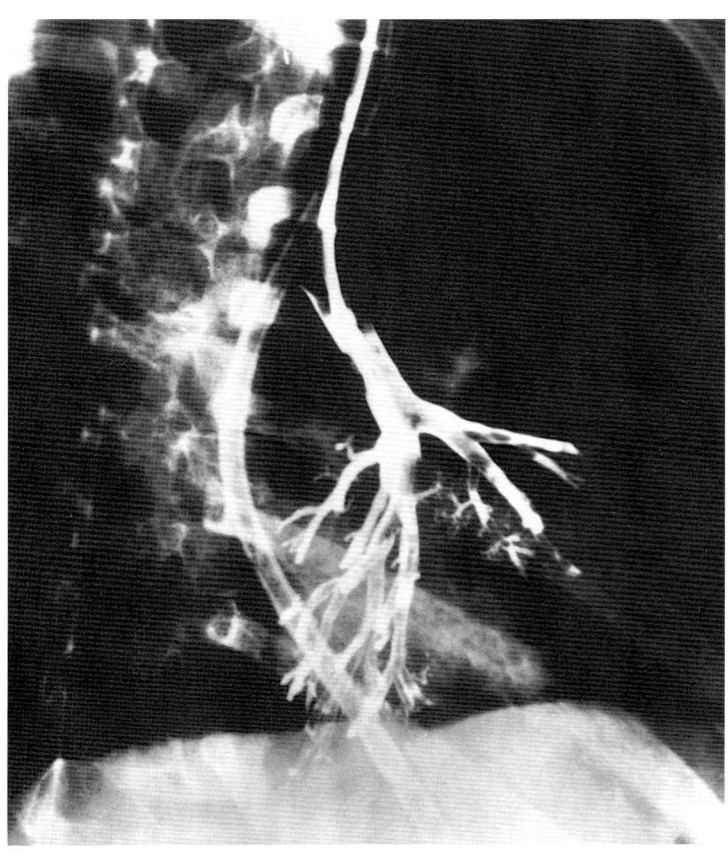

9. Pleural Diseases

9. Pleural Diseases

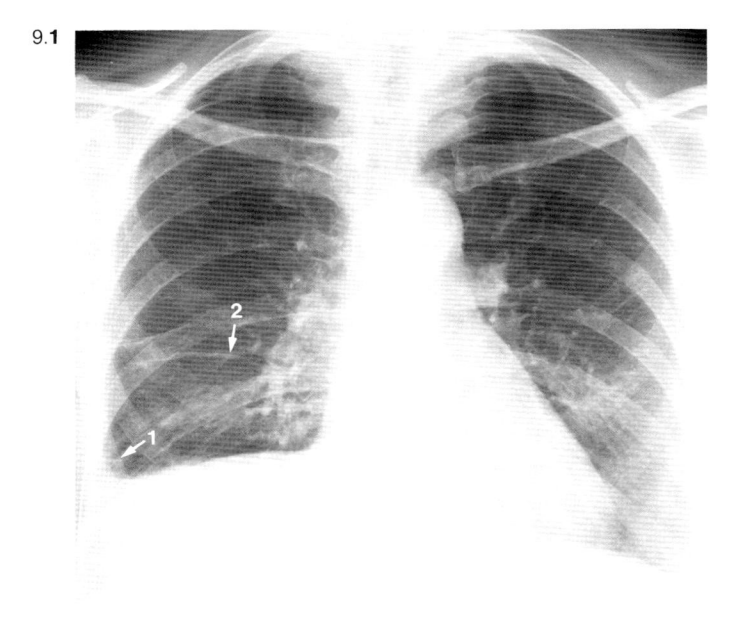

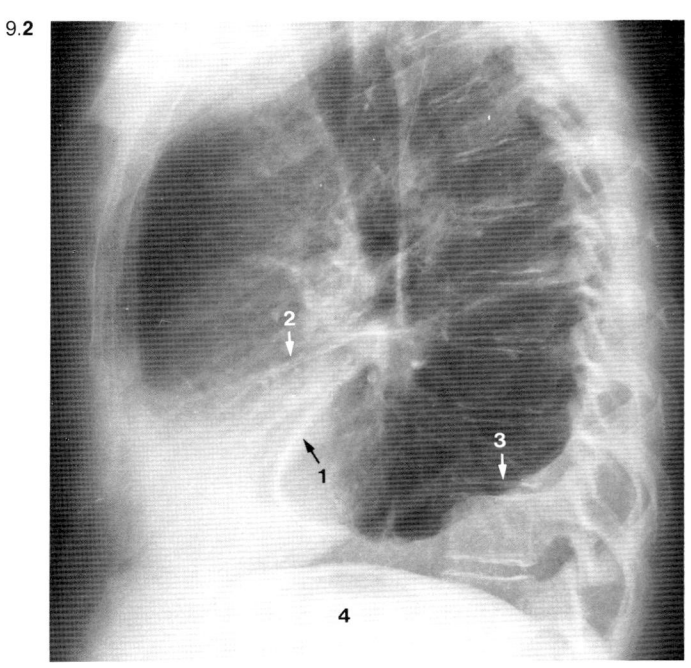

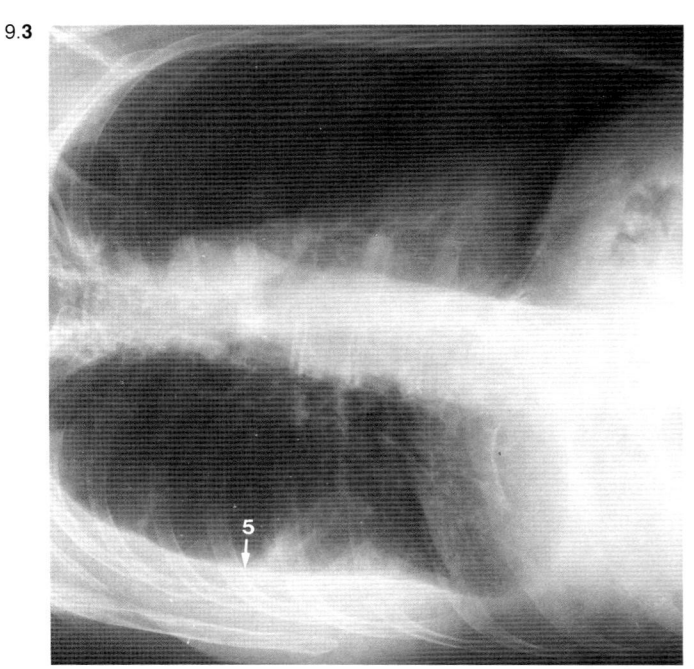

Pleural Effusions

The normal pleural space contains 15 mL of fluid which facilitates the respiratory motion of the two layers of pleura against each other. Pleural effusions can be exudative or transudative and contain pus, blood, chyle, bile, or cerebrospinal fluid. Small amounts of pleural fluid can be seen on decubitus films (less than 10 mL). Obliteration of the posterior costophrenic sulcus occurs with 50–75 mL, and a meniscus in the lateral costophrenic sulcus becomes visible with at least 150 mL of fluid. One hemithorax can accommodate up to 6 L of fluid. The distribution of fluid in the pleural space depends on gravity, capillary forces, pleural adhesions, and potential pulmonary pathology, e.g., atelectasis.

References: 96, 128.

Fig. 9.1 Pleural effusion with meniscus in lateral costophrenic sulcus (1), minor fissure (2).

Fig. 9.2 **Pleural fluid in posterior costophrenic sulcus.** Effusion in major fissure (1), minor fissure (2), obscuration of right posterior costophrenic sulcus (3), gastric air bubble under left hemidiaphragm (4).

Fig. 9.3 Right lateral decubitus view. Mobile pleural effusion layers along lateral aspect of rib cage.

Fig. 9.4 **Bilateral pleural effusions on supine CT.** Bilateral crescentic opacities in posterior aspect of both pleural cavities. Note pleural fluid in phrenicovertebral sulcus, posterior to liver.

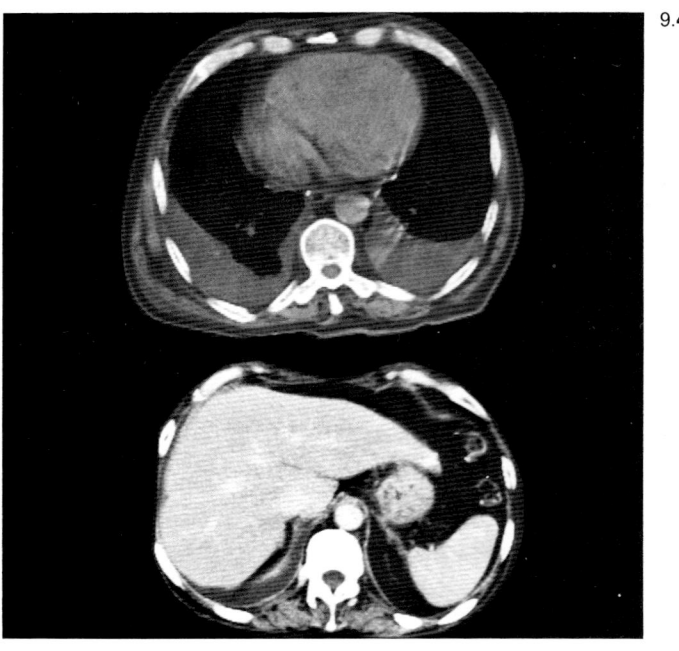

Fig. 9.5 **Large parapneumonic pleural effusion.**
53-year-old patient with high fever. Line of Ellis–Damoiseau (1), fluid in major fissure (2), descending thoracic aorta (3).

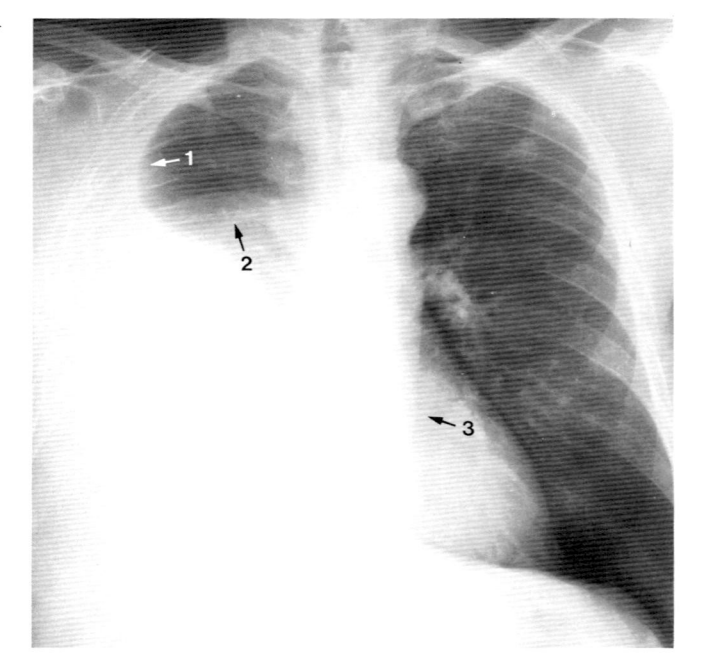

Fig. 9.6 **Pleural carcinomatosis due to breast cancer.**
Ellis–Damoiseau line (1), effusion in major fissure (2) and minor fissure (3). Left mastectomy.

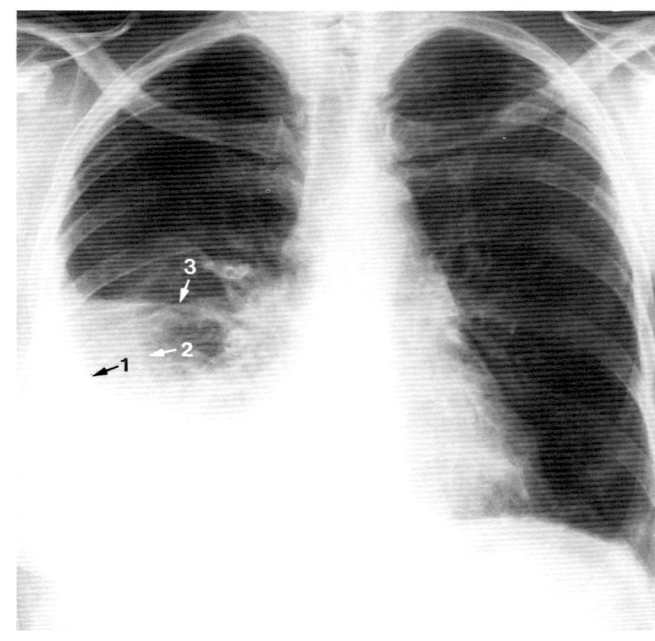

Fig. 9.7 a, b **Pleural carcinomatosis due to bronchogenic carcinoma in left lower lobe.**
65-year-old patient with marked dyspnea at initial presentation. Complete opacification of left hemithorax with cardiomediastinal shift to the right. After thoracentesis, hydropneumothorax (1) and central tumor mass become visible.

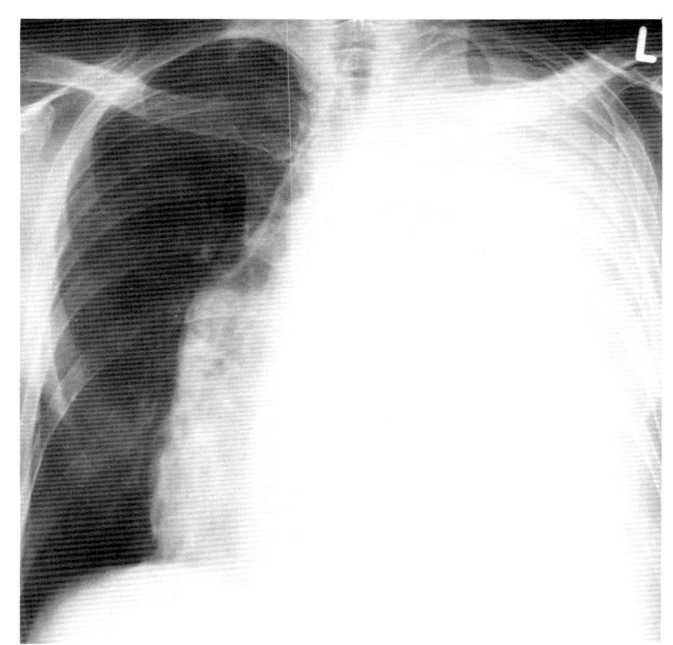

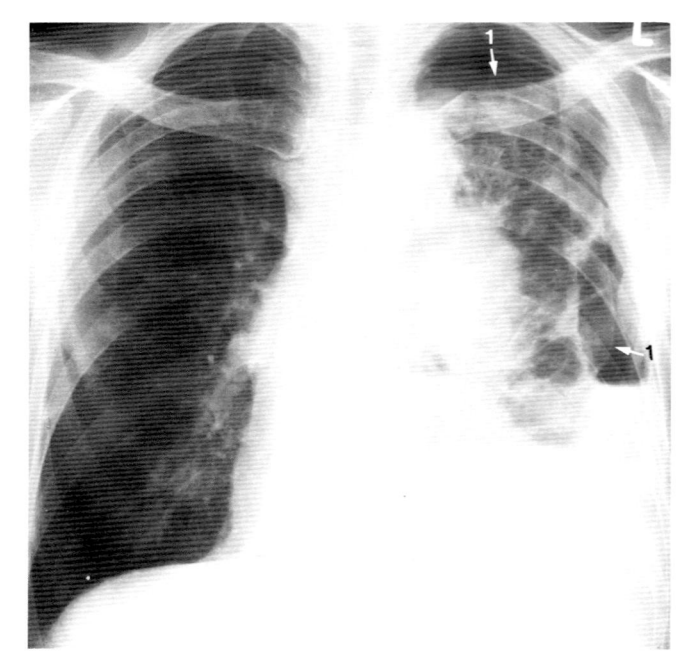

9. Pleural Diseases

Subpulmonic Effusions, Intrafissural Collections of Fluid, Loculated Effusions

These are atypical presentations of pleural pathology due to adhesions or regional pulmonary atelectasis or scarring.

Fig. 9.**8 a, b** **Subpulmonic effusion.**
Elevation of left lung base with lateral deviation of apex of curvature (1). No meniscus in lateral costophrenic sulcus visible. In supine position, the effusion layers posteriorly (**b**).

Fig. 9.**9 a, b** **Fluid loculated in major fissure.**
Patient with left ventricular failure. Lateral meniscus (1), fluid in superior accessory fissure, fluid in major fissure (3). Elliptical configuration is typical for intrafissural loculated effusions. Posterior meniscus (4).

Fig. 9.**10 a, b** **Encapsulated effusion in major fissure, so-called vanishing tumor.**
Patient with left ventricular failure.

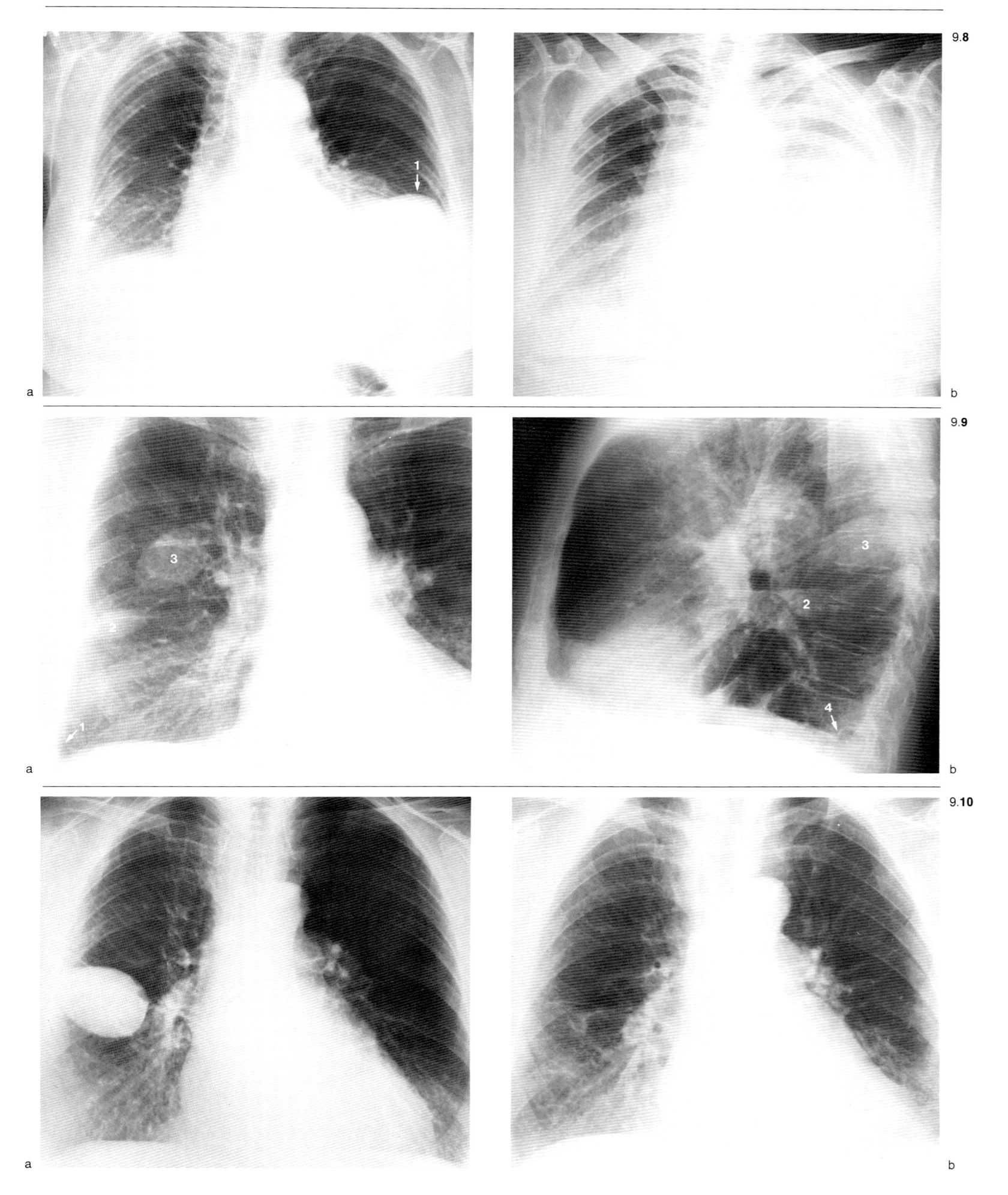

Pleural Effusions 221

9.8

9.9

9.10

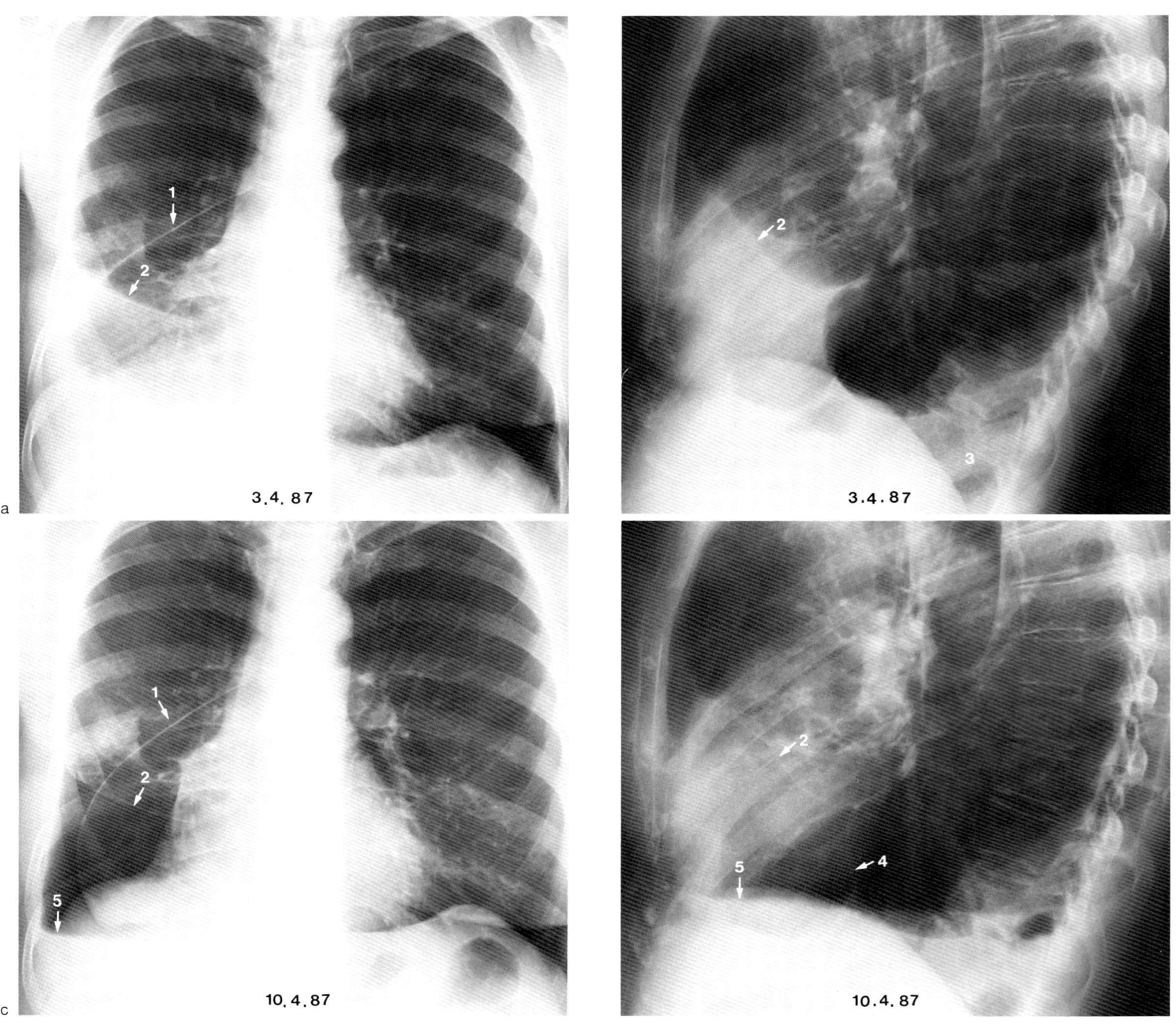

Fig. 9.**11 a–d** Pleural effusion accompanying lymphangitic carcinomatosis due to metastatic carcinoma of the breast in a 44-year-old patient. Occlusion of middle lobe bronchus by tumor. Pleural fluid in major fissure (1). Inferior border of upper lobe (2); posterior pleural effusion with meniscus (3). After thoracentesis (**c, d**), hydropneumothorax with gas-fluid level (5). Anterior contour of lower lobe (4). Trapped lung does not reexpand due to occlusion of the middle lobe bronchus, loss of compliance of lung, and pleural thickening.

Fig. 9.12 **Loculated pleural hematoma after cardiac transplant.**
CT scan shows loculated collection of pleural fluid in left hemithorax, posterolateral to descending aorta.

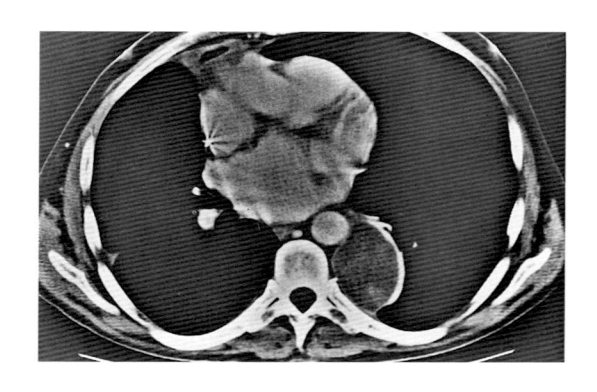

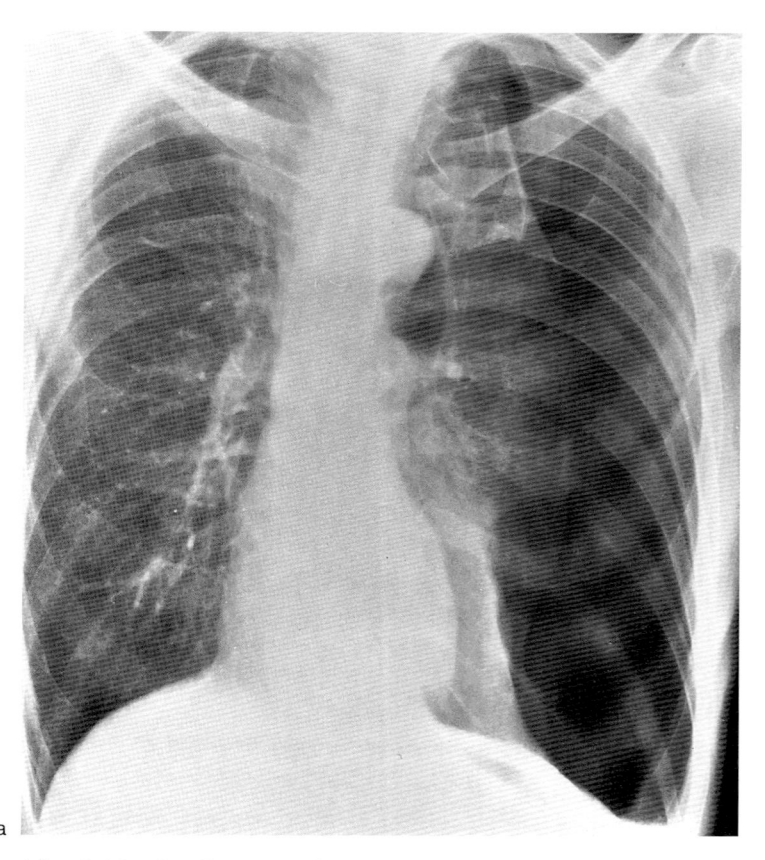

Fig. 9.13 a, b **Reexpansion pulmonary edema.**
a Initial chest radiograph shows large left-sided tension pneumothorax. b After chest tube insertion and rapid evacuation of pneumothorax, pulmonary edema develops.

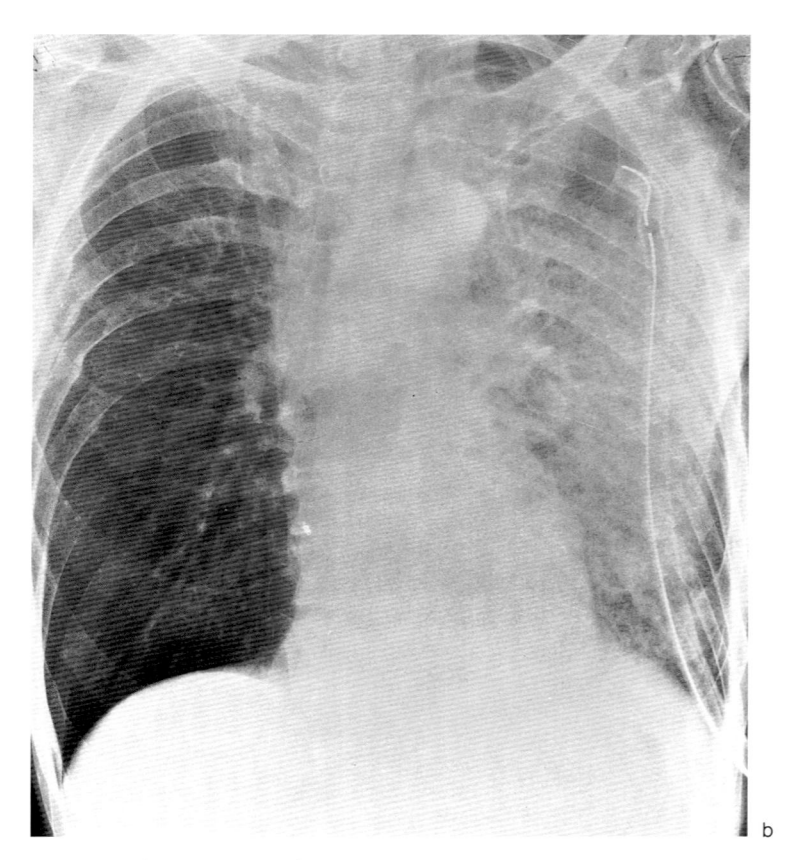

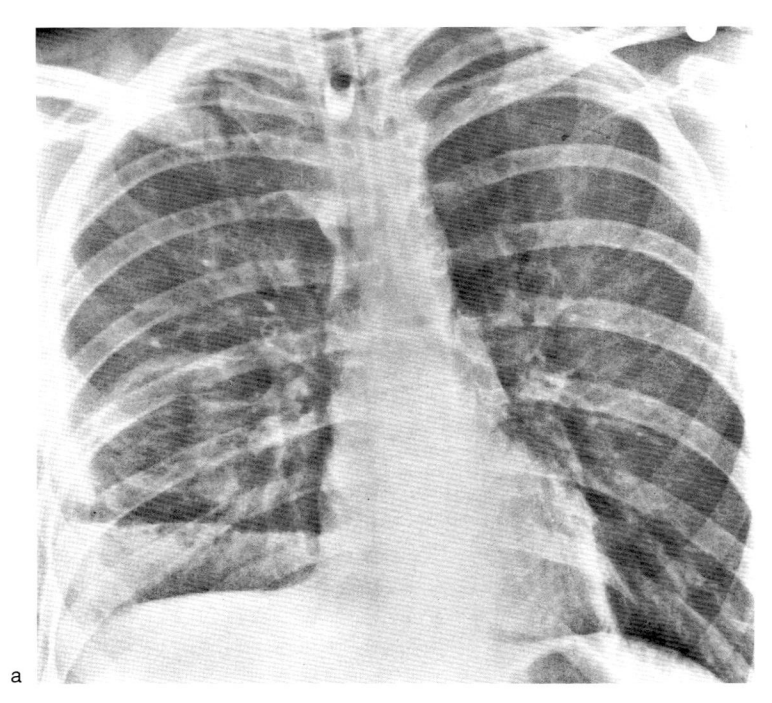

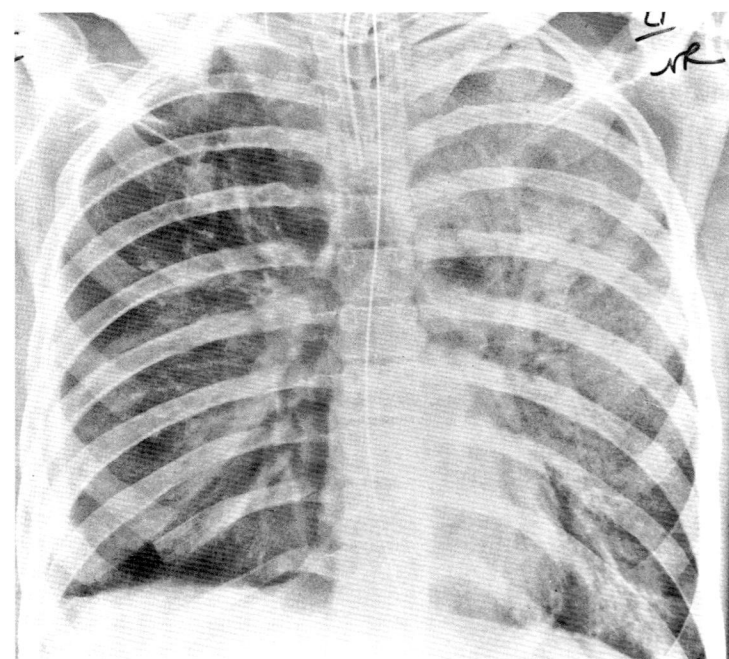

Fig. 9.**14 a, b** **Posttraumatic bronchopleural fistula with aspiration.**
a Initial chest radiograph shows right-sided air-fluid level.
b Follow-up reveals extensive consolidation of left lung concomitant with disappearance of right hydropneumothorax.

Rounded Atelectasis

Rounded atelectases are found in conjunction with organizing pleuritis and pleural thickening due to previous asbestos exposure (80%). Rounded atelectases can also form in the wake of any pleural effusion. They are usually found in the lower lobes, lingula, or middle lobe. They probably form when a portion of the lung parenchyma curls and the surrounding lung encases the airless part. Radiologically, these masses are located peripherally, are elliptical in shape, and are connected to the hilus by bronchi and vessels which form a characteristic comet-tail.

References: 65, 159.

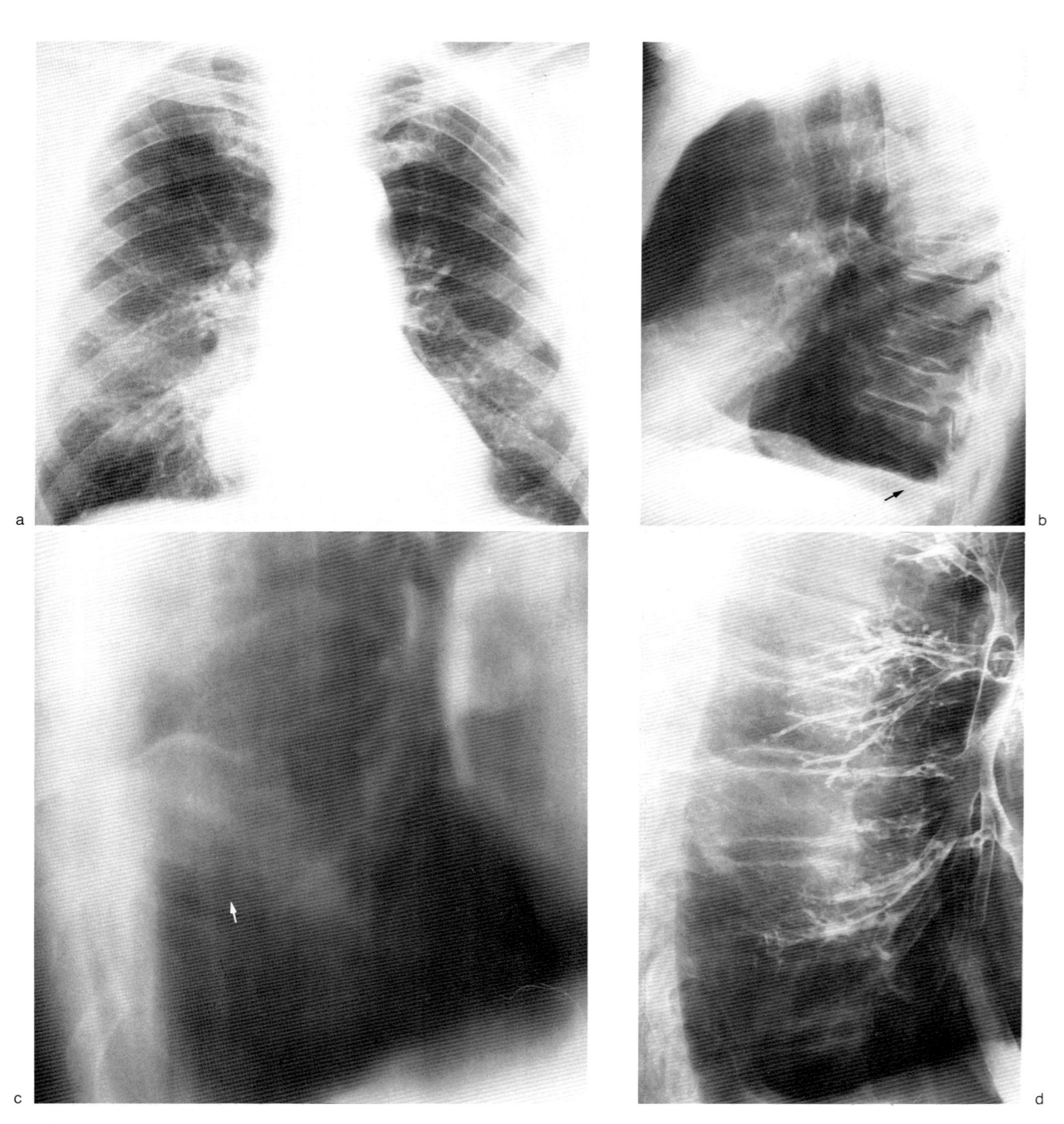

Fig. 9.15a–d **Rounded atelectasis.**
On frontal radiograph (**a**) right paracardiac mass is seen. On lateral projection, mass produces increased opacification superimposed over lower thoracic spine (**b**). Pleural scar (white arrow). Linear tomogram (**e**) confirms the mass and demonstrates the characteristic comet-tail (black arrow). Bronchogram confirms arcuate course of bronchi supplying rounded atelectasis.

Spontaneous Pneumothorax

The most common causes of a spontaneous pneumothorax are intrapleural apical blebs or subpleural bullae. The initial episode occurs in the third decade of life; chances of recurrence are 30% on the ipsilateral side and 10% on the contralateral side.

Other, less common causes of spontaneous pneumothorax include interstitial lung diseases like histiocytosis or lymphangioleiomyomatosis, tuberculous cavities, lung abscesses, and rarely pulmonary metastases from osteogenic sarcoma or primary bronchogenic carcinoma.

On upright radiographs, the most reliable sign of a pneumothorax is the white visceral pleural line. A large pneumothorax is characterized by a completely atelectatic lung, retracted towards the hilus. A tension pneumothorax results in a cardiomediastinal shift to the opposite side as well as inversion of the diaphragm.

References: 79.

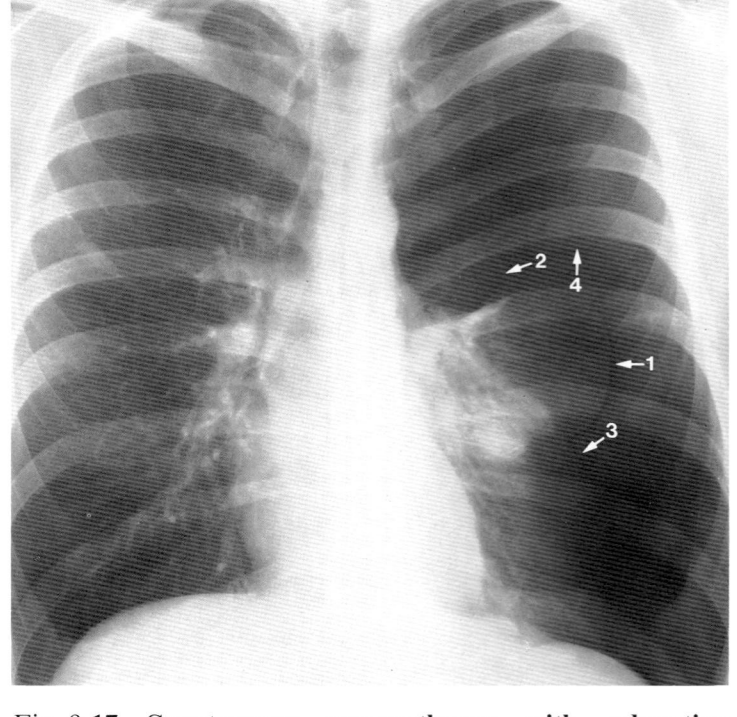

Fig. 9.17 **Spontaneous pneumothorax with relaxation atelectasis.**
26-year-old patient with two previous episodes of pneumothorax. Visceral pleural line (1), bullae (2, 3), rib (4).

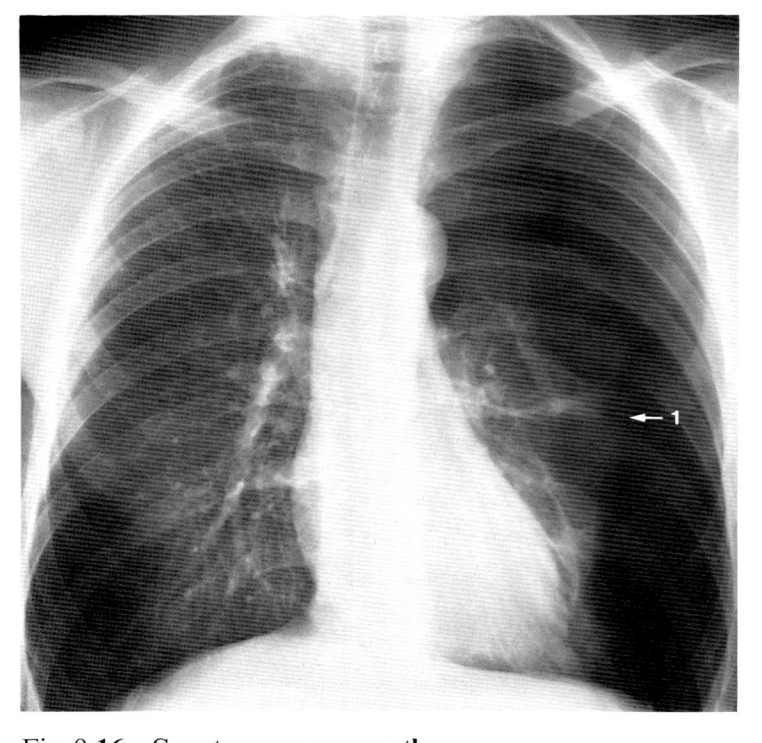

Fig. 9.16 **Spontaneous pneumothorax.**
18-year-old patient with sudden chest pain. Hyperlucency of left hemithorax, visceral pleural line (1), right apical pleuroparenchymal scarring. Mild tracheal deviation to the right.

Fig. 9.18 a–d **Spontanteous pneumothorax.**
76-year-old patient treated initially conservatively (a); due to persistent air leak (b), chest tube drainage became necessary (c). After 2 months (d), pneumothorax has disappeared. Visceral pleural line (1), medial scapular margin (2), lower lobe atelectasis (3), residual basilar pneumothorax.

Fig. 9.19 a, b **Pneumothorax.**
64-year-old emphysematous patient with acute chest pain. Initial chest film shows moderate left pneumothorax (a) which over the next 2 h increases (b), necessitating chest tube drainage. Visceral pleural line (1), displaced anterior junction line (2); emphysema is present and results in a paucity of pulmonary vascular structures.

Spontaneous Pneumothorax 227

a 14.3.59

b 19.3.59

c 21.3.59

d 12.5.59

9.18

a

b

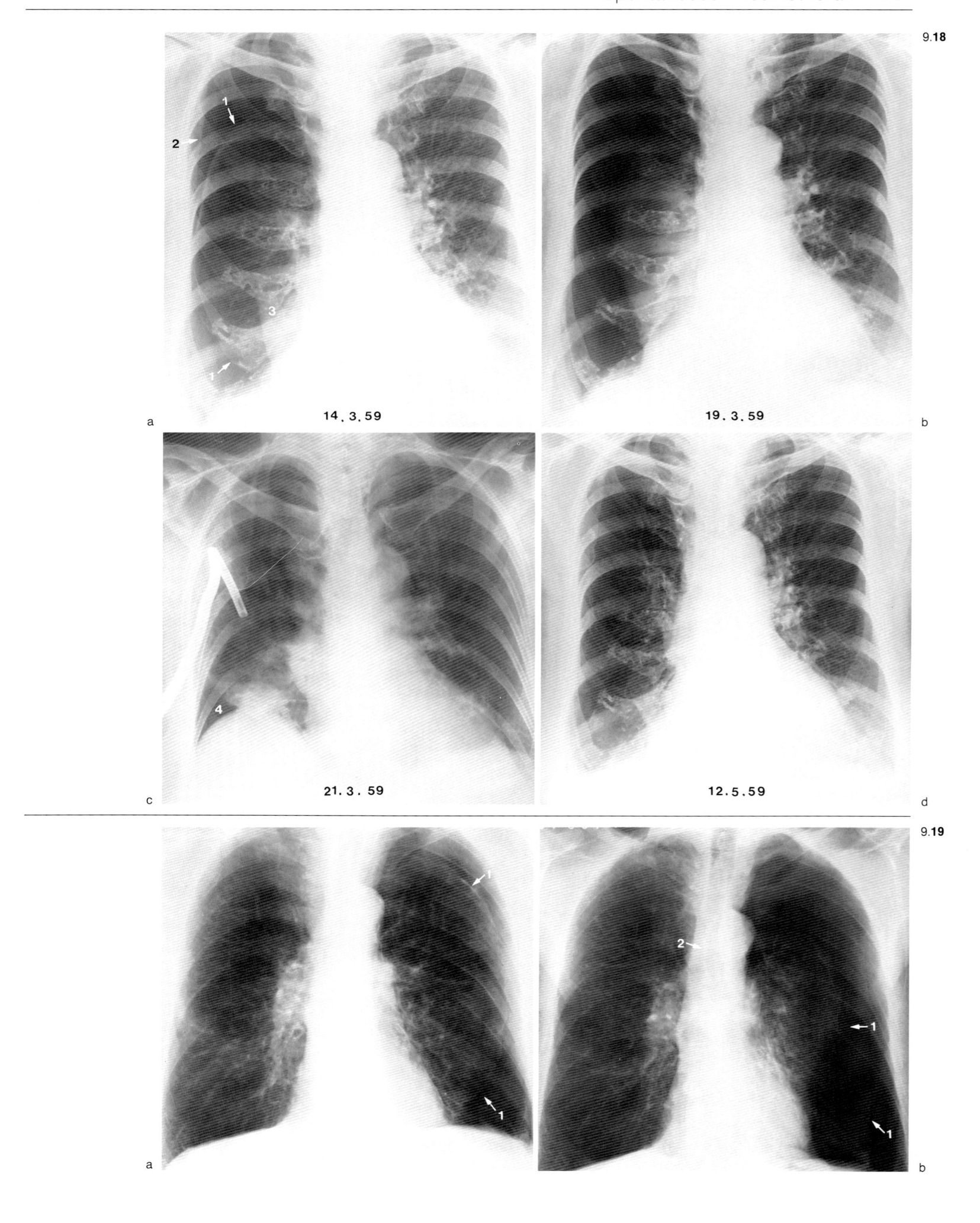

9.19

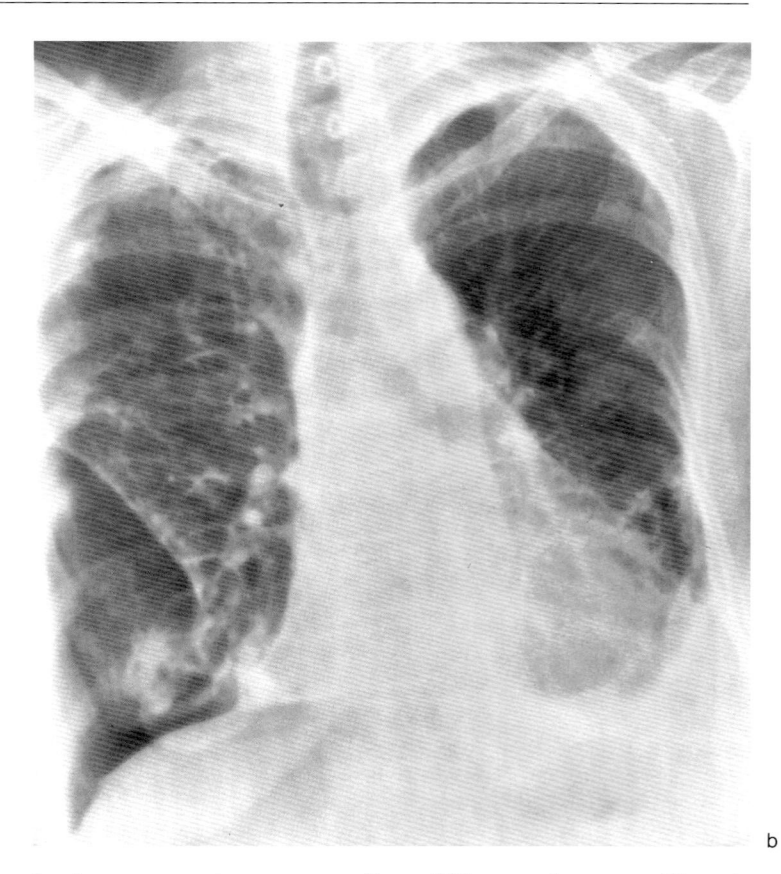

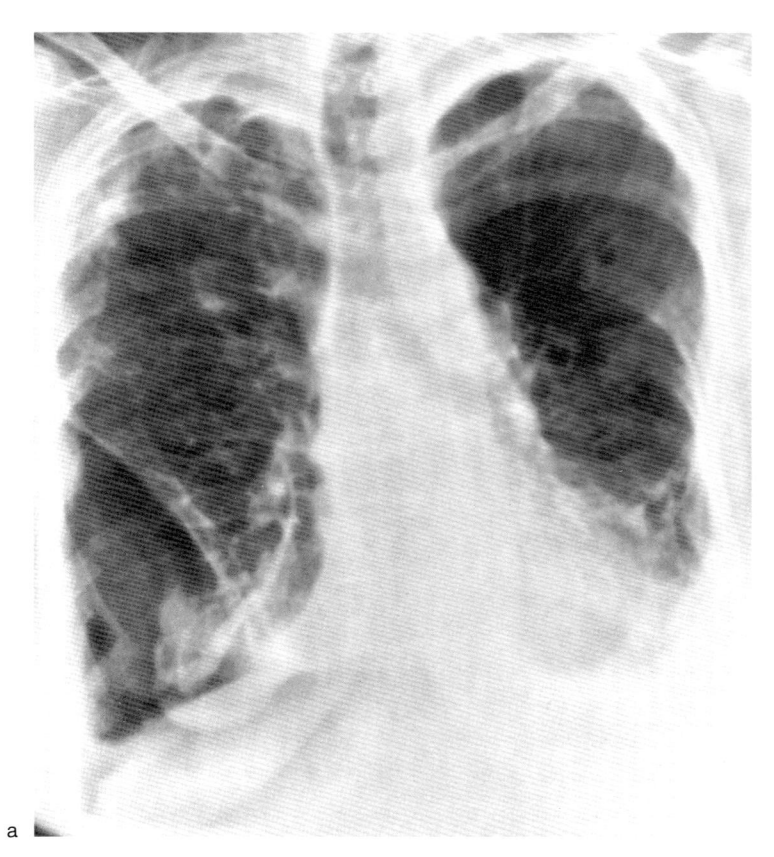

Fig. 9.20 a, b **Chronic hydropneumothorax in patient with rheumatoid arthritis.**
a Initial chest radiograph shows a loculated right basilar hydropneumothorax as well as diffuse pulmonary fibrosis and left-sided pleural fluid. b Chest radiograph taken 6 months later shows no change in the hydropneumothorax.

Pleural Thickening

Pleural thickening results from previous inflammation, traumatic hemothorax, or asbestos exposure. Symphysis of the visceral and parietal pleura precludes any respiratory motion; deformation of the peripheral lung parenchyma during respiration substitutes for the lack of pleural motion.

Pleura peels can reach a thickness of several centimeters. Once a thickness of 2 cm is exceeded, chronic, encapsulated pleural fluid has to be considered.

References: 40, 96.

Fig. 9.21 **Apical pleural cap.**
Note scalloped border towards the lung as well as apical blebs in close proximity to the thick pleura. These apical findings result from gravitational stress on the lung rather than from previous granulomatous disease.

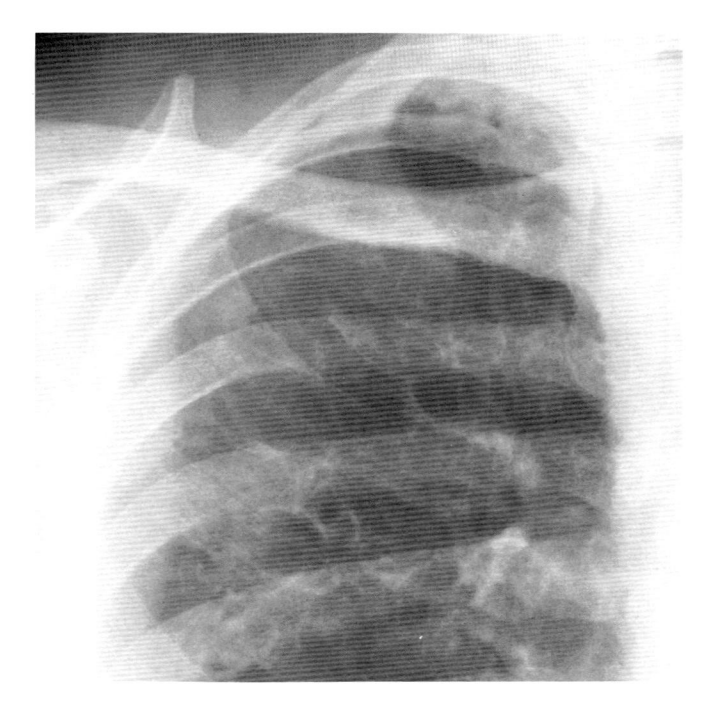

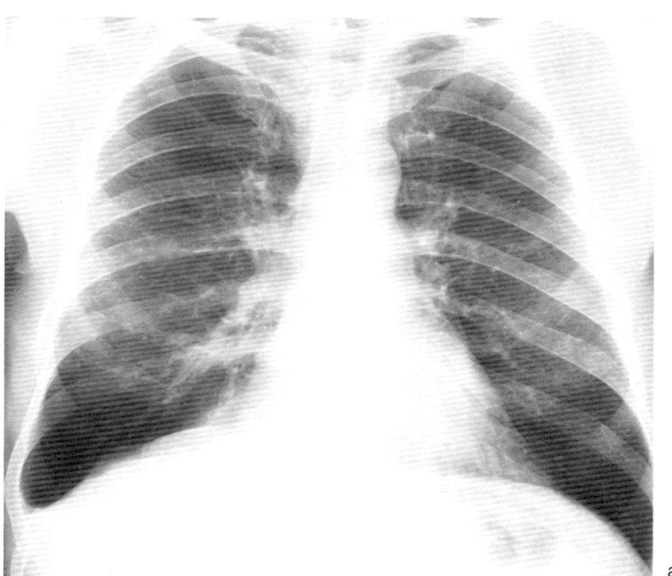

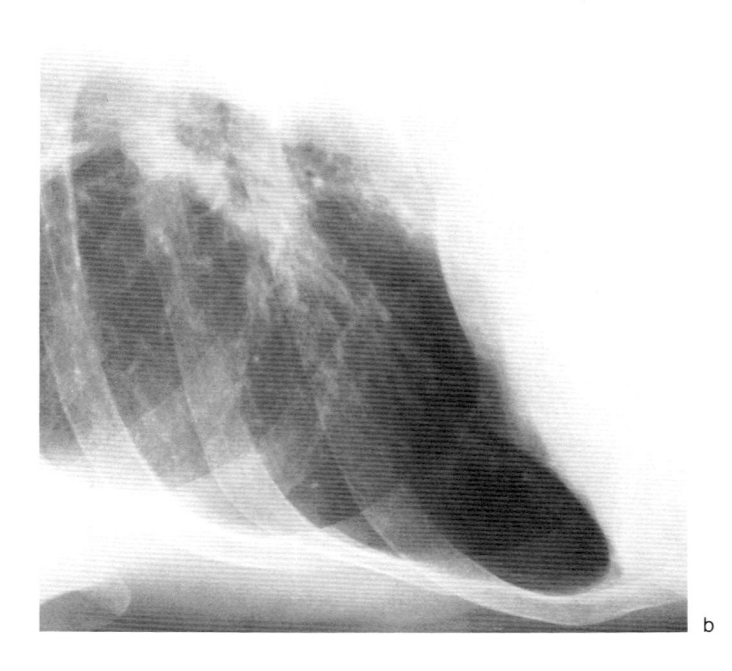

Fig. 9.22 a, b **Basilar pleural scarring.**
Right costophrenic sulcus is blunted. Decubitus film does not reveal any free pleural effusion.

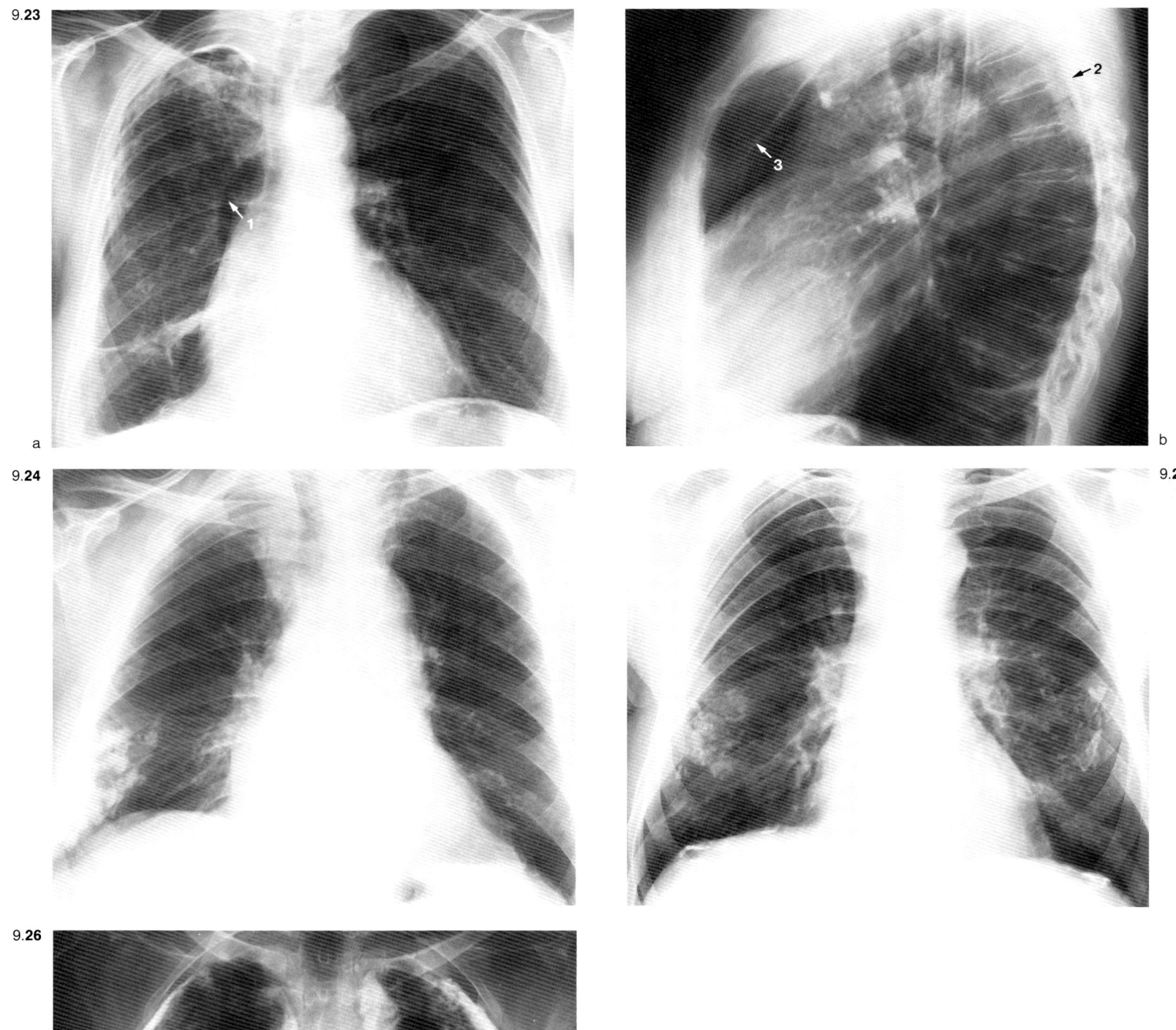

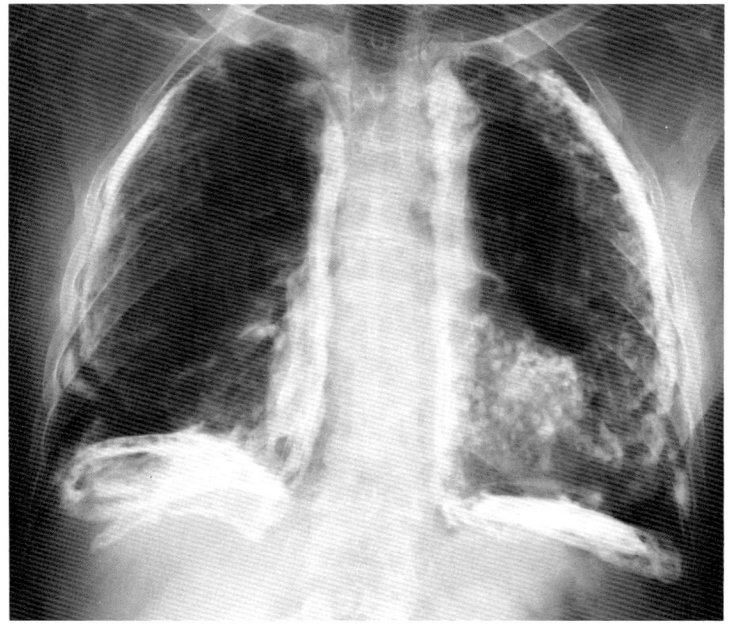

Fig. 9.23 a, b Pleural peel due to previous tuberculosis.
Apicoposterior pleural thickening and calcification (2), calcification of anterior pleura (3), herniation of anterior segment of left upper lobe into right hemithorax, anterior junction line (1).

Fig. 9.24 Calcified pleural hematoma.

Fig. 9.25 Asbestos-related calcified pleural plaques, involving diaphragmatic and parietal costal pleura in lower half of chest.

Fig. 9.26 Severe pleural calcification after asbestos exposure.
Heavy calcification of mediastinal, diaphragmatic, and costal pleura.

Plombage, Oleothorax

Prior to the era of antituberculous chemotherapy, different procedures were used to compress tuberculous cavities and thus facilitate their healing. Such procedures included therapeutic pneumothorax, thoracoplasty, and plombage with lucite balls or oil. The sequelae of these procedures are still occasionally found in elderly patients.

Fig. 9.27 **Oleothorax (plombage) with calcified rim.** Note right apical pleural-parenchymal scarring.

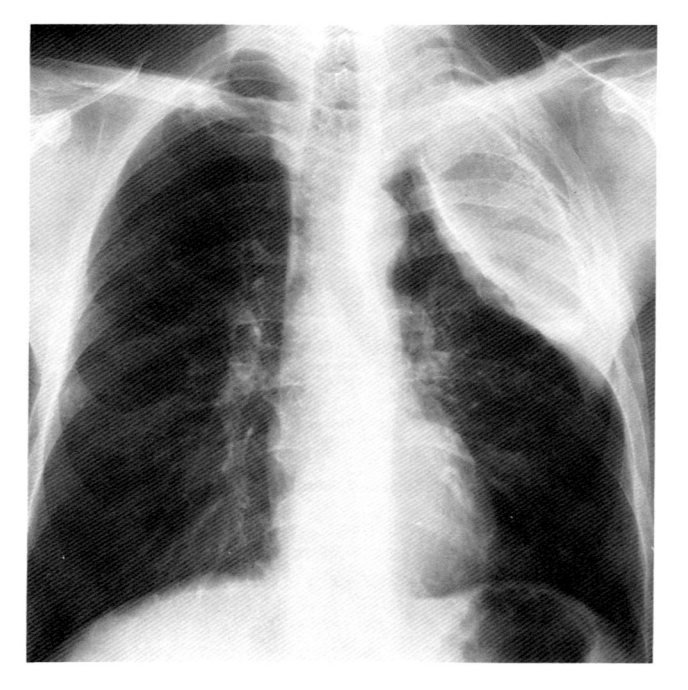

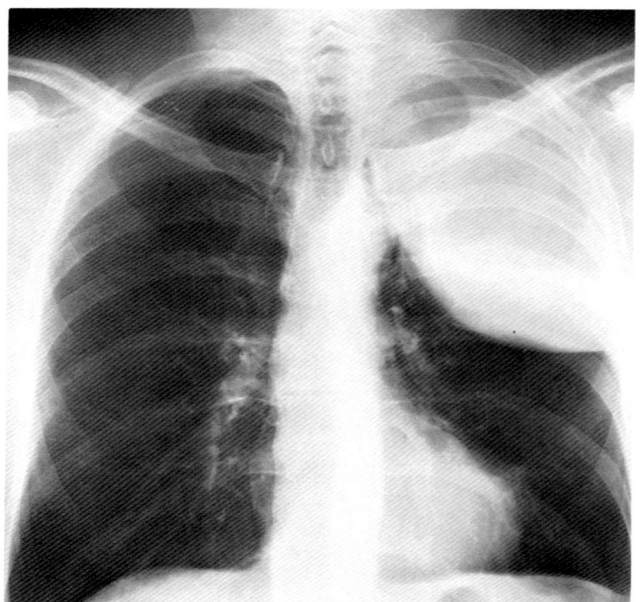

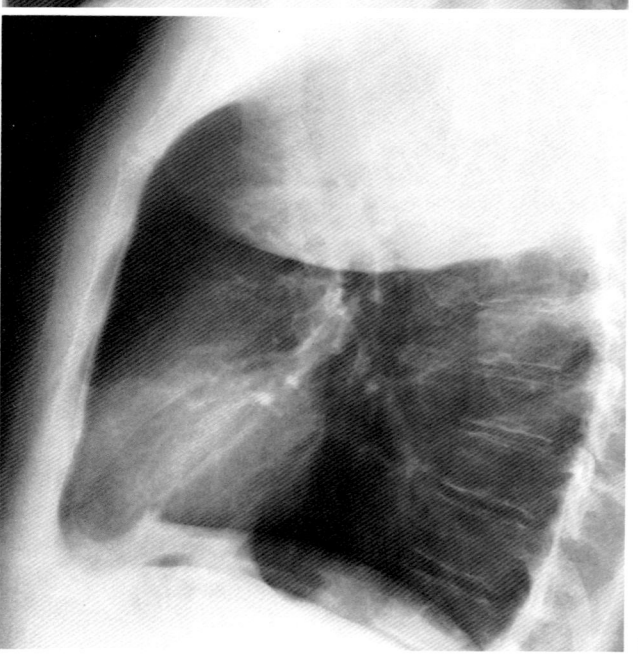

Fig. 9.28 a, b **Oleothorax (plombage) with compression of left upper lobe.**

232   9. Pleural Diseases

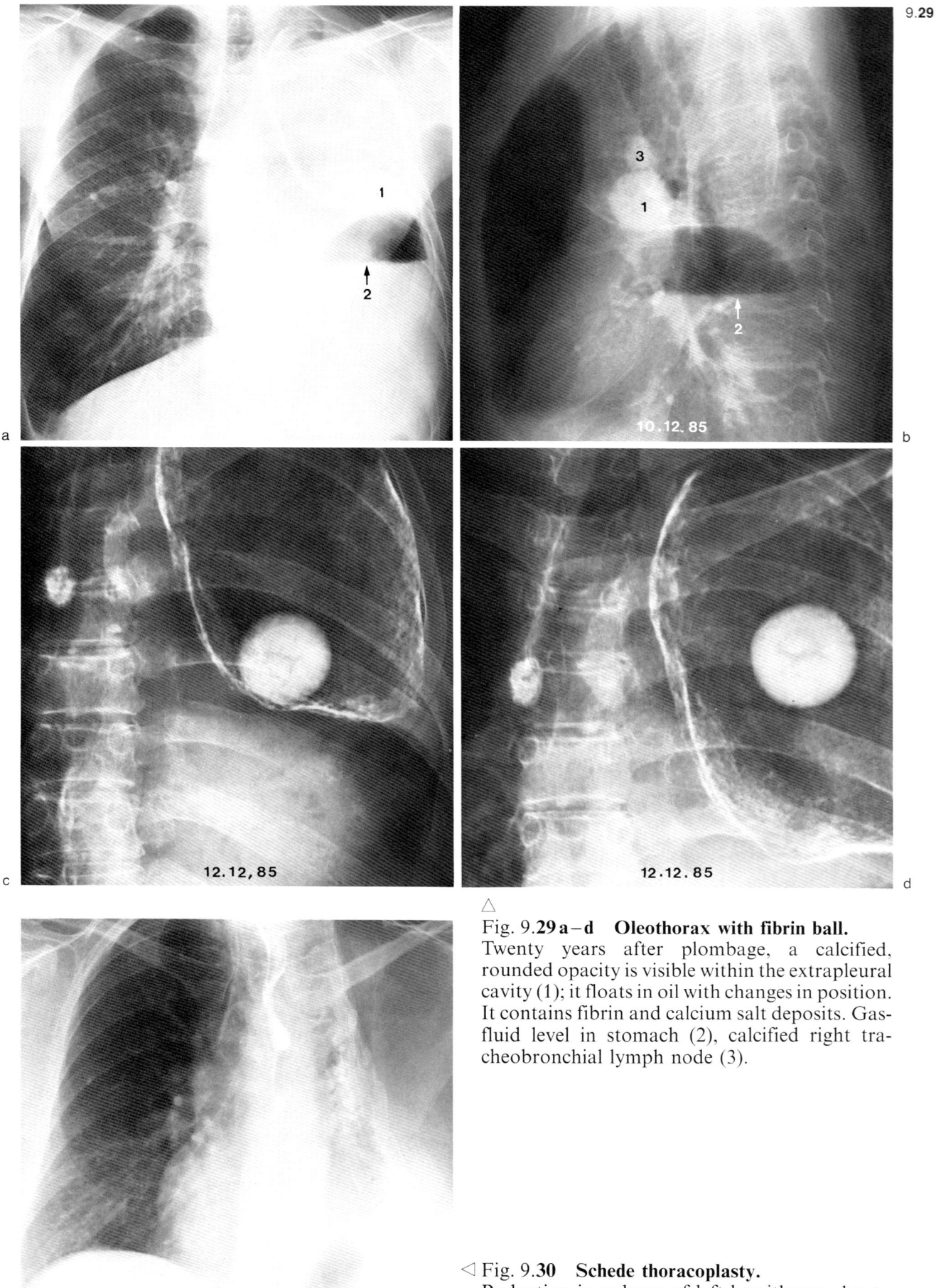

Fig. 9.29 a–d   **Oleothorax with fibrin ball.**
Twenty years after plombage, a calcified, rounded opacity is visible within the extrapleural cavity (1); it floats in oil with changes in position. It contains fibrin and calcium salt deposits. Gas-fluid level in stomach (2), calcified right tracheobronchial lymph node (3).

Fig. 9.30   **Schede thoracoplasty.**
Reduction in volume of left hemithorax due to resection of ribs. Extensive calcification in pleura and in regenerated periosteal rib remnants; left hemidiaphragm elevated.

Malignant Pleural Mesothelioma

This is a rare tumor with an incidence of 1–2 cases per million per year. Between 50% and 80% of these patients have documented asbestos exposure. The tumor spreads along the pleura; it results in pleural effusion, circumferential pleural thickening, or multiple pleural tumors. The lung becomes encased. The mediastinum, the chest wall, and the diaphragm can be involved.

References: 27, 93.

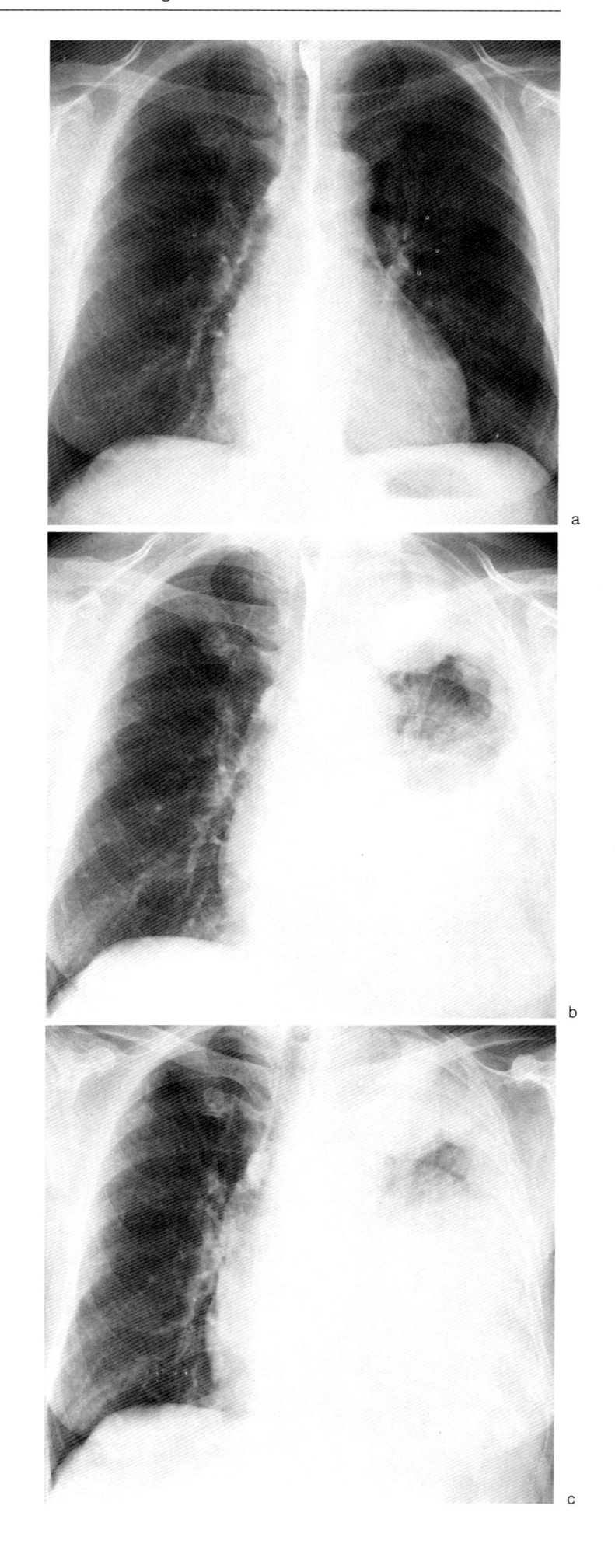

Fig. 9.**31 a–c Malignant pleural mesothelioma.**
67-year-old patient with history of asbestos exposure 20 years prior to current admission. Polycyclic pleural thickening with accompanying pleural effusion (**b, c**) with encasement of left lung. Radiograph taken 2 months prior to current admission was normal.

9. Pleural Diseases

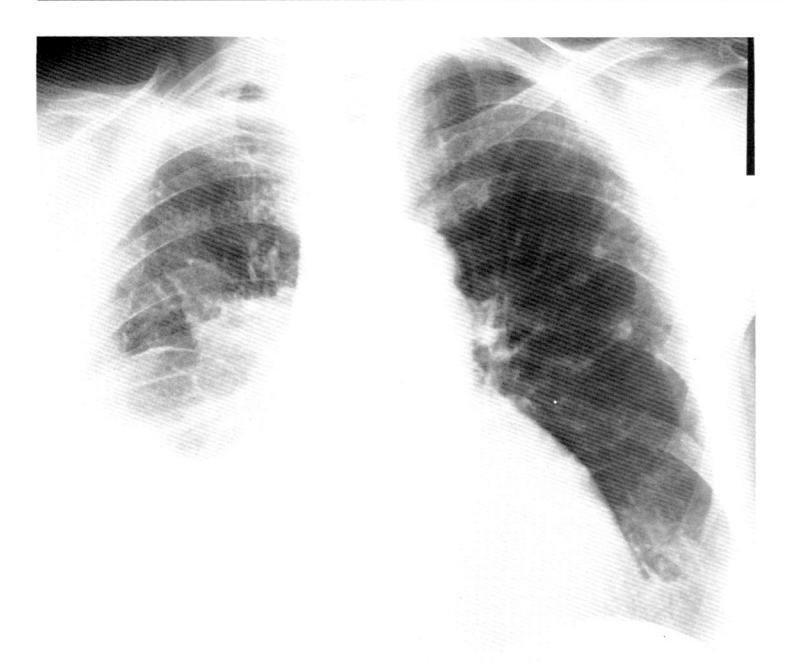

Fig. 9.**32 a, b Malignant pleural mesothelioma.**
75-year-old patient. No definite asbestos exposure elicited. Pleural plaques are visible in left hemithorax along lateral aspect of rib cage. Right basilar pleural effusion with relaxation atelectasis of right lower lobe, best seen on CT.

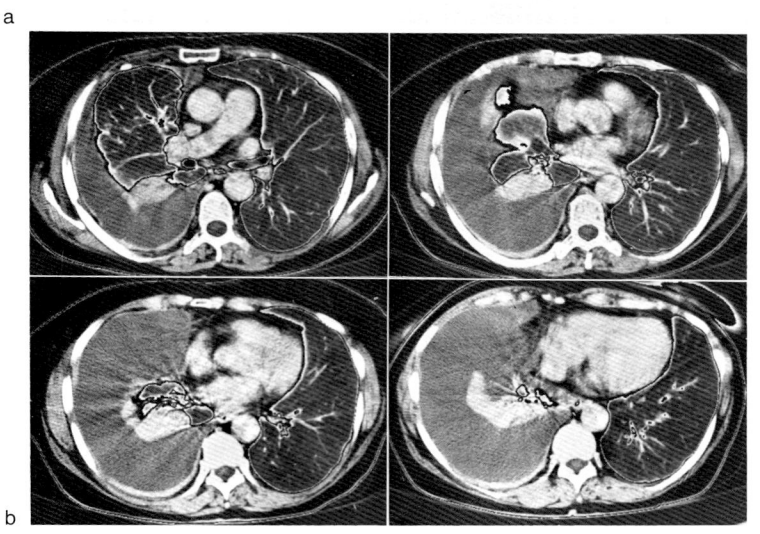

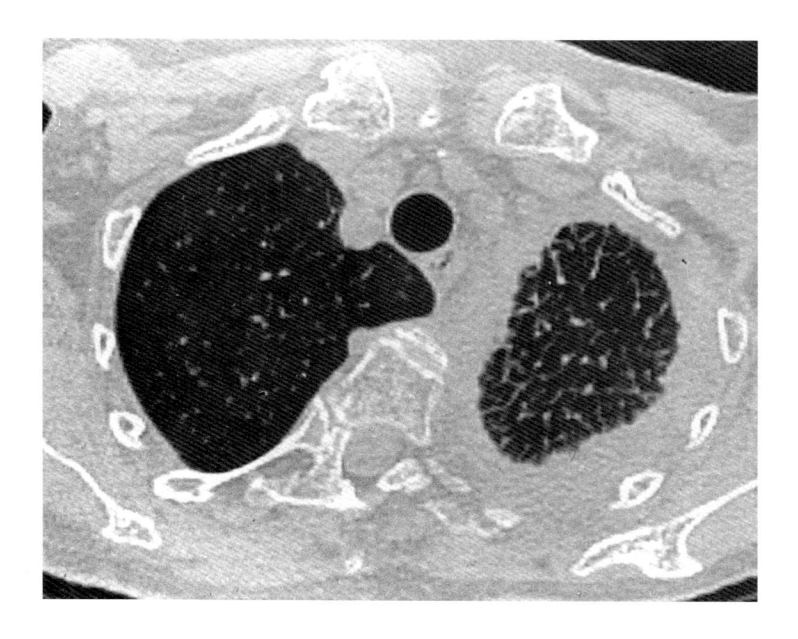

Fig. 9.**33 Malignant mesothelioma.**
CT scan shows a left-sided pleural rind encasing the left lung, with thickening of interlobular septa, likely due to tumor infiltration.

Fig. 9.34 **Malignant mesothelioma.**
Coronal T2-weighted MR scan shows massive right pleural effusion producing mediastinal sthift to the left side and inversion of right hemidiaphragm.

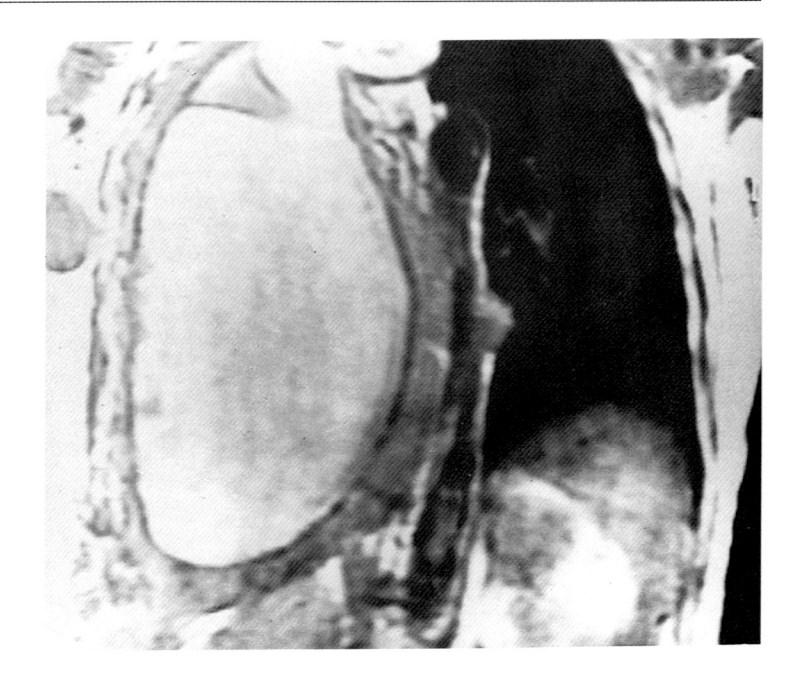

Fig. 9.35 **Fibrous tumor of pleura (benign fibrous mesothelioma).**
CT scan shows a large mass in left hemithorax, which displaces the left atrium to the right and does not conform to any intrapulmonary lobe or segment.

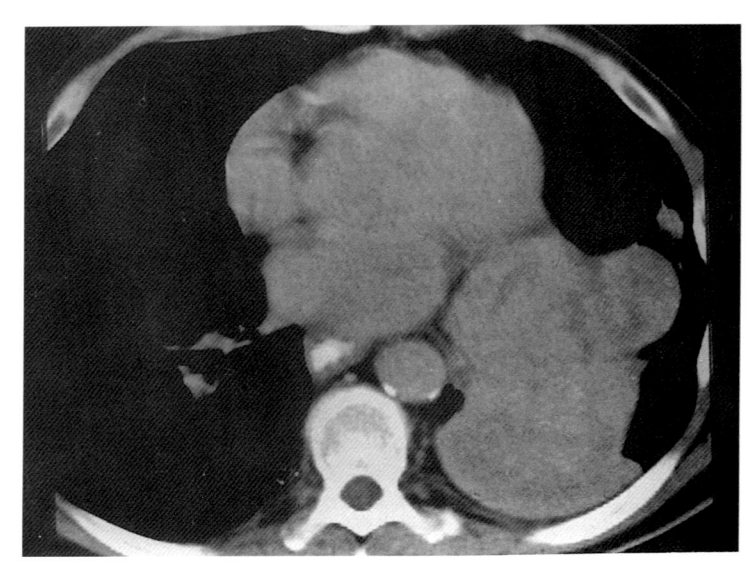

Fig. 9.36 **Fibrous tumor of pleura (benign fibrous mesothelioma).**
CT scan shows large retrosternal mass that mimics an anterior mediastinal mass but actually originates from the mediastinal pleura.

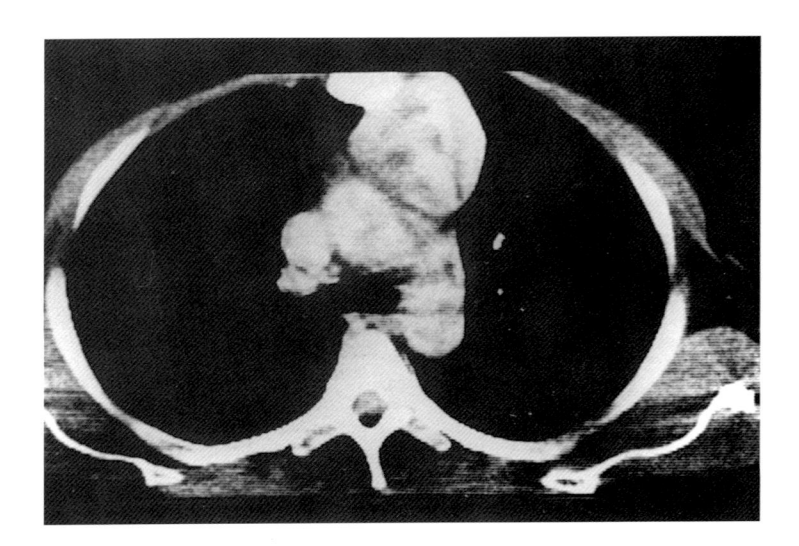

10. Mediastinum

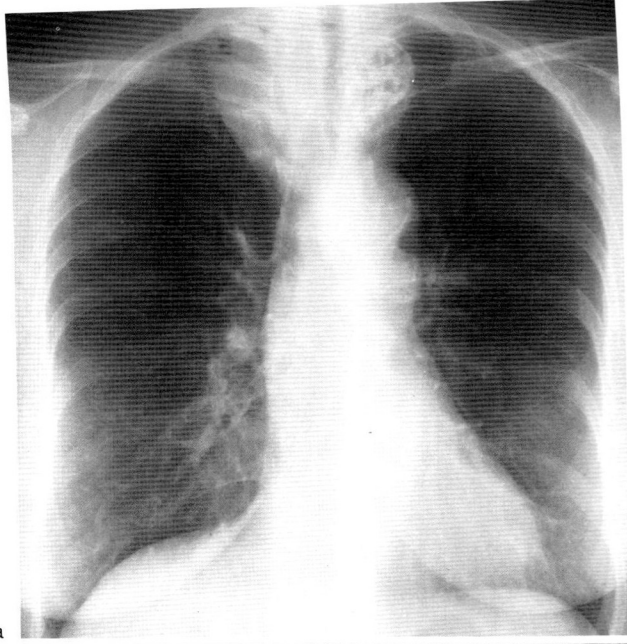

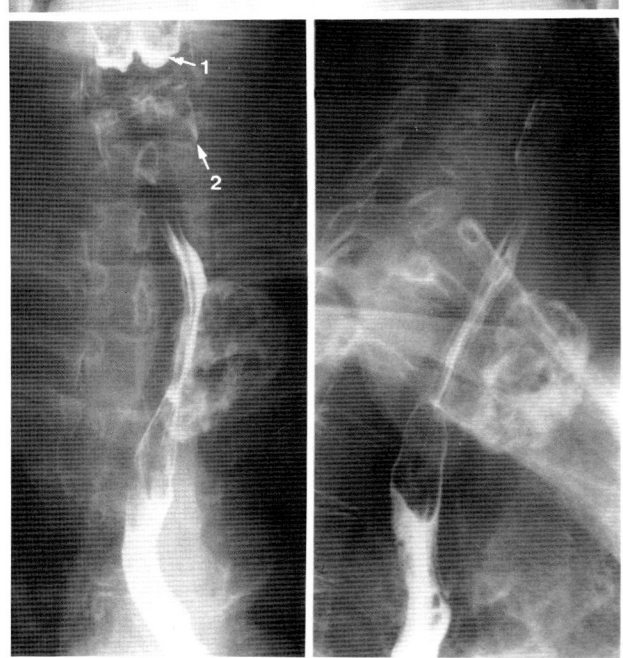

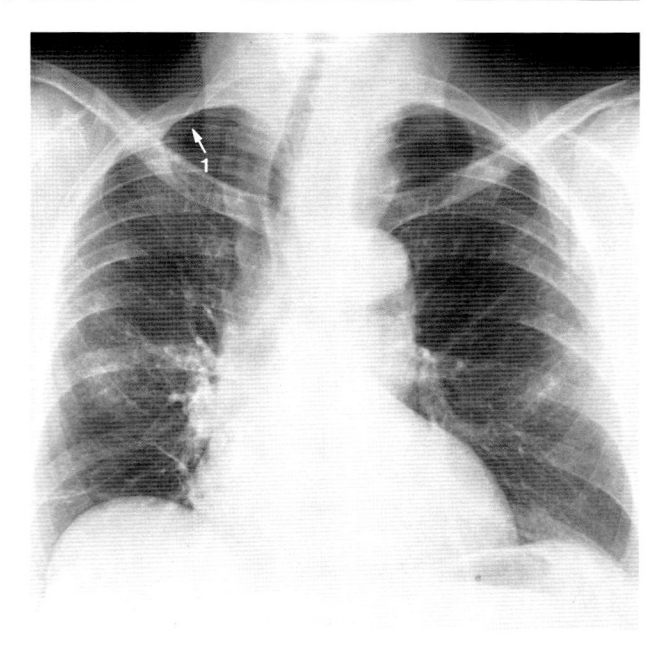

Goiters

Goiters result from enlargement of the thyroid gland due to cysts, hormone-producing parenchyma, or neoplastic tissue. Only 3% of goiters have an intrathoracic component. Of these, 80% are retrosternal and 20% posterior descending, located dorsal to the trachea and esophagus.

On plain chest radiographs, intrathoracic goiters result in widening of the superior mediastinum with displacement and narrowing of the trachea. CT and radionuclide scanning can demonstrate the goiter. Functioning and nonfunctioning parts of the goiter can be displayed with radionuclide studies.

References: 70.

◁ Fig. 10.1 a, b **Goiter.**
69-year-old patient with a known, decade-old history of goiter. Large superior mediastinal mass narrowing the trachea. Calcified nodular adenoma in left lobe of thyroid gland. Esophageal displacement present. Vallecula (1), piriform sinus (2).

◁ Fig. 10.2 **Goiter.**
Superior mediastinal mass with tracheal deviation to the right. Cervical rib (1).

Fig. 10.3 **Goiter with calcified left adenoma.** Tracheal displacement to right side with flattening of left aspect of tracheal wall. Calcifications and low attenuation region in left adenoma.

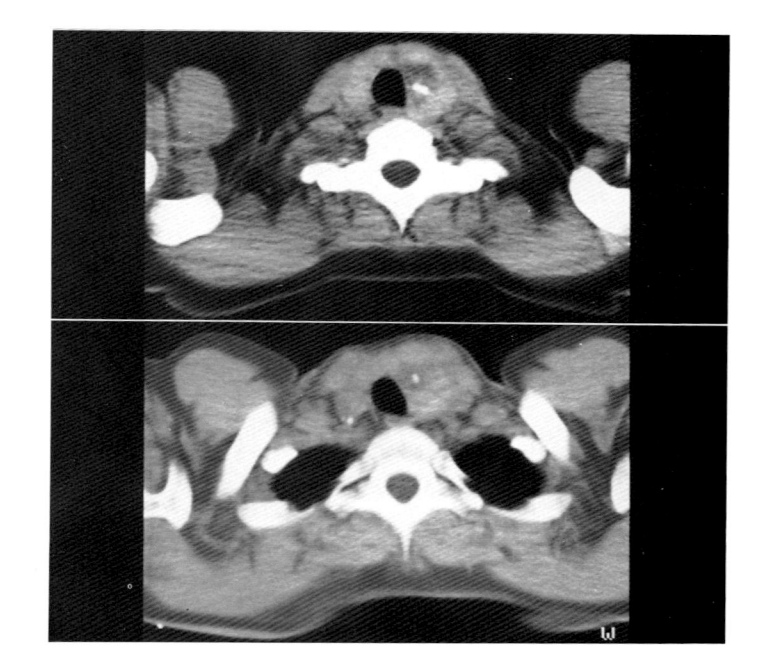

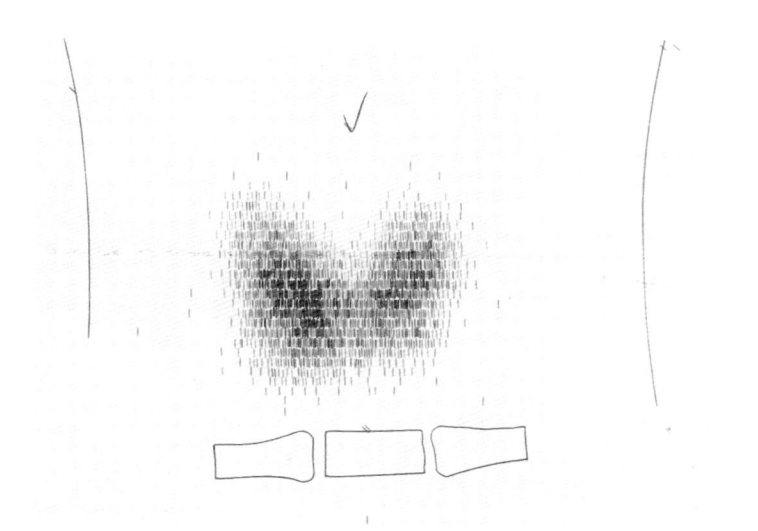

Fig. 10.4 Thyroid scan with technetium-99m. Normal thyroid gland.

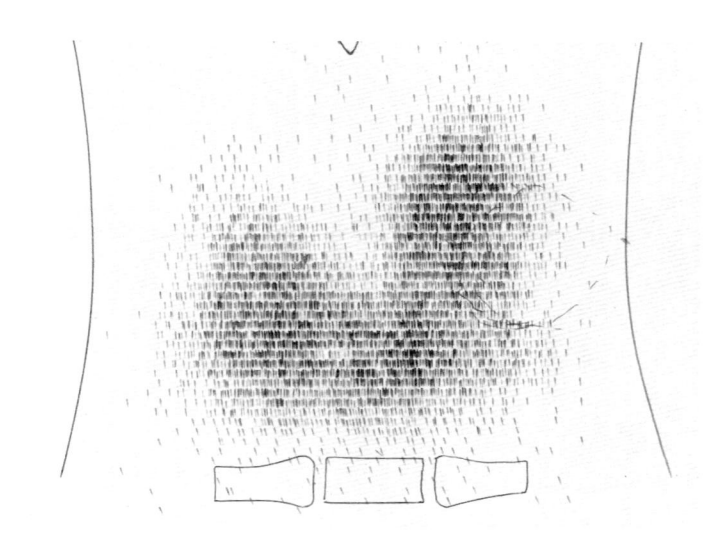

Fig. 10.5 **Diffuse goiter with cold nodule in left lobe.**

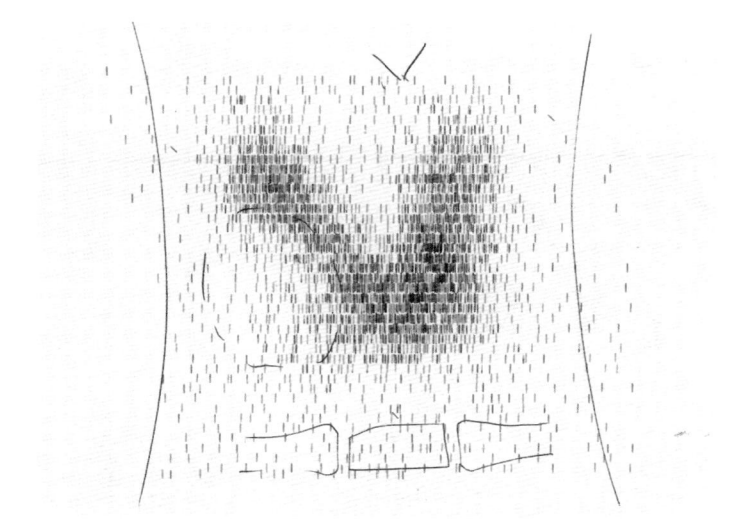

Fig. 10.6 **Cold nodule in right lobe of thyroid gland.**

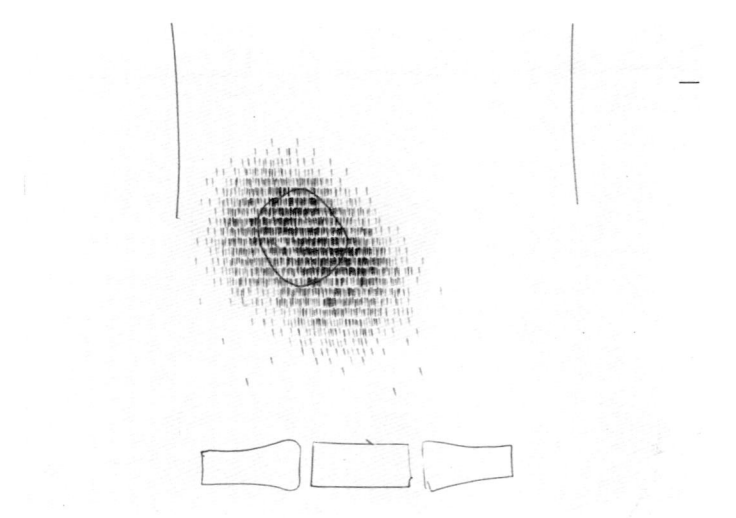

Fig. 10.7 Hyperfunctioning adenoma with lack of activity in the suppressed, normal thyroid gland.

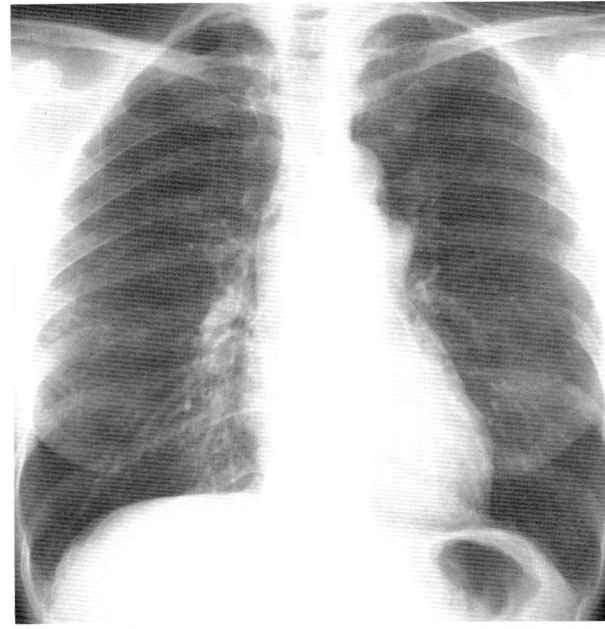

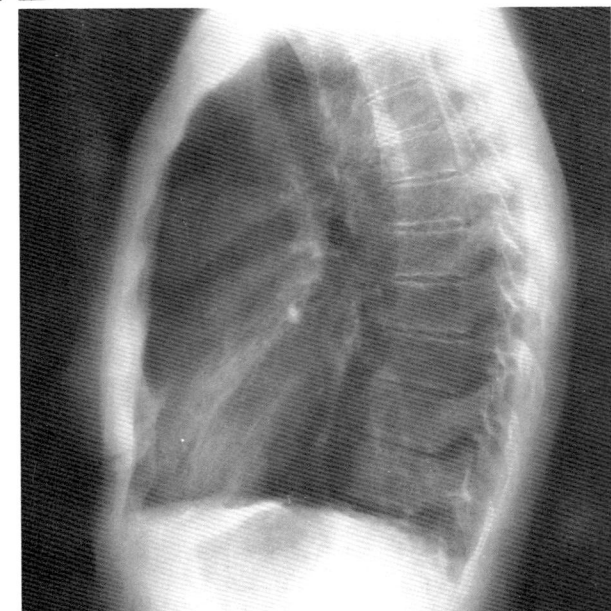

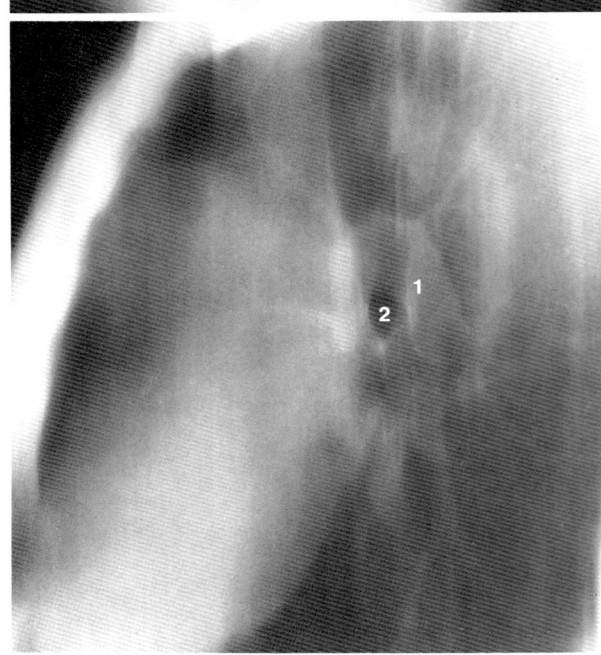

Thymic Hyperplasia and Thymoma

The thymus plays an important role in the development of cellular immunity. At birth, it weighs 15 g and increases in weight until puberty when it reaches a weight of 30 g. Then it is gradually replaced by fat, the so-called thymic involution. True thymic hyperplasia is seen in Graves disease, as a rebound after stress, or in remission after the treatment of lymphoma or leukemia in children and adolescents. The thymus is histologically normal in these conditions. The thymic hyperplasia described in 60–70% of patients with myasthenia gravis is different since it involves primarily the cortex and its lymphoid follicles.

Within the thymus or its mostly fatty replaced residue, tumors and cysts can form: Thymomas of the lymphoepithelial or spindle-cell variety, carcinoids, carcinomas, lymphomas, teratomas, lipomas, liposarcomas, and cysts can be found.

Thymomas are associated with myasthenia gravis in 50% of cases; conversely, 15% of myasthenics harbor a thymoma. Red cell aplasia and hypoglobulinemias can be associated with spindle-cell thymomas. Carcinoids can produce adrenocorticotropic hormone (ACTH) and be associated with Cushing syndrome.

Fig. 10.8 a–c **Thymoma.**
63-year-old patient with myasthenia gravis and proven thymoma. Frontal chest film shows mass superimposed on main pulmonary artery segment; it causes an extra convexity lateral to the descending aorta, overlying the aortic-pulmonic window.
The lateral view and the lateral tomogram show the retrosternal, anterior, mediastinal mass. Left pulmonary artery (1) with epibronchial course in relation to left mainstem bronchus (2).

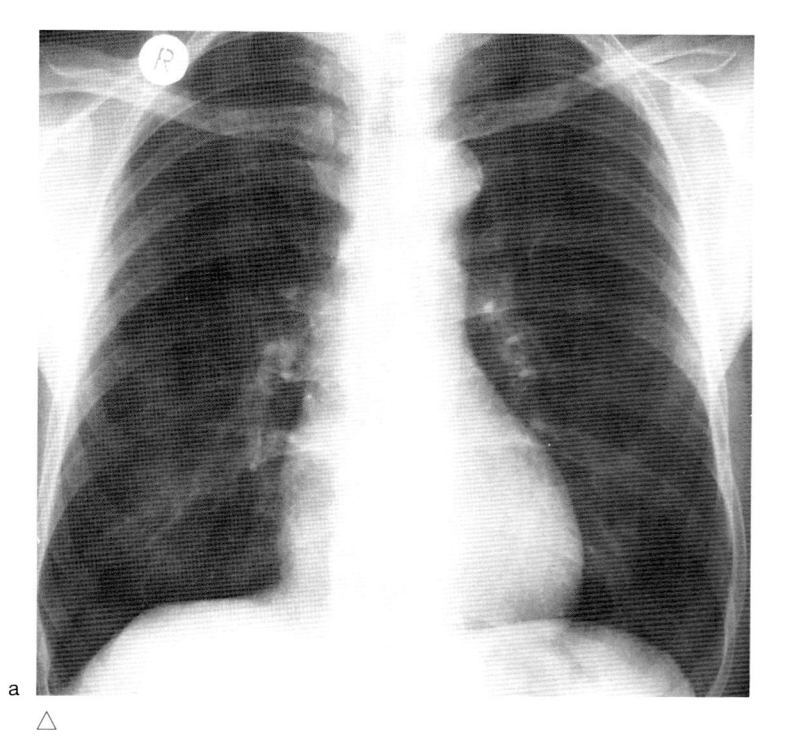

Fig. 10.9 a, b Small thymoma.
16-year-old, asymptomatic person. Incidental retrosternal mass seen only on lateral chest radiograph (1).

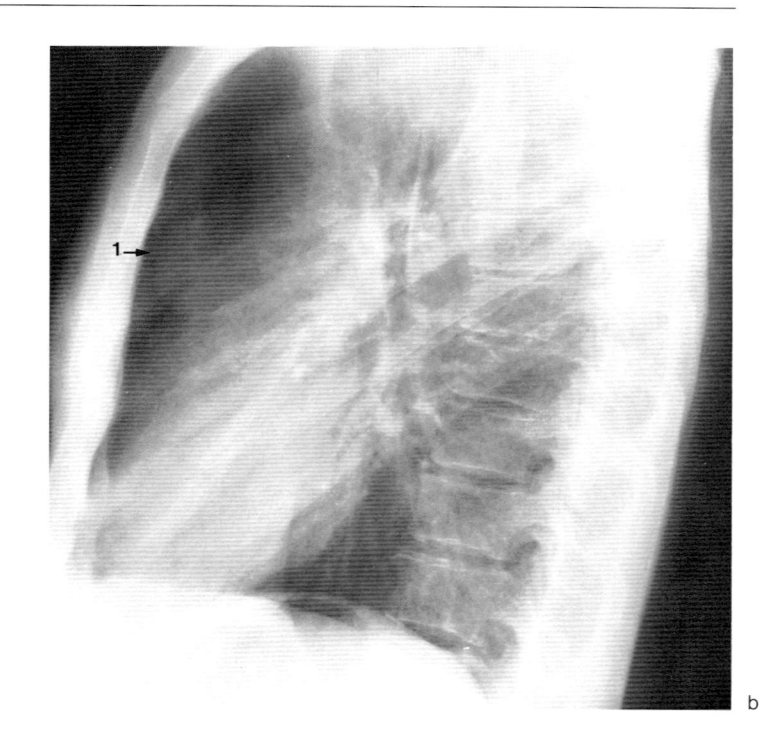

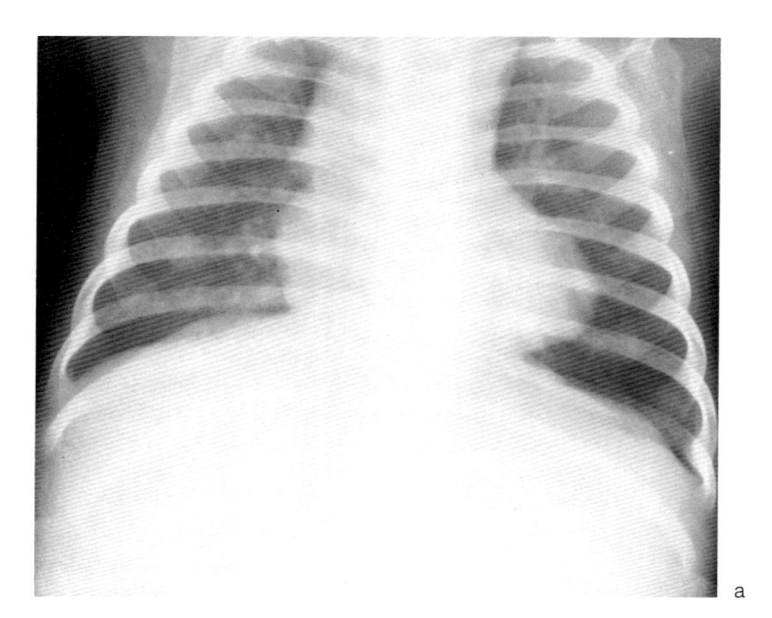

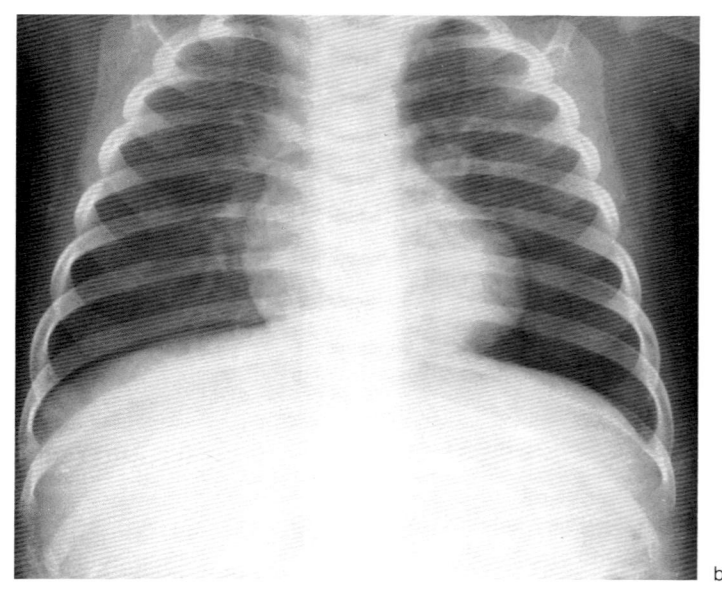

Fig. 10.10 a, b Thymic hyperplasia.
Nine-month-old child with stridor and large thymus. After low-dose radiotherapy, the thymus decreases in size. This type of therapy is not used anymore.

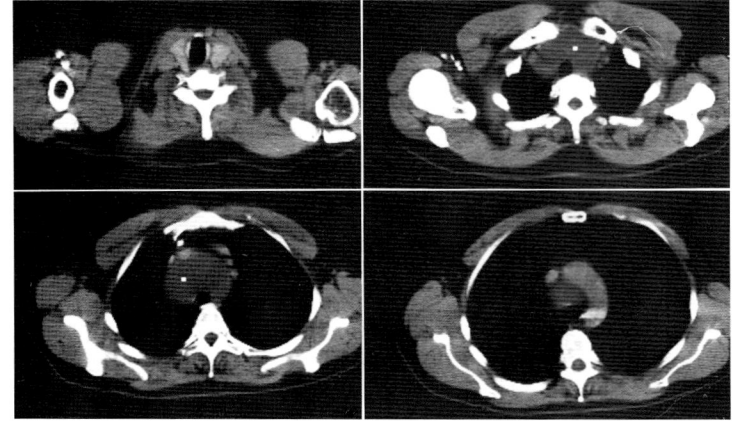

Mediastinal Cysts and Lymphangiomas

Fig. 10.11 a–c   Bronchogenic cyst.
56-year-old patient with stridor and dysphagia. Superior mediastinal widening and posterior tracheal deviation. Note curvilinear imprint on anterior tracheal wall seen on lateral view (1). Mass projects over tracheal air column (2). Posterior tracheal wall (3), lateral border of scapula (4). CT scan demonstrates hypoattenuating, smoothly marginated, peritracheal mass, which displaces the aortic arch branches.

Fig. 10.**12 a, b Dermoid cyst.**
21-year-old, asymptomatic patient. A previous chest radiography taken 5 years prior to current film. Subcarinal mass, projecting to the right and posterior to left atrium.

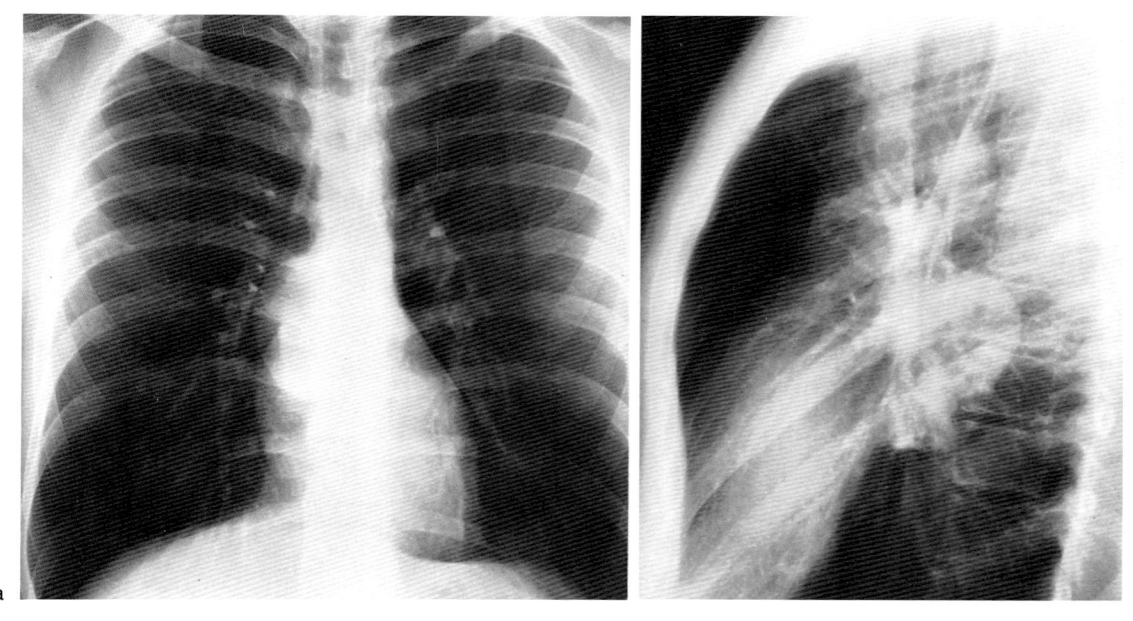

Fig. 10.**13 a, b Lymphangioma.**
6-year-old girl presenting with dyspnea. Marked mediastinal widening impinging upon adjacent lung. Trachea slightly displaced to the left and posteriorly but not narrowed (1), indicating that the mass is soft and pliable. Lymphangioma encompasses in this case all mediastinal compartments.

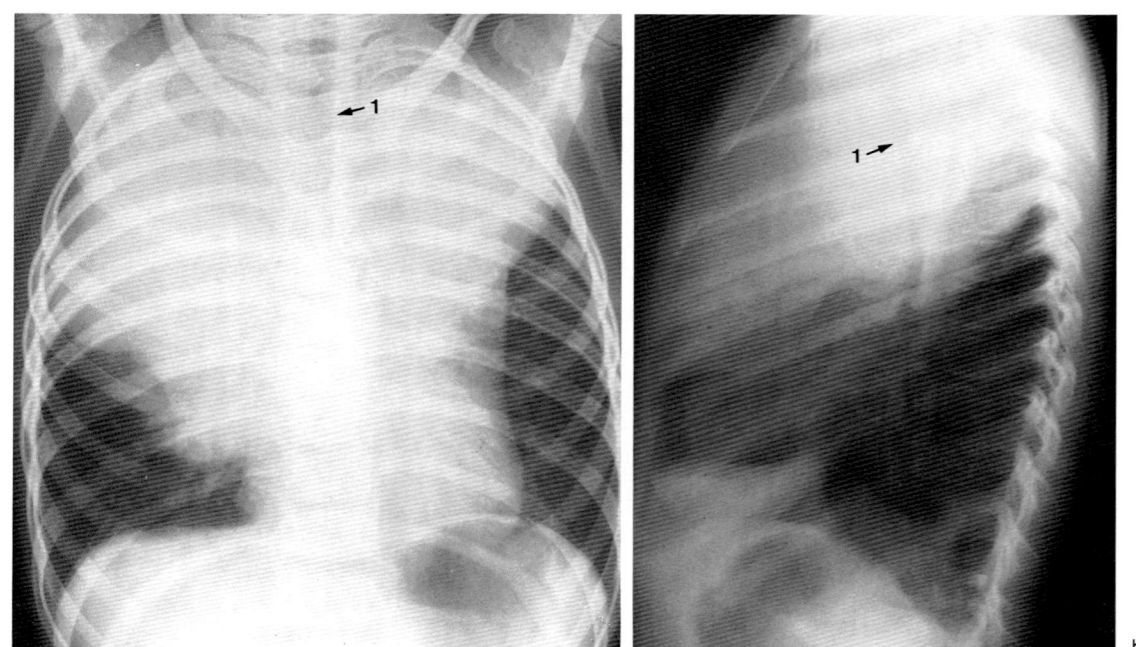

Fig. 10.**14 Cystic lymphangioma.**
53-year-old woman with mild dysphagia. Smoothly marginated right-sided, superior mediastinal mass. Calcified left paratracheal nodes (1) as an incidental finding.

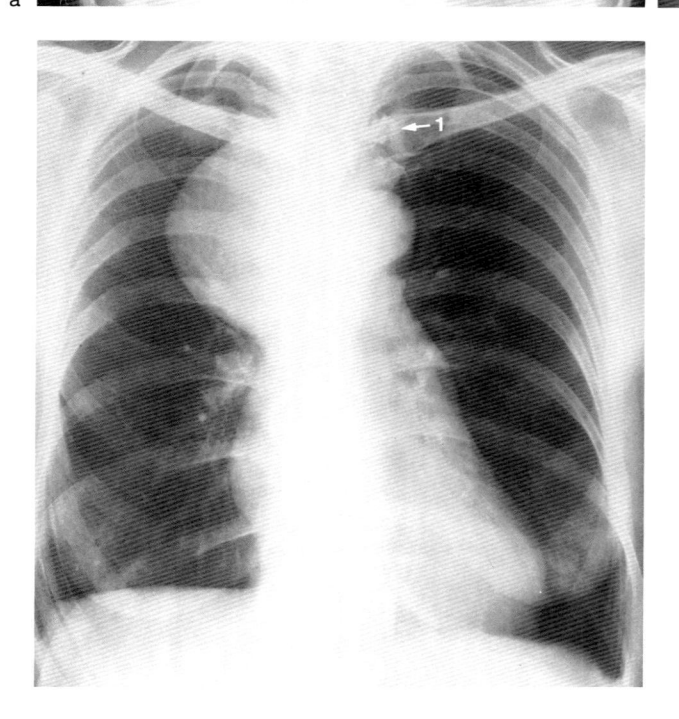

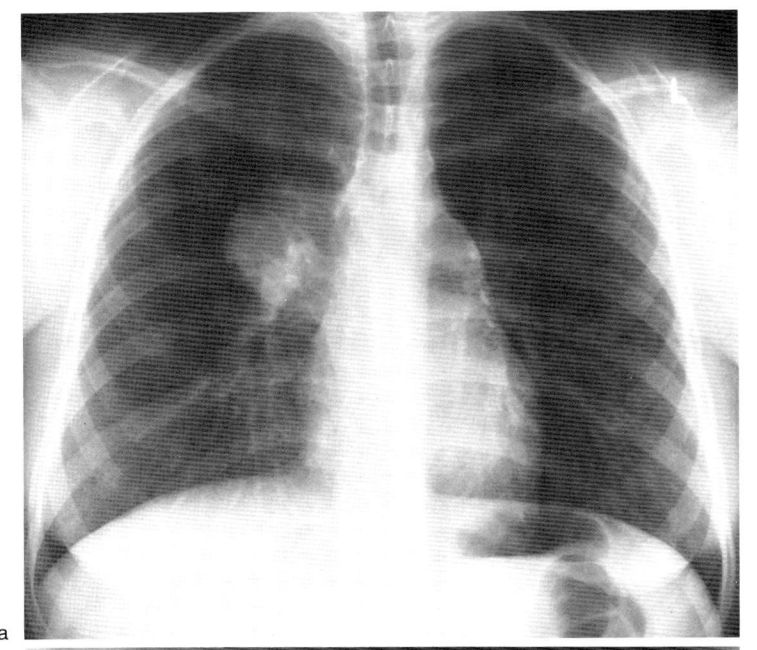

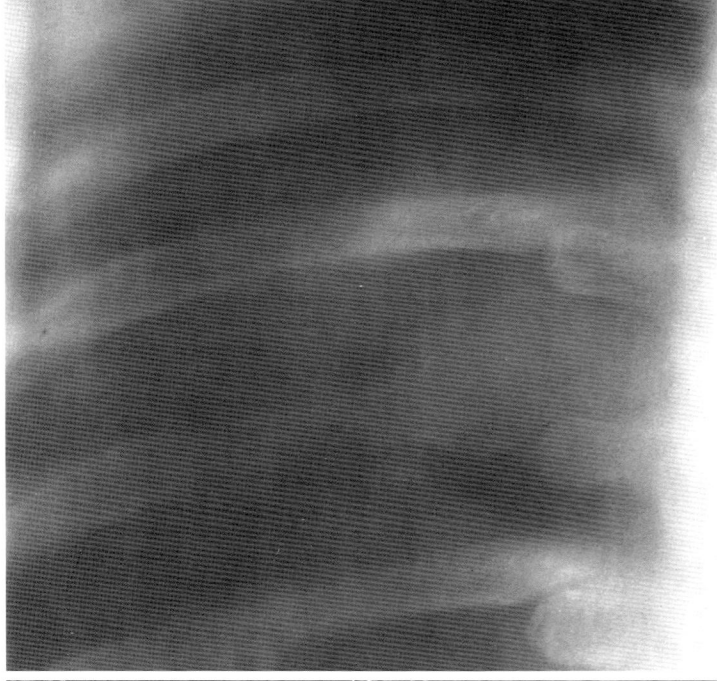

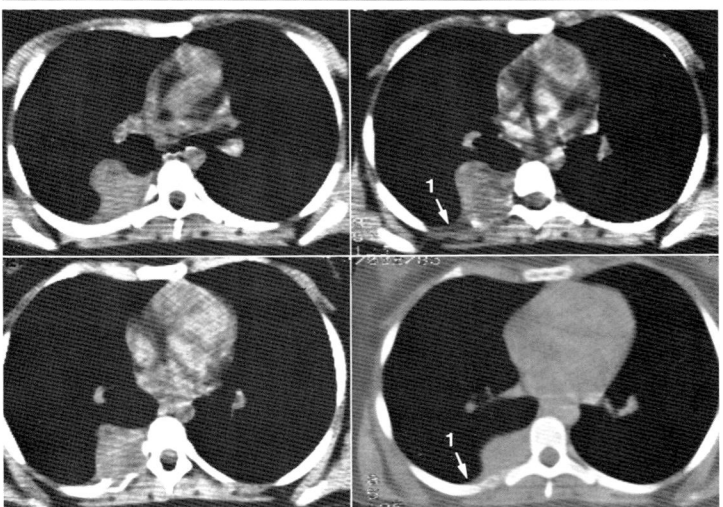

Fig. 10.15 a–c Neuroblastoma.
13-year-old patient with back pain.
Large, posterior, right, paravertebral mass projects over right hilus. Note focal destruction of rib. Extrapulmonary, paraspinal mass forms an obtuse angle of interface with the adjacent chest wall.

Fig. 10.16 a, b Schwannoma. ▷
11-year-old patient.
Smoothly marginated, left, paravertebral mass which obliterates the contour of the descending aorta and widens the left paraspinal stripe.

Fig. 10.17 a, b Ganglioneurofibroma. ▷
4-year-old patient with weight loss.
Marked widening of left paraspinal region, best appreciated on overpenetrated view of the chest.

Fig. 10.18 a, b Neurinoma. ▷
44-year-old patient with segmental neuralgia in dermatome T6. Left paravertebral mass projecting lateral to aortic arch into left hemithorax.

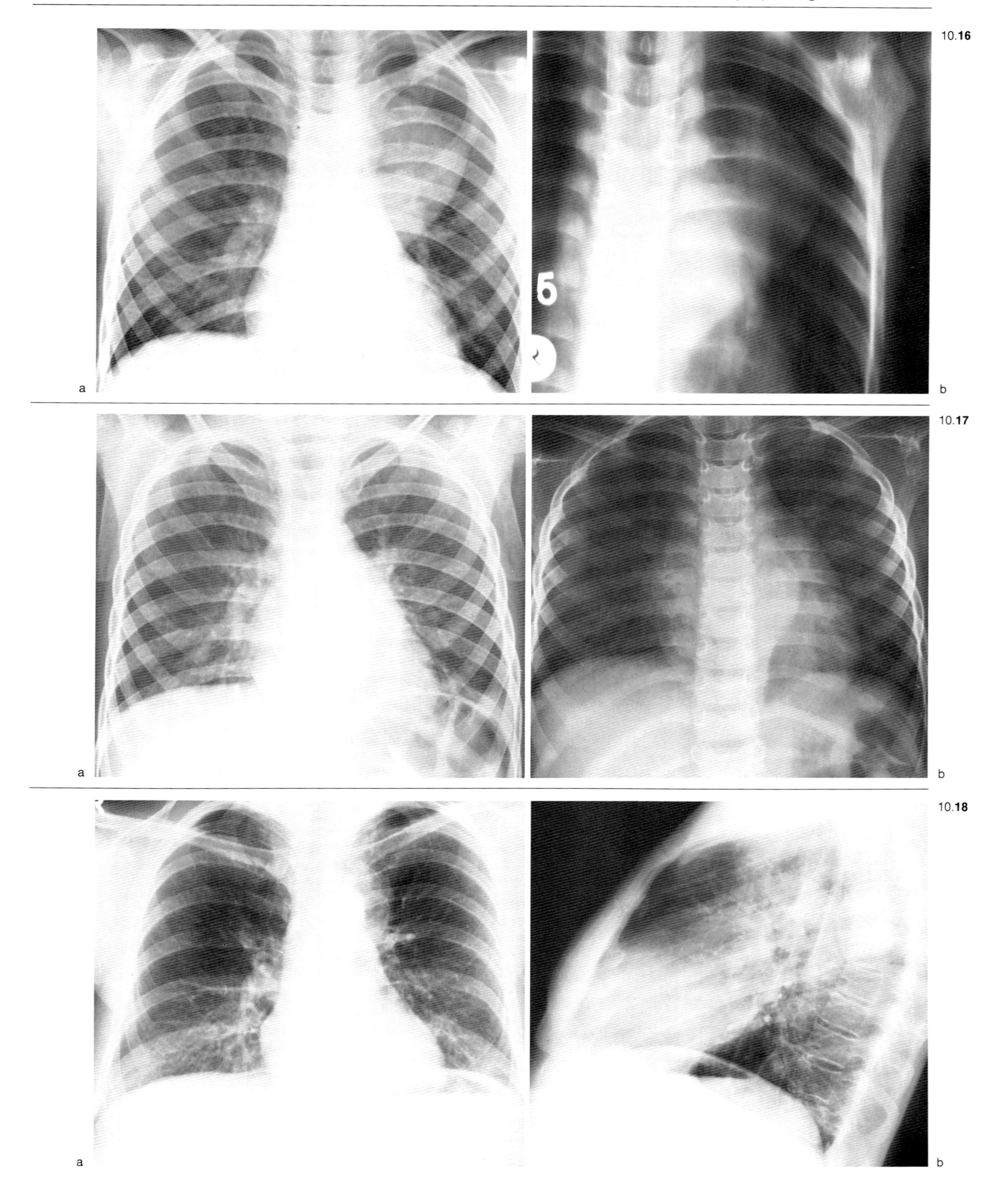

Mediastinal Cysts and Lymphangiomas 245

10.16

10.17

10.18

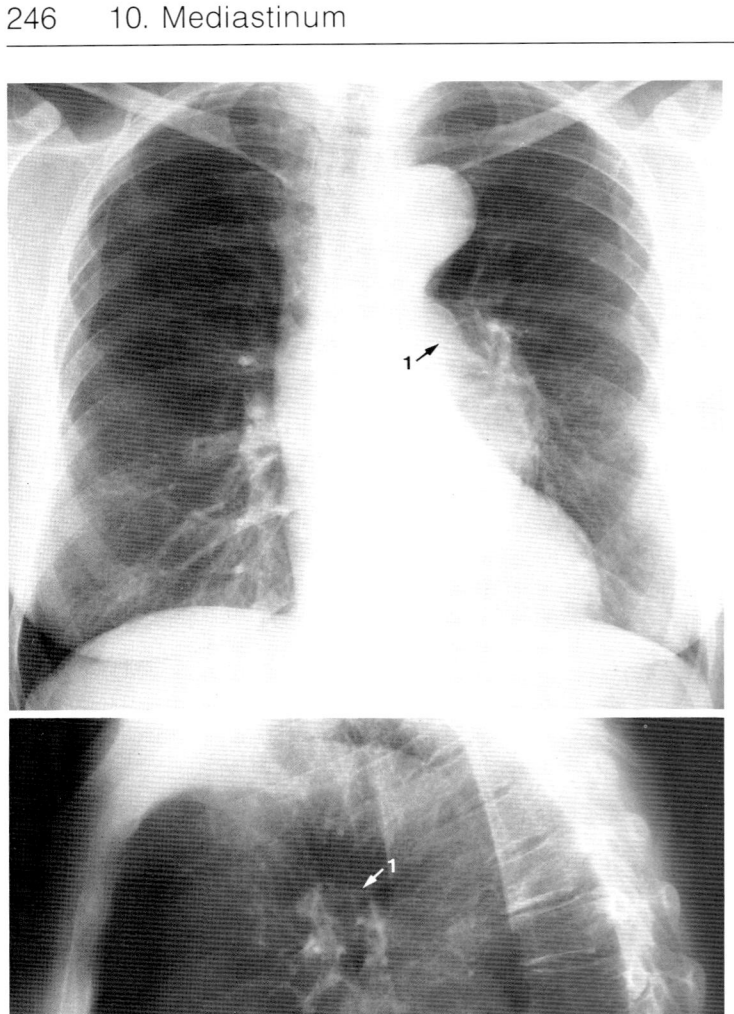

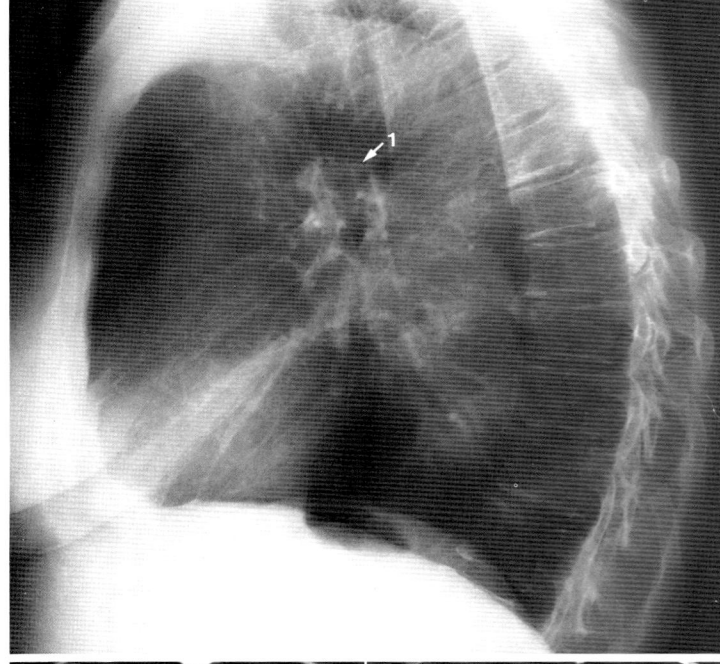

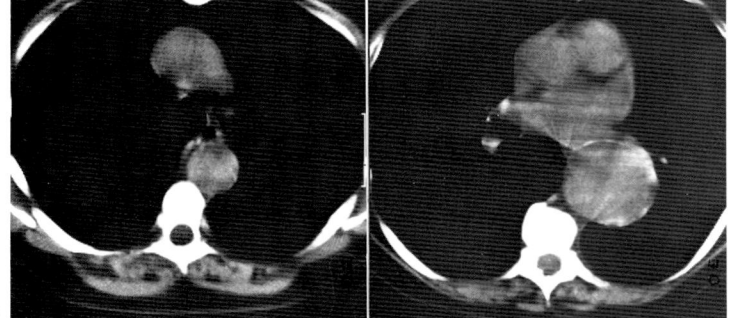

Thoracic Aorta

Dilatation or elongation of the thoracic aorta produces contour abnormalities of the mediastinum which can be clarified by CT, MRI, or angiography.

Fig. 10.**19 a–c Aneurysm of the descending thoracic aorta.** 71-year-old hypertensive patient with recent onset of dysphagia. Marked elongation with fusiform descending aortic aneurysm that has a shell-like calcific rim (1).

Fig. 10.**20 a, b Patient with Marfan syndrome, cystic medial necrosis, annuloaortic ectasia, and aortic regurgitation.**
a Coronal T1-weighted MR scan shows marked dilatation of the ascending aorta as well as dilatation of the left ventricle. **b** Axial T1-weighted MR scan demonstrates marked dilatation of the ascending aorta, which compresses the left atrium, the superior vena cava, and the main pulmonary artery.

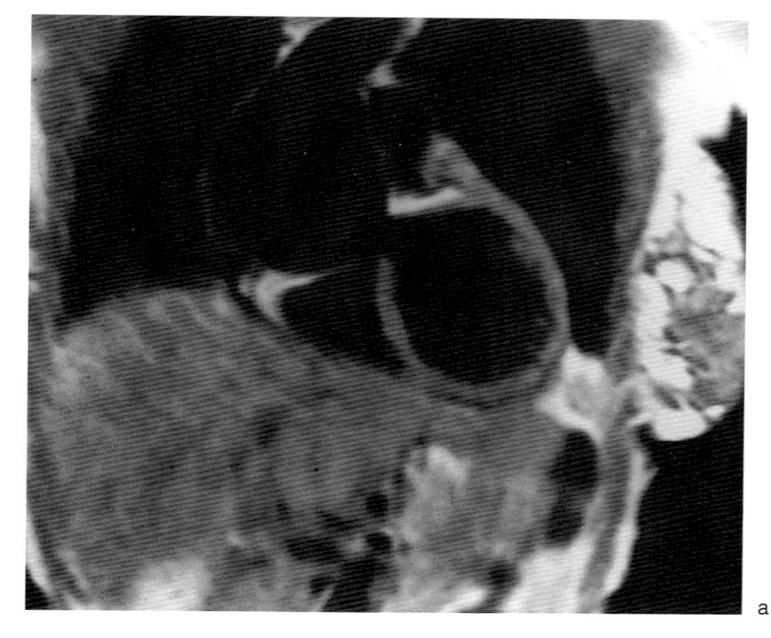

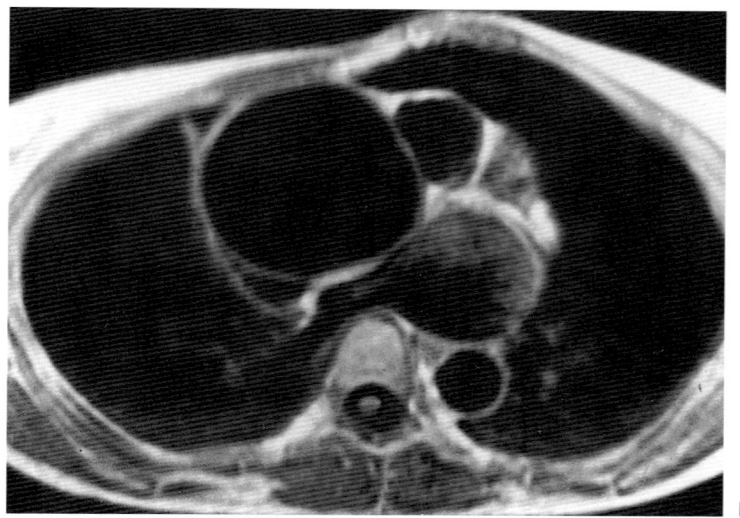

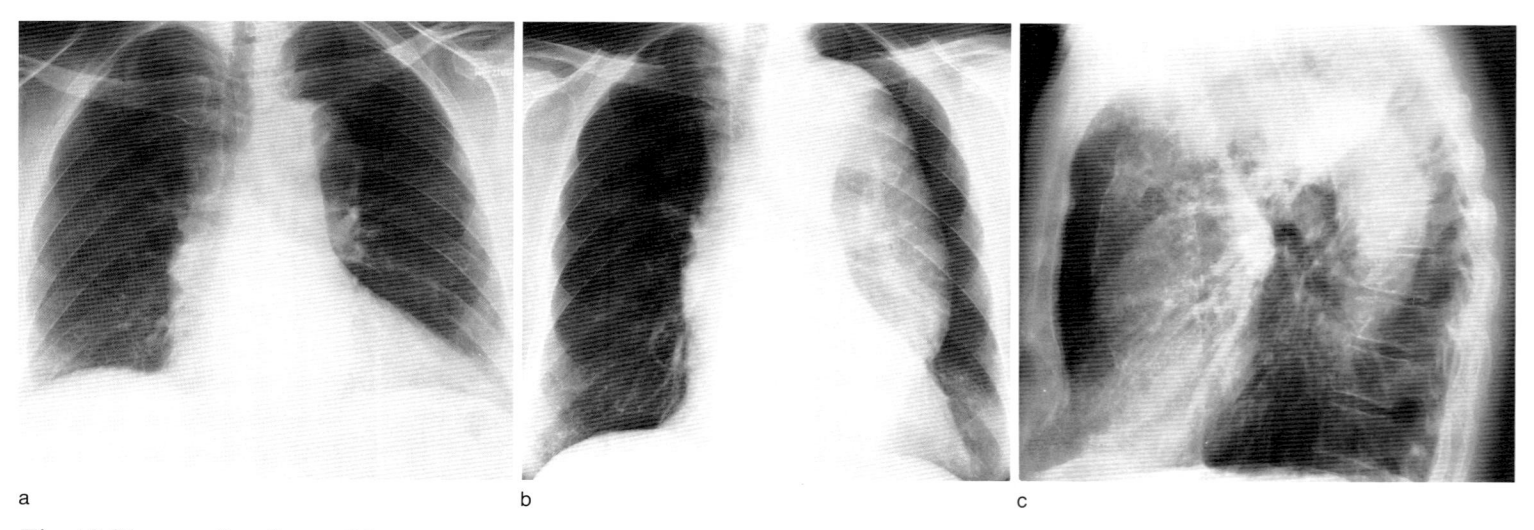

Fig. 10.**21 a–c Luetic aortitis.**
Positive VDRL test result. Isolated calcification of ascending aorta and generalized dilatation of entire thoracic aorta (**b, c**). Previous film taken 20 years prior to current examination shows only mild ectasia of aorta.

248   10. Mediastinum

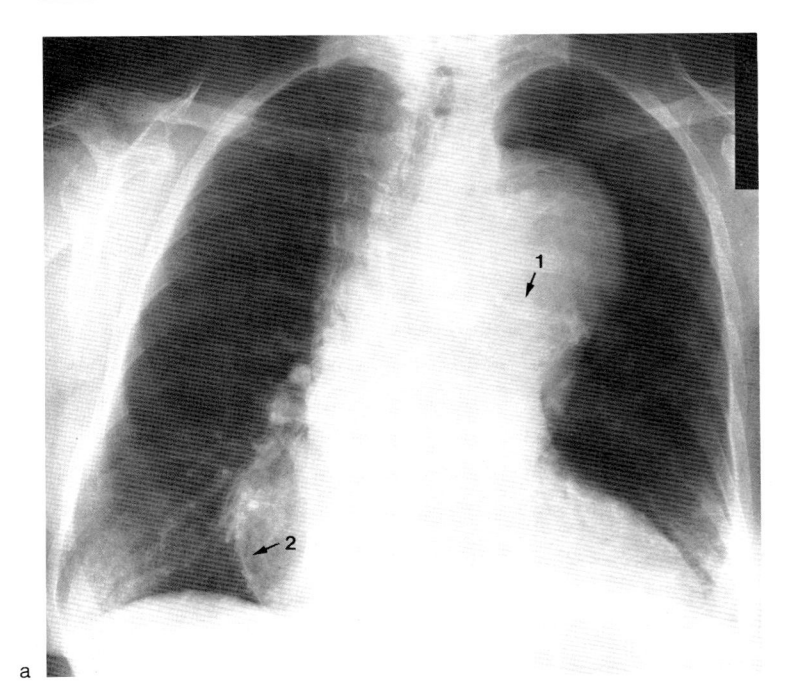

Fig. 10.22 a–c **Ruptured thoracic aortic aneurysm.**
63-year-old hypertensive patient. Initial film (**a**) shows generalized aneurysm of aortic arch and descending aorta. Calcifications are seen in the arch (1) and descending aorta (2). Trachea is markedly displaced to the right. An acute episode of chest pain and hypotension brought the patient to the hospital. Chest radiograph at admission (**b**) shows further dilatation of aorta, increased rightward tracheal deviation, and new left pleural effusion (3). CT confirms the left pleural effusion. Parietal thrombus present in the abdominal extension of the thoracic aneurysm.

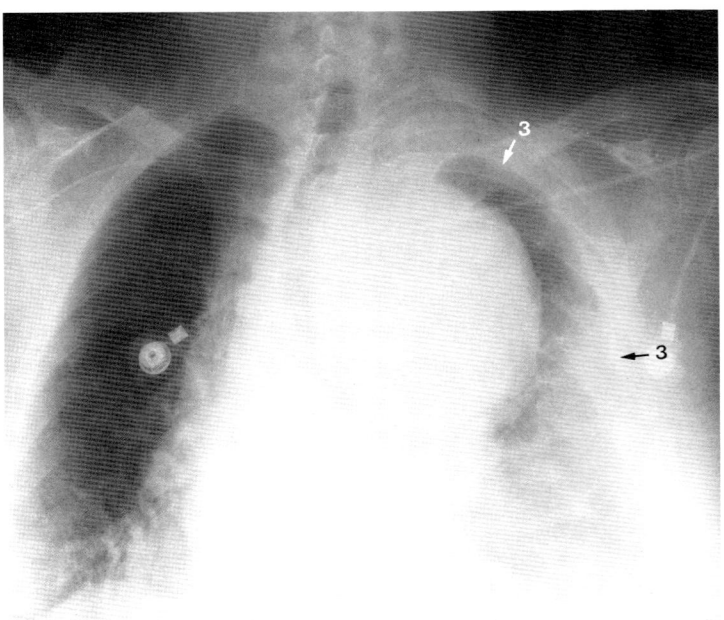

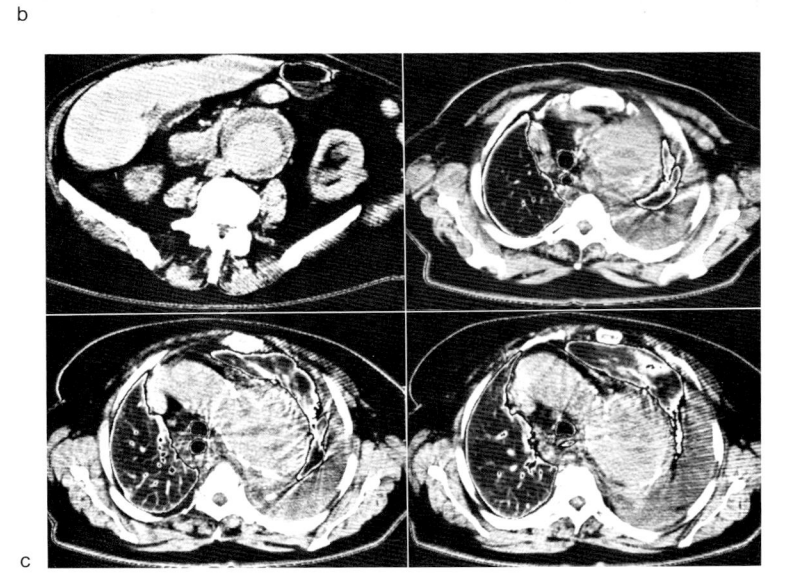

Fig. 10.23 a–c **Double aortic arch.**
Right (1) and left-sided aortic arch. The right arch is larger and higher in position. The trachea and esophagus are impinged upon from the right side and posteriorly (3). The descending thoracic aorta is tortuous and descends on the left before swinging to the right (4).

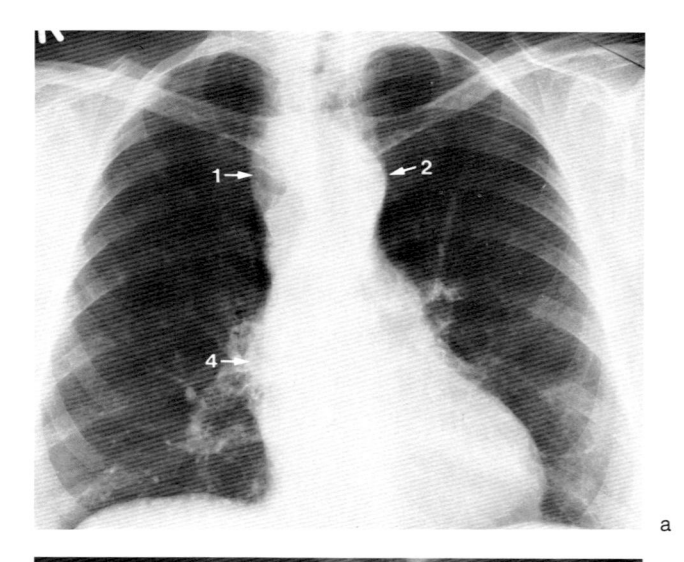

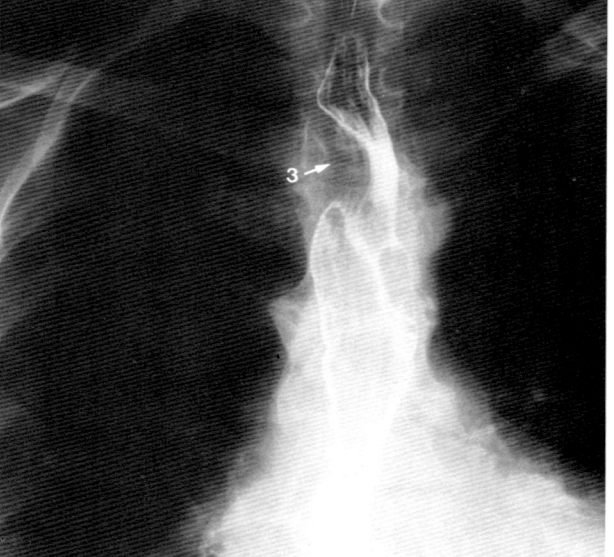

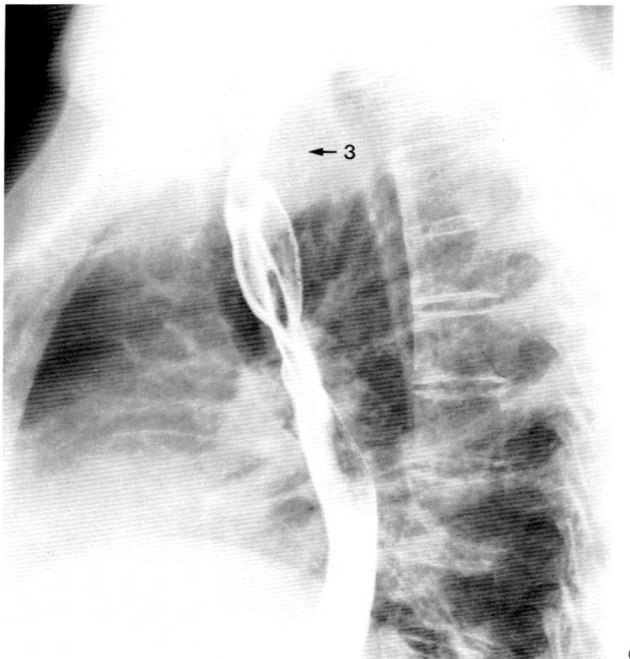

250   10. Mediastinum

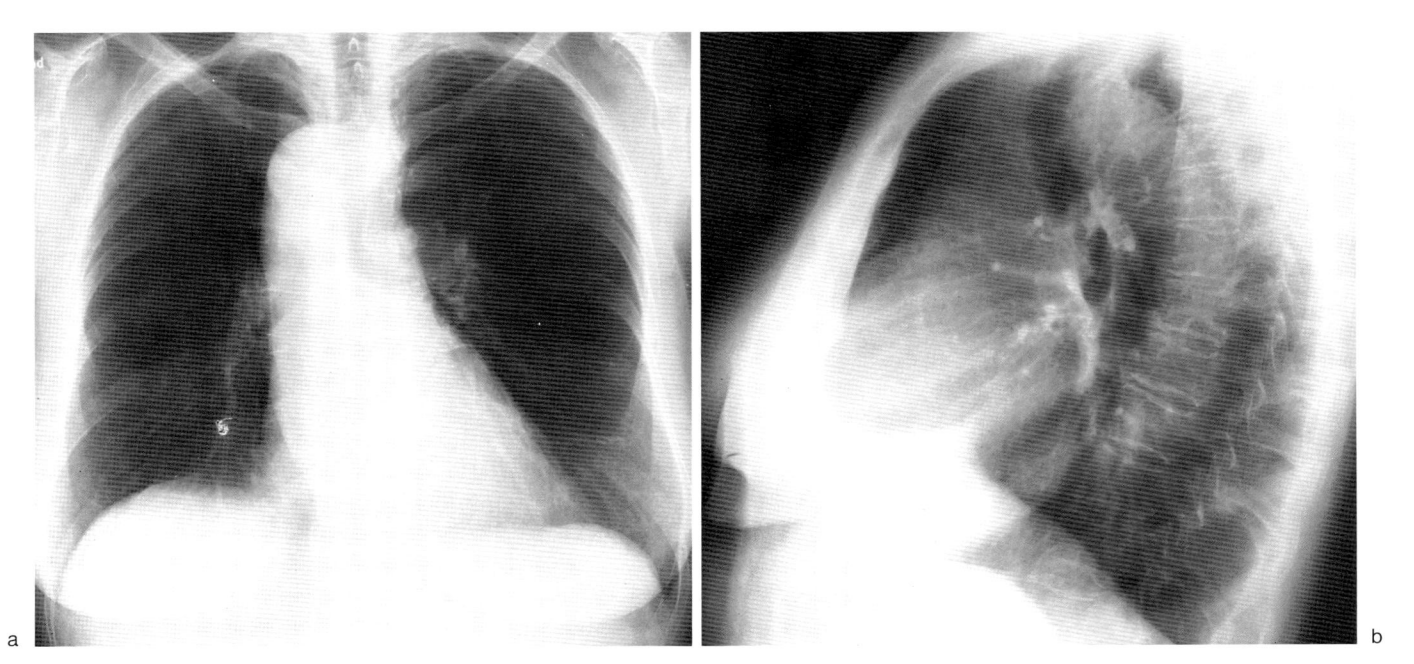

Fig. 10.24 a, b   **Right-sided aortic arch.**
Aorta descends on the right. Note posterior tracheal imprint.

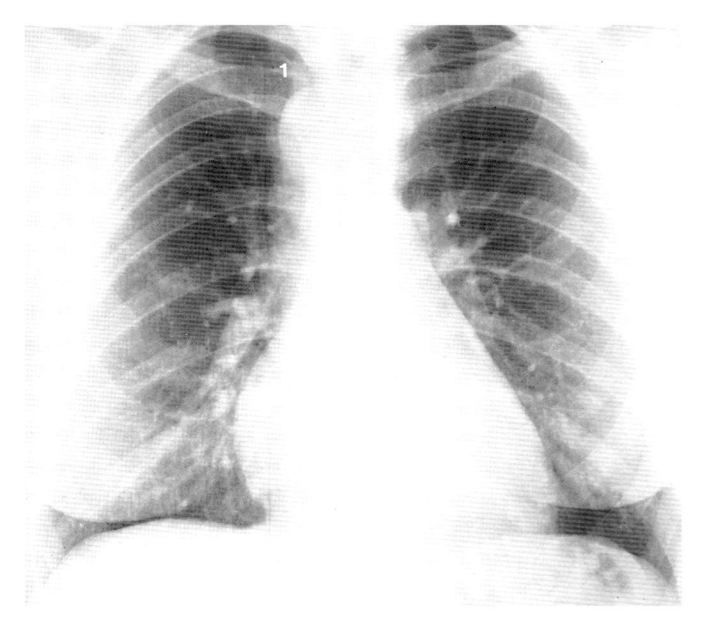

Fig. 10.25   **Right-sided aortic arch (1).**
Descending aorta on right side.

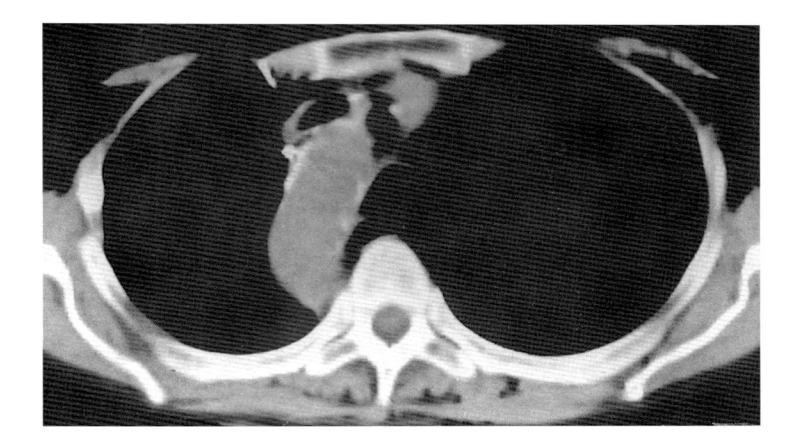

Fig. 10.26   **Right-sided aortic arch with mirror-image branching.**
CT scan shows right-sided arch without prevertebral, retrotracheal, vascular component.

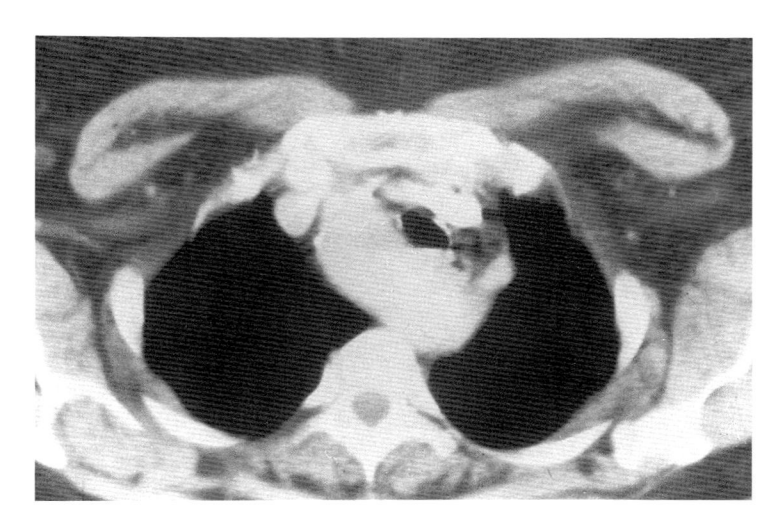

Fig. 10.27   **Right-sided aortic arch with aberrant left subclavian artery.**
CT scan demonstrates right arch with large retrocardiac component formed by so-called Kommerell diverticulum.

Fig. 10.**28** **Left-sided aortic arch.**
Calcified arteriosclerotic plaques in brachiocephalic artery (1) and descending aorta (2).

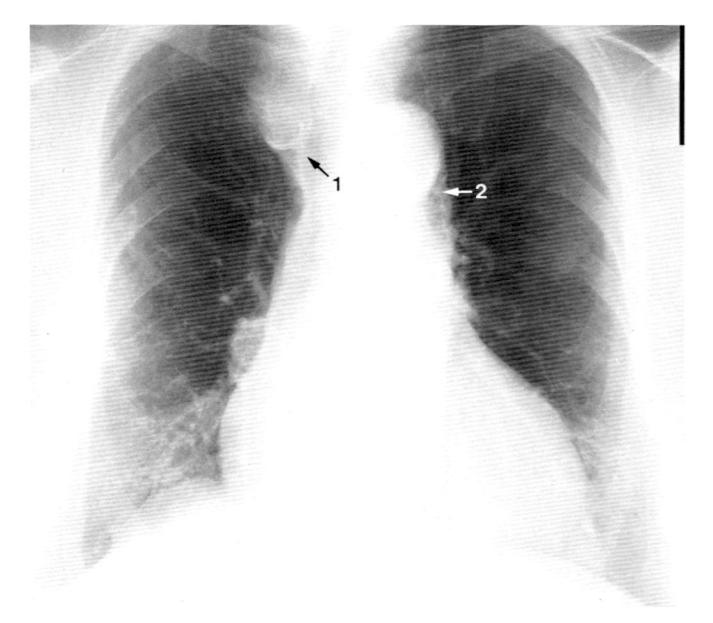

Fig. 10.**29 a, b** **Extensive calcific arteriosclerosis of aorta in hypertensive patient.**

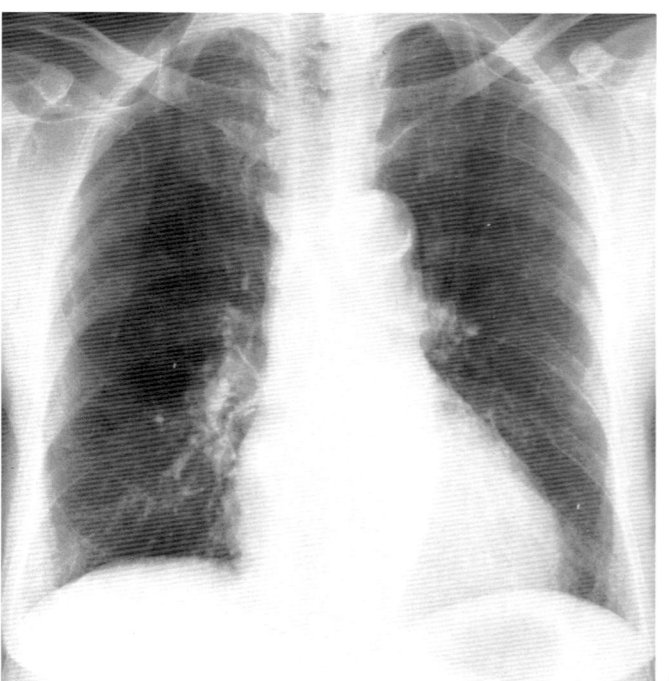

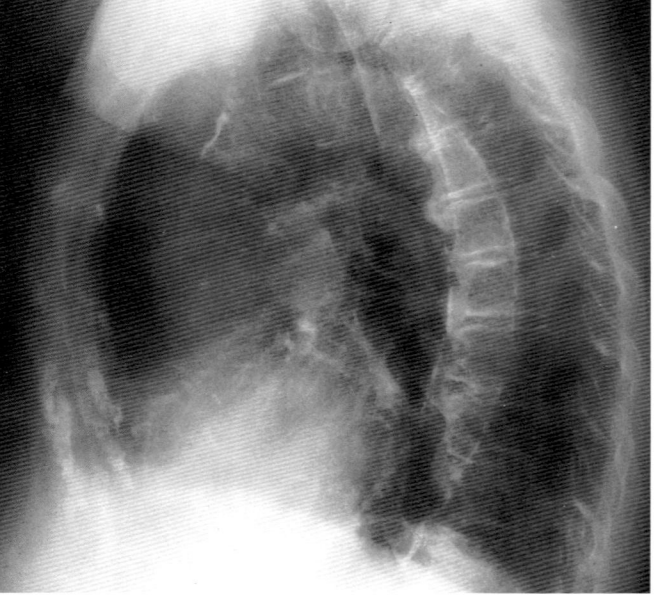

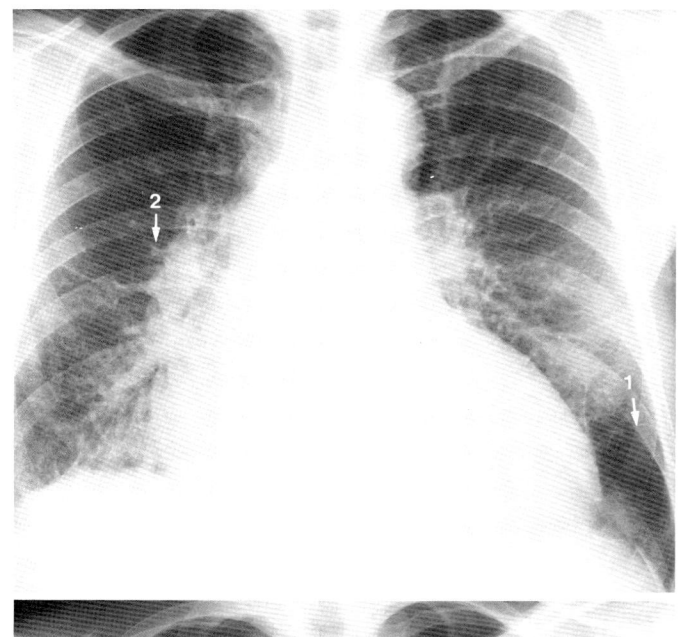

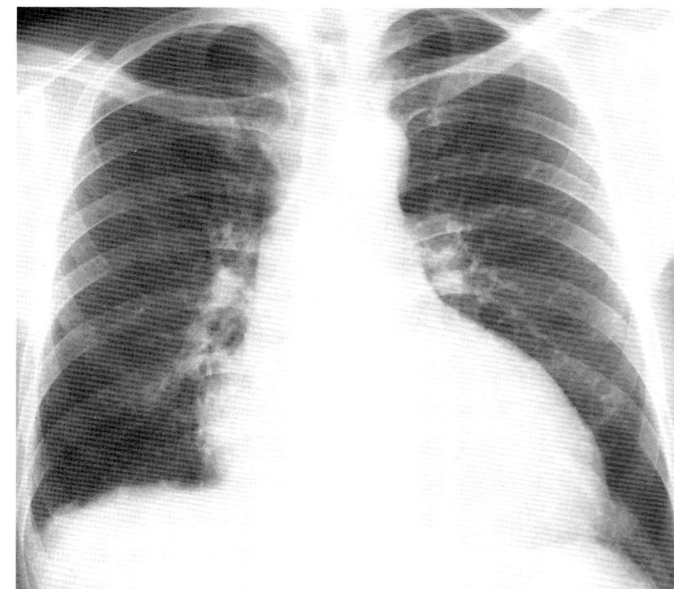

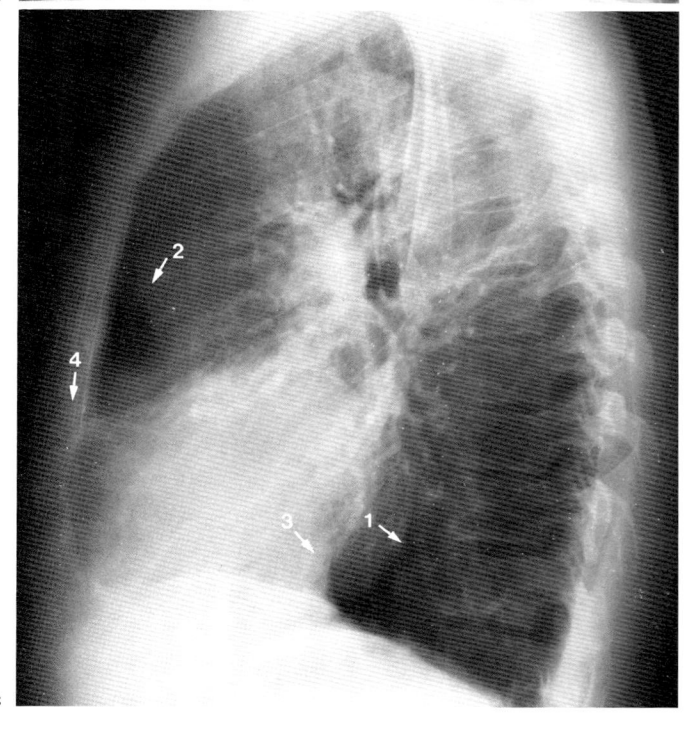

Cardiac Diseases

Aortic Valvular Disease, Ventricular Aneurysms

Aortic stenosis and regurgitation lead to an increase in afterload and preload, respectively, and to left ventricular hypertrophy and dilatation. Eventually, left ventri cular failure ensues, particularly if a critical cardiac weight of 500 g is exceeded. Ventricular aneurysms result after fibrosis of the infarcted myocardium and lead to dyskinetic or paradoxical motion of the left ventricle. They tend to occur at the left ventricular apex or along the left lateral ventricular wall. Subendocardial, thin, curvilinear calcifications can occur in the wall of such ventricular aneurysms.

Pseudoaneurysms of the left ventricle represent contained myocardial perforations. They account for 5% of ventricular aneurysms and project posteriorly rather than laterally.

The aneurysms can lead to left ventricular failure, arrhythmia, or thromboemboli. False aneurysms, on the other hand, can perforate since they are contained only by pericardium.

Fig. 10.30 a–c **Combined aortic valvular stenosis and regurgitation.**
33-year-old patient with a history of rheumatic fever at age 13 years. He had undergone a previous valve repair. On admission (**a**), signs of left ventricular failure are present with cardiomegaly, pulmonary vascular engorgement, and interstitial edema with Kerley A (2) and B (1) lines. After diuresis (**b, c**), persistent enlargement of the cardiac silhouette with left ventricular configuration (1); dilatation of ascending aorta (2), junction of inferior vena cava with right atrium (3), sternal wire suture (4).

Cardiac Diseases   253

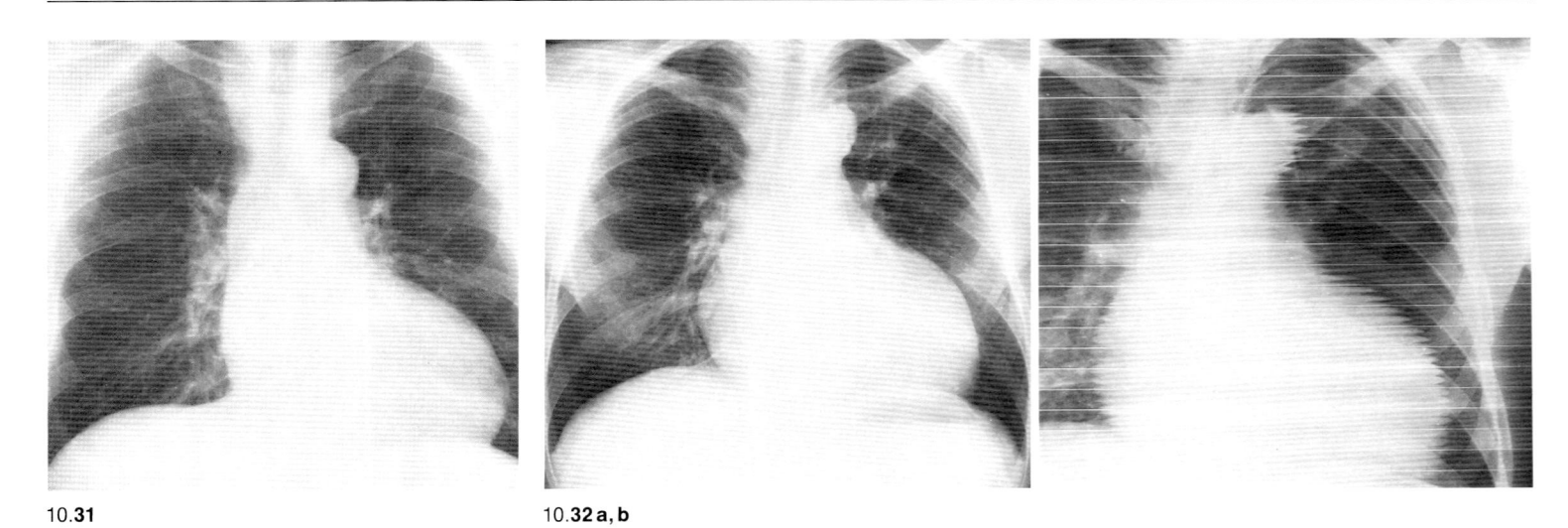

Fig. 10.**31** **Left ventricular enlargement in hypertensive patient.**

Fig. 10.**32 a, b** **Aortic regurgitation.**
Increased pulsations of ventricle and aorta with kymography.

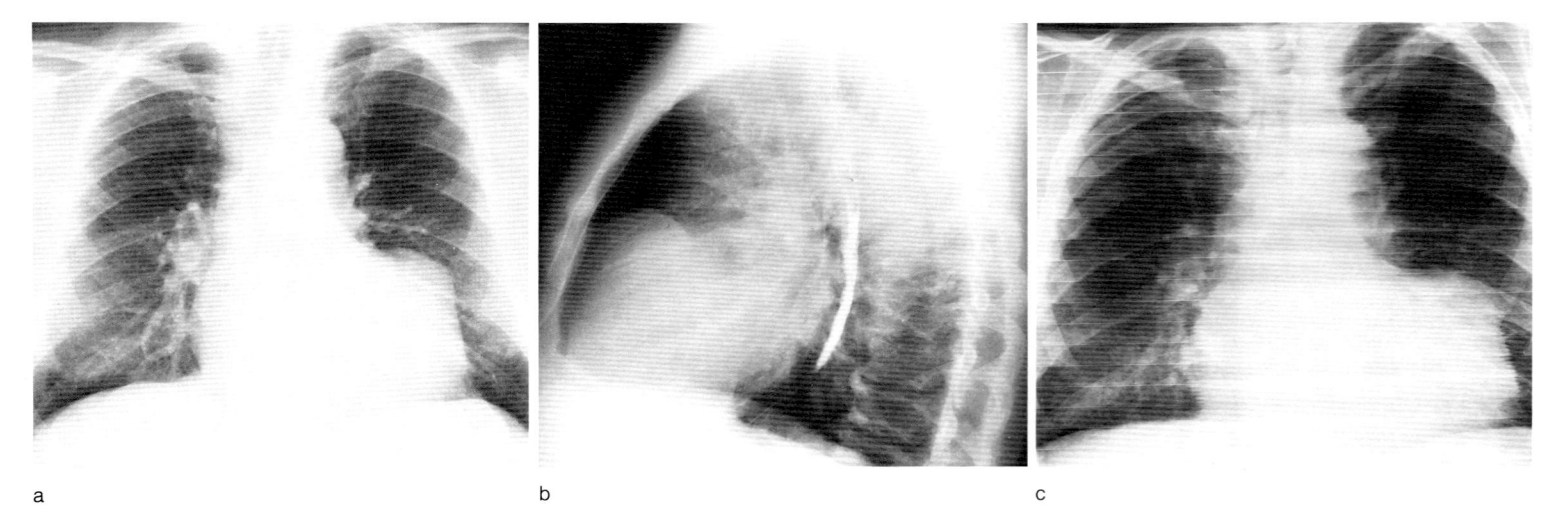

Fig. 10.**33 a–c** **Ventricular aneurysm.**
Added convexity to left ventricular contour. Lack of pulsation of aneurysm with kymography.

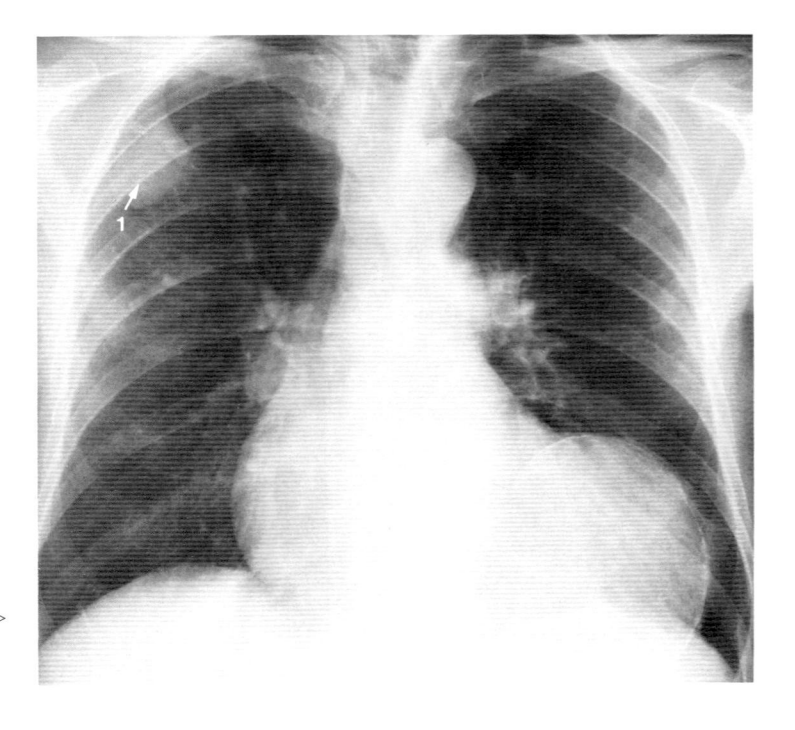

Fig. 10.**34** **Calcified ventricular aneurysm,** 3 years after a massive anterior wall myocardial infarction. In addition, a bronchogenic carcinoma in the right upper lobe is present.

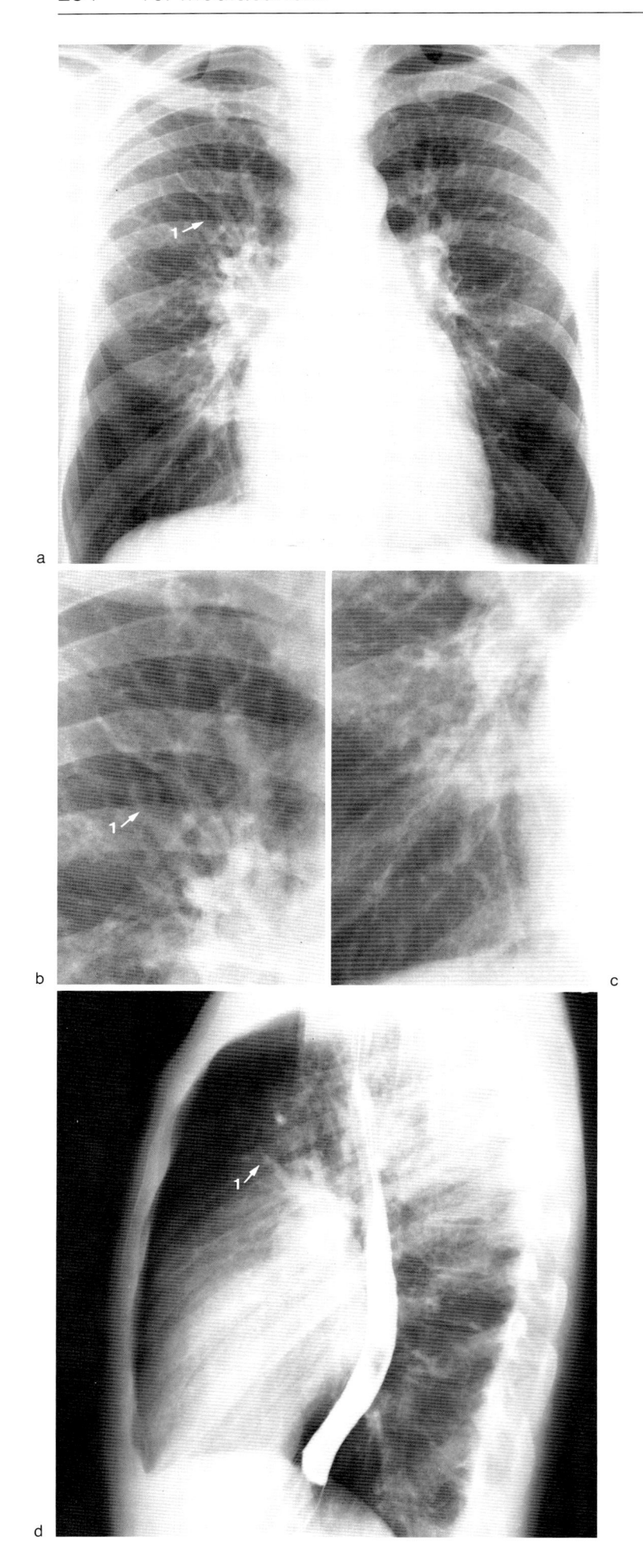

Mitral Valve Disease

Mitral valve stenosis or regurgitation are among the most common valvular defects. The most frequent etiology is rheumatic fever with carditis. Regurgitation can also be seen with rupture of the chordae tendineae, papillary muscle dysfunction, myxomatous degeneration of the mitral valve obstructive cardiomyopathy and mitral annulus calcification. Left atrial enlargement, right ventricular enlargement, and subsequent levorotation of the heart combine to produce the so-called mitral configuration.

Fig. 10.35 a–d **Mitral stenosis.**
26-year-old patient with a history of rheumatic fever at age 8 years who presented with dyspnea, diastolic murmur, and split second heart sound. Dilated pulmonary artery segment, left atrial appendage, and encroachment upon retrocardiac and retrosternal spaces in the lateral projection. Marked cephalization of pulmonary vascular flow (1).

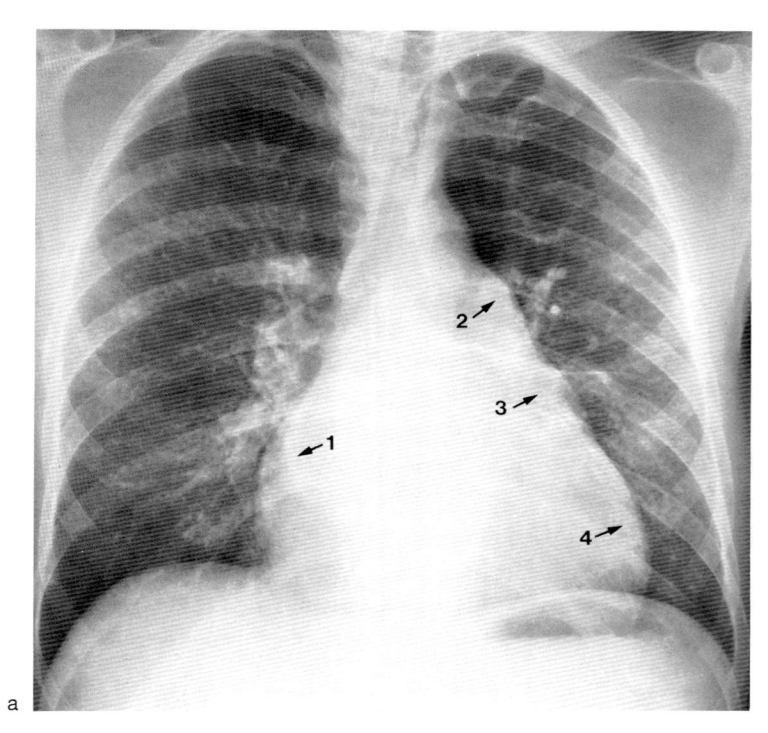

Fig. 10.**36 a, b** **Combined mitral stenosis and regurgitation.** 38-year-old patient with exertional dyspnea and minor hemoptysis of 10 year duration.

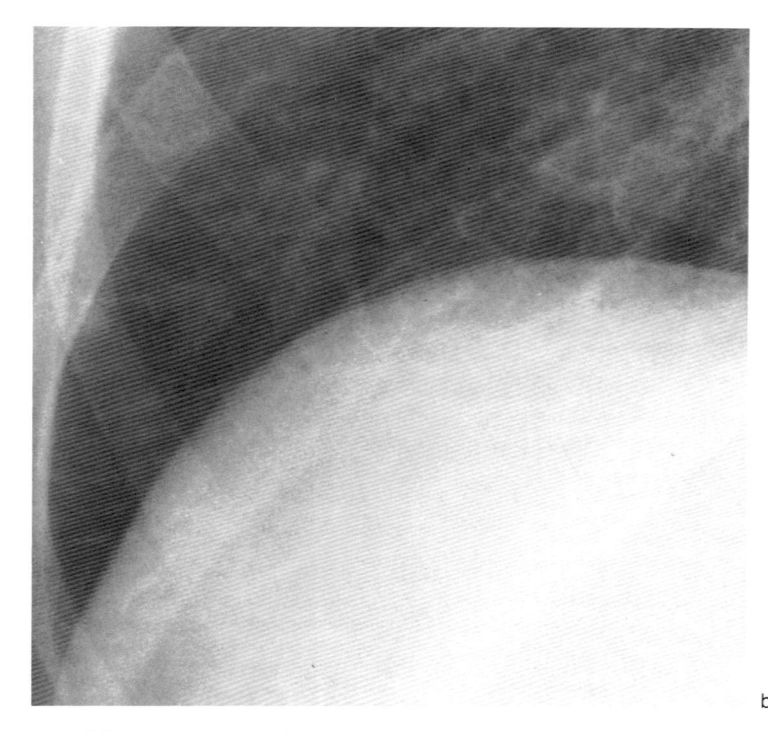

Double contour (1) formed by left atrium, dilated pulmonary artery segment (2), dilated left atrial appendage (3), enlarged left ventricle (4). Kerley B lines visible in lateral costophrenic sulcus.

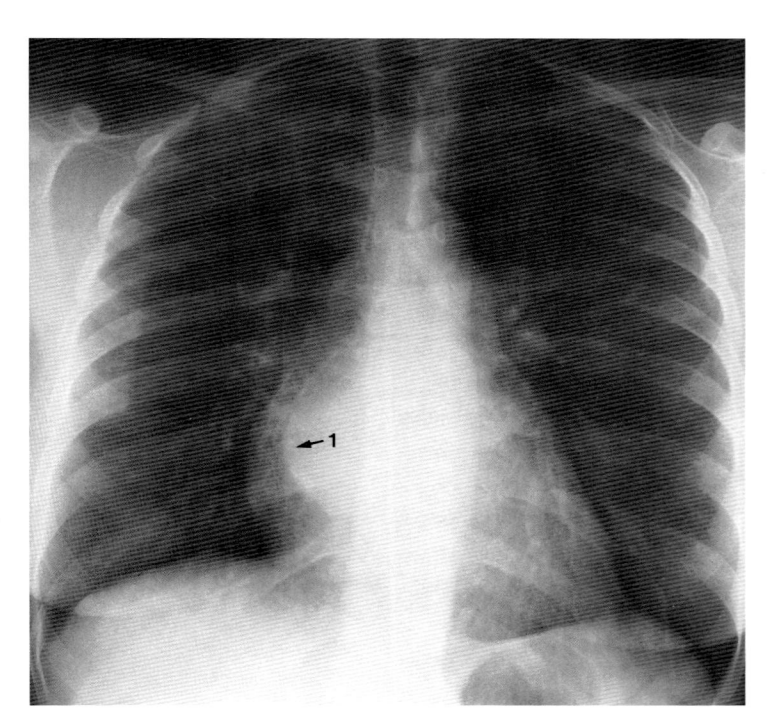

Fig. 10.**37** **Mitral stenosis.**
Clearly visible double contour formed by enlarged left atrium (1).

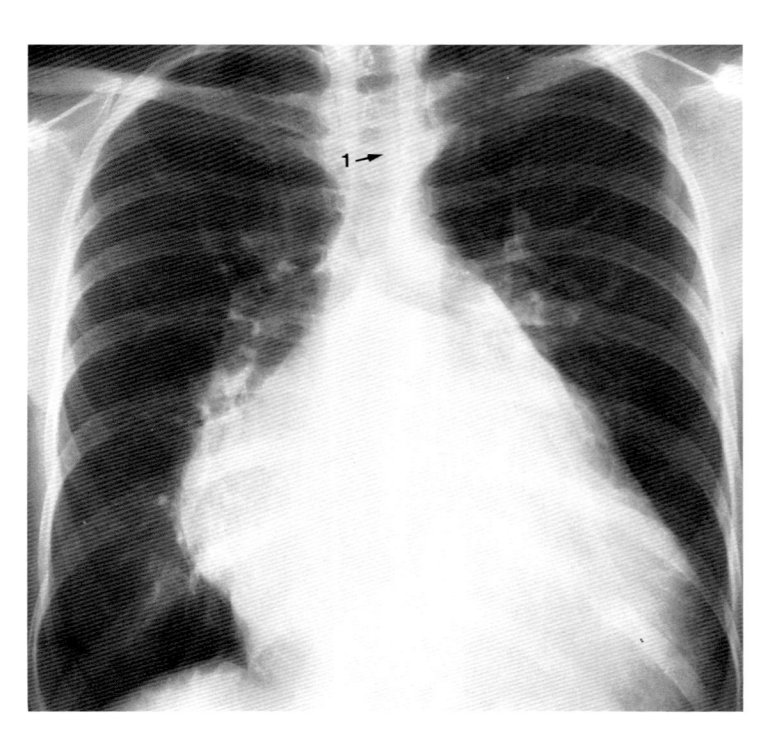

Fig. 10.**38** **Combined mitral stenosis and regurgitation.**
Enlarged cardiac silhouette. Left atrium forms the border on the right side. Note elevation of left mainstem bronchus and widened tracheal angle of bifurcation. Left atrial appendage also enlarged. Right paraesophageal stripe (1).

Septal Defects

The most common congenital heart disease at birth is ventricular septal defect (VSD). In adults, atrial septal defect (ASD) is more common, since VSD are usually recognized earlier. These defects result in a left to right shunt with hypercirculation in the pulmonary vascular bed, dilatation, and recruitment of all the pulmonary vessels. In ASD, the right atrium and the right ventricle are enlarged. In VSD, the left atrium, left ventricle, and later the right ventricle are dilated. Initially, the pulmonary arterial pressure is not elevated, even in the face of a large shunt. In the later stages, pulmonary arterial hypertension and right ventricular hypertrophy supervene as Eisenmenger reaction.

On chest radiographs, a left-to-right shunt of more than 1.5:1 can become visible, and it is easy to recognize if levels of 2:1 are exceeded.

Small defects in the muscular portion of the ventricular septum (morbus Roger) are inconsequential. ASD can be of the ostium primum, ostium secundum, or sinus venosus variety.

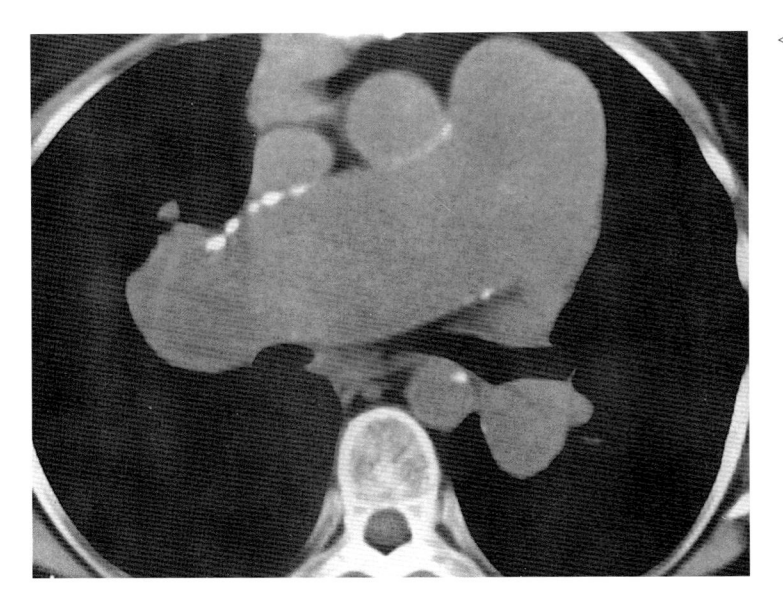

Fig. 10.39 **Patient with atrial septal defect and pulmonary arterial hypertension due to Eisenmenger reaction.**
CT scan shows marked dilatation of main pulmonary artery as well as right and left pulmonary arteries. Note calcifications in the wall of right pulmonary artery.

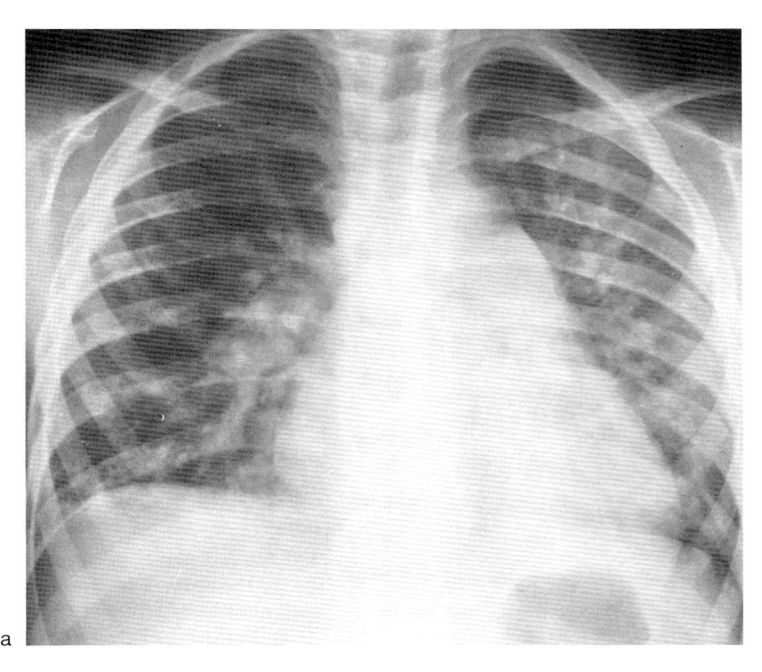

Fig. 10.40 a, b **Ostium secundum ASD.**
7-year-old patient. Cardiomegaly, dilated main pulmonary artery segment, and balanced increased flow throughout pulmonary vessels. Four years after surgical repair, normal cardiopulmonary structures, with near normal pulmonary vascularity (b).

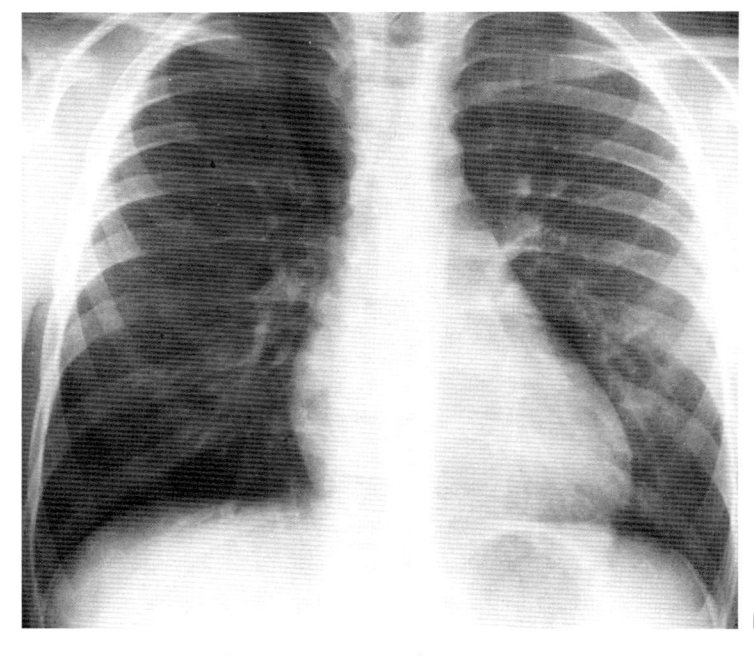

Cardiac Diseases 257

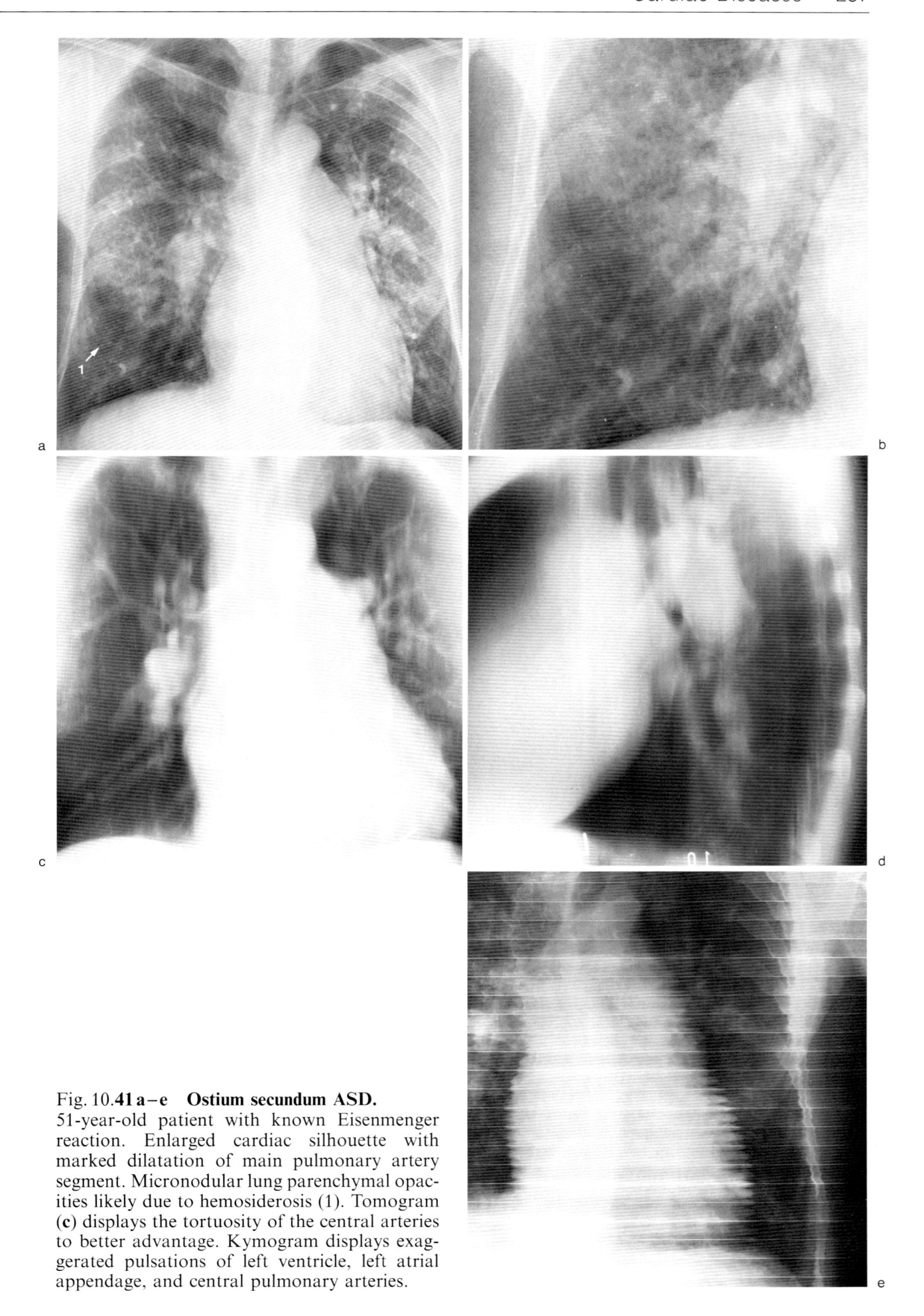

Fig. 10.**41 a–e Ostium secundum ASD.**
51-year-old patient with known Eisenmenger reaction. Enlarged cardiac silhouette with marked dilatation of main pulmonary artery segment. Micronodular lung parenchymal opacities likely due to hemosiderosis (1). Tomogram (**c**) displays the tortuosity of the central arteries to better advantage. Kymogram displays exaggerated pulsations of left ventricle, left atrial appendage, and central pulmonary arteries.

Tetralogy of Fallot, Patent Ductus Arteriosus, Coarctation of the Aorta

Tetralogy of Fallot is the most common cyanotic congenital heart defect encountered beyond childhood. It consists of a VSD, overriding aorta, infundibular pulmonic stenosis, and right ventricular hypertrophy. The severity of the malformation is determined by the degree of pulmonic stenosis.

Patent ductus arteriosus results in a left to right shunt. Only the left atrium, left ventricle, and aorta together with the pulmonary arteries and veins enlarge. The right ventricle enlarges only after the Eisenmenger reaction ensues.

Coarctation of the aorta leads to narrowing of the aorta distal to the take-off of the left subclavian artery, at the insertion of the ligamentum arteriosum (postductal coarctation). Rarely, the coarctation can be found proximal to the insertion of the ligamentum arteriosum (preductal coarctation).

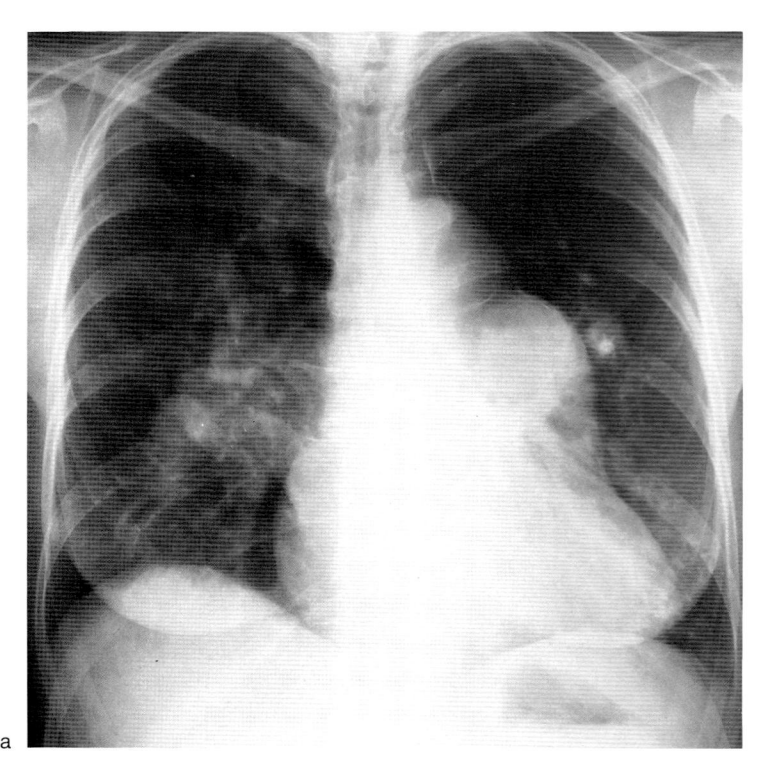

Fig. 10.**42 a, b Patent ductus arteriosus.**
55-year-old patient presents with cyanosis, likely due to Eisenmenger reaction. Marked dilatation of main pulmonary artery segment and central pulmonary arteries as well as aorta. Note thin shell of calcium outlining main pulmonary artery segment that represents definite evidence of pulmonary arterial hypertension.

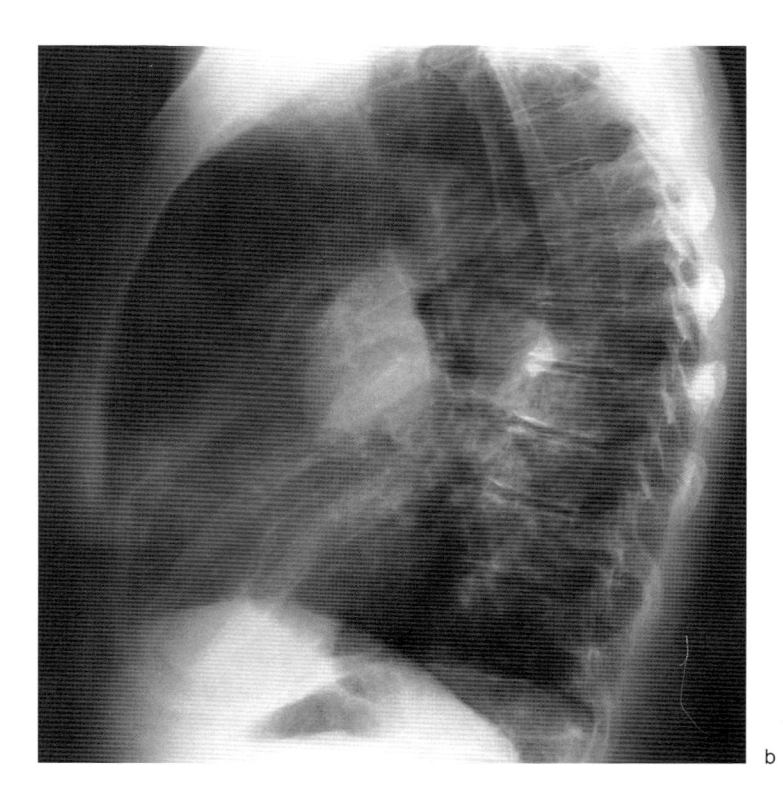

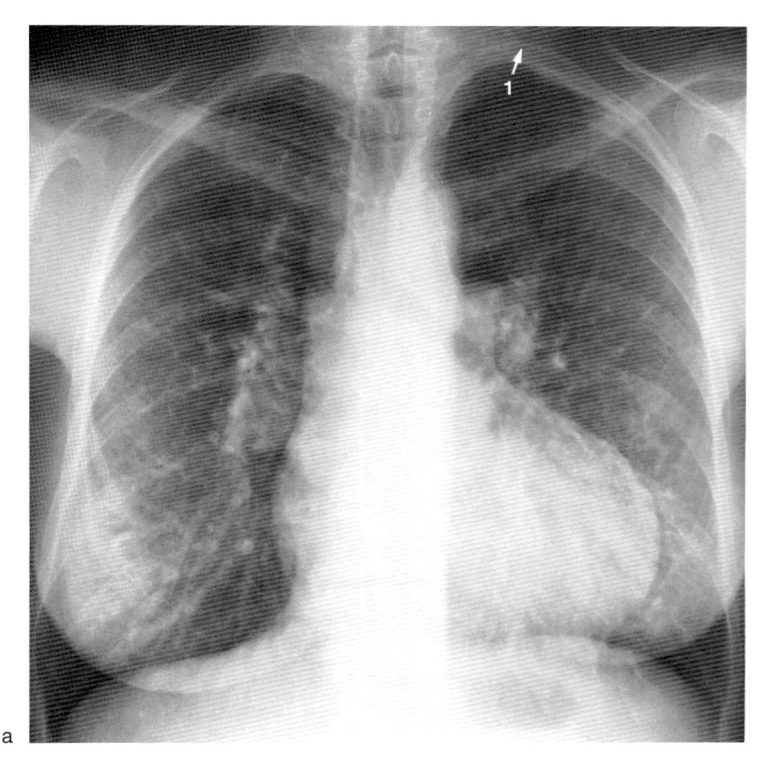

Fig. 10.**43 a, b Tetralogy of Fallot.**
39-year-old patient with long-standing history of cyanosis and finger clubbing. Boot-shaped heart due to right ventricular enlargement, levorotation of cardiac silhouette and elevation of cardiac apex. Deep cardiac waist due to infundibular stenosis. Left cervical rib (1).

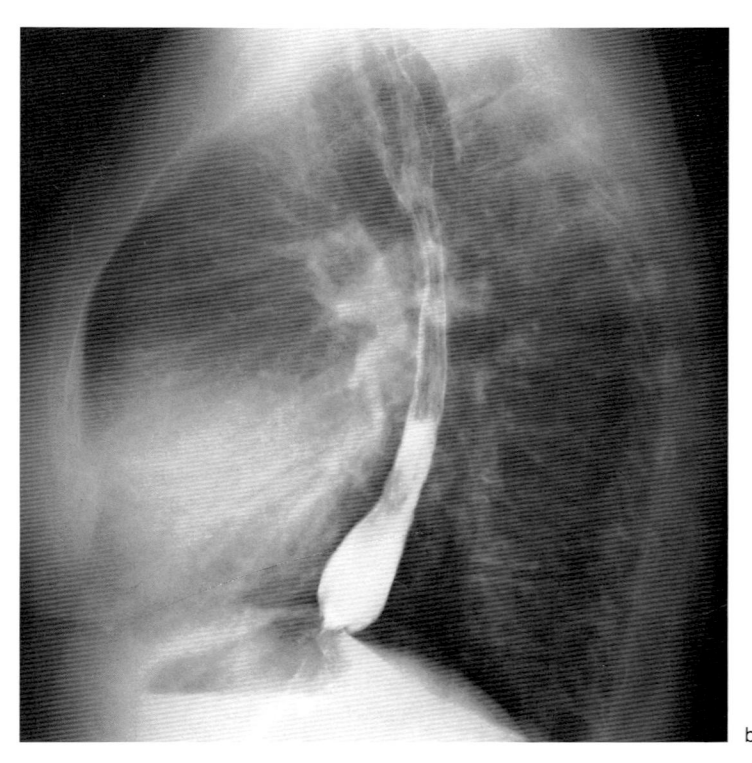

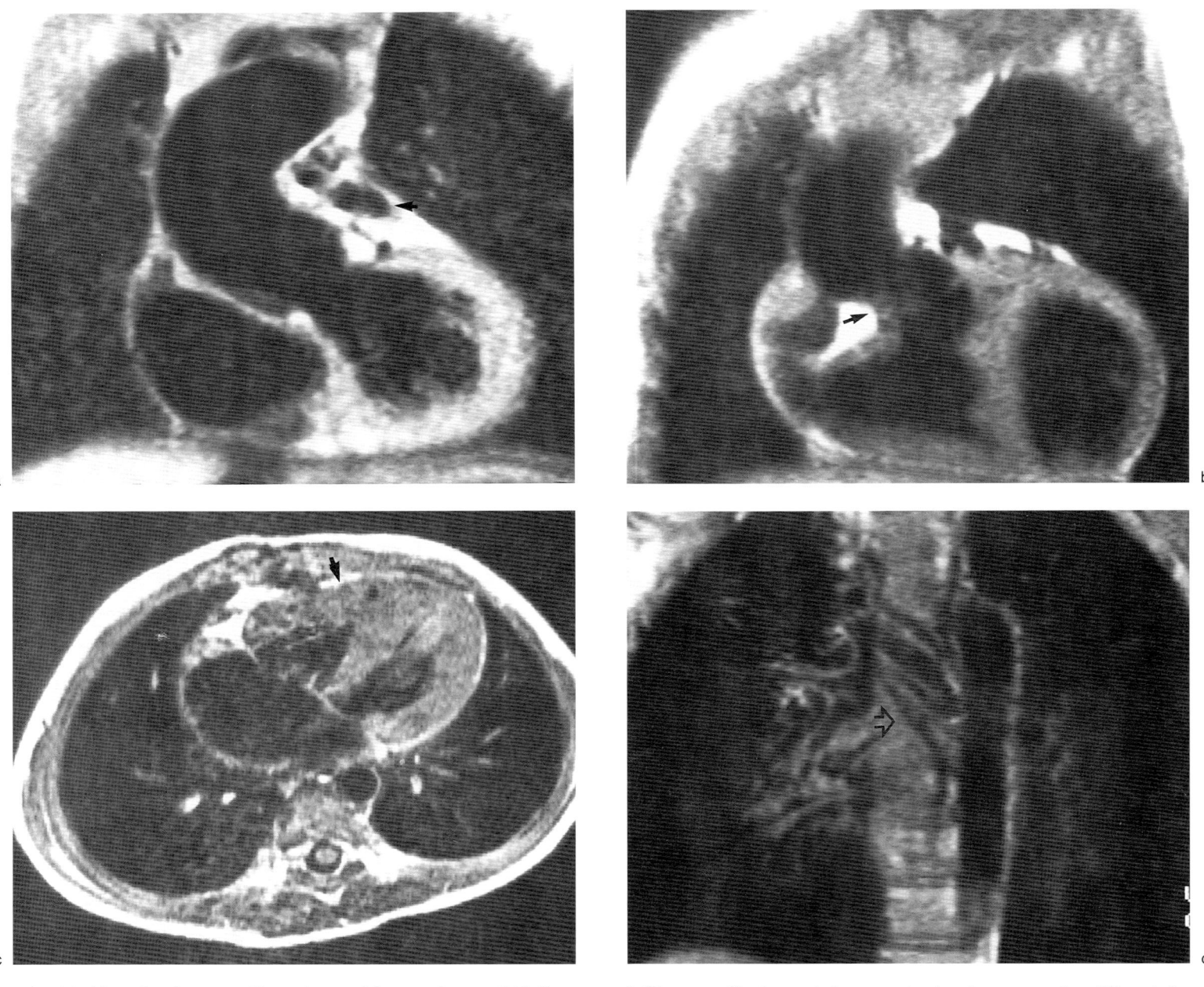

Fig. 10.44 a–d **3-year-old patient with tetralogy of Fallot. a** Coronal MR scan shows a dilated ascending aorta and a markedly narrowed main pulmonary artery segment (arrow). **b** Coronal MR scan demonstrates overriding aorta which connects also with the right ventricle (arrow). **c** Axial MR scan displays right ventricular hypertrophy. The right ventricular myocardium (arrow) exceeds the thickness of the left ventricle. **d** Coronal MR scan demonstrates marked dilatation of bronchial arteries, which supply oligemic lung.

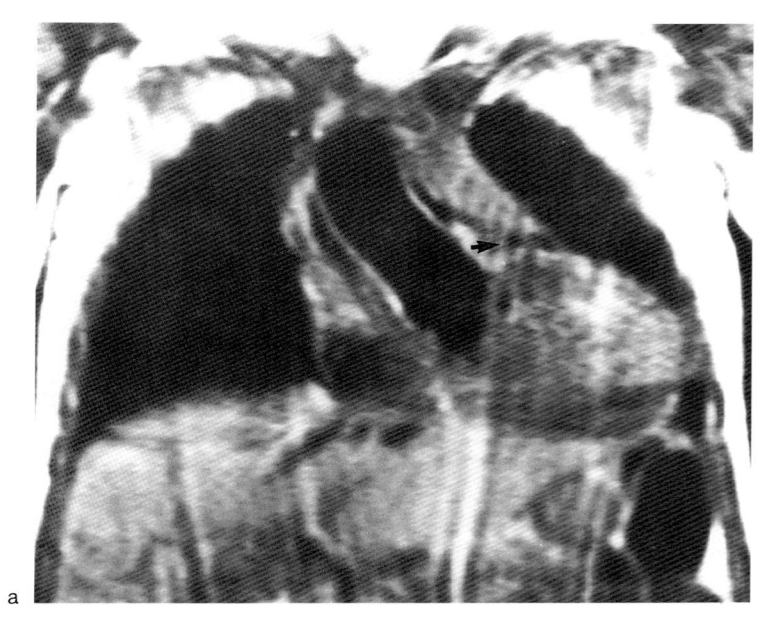

Fig. 10.**45 a, b**   **10-month-old patient with tetralogy of Fallot.**
a Coronal MR scan shows dilated ascending aorta and hypoplastic main pulmonary artery (arrow). **b** Coronal MR scan shows right-sided aortic arch with dilated bronchial artery (arrow).

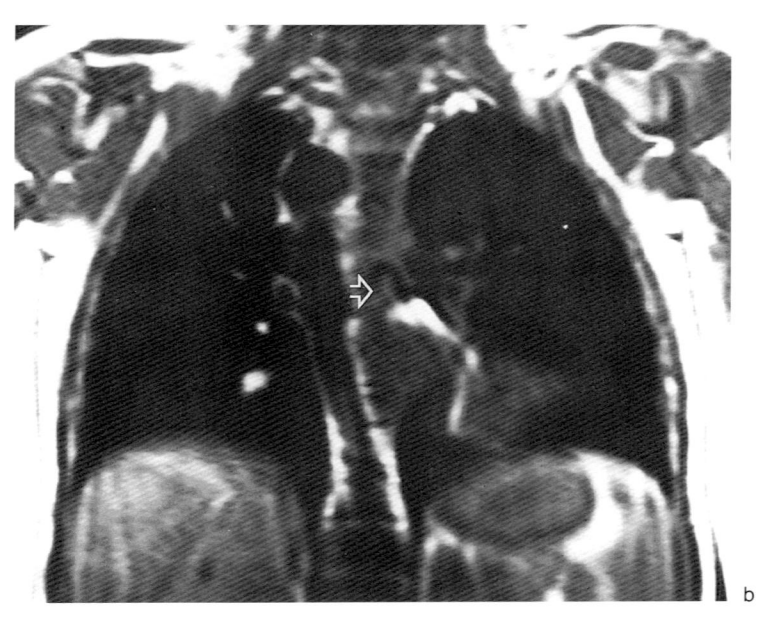

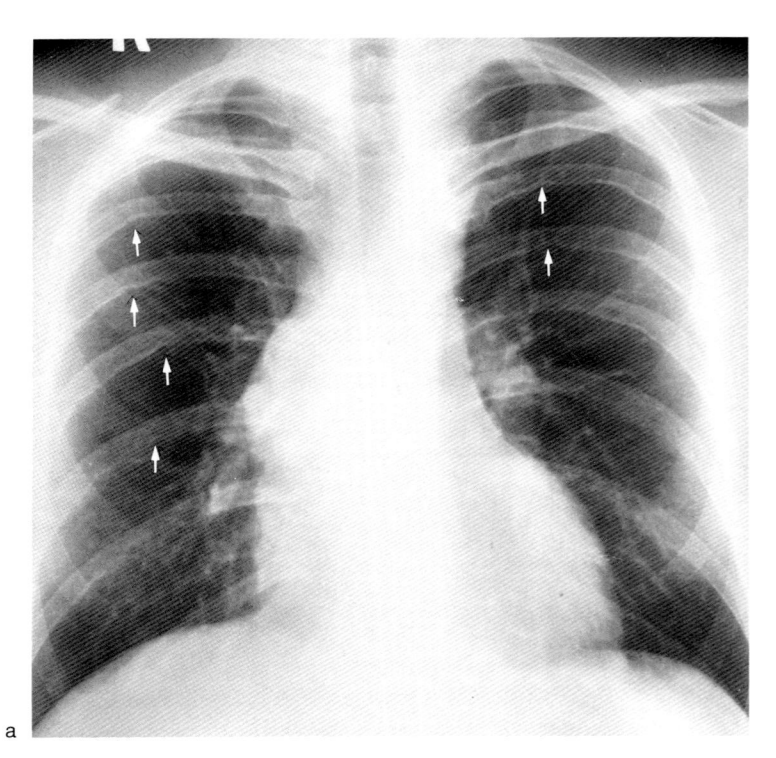

Fig. 10.**46 a, b**   **Coarctation of aorta.**
23-year-old patient with upper extremity arterial hypertension. Low rounding of left ventricle, nonexistent aortic arch, rib notching. Aortogram reveals isthmic stenosis (1) and dilated left internal mammary artery (2). Right subclavian artery not opacified due to manual compression.

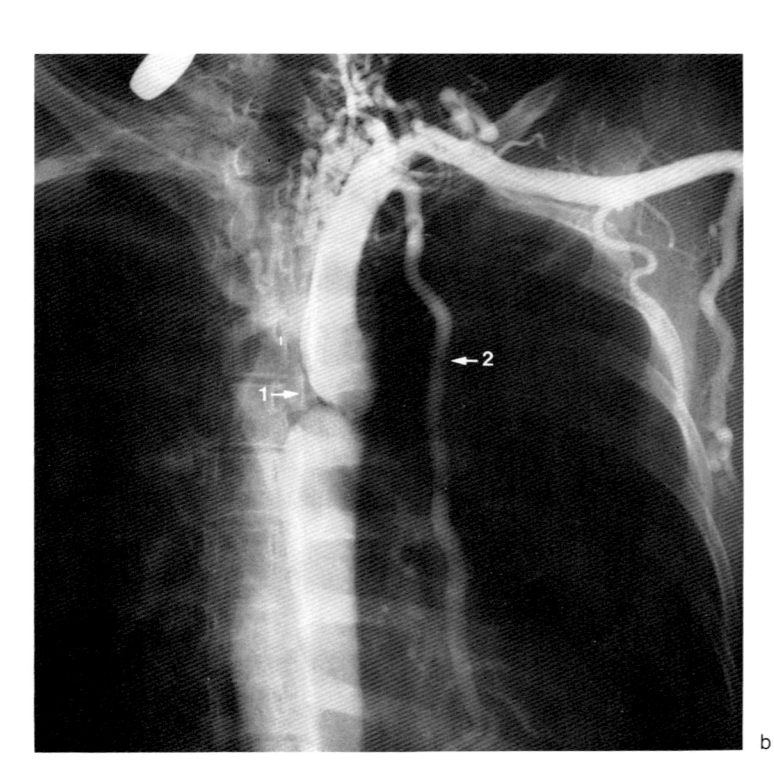

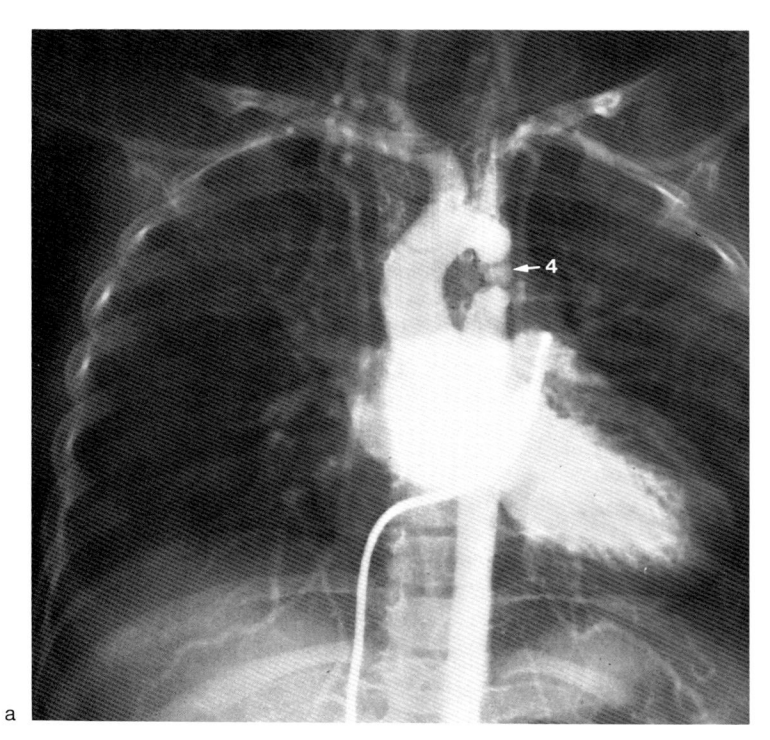

Fig. 10.**47 a, b** **Coarctation of aorta.**
11-year-old patient with upper extremity arterial hypertension. Catheter in main pulmonary artery with opacification of left atrium, ventricle, and aorta. Isthmic stenosis (4).

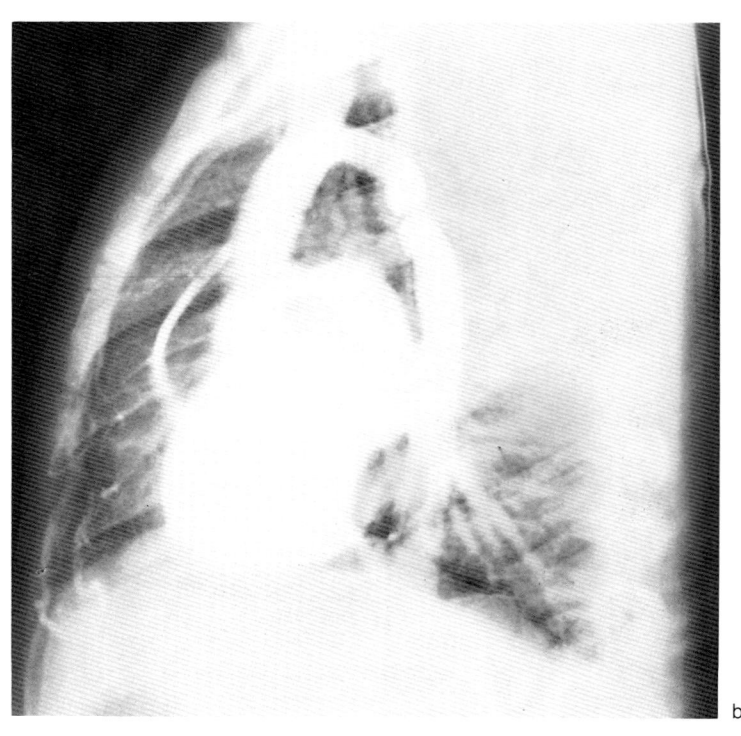

Pericardial Disease

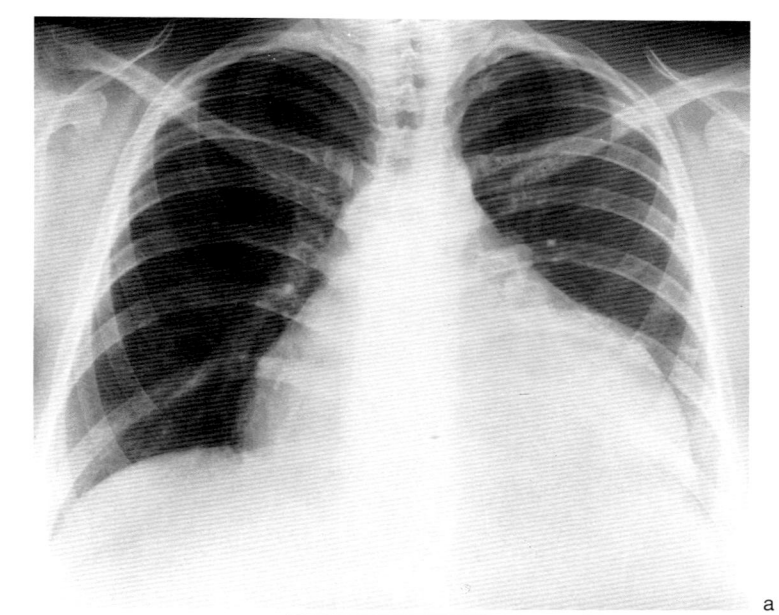

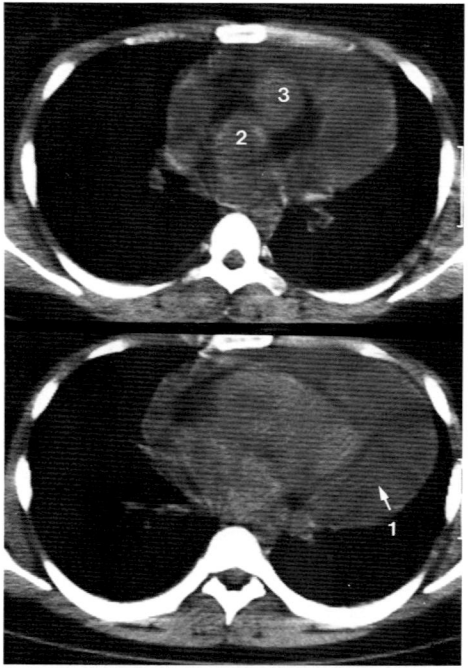

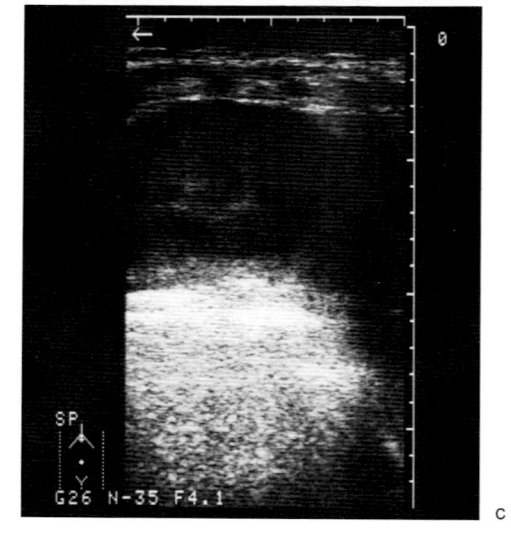

Fig. 10.**48 a–c** **Pericardial effusion.**
16-year-old with non-Hodgkin lymphoma and pericardial involvement as first manifestation. Marked enlargement of cardiac silhouette with pulmonary oligemia. CT scan shows low attenuation pericardial effusion (1) surrounding heart and outlining epicardial fat, ascending aorta (2), pulmonary artery (3). Cardiac ultrasound shows echo-free zone anterior to heart and posterior to pericardial echo.

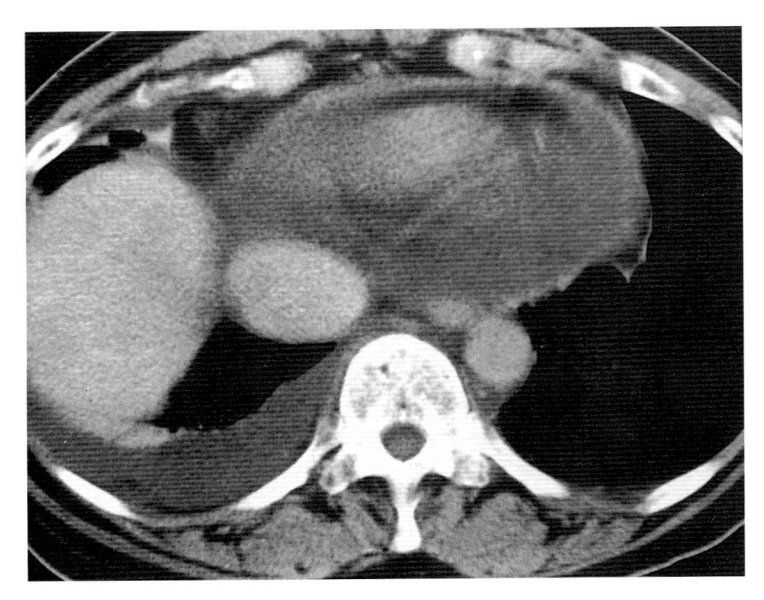

264   10. Mediastinum

Fig. 10.**49** **Pericardial effusion causing tamponade.**
CT scan shows pericardial fluid in inferior pericardial recess with dilatation of inferior vena cava. Right pleural effusion is also present.

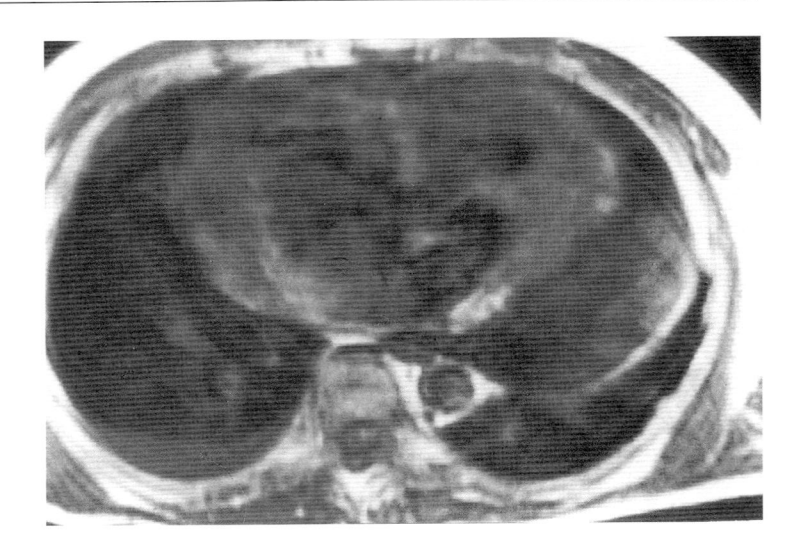

Fig. 10.**50** **Large pericardial effusion in patient with right ventricular failure.**
MR scan shows a low signal space surrounding the heart and bulging into left hemithorax.

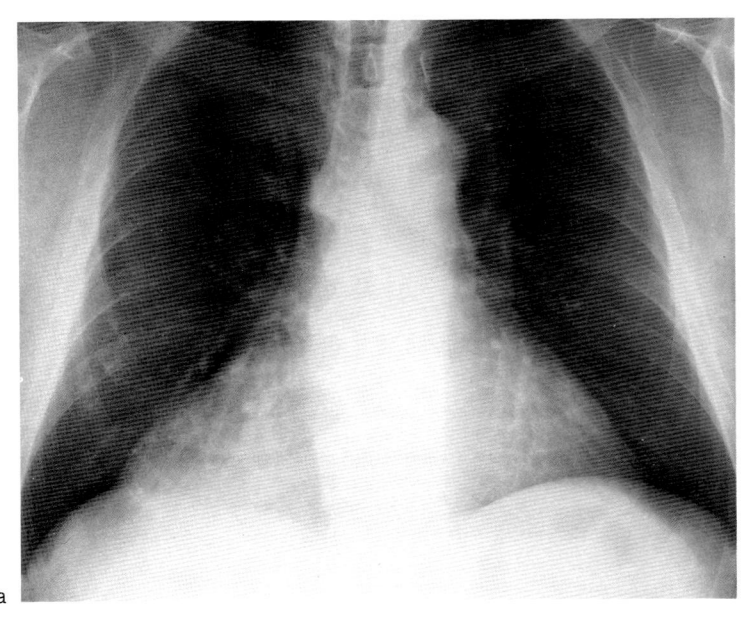

Fig. 10.**51 a, b** **Pericardial cyst.**
Mass in right cardiophrenic sulcus. CT scan shows fluid-filled cystic structure and compression atelectasis of right lower lobe.

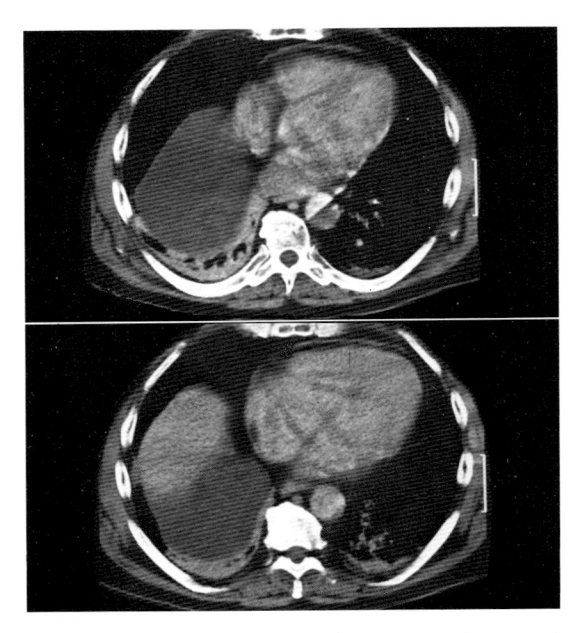

Fig. 10.**52 Pericardial cyst.**
Asymptomatic person with incidental finding on chest radiograph. CT scan demonstrates a large cystic structure in left cardiophrenic sulcus.

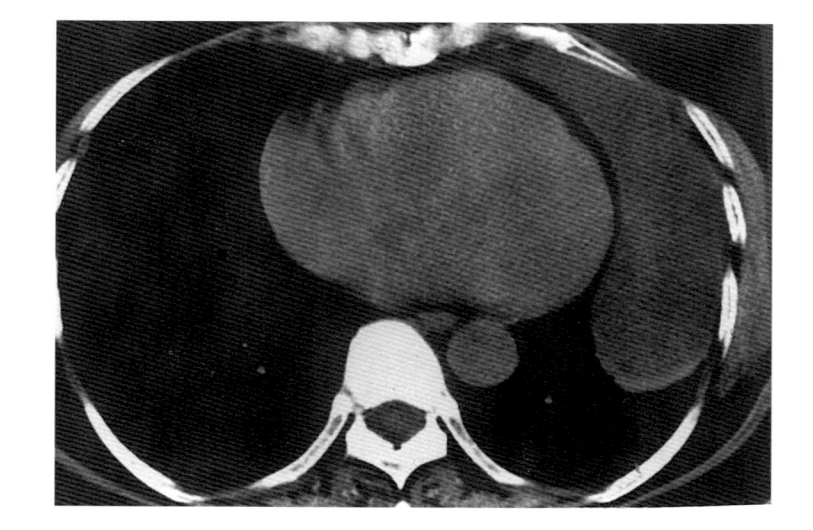

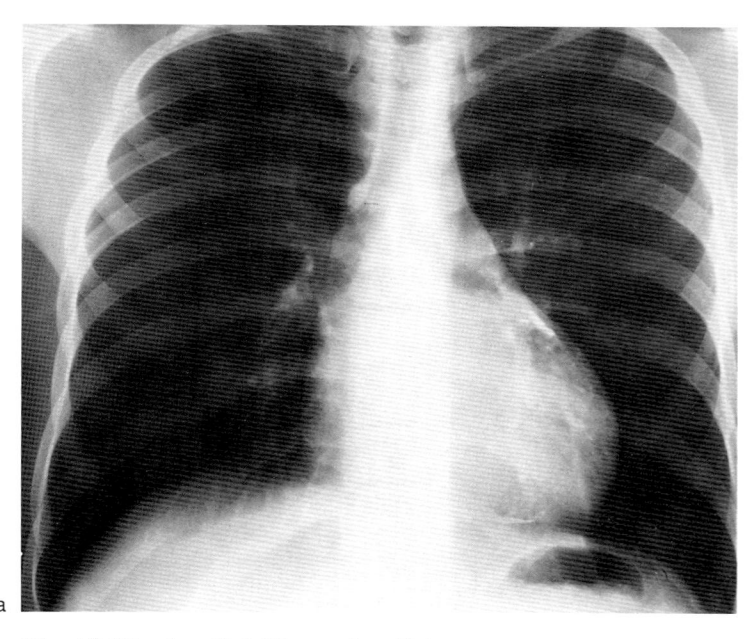

Fig. 10.**53 a, b   Calcific pericarditis.**
Thick, curvilinear, pericardial calcification surrounding almost the entire left ventricle.

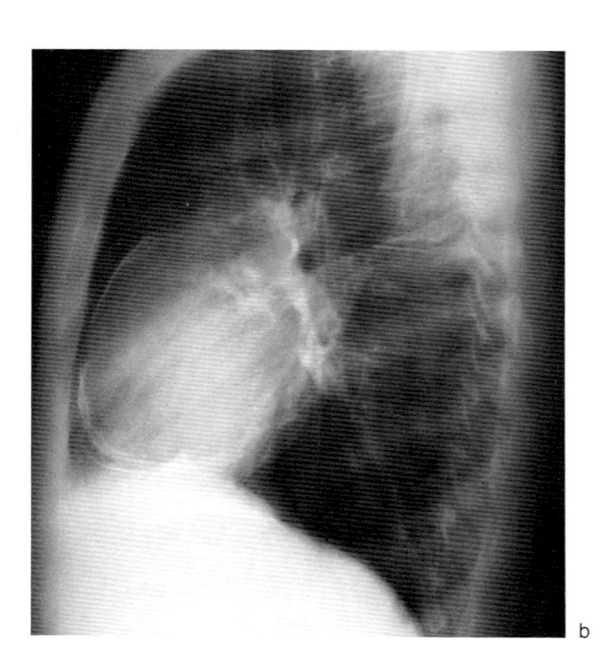

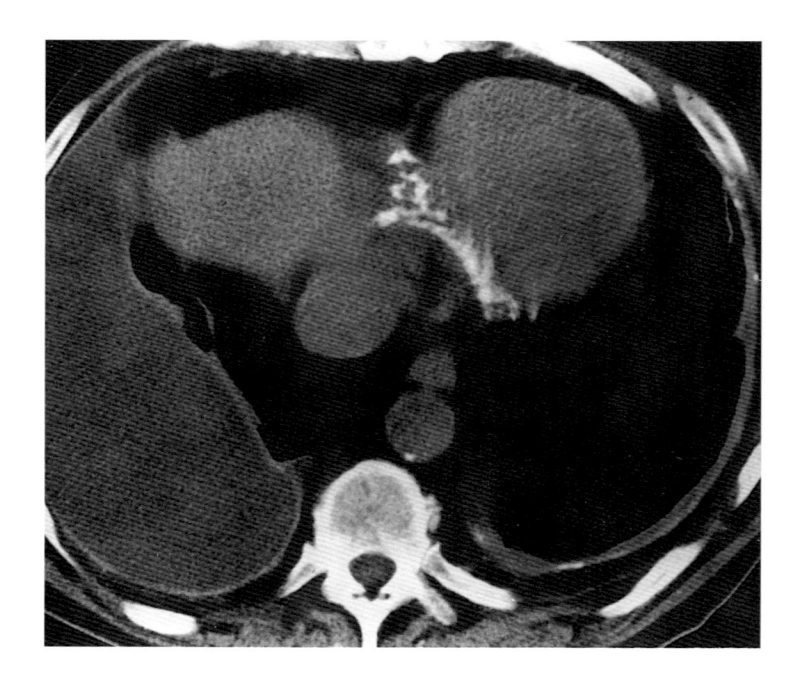

Fig. 10.**54   Calcific pericarditis.**
CT scan shows calcifications in atrioventricular groove. Incidental note is made of a large chronic right pleural effusion. Patient has rheumatoid arthritis.

11. Diaphragm

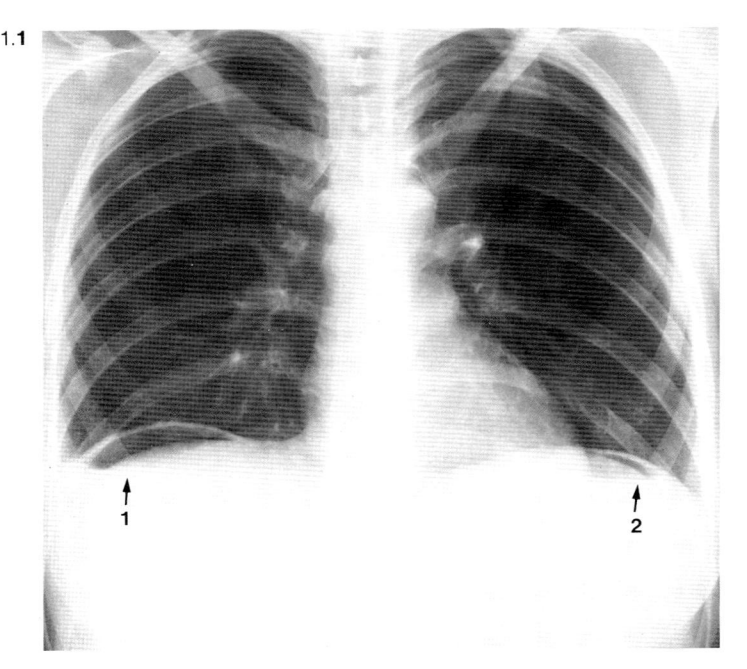

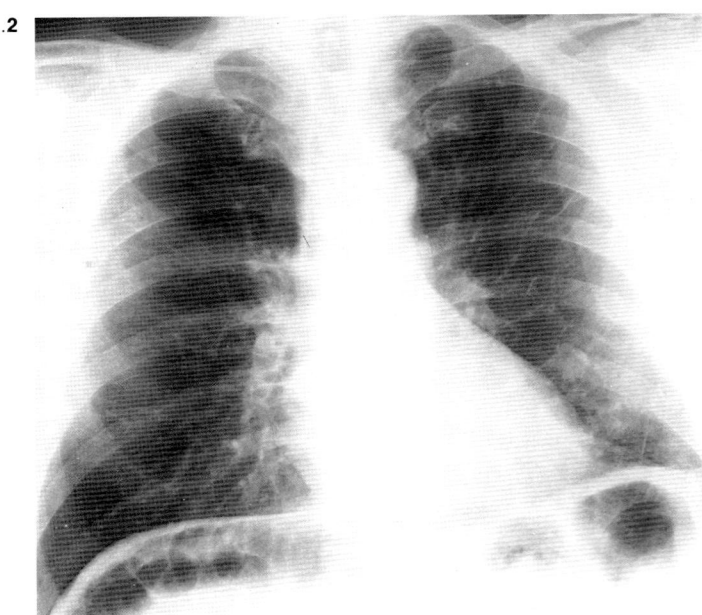

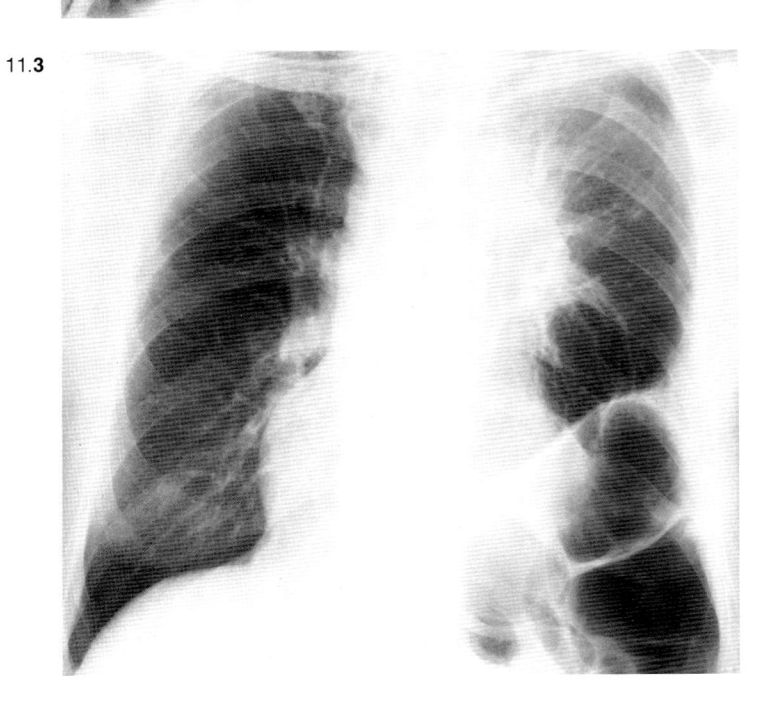

Diaphragm Anomalies

◁ Fig. 11.1 **Pneumoperitoneum.**
Note free intraperitoneal gas underneath right hemidiaphragm, gas-fluid level (1) indicating ascites as well as gas separating stomach fundus and spleen from diaphragm (2).

◁ Fig. 11.2 **Chilaiditi syndrome.**
Colon interposed between liver and right hemidiaphragm. Left lower lobe pneumonia also present.

Fig. 11.3 **Paralyzed left phrenic nerve due to invasion by bronchogenic carcinoma.**
Note left hilar enlargement, left upper lobe atelectasis, and marked elevation of left hemidiaphragm.

Fig. 11.4 **Abdominal situs inversus.**
Stomach bubble seen under right hemidiaphragm. Left hemidiaphragm is lower in position due to the weight of the heart. Right hemidiaphragm is not higher because of pressure effect of liver, as this case with a left-sided liver illustrates.

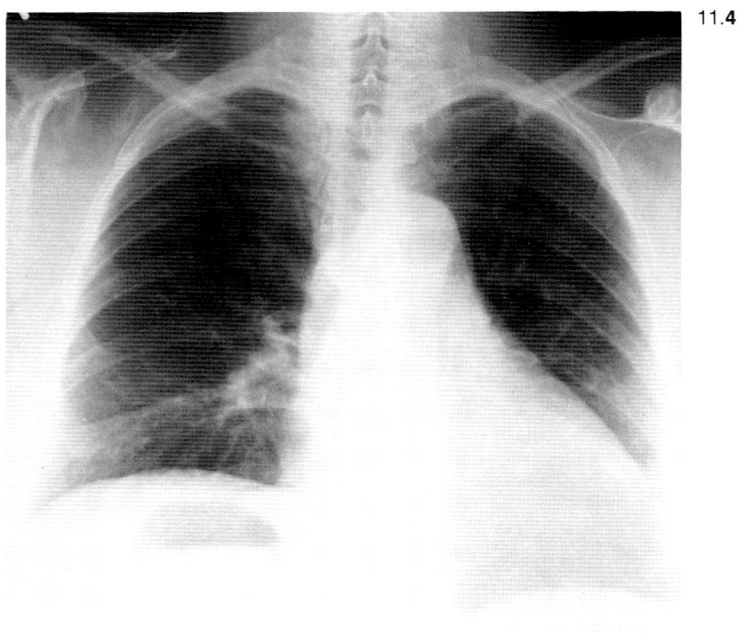

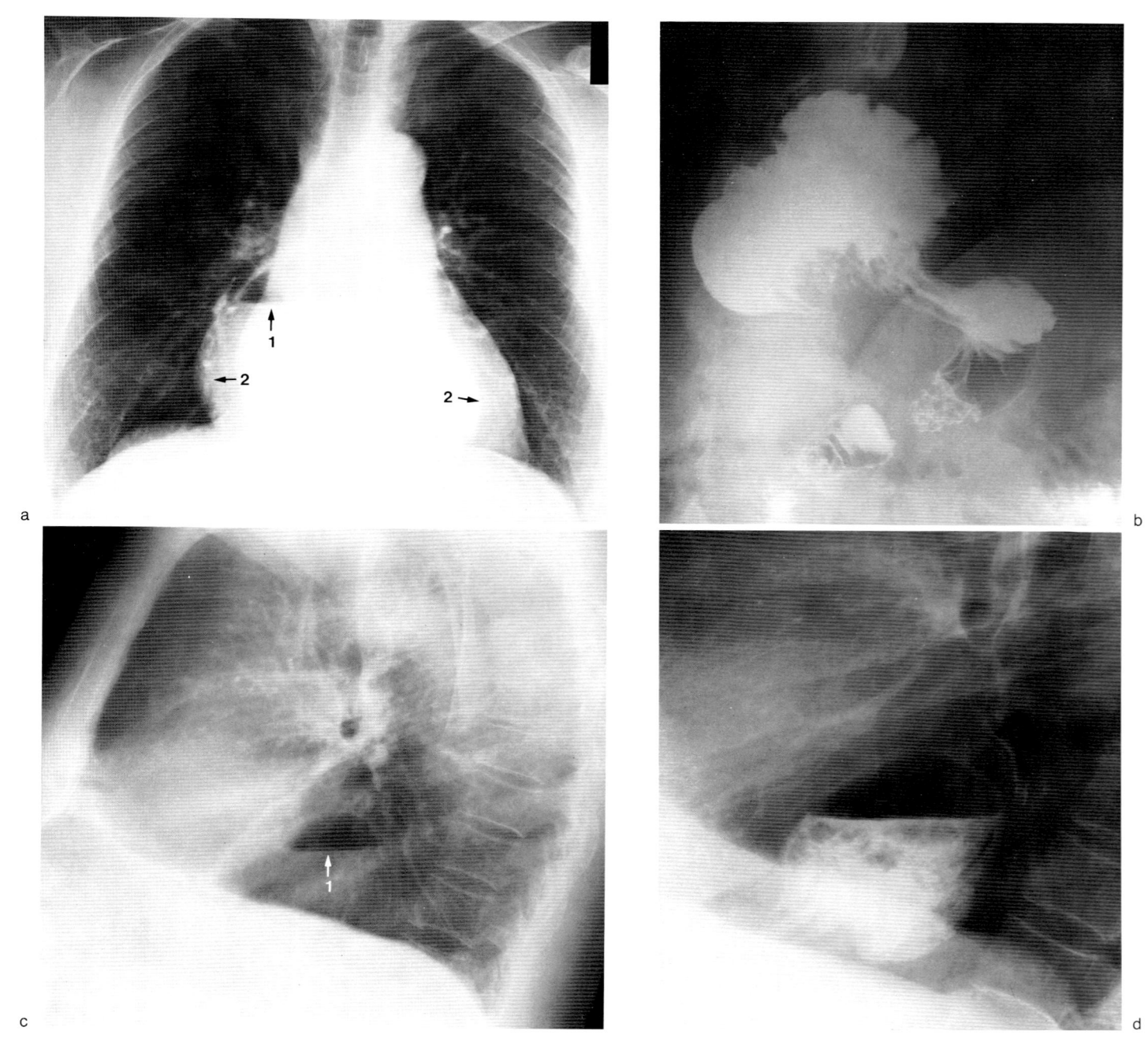

Fig. 11.5 a–d **Hiatal hernia.**
Note gas-fluid level (1) and double contour formed by stomach (2). Barium study confirms diagnosis.

270   11. Diaphragm

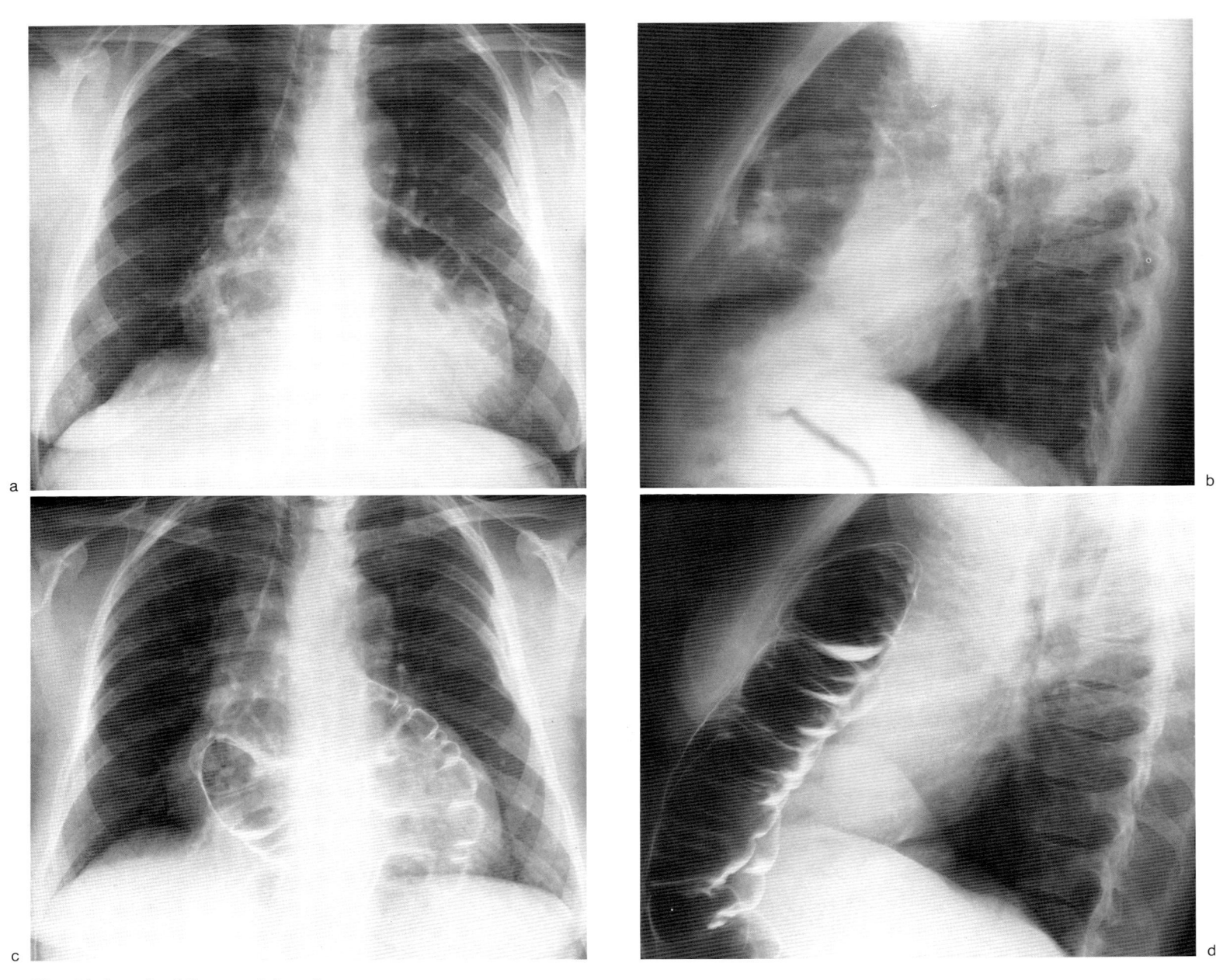

Fig. 11.6 a–d   **Morgagni hernia.**
Transverse colon seen in retrosternal location. Bowel enters the chest through right sternocostal triangle.

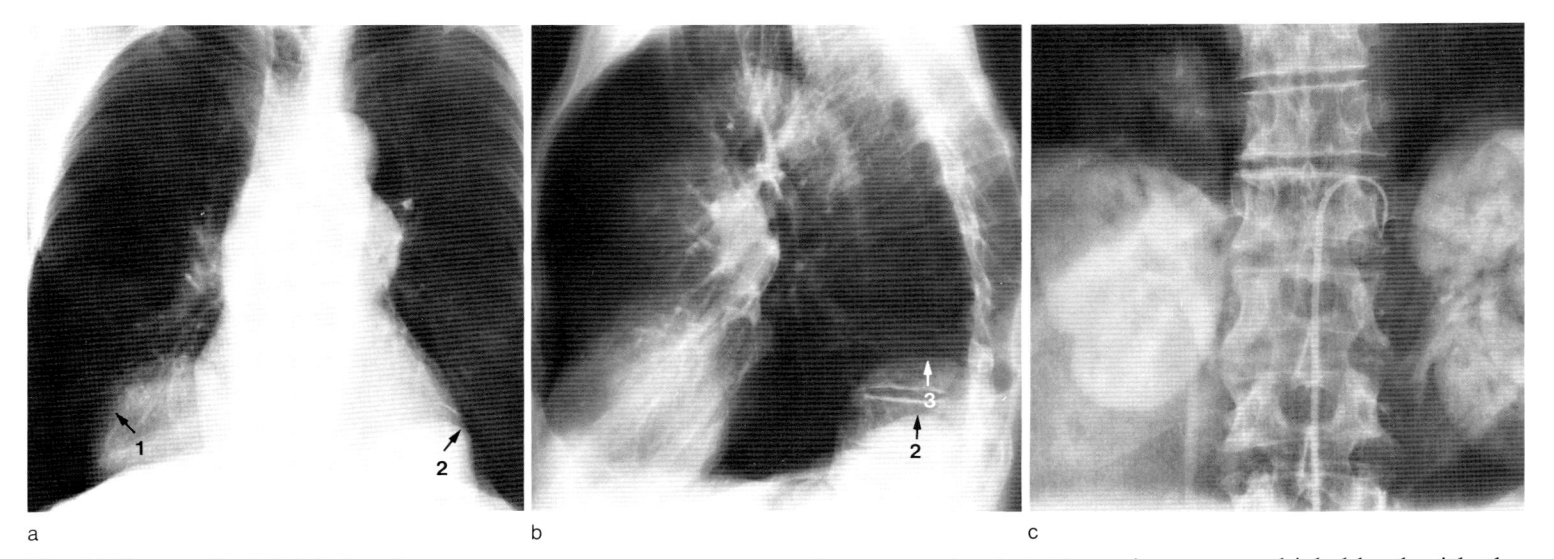

Fig. 11.7 a–c   **Bochdalek hernia.**
Bilateral, partially intrathoracic kidneys; both kidneys produce posterior intrathoracic masses which blend with the diaphragm (1, 2, 3).

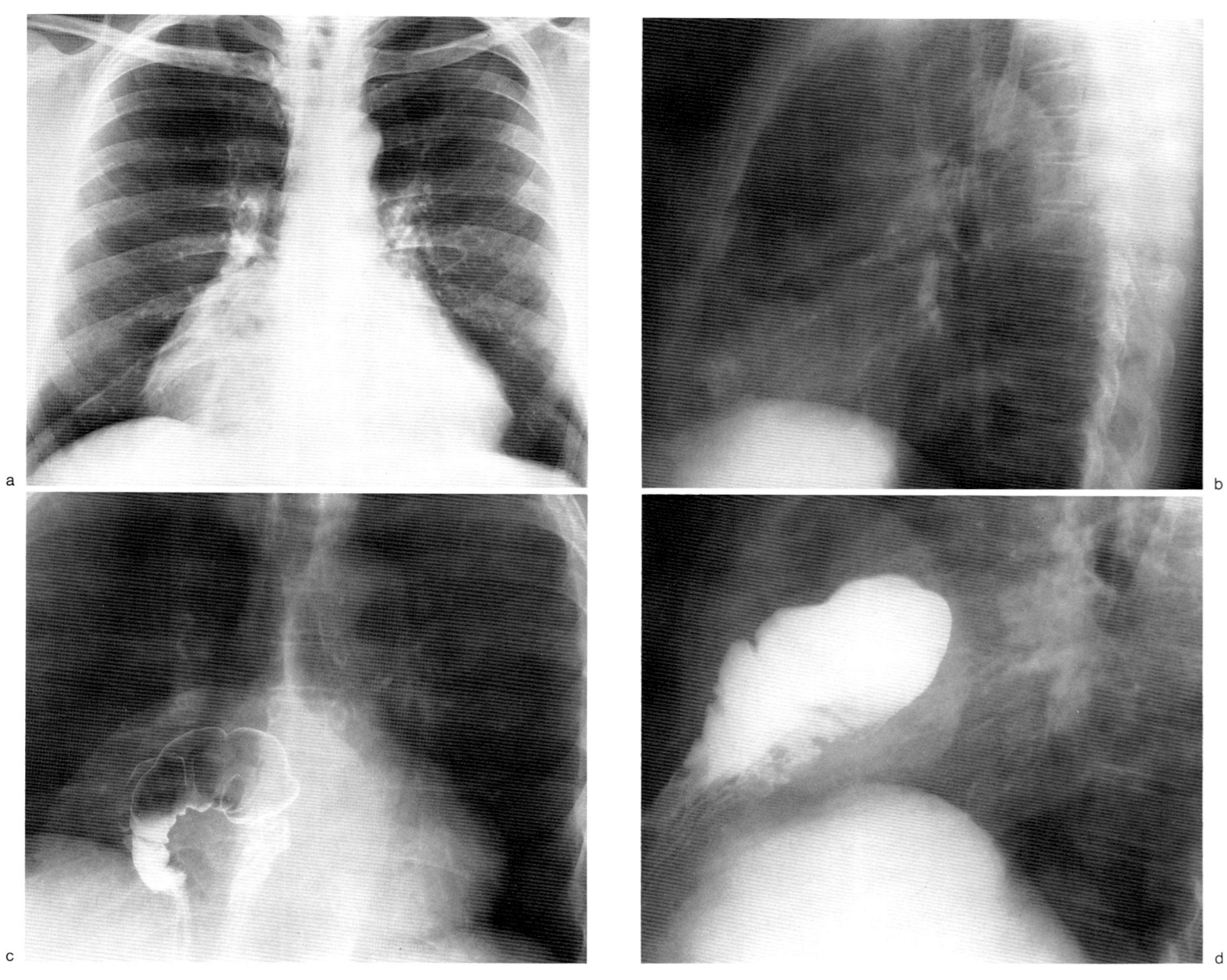

Fig. 11.8 a–d   Morgagni hernia.
Mass in right cardiophrenic sulcus. Lateral view shows retrosternal, gas-filled mass. Barium enema confirms intrathoracic location of colonic loop.

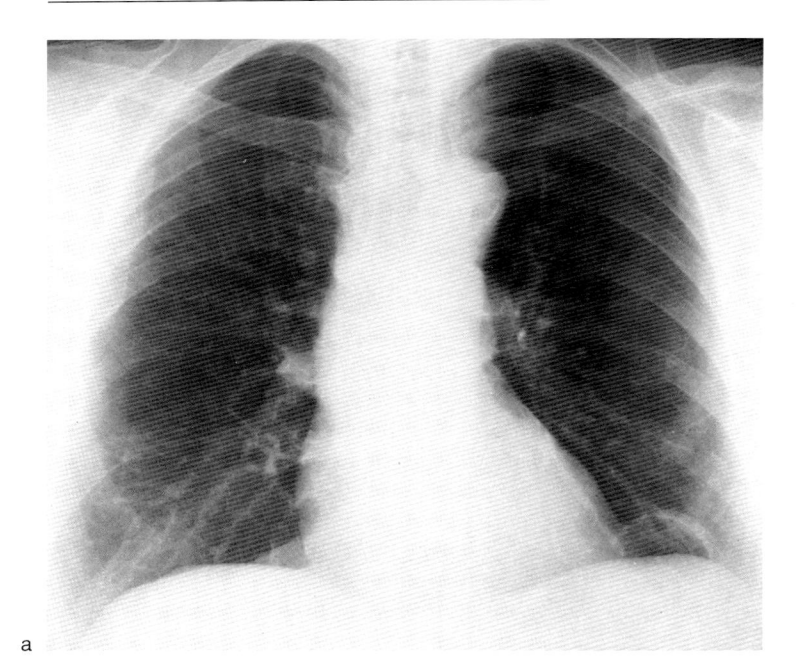

Fig. 11.9 a, b Traumatic rupture of left hemidiaphragm. Patient presented 3 years after severe abdominal trauma. Crescentic lucency seen above contour of left hemidiaphragm. On subsequent lateral film, lucency fills in. Splenic flexure herniates through diaphragmatic defect into left hemithorax.

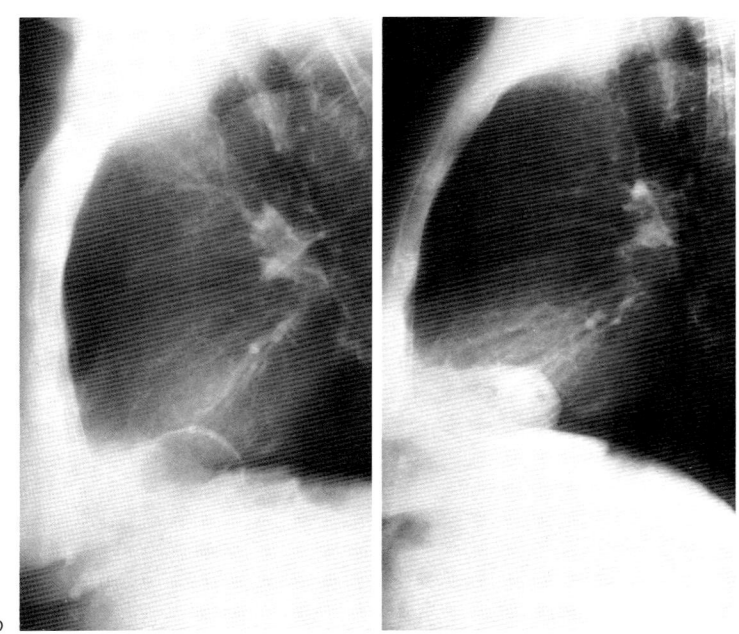

# 12. Diseases of the Chest Wall

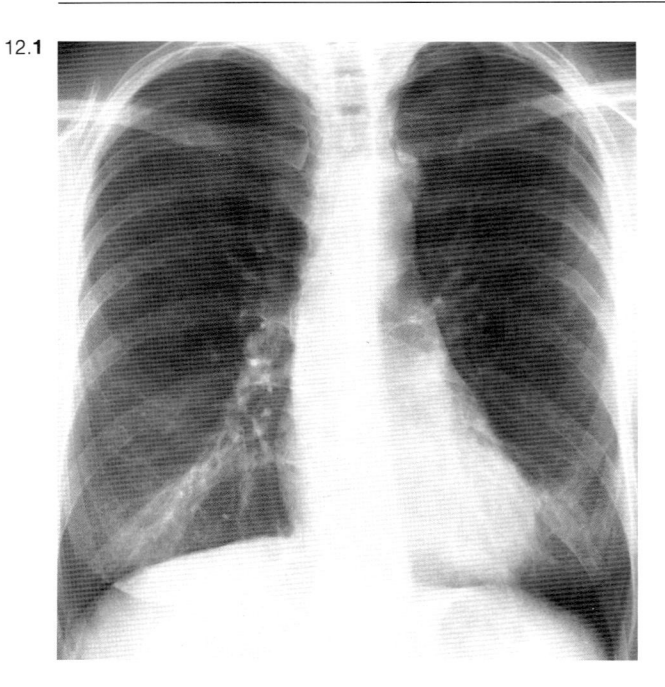

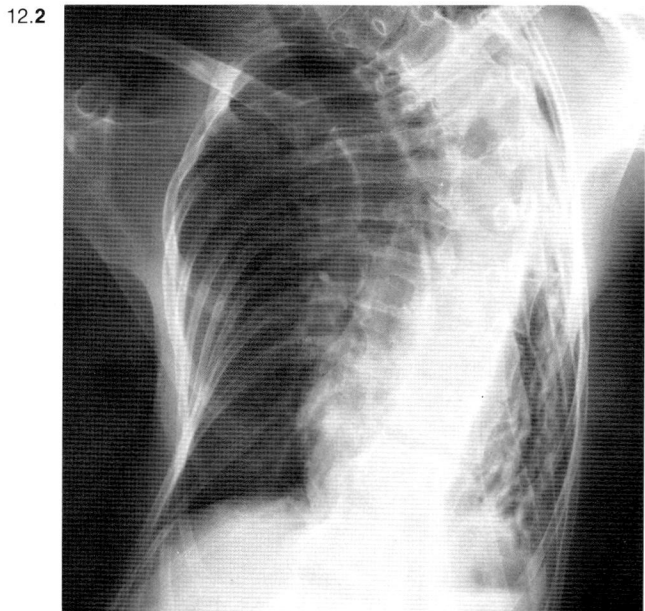

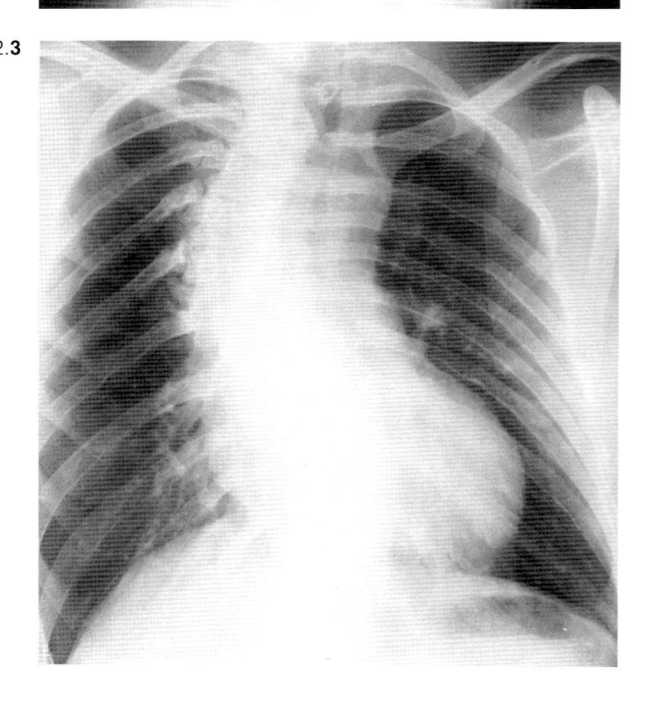

Thoracic Skeleton

◁ Fig. 12.1 **Mild scoliosis.**

◁ Fig. 12.2 **Marked paralytic scoliosis with deformity of the left hemithorax, due to early childhood brain damage.**

◁ Fig. 12.3 **Scoliosis due to neurofibromatosis.** Note rib notching.

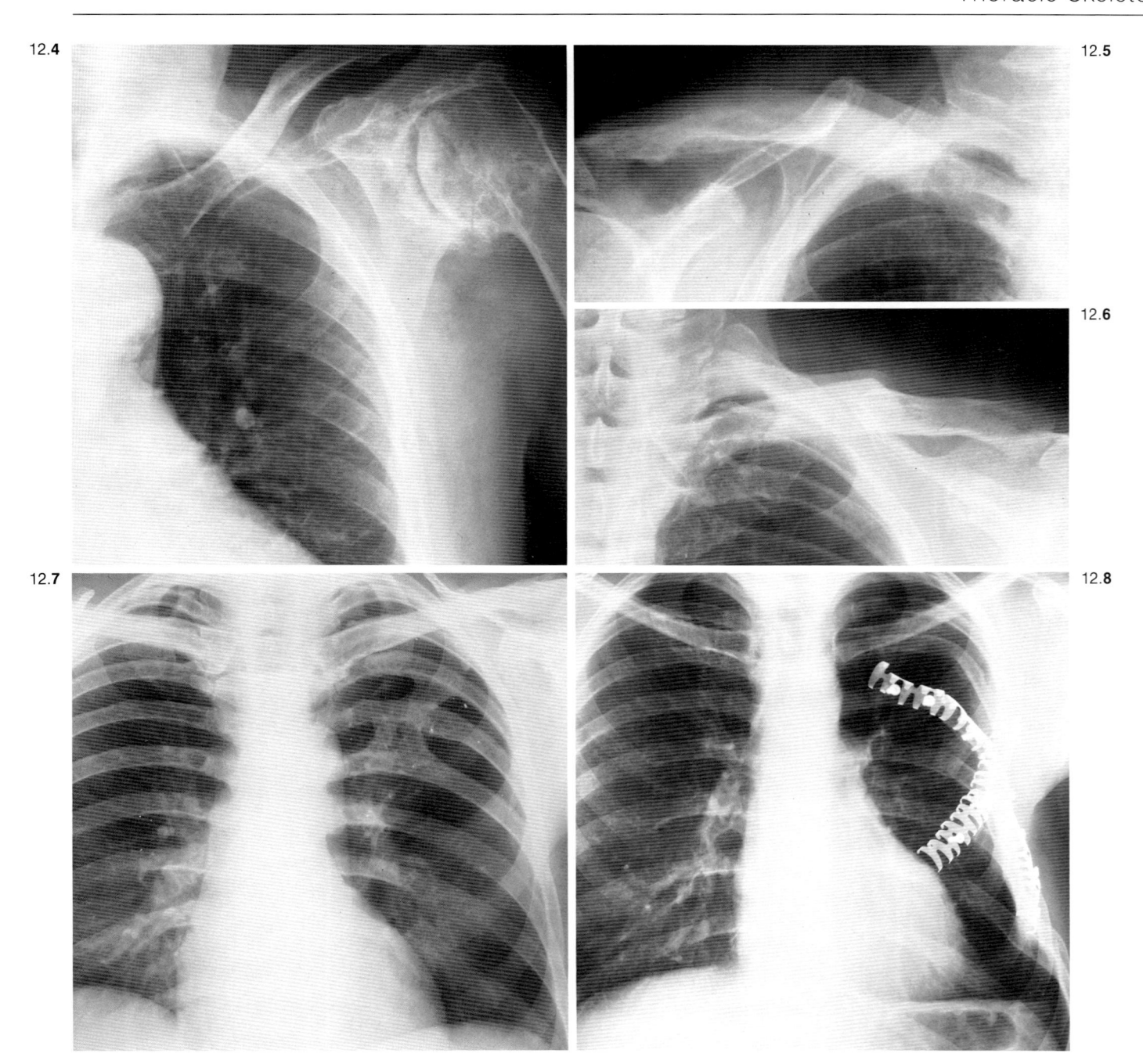

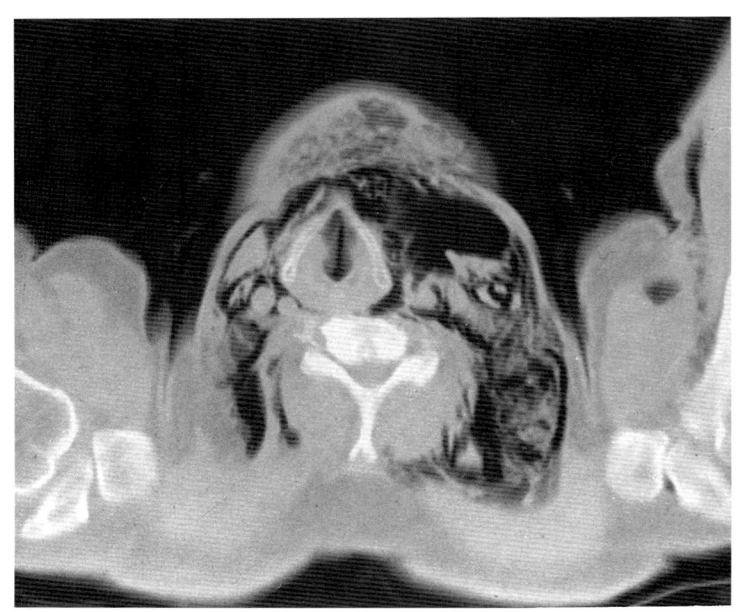

Fig. 12.4 **Posttraumatic osteoarthrosis of left should joint subsequent to an old left subcapital humeral fracture.**

Fig. 12.5 **Paget's disease.**
Deformity, cortical thickening, and sclerosis of right clavicle.

Fig. 12.6 **Old healed clavicular fracture.**

Fig. 12.7 **Posttraumatic fusion of several left-sided posterior ribs.**

Fig. 12.8 **Posttraumatic flail chest with open reduction and internal fixation of unstable hemithorax.**

Fig. 12.9 Extensive subcutaneous emphysema in patient with anastomotic leak after esophageal surgery. CT scan shows a large amount of gas in the soft-tissue planes of the neck, surrounding the larynx and the carotid sheath.

276   12. Diseases of the Chest Wall

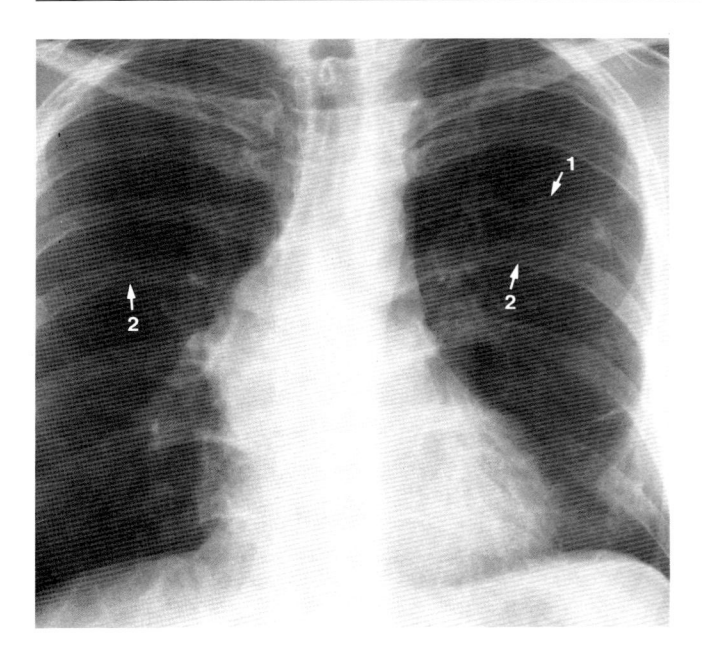

Fig. 12.**10**   **Rib resection.**
Regeneration of bone in periosteal remnant (1). Rib notching (2) due to coarctation of aorta.

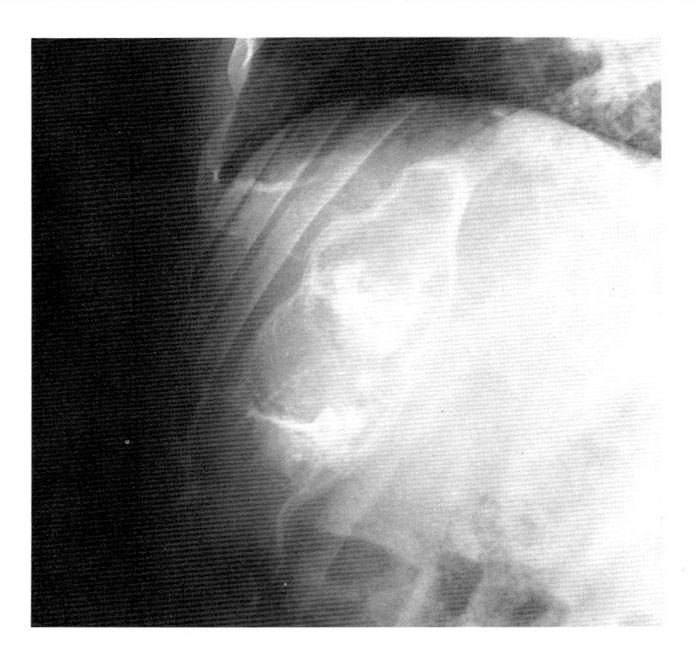

Fig. 12.**11**   **Enchondroma of rib, biopsy proven.**

Fig. 12.12 a–d Lymphoblastic lymphoma involving rib.
70-year-old patient. Extrapleural mass (1) and destruction of anterior aspect of third rib on the right (**a**). After chemotherapy, the mass shrinks, and the destroyed rib recalcifies (**b**). Right axillary, pretracheal, and prevascular lymph nodes are visible on CT scans (**c, d**).

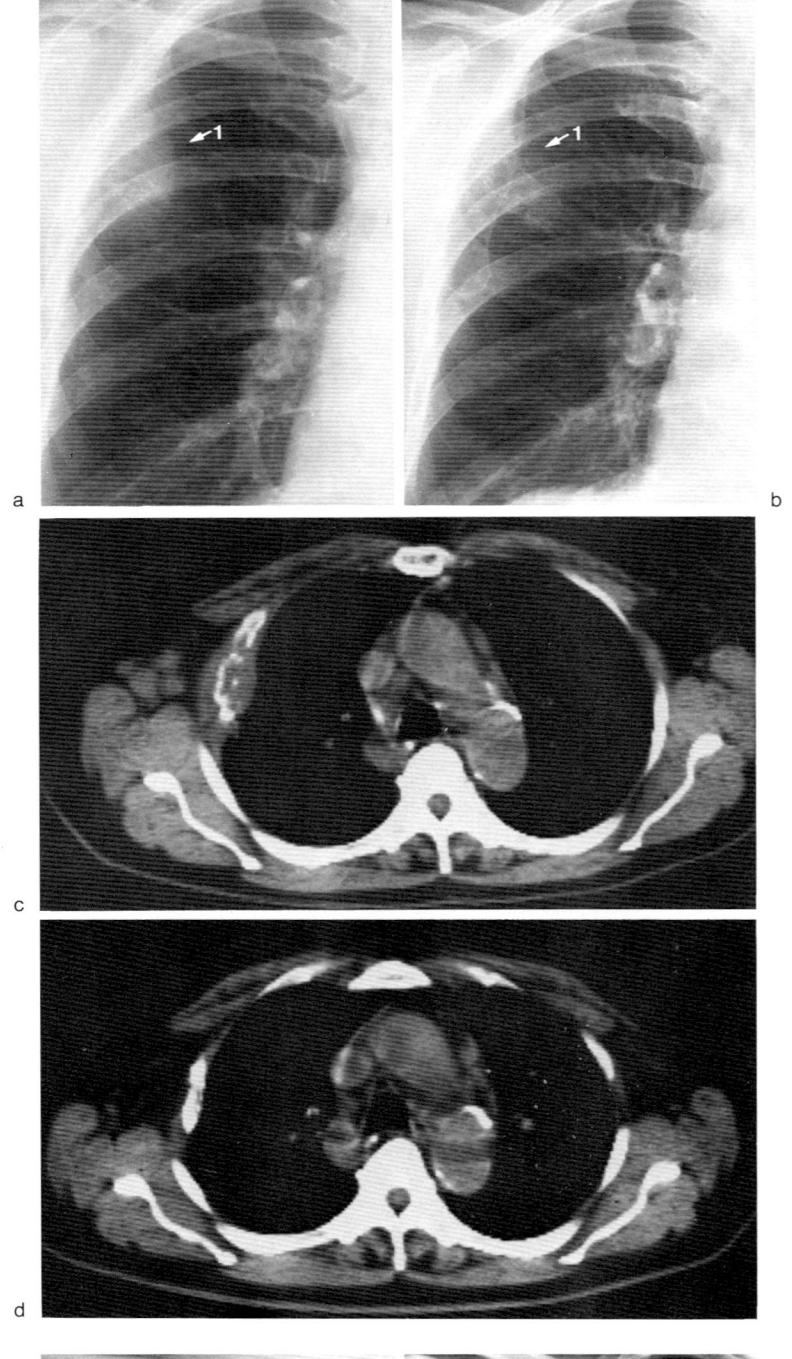

Fig. 12.13 a, b Rib metastases from renal cell carcinoma.
47-year-old patient. Osteolytic destruction, posterior aspect of fifth right rib (1). After radiation therapy, recalcification of destroyed rib is apparent (**b**).

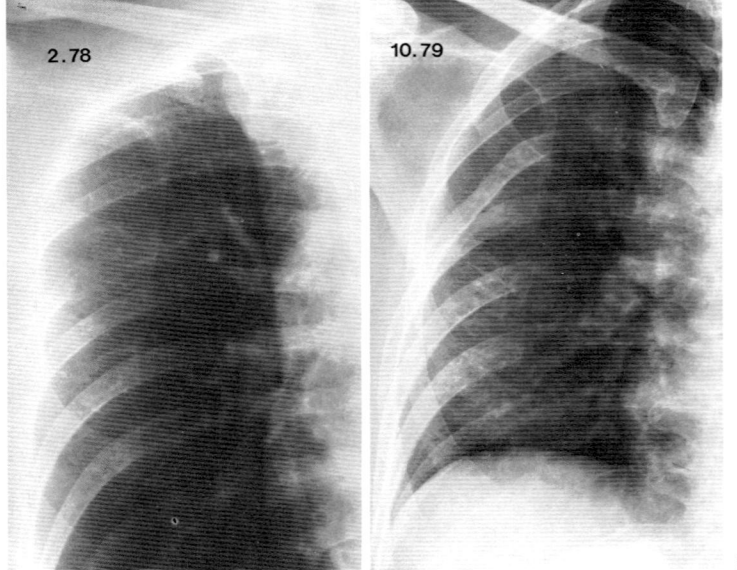

278   12. Diseases of the Chest Wall

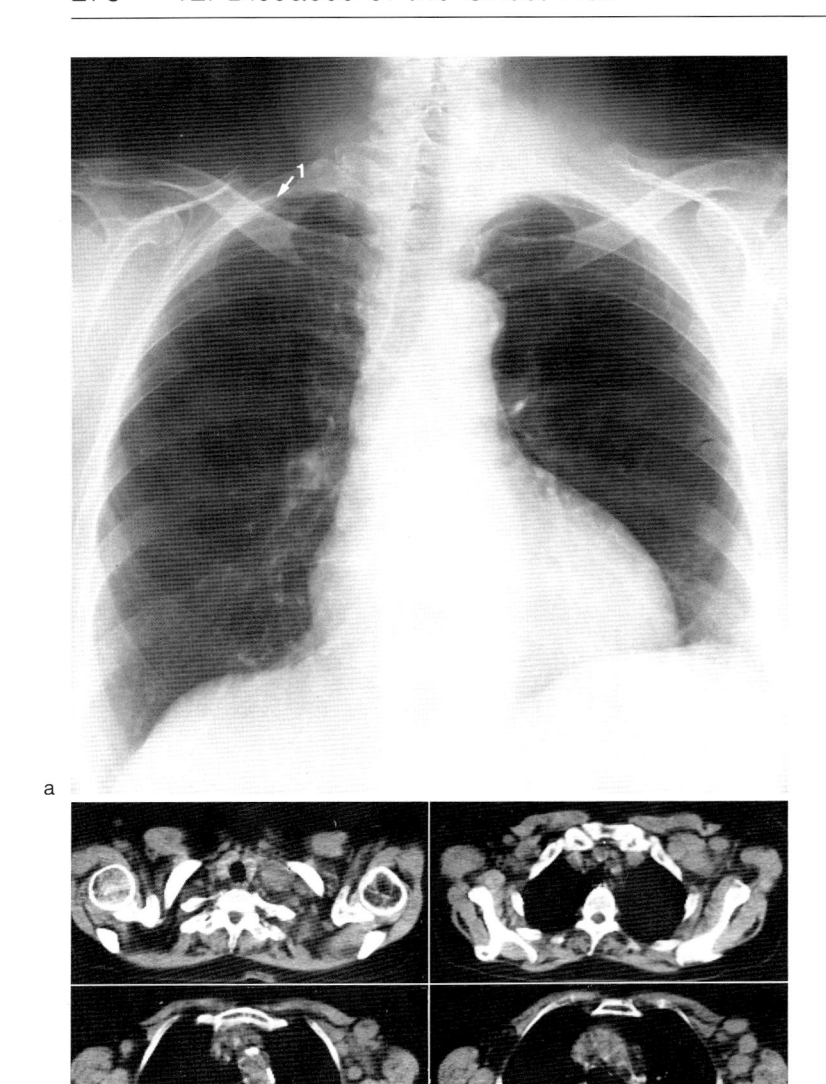

Fig. 12.**14 a, b   Hodgkin lymphoma with enlarged left supraclavicular and axillary lymph nodes.**
Clavicular companion shadow (1) is obliterated on the left side. CT scan demonstrates supraclavicular, infraclavicular, and axillary lymph node enlargement.

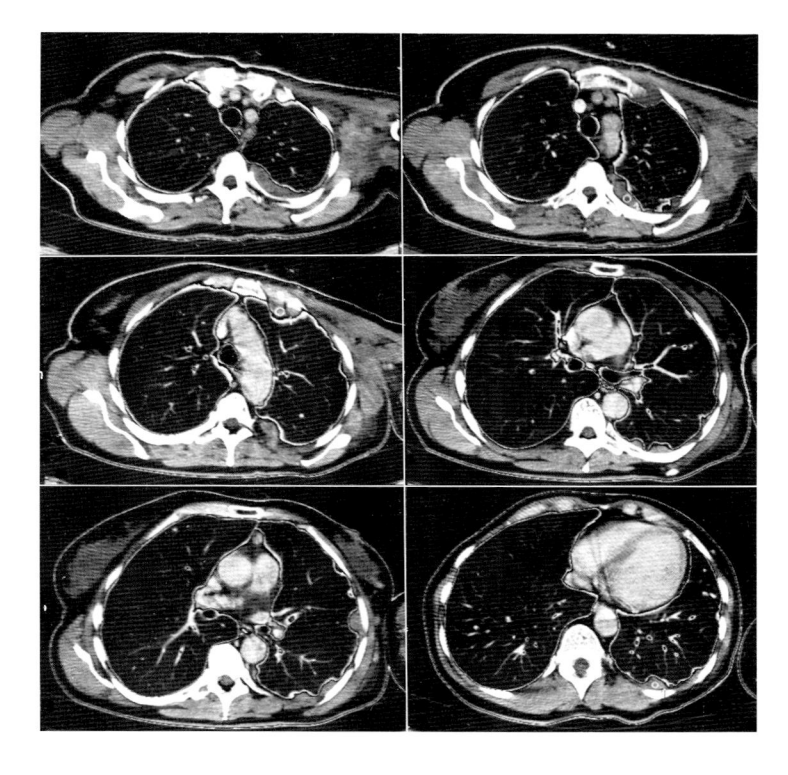

Fig. 12.**15   Breast cancer with chest wall recurrence.**
60-year-old patient, 6 years after left radical mastectomy. CT scan demonstrates enlarged left axillary and infraclavicular lymph nodes, pleural carcinomatosis, and chest wall tumor infiltrating left pectoralis muscle group.

Chest Wall Soft-Tissue Abnormalities

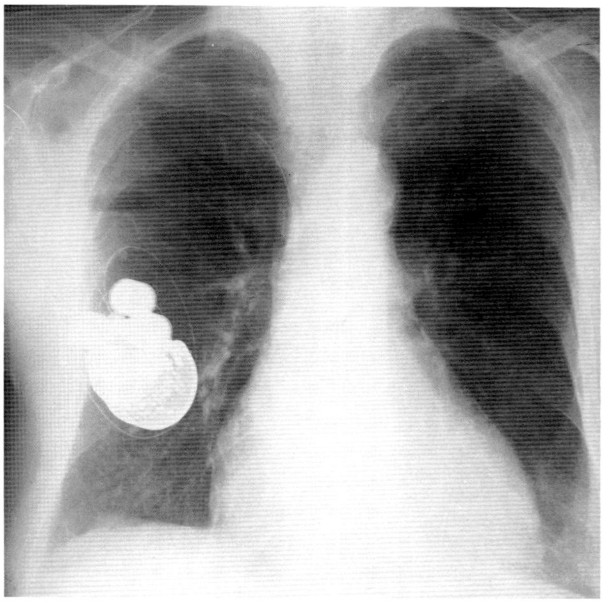

Fig. 12.**16** **Pacemaker battery pack with infected subcutaneous pouch.** Note gas-fluid level.

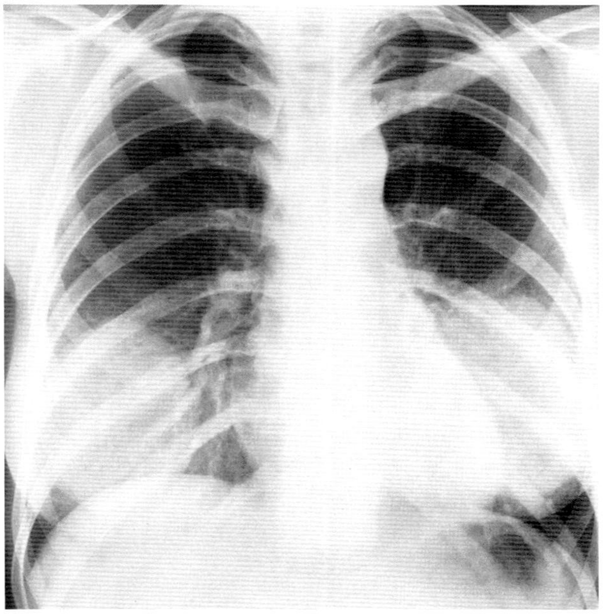

Fig. 12.**17** **Bilateral augmentation mammoplasty with silicon implants.**

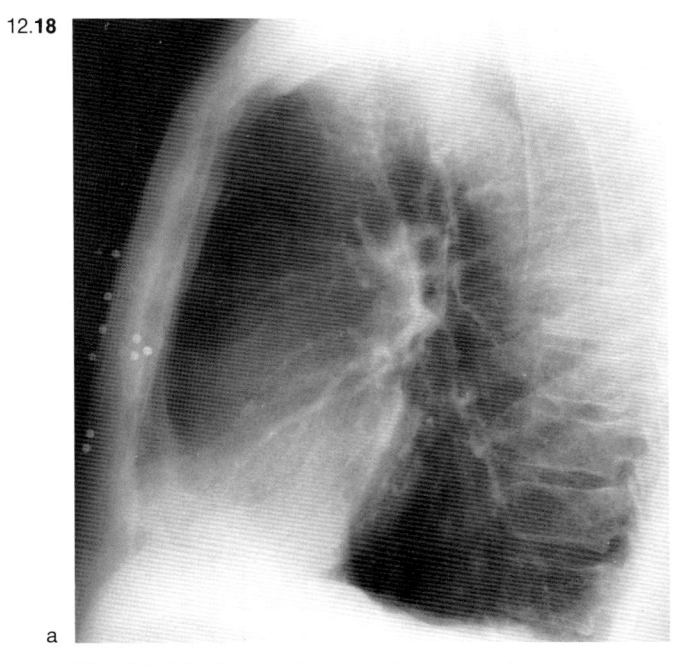

Fig. 12.**18 a, b**   Pellets in right anterior chest wall.

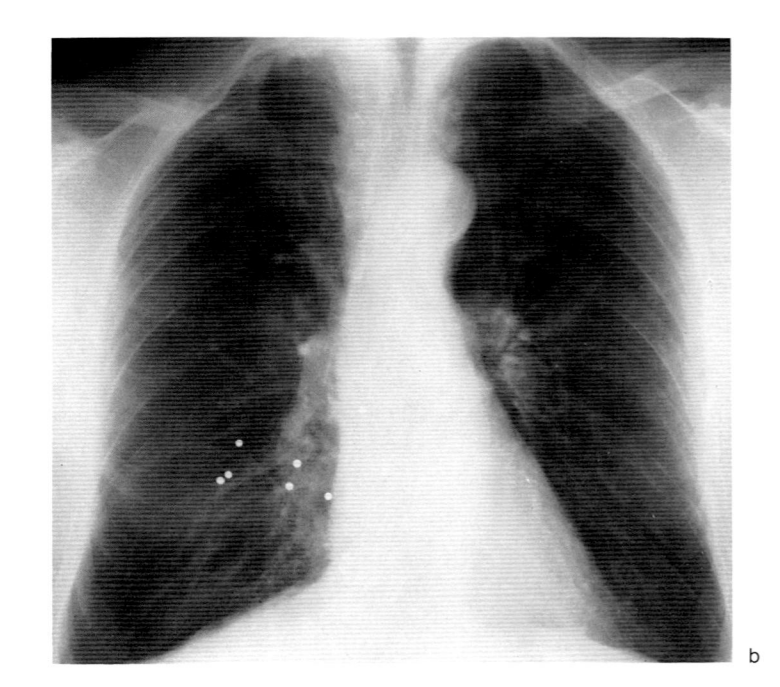

280   12. Diseases of the Chest Wall

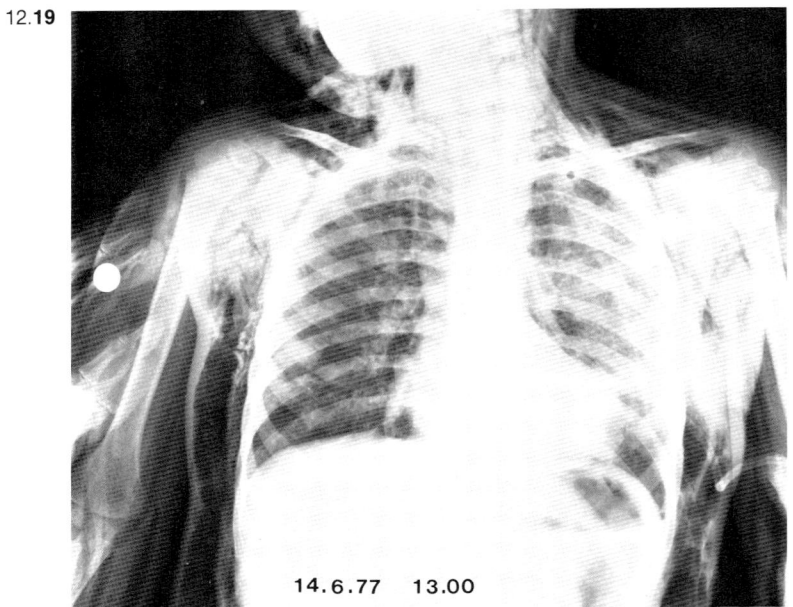

Fig. 12.19 Extensive subcutaneous emphysema, deep cervical emphysema, and pneumomediastinum in patient after repair of aortic aneurysm.

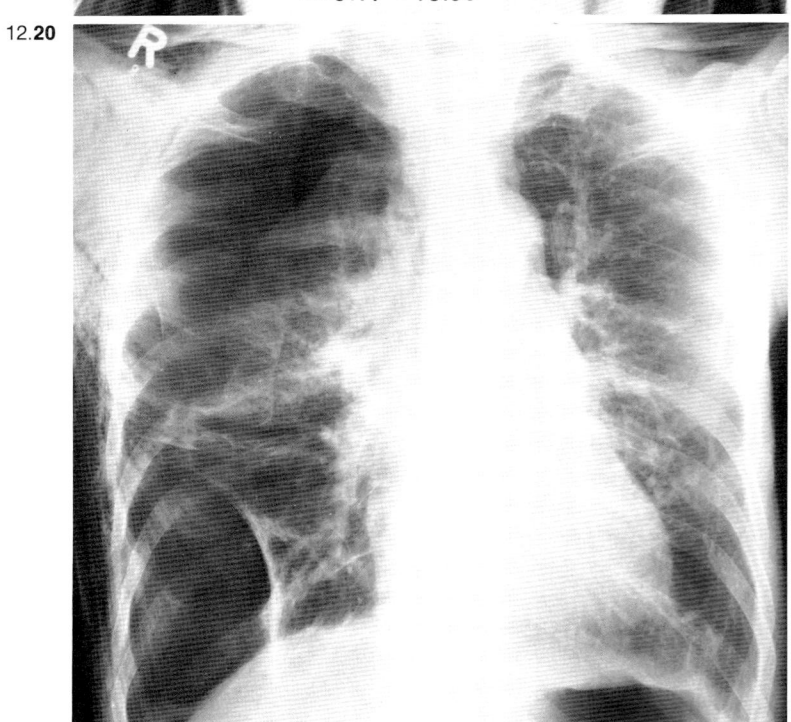

Fig. 12.20 Subcutaneous emphysema in patient with spontaneous pneumothorax.
Note outline of pectoralis muscle fibers.

Fig. 12.21 Deep cervical emphysema after spontaneous pneumothorax.
Pneumomediastinum. Note air outlining esophagus, aortic arch branches, and interstices of neck.
▽

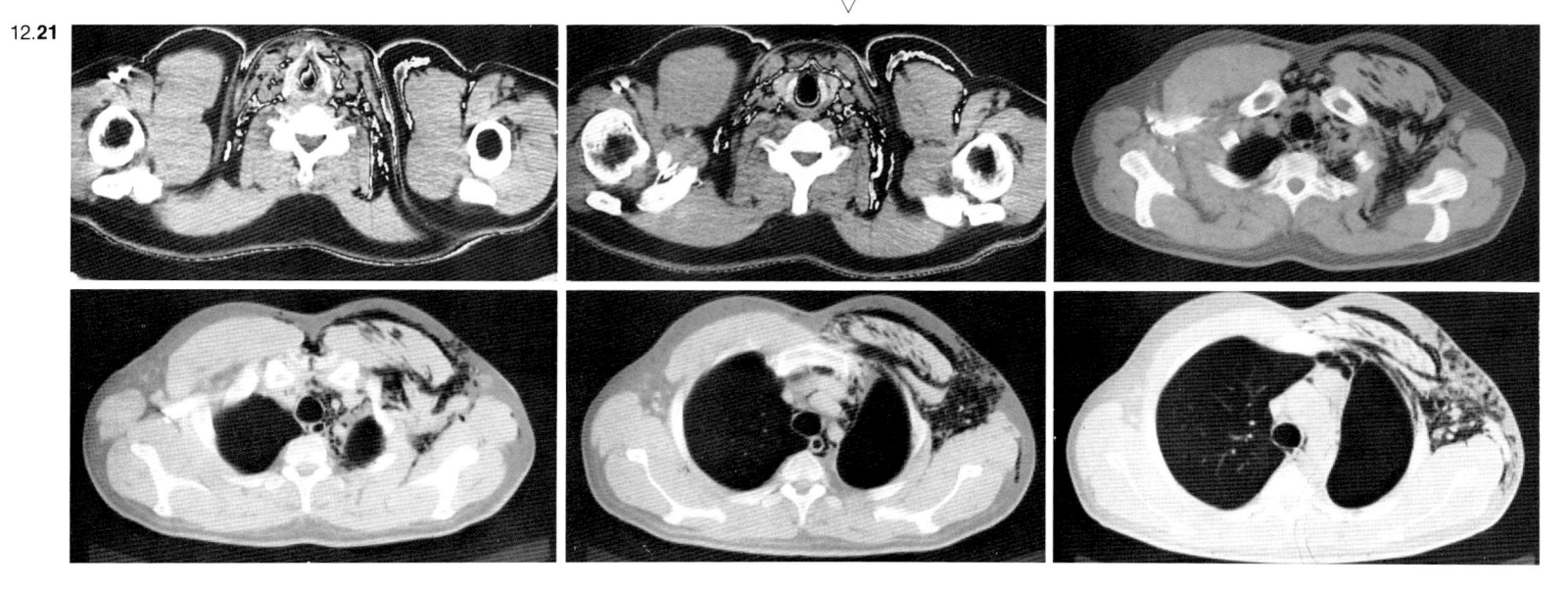

References

1. Aberle, D. R., G. Gamsu, C. S. Ray, I. M. Feuerstein: Asbestosis-related pleural and parenchymal fibrosis: detection with high-resolution CT. Radiology 166 (1988) 729
2. Aberle, D. R., J. P. Wiener-Kronish, W. R. Webb, M. A. Matthay: Hydrostatic versus increased permeability pulmonary edema: diagnosis based on radiographic criteria in critically ill patients. Radiology 168 (1988) 73
3. Alderson, P. O., E. C. Martin: Pulmonary embolism: diagnosis with multiple imaging modalities. Radiology 164 (1987) 297
5. Amin, R.: Complete regression of pulmonary metastases from malignant melanoma of the vulva following therapy with tamoxifen. Brit. J. Radiol. 59 (1986) 171
6. Assmann, H.: Frühinfiltrat. Ergebn. ges. Tuberk.- u. Lung.-Forsch. 1 (1930) 1115–194
7. Austrian, R.: Pneumococcal pneumonia and pneumococcal vaccine. Mt Sinai J. Med. 48 (1981) 532–538
8. Ayvazian, L.: Diagnostic aspects of pleural effusion. Bull. N.Y. Acad. Med. 53 (1977) 532
9. Ball, J. B., A. V. Proto: The variable appearance of the left superior intercostal vein. Radiology 144 (1982) 445
10. Barnes, P., T. Verdegem: Chest roentgenogram in pulmonary tuberculosis. New data on and old test. Chest 94 (1988) 316
11. Baum, G. L.: Pulmonary calcification. Amer. Rev. resp. Dis. 99 (1966) 296
12. Baum, G. L.: Textbook of Pulmonary Diseases. Little Brown & Co., Boston 1974
13. Behrend, H., M. Rupec: Die Aussagekraft der Kveim-Reaktion in der Diagnostik der Sarkoidose. Z. Erkr. Atm.-Org. 149 (1977) 122
14. Beitzke, A., G. Gypser, W. D. Sager: Scimitarsyndrom. Fortschr. Röntgenstr. 136 (1982) 265
15. Bergin, C. J., N. L. Müller: CT of interstitial lung disease: diagnostic approach. Amer. J. Roentgenol. 148 (1987) 9
16. Bergin, C., V. Roggli, C. Coblentz et al.: Secondary pulmonary lobule: normal and abnormal CT appearances. Amer. J. Roentgenol. 151 (1988) 21
17. Berkmen, J.: Radiologic aspects of intrathoracic sarcoidosis. Semin. Roentgenol. 20 (1985) 356
18. Black, L. F.: The pleural space and pleural fluid. Mayo Clin. Proc. 47 (1972) 493
19. Blaha, H.: Die Lungentuberkulose im Röntgenbild. Springer, Berlin 1976
20. Bloomfield, J. A.: Protean radiological manifestations of hydatid infestation. Aust. Asian. Radiol. 10 (1966) 330–343
21. Boeck, C.: Nochmals zur Klinik und zur Stellung des „benignen Miliarlupoid". Arch. Dermatol. Syph. 121 (1916) 707
22. Bohlig, H.: Lunge und Pleura, 2. Aufl. Thieme, Stuttgart 1975
23. Bohlig, H.: Die Bedeutung der Herdwanderung für das Erscheinungsbild klein-fleckiger Lungenerkrankungen am Beispiel der Silikose. Radiologe 19 (1979) 486
24. Bohlig, H., E. Hain, H. Valentin, H. J. Woitowitz: Die Modifikation der Internationalen Staublungenklassifikation für die arbeitsmedizinischen Vorsorgeuntersuchungen staubgefährdeter Arbeitnehmer usw. – Arbeitsmed. aktuell 10. Lieferung, F
25. Bohlig, H., E. Hain, H. Valentin, H. J. Woitowitz: Die Weiterentwicklung der Internationalen Staublungenklassifikation und ihre Konsequenzen f. d. arbeitsmed. Vorsorgeuntersuchungen. (ILO 1989/BRD), Prax. Pneumol. 35 (1981) 1134–1139
26. Brecht, G., Th. Harder: Aortenaneurysma und Aortendissektion. Computertomographie – Angiographie – Sonographie. Fortschr. Röntgenstr. 135 (1981) 388
27. Brenner, J., P. P. Sordillo, G. B. Magill, R. B. Goldbey: Malignant mesothelioma of the pleura: review of 123 patients. Cancer 49 (1982) 2431–2435
28. Buckwalter, K. A., B. H. Gross, R. J. Hermandez: Bolus dynamic computed tomography in the evaluation of pulmonary sequestration. CT 11 (1987) 335
29. Buhlmann, A. A.: Lungenemphysem, Einteilung nach klinischen, röntgenologischen und funktionellen Gesichtspunkten. Münch. med. Wschr. 116 (1974) 1627
30. Burgener, F. A.: Die Röntgenmanifestation der disseminierten Histiocytosis X beim Erwachsenen. Fortschr. Röntgenstr. 126 (1977) 466
31. Calenoff, L., G. D. Kruglik, A. Woodruff: Unilateral pulmonary edema. Radiology 126 (1978) 19
32. Cervantes-Perez, P., A. H. Toro-Perez, P. Rodrigucz-Jurado: Pulmonary involvement in rheumatoid arthritis. Amer. med. Ass. 243 (1980) 1715
33. Chalmers, A. G., J. Wyatt, P. J. Robeinson: Computed tomographic and pathological findings in pulmonary alveolar microlithiasis. Brit. J. Radiol 59 (1986) 408
34. Chang, C. H.: The normal roentgenographic measurement of the pulmonary artery in 1085 cases. Amer. J. Roentgenol 87 (1962) 929
35. Chintapalli, K., M. K. Thorsen, D. L. Olson et al.: Computed tomography of pulmonary thromboembolism and infarction. J. Comput. assist. Tomogr. 12 (1988) 553
36. Christ, F., R. Janson, C. Engel: Zwerchfellverletzungen aus radiologischer und klinischer Sicht. Fortschr. Röntgenstr. 135 (1981) 301
37. Christensen, E. E., G. W. Diezt: The supraclavicular fossa. Radiology 118 (1976) 37–39
38. Davis, L. A.: The vertical fissure line. Amer. Roentgenol. 84 (1960) 451–453
39. Deutsche Forschungsgemeinschaft: Forschungsbericht Chronische Bronchitis und Staubbelastung am Arbeitsplatz. Forschungsbericht Chronische Bronchitis, Teil 2. Boldt, Boppard 1975, 1981
40. Dihlmann, W.: Beitrag zur Pleurakuppenschwiele. Fortschr. Röntgenstr. 122 (1975) 461
41. Doerr, W.: Spezielle pathologische Anatomie, Bd. XVI. Springer, Berlin 1983
42. Esser, C.: Der Hilus des Erwachsenen im Röntgenbild. Pneumol. 23 (1969) 743
43. Euler, M. S. V., G. Liljestrand: Observations on the pulmonary arterial blood pressure in the cat. Acta physiol. scand 12 (1946) 301–320
44. Fauci, A., S. Wolff: Wegener's granulomatosis. – Studies in eighteen patients and a review of the literature. Medicine (Baltimore) 52 (1973) 535
45. Felson, B.: The lobes and interlobar pleura. Fundamental roentgen considerations. Amer. J. med. Sci. 230 (1955) 572
46. Felson, B.: Chest Roentgenology. Saunders, Philadelphia 1973.
47. Fildermann, A. E., C. Shaw, R. A. Matthay: Lung cancer, part I: etiology, pathology, natural history, manifestations, and diagnostic techniques. Invest. Radiol. 21 (1986) 80
48. Fiore, D., P. R. Biondetti, F. Sartori et al.: The role of computed tomography in the evaluation of bullous lung disease. J. Comput. assist. Tomogr. 6 (1982) 105–108
49. Fleischer, F. G., A. O. Hampton, B. Castleman: Linear shadows in the lungs (interlobar pleuritis, atelectasis and healed infarction). Amer. J. Roentgenol. 46 (1941) 610
50. Fon, G. T., M. E. Bein, A. A. Mancuso et al.: Computed tomography of the anterior mediastinum in myasthenia gravis. Radiology 142 (1982) 135
51. Foster, W. L. jr., P. C. Pratt, V. L. Roggli, J. D. Godwin, R. A. Halvorsen: Centrilobular emphysema: CT-pathologic correlation. Radiology 159 (1986) 27
52. Foster, W. L., P. C. Pratt, V. L. Roggli et al.: Centrilobular emphysema: CT-pathologic correlation. Radiology 159 (1986) 27
53. Fraser, R. G. J. A. Pare: Synopsis of Diseases of the Chest. Saunders, Philadelphia 1983
54. Freimann, D. G.: The pathology of sarcoidosis. Semin. Roentgenol. 20 (1985) 327
55. Fuchs, W. A., E. Voegli: Röntgendiagnostik der Lunge. Huber, Bern 1973
56. Gamsu, G., W. R. Webb, P. Sheldon et al.: Nuclear magnetic resonance imaging of the thorax. Radiology 147 (1983) 473
57. Gloor, F., T. Wegmann: Pathologie und Klinik der einheimischen Systemmykosen. Chemotherapy 22 Suppl 1 (1976) 31
58. Gomes, M., P. Bernatz: Arteriovenous fistulas: a review and ten-year experience at the clinics. Mayo Clin. Proc. 45 (1970) 81
59. Good, C. A.: Radiologic appraisal of solitary pulmonary nodules. Minn. Med. 45 (1962) 157
60. Greene, R.: Adult respiratory distress syndrome: acute alveolar damage. Radiology 163 (1987) 57

61. Greenspan, R. H.: Die Röntgendiagnostik der Lungenembolie – In Fuchs. E. Voegli: Aktuelle Probleme der Röntgendiagnostik, Bd. II: Röntgendiagnostik der Lunge. Huber, Bern, 1973
62. Günther, D., G. Müller: Der Lobus venae azygos und seine klinische Bedeutung. Fortschr. Röntgenstr. 132
63. Gullota, W. H. Wenzl: Posttraumatische Lungenhaematome und Pneumatozelen. Fortschr. Röntgenstr. 121 (1974) 35
64. Hamper, U. M., E. K. Fishmann, N. F. Khouri et al.: Typical and atypical CT manifestations of pulmonary sarcoidosis. J. Comput. assist. Tomogr. 10 (1986) 928
65. Hanke, R., R. Kretschmar: Die Rundatelektase. Fortschr. Röntgenstr. 138 (1983) 151
66. Hauptverband der gewerblichen Berufsgenossenschaften, Bonn: Das Berufskrankheitengeschehen. Eine exemplarische Darstellung über ausgewählte Berufskrankheiten. Sutter, Essen 1985
67. Heerfordt, C. E.: Über eine „febris uveo-parotidea subchronica" an der glandula parotis und der uvea des Auges lokalisiert u. häufig mit Paresen cerebrospinaler Nerven kompliziert. Arch. Ophth. 70 (1909) 254
68. Heilmeyer, L., F. Schmid: Die progressive Lungendystrophie. Dtsch. med. Wschr. 81 (1956) 1293
69. Heitzmann, E. R.: The Lung. Mosby, St. Louis 1973
70. Heitzmann, E. R.: The Mediastinum. Radiologic Correlation with Anatomy and Pathology. Mosby, ST. Luis 1977
71. Heitzmann, E. R.: Bronchogenic carcinoma: radiologic-pathologic correlations. Semin. Roentgenol. 12 (1977) 165
72. Heitzmann, E. R.: The Lung, Radiologic-pathologic Correlation. Mosby, St. Louis 1984
73. Heitzmann, E. R., D. M. Panicek, S. A. Randall et al.: Continuum of pulmonary developmental anomalies. Radiographics 7 (1987) 747
74. Henvin, A.: Postmortem demonstration of abnormal deep pulmonary lymphatic pathways in lymphangitic carcinomatosis. Cancer 33 (1974) 1598
75. Heron, C. W., A. L. Poszniak, G. J. S. Hunter et al.: Case report: Anomalous systemic venous drainage occurring in association with the hypogenetic lung syndrome. Clin. Radiol. 39 (1988) 446
76. Heymer, R., G. Benz-Bohm, G. Arnold: Röntgenbefunde bei kongenitalen zystischen Lungenveränderungen im Säuglingsalter. Fortschr. Röntgenstr. 137 (1984) 451
77. Hofner, W. W., W. Küster, P. Plötzlo: Intrapulmonale Veränderungen bei M. Hodgkin. Fortschr. Röntgenstr. 130 (1979) 144
78. Hunninghake, G. W., A. S. Fauci: Pulmonary involvement in the collagen vascular diseases. Amer. Rev. resp. Dis. 119 (1979) 471
79. Huzly, A.: Der Spontanpneumothorax. Therapiewoche 19 (1969) 387
80. Huzly, A.: Bronchiektasen. In Hornborstel, H., W. Kaufmann, W. Siegenthaler: Innere Medizin in Praxis und Klinik, Bd. I. Thieme, Stuttgart 1973 (S. 3)
81. Huzly, A., F. Böhm: Bronchus und Tuberkulose. Thieme, Stuttgart 1955
82. Iwai, K., G. Shindo, H. Hajikano, H. Tajima, M. Morimoto et al.: Intralobar pulmonary sequestration, with special reference to developmental pathology. Amer. Rev. resp. Dis. 107 (1973) 911
83. Jonson, D. H. M.: Pulmonary aspergilloma. Brit. J. clin. Pract. 31 (1977) 207
84. Jüngling, O.: Ostitis tuberculos multiplex cystica (eine eigenartige Form der Knochentuberkulose). Fortschr. Röntgenstr. 27 (1919–1921) 375
85. Kantor, H. G.: The many radiologic faces of pneumococcal pneumonia. Amer. J. Roentgenol. 137 (1981) 1213–1220
86. Kauffmann, G. W., W. Vogel, K. H. Rühle, H. H. Friedburg et al.: Verlaufsbeobachtungen bei überlebter Schocklunge. Fortschr. Röntgenstr. 138 (1983) 292
87. Kaufmann, R. A.: Calcified postinflammatory pseudotumor of the lung. J. Comput. assist. Tomogr. 12 (1988) 653
88. Keast, T. E.: The aortic-pulmonary stripe. Amer. J. Roentgenol. 116 (1972) 107
89. Küster, W., W. Hofner, L. Wicke, L. Kühböck: Varizellenpneumonie bei Morbus Hodgkin. Radiologe 18 (1978) 398
90. Kuriyama, K., R. G. Gamsu, C. E. Stern, R. Cann et al.: CT-determined pulmonary artery diameters in prediciting pulmonary hypertension. Invest. Radiol. 19 (1984) 16
91. Kyser, P. L., B. L. McComb, W. F. Bennet: CT evidence of calcification within a small cell carcinoma of the lung. Comput. Radiol. 10 (1986) 107
92. Lange, S.: Radiologische Diagnostik der Lungenerkrankungen. Thieme, Stuttgart 1986
93. Lange, S., W. Anhuth: Das maligne Pleuramesotheliom. Fortschr. Röntgenstr. 141 (1984) 402
94. Lange, S., C. Minck: Die Lymphangiosis carcinomatosa der Lungen bei metastasierten Mammacarcinomen. Fortschr. Röntgenstr. 140 (1983) 411
95. Langer, R., M. Langer, K. A. Schumacher: Darstellbarkeit intrapulmonaler a. v. Shunts unter besonderer Berücksichtigung der Computertomographie. Fortschr. Röntgenstr. 136 (1982) 563
96. Light, R. W.: Pleural Diseases. Lea & Febiger, Philadelphia 1983
97. Loddenkemper: Die Lungentuberbkulose – eine vergessene Krankheit? Dtsch. Ärztebl. 87 (1990) 194
98. Löfgren, S., H. Lundbäck: The bilateral hilar lymphoma syndrome. A study of the relation to age and sex in 212 cases. Acta med. scand. 142 (1952) 259
99. Mahoney, M. C., R. T. Shipley: Neofissure after right upper lobectomy. Radiology 166 (1988) 721
100. Mann, H., S. V. Karwande: New proposed staging system for lung cancer. Semin. US CT MB 9 (1988) 34
101. McDonald, C. J., R. A. Castellino, N. Blank: The aortic nipple. Amer. J. Roentgenol. 116 (1972) 107–109
102. Mc Loud, T. C., G. R. Epler, T. V. Colby, E. A. Gaensler, C. B.Carrington: Bronchiolitis obliterans. Radiology 159 (1986) 1
103. McLoud, Th. C., L. Kalisher, P. Stark, R. Greene: Intrathoracic lymph node metastases from extrathoracic neoplasma. Amer. J. Roentgenol. 131 (1978) 403
104. Milne. E. N. C.: Die röntgenologische Diagnose der Linksinsuffizienz. In Fuchs, W., E. Vögeli: Röntgendiagnostik der Lunge. Huber, Bern 1973 (S. 33)
105. Milne, E.: Some new concepts of pulmonary blood flow and volume. Radiol. Clin. N. Amer 16 (1978) 515
106. Mittermayer, Ch.: Perfusionsstörungen. In Doerr, W.: Spezielle pathologische Anatomie, Bd. XVI. Springer, Berlin 1983
107. Morgan, M. D. L., D. M. Denison, B. Strickland: Value of computed tomography for selecting patients with bullous lung disease for surgery. Radiology 164 (1987) 589
108. Moser, E. S. jr., A. V. Proto: Lung torsion: case report and literature review. Radiology 162 (1987) 639
109. Müller, H. E.: Die erregerspezifischen Laboratoriumsmethoden zur Diagnostik der Tuberkulose. Dtsch. med. Wschr. 108 (1983) 63
110. Müller, K. H.: In Doerr, W.: Lungentumoren. Spezielle pathologische Anatomie, Bd. XIV. Springer, Berlin 1983
111. Müller, W.: Die pathologische Anatomie des Mediastinums. Prax. Klin. Pneumol 8 (1969) 513
112. Munk, P. L., N. L. Müller, R. R. Miller, D. N. Ostrow: Pulmonary lymphatic carcinomatosis: CT and pathologic findings? Radiology 166 (1988) 705
113. Murray, J. F.: The normal Lung: the Basis for Diagnosis and Treatment of Disease. Saunders, Philadelphia 1976
114. Mussshoff, K., K. Wurm, H. Reindell, E. Doll: Differentialdiagnose der Sarkoidose. Radiologe 8 (1968) 127
115. Naidich, D. P., D. I. Mccauley, N. F. Khouri et al.: Computed tomography of bronchiectasis. J. Comput. assist. Tomogr. 6 (1982) 437–444
116. Neufang, K. F., D. Beyer: Diagnostische Wertigkeit pleuromediastinaler Linien für die Röntgennativuntersuchung des Mediastinums (Teil I). Röntgenblätter 33 (1980) 257
117. Ominsky, S., H. S. Berinson. The suprasternal fossa. Radioloy 122 (1977) 311–313
118. Ort, S., J. L. Ryan, G. Barden, N. Désopo: Pneumococcal pneumonia in hospitalized patients: clinical and radiological presentations. J. Amer. med Ass. 249 (1983) 214–218
119. Osborne, D., P. Vock, J. D. Godwin et al.: CT identification of bronchopulmonary segments: fifty normal subjects. Amer. J. Roentgenol. 142 (1984) 47–52
120. Peuchot, M., H. I. Libshitz: Pulmonary metastatic disease: radiologic-surgical correlation. Radiology 164 (1987) 719
121. Pfister, R. C., S. O. Kook, J. T. Ferucci: Retrosternal density – radiographic evaluation of the retrosternal premediastinal space. Radiology 96 (1970) 317
122. Proto, A.: CT-analysis of the pulmonary nodule. Radiology 149 (1983) 42
123. Proto, A. V., E. S. Moser jr.: Upper lobe volume loss: divergent and parallel patterns of vascular reorientation. Radiographics 7 (1987) 875
124. Rassiga, A. L.: Advances in adult non-Hodgkin's lymphoma: current concepts of classification, diagnosis and management. Arch. intern. Med. 140 (1980) 1647
125. Rauber, K., S. Tuengerthal, H. Riemann: Die digitale Subtraktionsangiographie der A. pulmonalis. Prax. Pneumol. 37 (1983) 295
126. Reid, L.: The Pathology of Emphysema. Lloyd-Luke, London 1967
127. Renner, R. R., A. P. Coccaro, E. R. Heitzmann, E. T. Dailey: Pseudonomas pneumonia: a prototype of hospital-based infection. Radiology 105 (1972) 555
128. Rigler, L. G.: An overview of diseases of the pleura. Semin. Roentgenol. 12 (1977) 265
129. Rogers, L. F., J. C. Osmer: Bronchogenic cyst: a review of 46 cases. Amer. J. Roentgenol. 91 (1964) 273
130. Rovner, A. J., J. L. Westcott: Pulmonary edema and respiratory insufficiency in acute pancreatitis. Radiology 118 (1976) 512
131. Rubin, S. A.: Radiology of immunologic diseases of the lung. J. thorac. Imag. 3/2 (1988) 21
132. Rudikoff, J. C.: The pulmonary ligament and subpulmonic effusion. Chest 80 (1981) 505–507
133. Savoca, C. J., H. M. Austin, H. I. Golberg: The right paratracheal stripe. Radiology 122 (1977) 295–301
134. Schermuly, W.: Röntgenologische und szintigraphische Befunde bei Sarkoidose-Patienten. Internist 23 (1982) 325–334
135. Schlungbaum, W., S. Lange: Bronchialtumoren. In Schinz, W. Frommhold, W. Dihlmann, H.-St. Stender: Lehrbuch der Röntgendiagnostik, Bd. IV/1. Thieme, Stuttgart 1968

136. Schmitz-Cliever: Über das Vorkommen des lobus venae azygos der linken Lungenseite. RöFo 72 (1950) 728
137. Scott, I. R., N. L. Müller, R. R. Miller, K. G. Evans, B. Nelems: Resectable Stage III lung cancer, surgical, and pathologic correlation. Radiology 166 (1988) 75
138. Seeliger, H. P. R., U. Vögtle-Junker: Die aktuelle Bedeutung der Systemmykosen in Mitteleuropa. Chemotherapy 22, Suppl. 1 (1976) 1
138a. Shermann, Neptune, Weichselbaum et al.: Unaggresive approach to merginaly resectable lung cancer. Cancer 41 (1978) 2040.
139. Shioya, S., M. Haida, Y. Ono, M. Fukuzaki et al.: Lung cancer: differentiation of tumor, necrosis, and atelectasis by means of T 1 and T 2 values measured in vitro. Radiology 167 (1988) 105
140. Siegelmann, S. S., E. A. Zerhouni et al.: CT of the solitary pulmonary nodule. Amer. J. Roentgenol. 135 (1980) 1
141. Siegelmann, S. S., N. F. Khouri, W. W Scott jr., F. P. Leo, U. M. Hamper: Pulmonary harmatoma: CT findings. Radiology 160 (1986) 313
142. Snider, G. L.: The concept of interstitial lung disease. Prax. Klin. Pneumol. 40 (1986) 240
143. Spencer, H.: Pathology of the lung, 4th ed. Pergamon Press, Oxford 1985
144. Stark, P.: Das adenoidzystische Karzinom (Zylindrom) der Trachea. Eine Analyse von 9 Fällen. Fortschr. Röntgenstr. 136 (1982) 131
145. Stark, P.: Die normale Anatomie der Lungenhili im Computertomogram. Fortschr. Röntgenstr. 137 (1982) 77
146. Stark, D. D., M. P. Federle, P. C. Goodman et al.: Differentiating lung abscess and empyema: radiography and computed tomography. Amer. J. Roentgenol. 141 (1983) 163
147. Statistisches Bundesamt Wiesbaden: Fachserie 12 Gesundheitswesen, Reihe 4. Kohlhammer, Stuttgart 1986
148. Staub, N. C.: New concepts about the pathophysiology of pulmonary edema. J. thorac. Imag. 3/3 (1988) 8
149. Stender, H. St., D. Saure: Röntgenuntersuchungstechnik der Lunge. Röntgenblätter 35 (1982) 158
150. Tew, J., L. Calenoff, B. S. Berlin: Bacterial or non bacterial pneumonia: accuracy of radiographic diagnosis. Radiology 124 (1977) 607–612
151. Thurlbeck, W. M., G. Simon: Radiographic appearance of the chest in Emphysema. Amer. J. Roentgenol. 130 (1978) 429
152. UICC: TMN-Atlas. Springer, Berlin 1985
153. Ulmer, W. T.: Die obstruktiven Atemwegserkrankungen. In Schiegk, H.: Handuch der inneren Medizin, Bd. IV/2. Springer, Berlin 1979
154. Vogel, M.: Mißbildungen und Anomalien der Lunge. In Doerr, W.: Pathologie der Lunge, Band I. Springer, Berlin 1983
155. Wagner, R. B., W. O. Crawfort jr., P. P. Schimpf: Classification of parenchymal injuries of the lung. Radiology 167 (1988) 77
156. Webb, W. R., G. Gamsu, D. D. Stark et al.: Magnetic resonance imaging of the normal and abnormal pulmonary hila. Radiology 152 (1984) 89
157. Wells, G. A.: Pulmonary edema and other acute causes of a butterfly pattern in the postoperative chest. Semin. Roentgenol. 23 (1988) 4
158. Westermark, N.: On the roentgen diagnosis of lung embolism. Acta radiol. (Stockh.) 19 (1938) 357–372
159. Woodring, H. H.: Round atelectasis. Radiology 31 (1987) 144
160. World Health Organization Report of an Expert Committee: Definition and diagnosis of pulmonaly disease with special reference to chronic bronchitis and emphysema in chronic cor pulmonale. Wld Hlth Org. Techn. Rep. Ser. 213 (1961) 14–19
161. Wynder, E., J. Moeschinsky, Spivak: Tobacco and alcoholconsumption in relation to the development of multiple primary cancers. Cancer 40 (1977) 1872
162. Yamashita, H.: Roentgenologic Anatomy of the Lung. Thieme, Stuttgart 1978
163. Zerhouni, E. A., F. P. Stitik, S. S. Siegelmann, D. P. Naidich et al.: CT of the pulmonary nodule: cooperative study.
164. Ziter jr., F. M. H., D. N. Bramwit, K. R. Hollomann, P. J. Conte: Calcified Mediastinal Bronchogenic Cysts. Radiology 93 (1969) 1025

Subject Index

A

Abdominal situs inversus 268
Abscess cavity 45, 46
Accessory fissure 14, 16
Acinar-nodose foci 58
Acini, air-containing 37
- fluid-filled 168
Acromion 8
Actinomycosis 71
Adenocarcinoma 126
- central bronchogenic 143
- coal workers' pneuomoconiosis 130
- tracheal 165
Adult respiratory distress syndrome, see ARDS
Aerobacter 31
AIDS, cystic *Pneumocystis carinii* pneumonia 42
- premature emphysema 96
- tuberculosis 49
Air alveologram 37
Air bronchogram 29
- ARDS 192–195
- aspiration pneumonia 37
- bronchoalveolar cell carcinoma 131
- Hodgkin disease 151
- pneumonia with parapneumonic effusion 31
- radiation pneumonitis 86
Air space consolidation 29
Air trapping 102, 164
Alcoholic cardiomyopathy 33
Alveolar microlithiasis 62, 63
Alveolitis 186
Anaplastic thyroid carcinoma, nodular metastases 156
Aneurysm, aortic 246, 248
- - ruptured 248
Angiograms 20
Angle of Louis 9
Anhydrosis 145
Ann Arbor staging of Hodgkin disease 149
Antiprotease deficiency 100
- bullous emphysema 100
α_1-Antitrypsin deficiency 92, 100
- bullous emphysema 100, 101
Aorta, ascending, see ascending aorta
- calcifications 251
- coarctation 258, 261, 262
- dilated 5
- on righthand side 250
- thoracic, see thoracic aorta
- tortuous 4, 30, 102
Aortic arch 2, 3, 7, 13, 18
- calcified 62, 248
- double 249
- radiation fibrosis 88
- right-sided 250
Aortic nipple 13
Aortic-pulmonic window 13, 18
- lymph node enlargement 64
Aortic regurgitation 247, 252, 253
Aortic valve, in MRI 25
Aortic valvular diseases 252
- stenosis 252
ARDS 192–195
- air bronchograms 192–195
- septic shock 195
Arrhythmia 252
Arteriovenous malformation, lung 214
Arthritis, rheumatoid 83
Asbestos-containing dust 122
Asbestos exposure 122, 123
- malignant pleural mesothelioma 233
- pleural calcification 230
- pleural thickening 229
- rounded atelectasis 225
Asbestosis 112, 122, 123
Ascending aorta 3
- dilatation 247
Aschoff's coarse nodules in apices 49
Aspergilloma 71
Aspergillosis 71
- pneumonia 71, 72
Aspergillus 71
Aspiration pneumonia 37
Atelectasis, causes 132
- central bronchogenic carcinoma 126, 132
- cicatrization 61
- lower lobe 46, 136
- lymphangitic carcinomatosis 160
- middle lobe 62, 133
- subsegmental 180
- upper lobe 134, 135, 136, 137, 138
Athletic individual, rib cage configuration 4
Atrial septal defect (ASD) 256, 257
Atrium, left, dilatation 177
- right, double contour 177
Axillary fold 2, 6
Azygoesophageal recess 31
Azygoesophageal stripe 12, 13, 26, 134, 165, 203
Azygos fissure 14–16
- CT scan 15
Azygos vein 15, 16, 19, 30, 147
- in CT 23
- in MRI 25

B

Barrel chest 93–95
Batwing pulmonary edema 174, 175
Bell-shaped chest 4
Berylliosis, multiple calcifications 42
Bifid rib 9
Bilateral pneumonia 38
Blastomyces dermatidis 71
Blebs, intrapleural 96
Blood transfusion, ARDS 192
Bochdalek hernia 270
BOOP 28, 108
Brachial plexus, tumor invasion 145
Breast cancer, chest wall recurrence 278
- lymphangitic carcinomatosis 160, 161, 222
- pleural carcinomatosis 219
- pulmonary metastasis 159
Bronchial atresia, congenital 216
Bronchial carcinoid, bronchus intermedius 164
Bronchiectasis(-es) 60, 104–107
- cylindrical 92, 104, 106
- cystic 104, 107
- saccular 104, 105
- - lower lobe 105
- sarcoidosis 69
- varicose 104
Bronchioles, respiratory 36
- terminal 36, 92
Bronchiolitis, necrotizing 36
- obliterans 103, 108
- - with organizing pneumonia, see BOOP
Bronchitis, chronic 108, 109
- recurrent 208
Bronchoalveolar cell carcinoma 131
Bronchogenic carcinoma 126–148
- adenocarcinoma 126
- apical 145
- asbestosis 122
- atelectasis 132–134
- central 126, 141–144, 148
- - atelectasis 132
- - esophagus involvement 148
- - hilar mass 141–144
- course 137, 138
- esophageal invasion 147, 148
- impaired venous return 147
- large cell 126
- paramediastinal extension 147

Bronchogenic carcinoma, peripheral 126–130
– – upper lobe 129
– phrenic nerve paralysis 268
– pleural carcinomatosis 219
– pneumonectomy 137
– radiotherapy 137, 138
– small cell 126
– squamous cell carcinoma 126
– TNM Classification 126
– WHO classification 126
Bronchogenic cyst(s) 206, 207, 242
– communicating 207
– radiologic features 206
– ring shadows 209, 210
Bronchogenic spread of tuberculosis 58
Bronchography 21, 22
– bronchioectases 104
Broncholithiasis 62
Bronchopleural fistula 224
Bronchopneumonia 28, 36, 39
Bronchus(-i) 21, 22
– intermedius 2
– – bronchial carcinoid 164
– upper lobe, see upper lobe bronchus
Bulla(-ae) 94–98
– subpleural 96
Bullous emphysema, see emphysema, bullous

C

Calcific pericarditis 265
Calcopherites 62
Canals of Lambert 36
Candida albicans 71
Candida pneumonia 73
Candidiasis 73
Carcinoma, bronchoalveolar cell 131
– in situ 126
Cardiac diseases 252–262
Cardiac silhouette, enlarged 168–170, 178, 179
– leftward rotation 5
Cardiomegaly 168–170
Cardiomyopathy, alcoholic 33
Cardiophrenic sulcus, obscured 171
Carditis, with rheumatic fever 254
Carnified lung 44
Carotid artery, in CT 23
– in MRI 24
Cavitary tuberculosis 49, 58
Cavitation, tuberculous 58, 59
Cavity, gas-containing, echinococcal disease 81
Cervical carcinoma, lymphangitic carcinomatosis 158
Cervical rib 9, 238
Check-valve mechanism, pneumothorax 188
Chest, increased sagittal diameter 5
– postoperative 200–203
– tomograms 19
– tube drainge 226
Chest wall 6–9
– diseases of 274–280
– soft-tissue abnormalities 279, 280
– tumor invasion 145
Chickenpox pneumonia 42, 43
– healed 42

Chilaiditi syndrome 268
Chondroma, pulmonary 163
Choriocarcinoma, testicular, pulmonary metastasis 157
Chyle 218
Cicatrization atelectasis 45, 86
Cigarette consumption 126
– emphysema 96
Classification, non-Hodgkin lymphoma 149
Clavicle, companion shadow 2, 4, 7, 8, 278
– sclerosis 275
Clavicular fracture 275
Clubbed finger 259
Coal workers' pneumoconiosis 112
– adenocarcinoma 130
Coarctation of aorta 258, 261, 262
Coccidioides immitis 70
Coccidioidomycosis 78–80
Collagen vascular diseases 83, 84
Colonic loop, intrathoracic location 271
Comet-tail, rounded atelectasis 225
Compensatory hyperexpansion 92
Computed tomograms (CT) 23
– azygos fissure 15
– bronchiectases 104
Congenital bronchial atresia 216
Congenital malformations 205–216
Conglomerate shadow, pneumoconiosis 118, 120
Consolidation, diffuse 39
– infraclavicular 49
– wedge-shaped areas 180
Cor pulmonale, emphysema 92
– fibrous tuberculosis 60
– sarcoidosis, stage IV 70
Coracoid process 2, 6, 8
Corona radiata 127
Coronary sinus 198
Costophrenic sulcus 2, 3
– blunted 93, 229
– – emphysema 93
– obscured 171, 218
– posterior 10
Costotransversal articulation 8
Cowden syndrome 163
Crescent sign, echinococcal disease 81
Cryptococcosis 70, 74
Cryptococcus neoformans 70
Cuffing, peribronchial 168
Cushing syndrome 240
Cyanosis, chronic, emphysema 94, 95
Cyst(s), bronchogenic, see bronchogenic cysts
– dermoid 243
– echinococcal 81
– mediastinal 206, 207
Cystic-adenomatoid malformation 208, 209
Cystic bronchiectasis 45

D

Dermoid cyst 243
Diaphragm 268–272
– anomalies 268–272
– flattening, emphysema 92, 93
– high 4
Diaphragmatic inversion 93
Diastolic murmur 254

Discoid atelectasis 183, 186
Diuretics therapy 172, 172
Double tracks sign, bronchiectases 104
Draining bronchus, tuberculous cavity 59
Dysphagia 242
Dyspnea, emphysema 94, 95
– progressive 120

E

Echinococcal cyst 81
Echinococcal disease 81, 82
Ectasia, annuloaortic 247
Ectocyst 81
Edema, of ankle 171
– pulmonary, see pulmonary edema
– subliminal interstitial 168
Eggshell calcifications, of lymph nodes 120
– pneumoconiosis 112, 113
– silicosis 113
Eggshell pattern, sarcoidosis 69
Eisenmenger reaction 256, 257
Ellis-Damoiseau line 219
Embolism, pulmonary, see pulmonary embolism
Emphysema 92–103
– basiliar 100
– bullous 70, 94–98
– – antiprotease deficiency 100
– – α_1-antitrypsin deficiency 100, 101
– – pleural adhesions 98
– – pneumothorax 94, 97, 98
– – sarcoidosis stage IV 70
– centriacinar 92
– cervical, deep 41
– – spontaneous pneumothorax 280
– cigarette consumption 96
– decreased markings 92
– distal acinar 92
– inceased markings 92
– paracinar 92
– paraseptal 92, 96
– pathological classification 92
– pericicatriceal 60, 92, 102
– pneumoconiosis 118, 120
– senile 92
– subcutaneous 41
– – pneumomediastinum 191
– – posttraumatic 189, 191
– – spontaneous pneumothorax 280
Enchondroma, of rib 276
Endocyst 81
Enophthalmus 145
Erythema nodosum 64
Esophagus, invasion by bronchogenic carcinoma 147, 148
– wall 13

F

Fat embolism syndrome 192
Fat pad, pericardial 10, 11
Fibroma 165
Fibrosis, cystic 108–110
– pulmonary, see pulmonary fibrosis
– radiation, see radiation fibrosis
Fibrous mesothelioma, benign 235
Fibrous postprimary tuberculosis 60, 61

Fissures, interlobar 14–16
– – thickened 168
Fistula, tracheoesophageal 148
Flail chest 190
Fold, axillary, see axillary fold
Foreign bodies, cause of atelectasis 132
Fungal diseases 71–80
Fungi, classification 71
Fungus ball 70, 72

G

Ganglioneurofibroma 244
Ghon focus 49
Glenoid fossa 8
Glomerulonephritis 85, 174
Goiter(s) 238, 239
– diffuse 239
– radionucleide scanning 238, 239
Golden S-sign 141
Gram-negative pneumonia 45
Granuloma, calcified 4, 34
– – primary 50
– eosinophilic 89
– mediastinal 77
– necrotizing 85
Graves disease 240
Ground glass opacification 40, 41
Gynecomastia 128

H

Hamartoma 163
Hampton hump 180
Hand-Schüller-Christian disease 89
Heart, boot-shaped 259
Heart failure, pulmonary edema 173
Hematoma, mediastinal 199
– pleural 190
– – calcified 230
Hemiazygos vein 16, 148
Hemidiaphragm, elevation after pneumonectomy 201
– left 9
– right 3, 9
– traumatic rupture 272
Hemopneumothorax 188, 191
Hemosiderosis 177, 178, 257
Hemothorax 190, 196
– posttraumatic 53
Hempotysis 214
Hiatal hernia 269
Hilar artery, enlargement 180
Hilar lymph node, enlargement 64
Hilar mass, central bronchogenic carcinoma 141–144
Hilar vascular structures 17
– cephalad retraction 60, 61, 102
Histiocytosis X 89, 90
Histoplasma capsulatum 70
Histoplasma pneumonia 75
Histoplasmosis 76, 77
– healed 76
– miliary 76
– multiple calcifications 42
Hodgkin disease, Ann Arbor classification 149
– nodular-sclerosing 151

Hodgkin lymphoma 149–152
– enlarged axillary lymph nodes 278
– enlarged supraclavicular lymph nodes 278
– Rye classification 149
Honeycomb pattern, subpleural 103
Horner syndrome 145, 146
Humeral head 7
Hyalin, in pleural plaques 122
Hydropneumothorax, pleural carcinomatosis 219
– rheumatoid arthritis 228
Hydrothorax, after pneumonectomy 200
Hyperkyphosis, rib cage configuration 5
Hyperelucent lung, Swyer-James syndrome 103
Hyperplasia, thymic 24, 241
Hypertension, arterial, of upper extremities 262
– calcific arteriosclerosis of aorta 251
– left ventricular enlargement 253
– pulmonary arterial 258
– – sarcoidosis stage IV 70
Hypogenetic lung syndrome 214
Hypovolemic shock, ARDS 192

I

ILO, classification of pneumoconiosis 112, 114–117
Immunocompromised host, fungal diseases 71
Industrial disease, asbestosis 122
Infections 27–90
Influenza pneumonia 39
Innominate vein, caudal displacement 147
Inorganic dust inhalation, pneumoconiosis 112
Intercostal spaces, asymmetric narrowing 5
– wide 93
Intercostal vein, left superior 13
Interlobar fissures 14–16
– thickened 168
International Labour Office, see ILO
Interstitial pneumonia 28, 40–42, 83
Intrapulmonary calcifications 62, 63
Intrapulmonary tension pneumothorax 94
Intrathoracic tumors, benign 163
– – doubling time 163
– unusual 163–165
Isthmic stenosis, 261, 262
– aortogram 261

J

Jugular vein, occlusion 147
Junction lines 12, 13

K

Kerley lines 177
– A line 168, 169, 172, 252
– B line 160, 168, 169, 172, 173, 252, 255
Kidneys, intrathoracic position 270
Kommerell diverticulum 250
Kveim test 64
Kymography 253, 257

L

Large cell carcinoma, lymph node involvement 136

Laryngeal tuberculosis 58
Left to right shunt, abnormal venous return 214
– patent ductus arteriosus 258
– septal defects 256
Left ventricular enlargement 253
Left ventricular failure 39, 168–170
– pleural effusion 220
– radiographic signs 168
Leiomyoma, benign metastasizing of uterus 150
– multiple 163
Leukemia, apsergillosis pneumonia 71
Lines, complications of 198
– subclavian 198
Lingula bronchus 19
Lingula, wedge-shaped opacity 182
Lobar pneumonia 28–35
– differential diagnosis 28
Lobe resection 202
Lofgren syndrome 64
Lower lobe, artery, in CT 23
– atelectasis 46
– bronchopneumonia 36
– pneumonia 29, 33
– segmental pulmonary artery 17
– veins 20
– vessels 17, 18
Luetic aortitis 247
Lung abscess(-es) 45–48
– differential diagnosis 45
– pus formation 45
Lung bud, accessory 210
Lung cancer, see bronchogenic carcinoma
Lung contusion, massive, ARDS 192
Lung gangrene 45
Lung lobe, atelectasis 132
Lung malformations 208, 214–216
– cystic-adenomatoid 208
– vascular 214–216
Lung margins 10
Lung parenchyma, cicatrization 60
– destruction 100
– – emphysema 92
Lung volume, decreased, postirradiation 86
– – Swyer-James snydrome 103
Lupus erythematodes 83–85
Lupus pernio 64
Lymph node enlargement, mediastinal 148
– sarcoidosis 64–69
Lymph node involvement, large cell carcinoma 136
– squamous cell carcinoma 133
Lymph node metastases, paratracheal 140
– pretracheal 141
– retrotracheal 140
Lymphadenitis, regional 49
– symptomatic 49
Lymphangioma 242, 243
– cystic 243
Lymphangitic carcinomatosis 160–162
– breast cancer 222
– cervical carcinoma 158
– pleural effusion 222
– primary tumor 160
Lymphangitis 49
Lymphoblastic lymphoma 154
– involving rib 277

M

Mach band 6, 10
Magnetic resonance imaging, see MRI
Main bronchus 19
– in CT 23
– in MRI 24
Major fissure 14
Malformations, vascular, of lung 214–216
Malignant lymphoma 149–155
– Ann Arbor staging 149
Mammoplasty, with silicon implants 279
Manubrium sterni 6, 9
Marfan syndrome 247
Maxillary sinusitis 85
Mediastinal cysts 242
Mediastinal shift, contralateral 164
Mediastinum 23–26, 238–265
– contour abnormalities, thoracic aorta changes 246
– contralateral shift 103, 188
– CT 23
– diplacement in pneumothorax 188
– herniation 106
– MRI 24–26
– obliteration, bronchogenic carcinoma 147
– paratracheal, widening, small cell carcinoma 140
– widening 238, 242
– – non-Hodgin lymphoma 154
– – T-cell lymphoma 154
Meiosis 145
Melting iceberg sign of Woesner 183
Meniscus sign, pleural effusion 218
Mesothelioma, benign fibrous 235
– malignant, asbestosis 122
Metastasis(-es), adrenal, small cell carcinoma 139
– nodular 156
– of rib 277
– therapy 158
Metastatic disease 156–162
Middle lobe, pneumonia 33
Miliary nodules, multiple 43
Miliary tuberculosis 49, 51–53
Minor fissure 14
Mitral regurgitation 254, 255
Mitral stenosis 177–180, 254, 255
– combined with regurgitation 255
– radiographic signs 177
Mitral valve disease 179, 254, 255
– stenosis 168
Monocle sign 17
Morbus Roger 256
Morgagni hernia 270, 271
MRI, coronal, mediastinum 25
– – Pancoast tumor 145
– sagittal, mediastinum 25
– tranverse 24, 26
Mucor 70
Mucormycosis 74
Mucus pus, cause of atelectasis 132
Multiple sclerosis 46
Muscle, sternocleidomastoid, see sternocleidomastoid muscle
Myasthenia gravis 240
Mycobacterium tuberculosis 49
Mycoplasma pneumonia 40

Mycosis, see fungal diseases
Myocardial infarction 174

N

Necrotizing bronchiolitis 36
Necrotizing pneumonia 45–48
– middle lobe, with abscess formation 47, 48
– upper lobe 48
Nephrectomy 158
Neuralgia, segmental 244
Neurinoma 164, 244
Neuroblastoma 244
Neurofibromaosis, cause of scoliosis 276
Nipple, aortic 13
– shadow 9
Nocardiosis 70
Nocturia 173
Nodular metastasis 156
Non-Hodgkin lymphoma 149, 153–155
– chemotherapy 154
– classification 149
– pericardial effusion 263
– rib involvement 277
Nucleus pulposus, calcified 9

O

Oleothorax 231, 232
Oligemia 180
Opacity(-ies), confluent, radiation pneumonitis 86
– – tuberculous pneumonia 54
– elliptical, interfissural effusions 220
– ground glass 40, 41
– irregular, pneumoconiosis 116, 117
– large, pneumoconiosis 118, 119
– linear from hilus 152
– linear and reticular 83–85
– micronodular, miliary tuberculosis 51–53
– miliary pattern, bronchitis obliterans 108
– – sarcoidosis 67
– near complete, Pancoast tumor 145
– nodular, Hodgkion disease 152
– oblique, linear, scarlike, radiation pneumonitis 86
– perihilar 173
– reticular, miliary tuberculosis 51–53
– reticulonodular 40
– reticulonodular, diffuse 63, 69
– – histiocytosis X 90
– round, pneumoconiosis 114
– streaky 39, 44
– tubular, paracardial 215
– wedge-shaped, lingula 182
Orthopnea 171, 172
Osteoarthrosis, posttraumatic 275
Osteoporotic patient, rib cage configuration
Ostium primum, ASD 256
Ostium secundum, ASD 256, 257
Overweight individual, rib cage configuration

P

Pacemaker battery 279
Paget's disease 275
Pancoast syndrome 145, 146
Pancoast tumor 145, 146

– destruction of vertebral bodies 145
– radiologic features 145
– shoulder/arm pain 145, 146
Pancreatic carcinoma, lymphangitis carcinomatosis 160
Papillary muscle, in MRI 25
Papilloma, squamous cell 163
Papillomatosis, tracheal 165
Parapneumonic effusion 31
Paraspinal line 12
Parotis 64
Patchy consolidation, lower lung 36
Patent ductus arteriosus 258
Pectoral veins 148
Pectus excavatum deformity 5
Pedal edema 173
Pedicle 6, 8
– superior vascular 15
Pellets, in chest wall 279
Pericardial cyst 264, 265
Pericardial disease 262–265
Pericardial effusions, collagen vascular diseases 83
– non-Hodgkin lymphoma 263
Pericarditis, calcific 265
Pericyst 81
Pleura 10–13
– apical 10
– calcification 113, 123
– interfaces 10
– parietal 10
– visceral 10
Pleural adhesions, bullous emphysema 98
Pleural calcification, asbestos exposure 230
Pleural caps 61
– apical 229
Pleural carcinomatosis, breast cancer 219
– bronchogenic carcinoma 219
Pleural diseases 218–235
Pleural effusion(-s) 33, 46, 218–224
– basiliar, posttraumatic 189
– bilateral 218
– biventricular failure 171
– collagen vascular disease 83
– exudative 218
– heart failure 173–175
– intrafissural collection of fluid 220
– left ventricular failure 168, 220
– loculated 220
– lymphangitic carcinomatosis 222
– malignant mesothelioma 234, 235
– parapneumonic 219
– pulmonary edema 174
– subpulmonic 220
– transudative 218
– tuberculous 49, 53
Pleural fibrosis, visceral 61
Pleural hematoma 190
– calcified 230
– loculated 223
Pleural mesothelioma, malignant 233–235
– – pleural effusion 234
Pleural peel 229, 230
– calcified 60
– emphysema 102
Pleural plaques, asbestosis 122, 123
– calcified 230
– hyalin containing 122

Subject Index

Pleural scarring, basilar 229
Pleural tail 127
– squamous cell carcinoma 128
Pleural thickening 229, 230
Plombage 231, 232
Pneumatocele(-s) 42
– traumatic 196
Pneumoconiosis 111–124
– classification, radiologic 112
– coal workers' 112
– conglomerate shadow 118
– irregular opacities 116, 117
– large opacities 118, 119
– round opacities, classification 114
– – profusion 114
– – size 114
– – types 114, 115
Pneumocystis carinii 70
– pneumonia 41
Pneumomediastinum 41, 191, 280
Pneumonectomy 200
– bronchogenic carcinoma 137, 138
– postoperative status 200
Pneumonia 28–48
– abscess formation 28
– air space 28–35
– anterobasal segment of lower lobe 33
– aspergillosis 71, 72
– aspiration 37
– bilateral 38
– Candida 73
– chickenpox 42, 43
– – healed 42
– chronic organizing 44
– Gram-negative 45
– Histoplasma 75
– interstitial 28, 40–42, 83
– lower lobe 29, 33
– lung segment involved 28
– middle lobe 33
– necrotizing 45–48
– – middle lobe, with abscess formation 47, 48
– – upper lobe 48
– with parapneumonic effusion 31, 32
4*Pneumocystis carinii* 41
– recurrent 210
– segmental consolidations 28
– – recurrent 28
– tuberculous 54, 55, 58
– – progressive 55
– upper lobe 31–35
– varicella 42, 43
Pneumoperitoneum 199, 268
Pneumothorax, bullous emphysema 94, 97, 98
– chest tube drainage 97
– after insertion of central venous line 199
– mediastinum displacement 188
– spontaneous, *see* spontaneous pneumothorax
– therapeutic 231
– traumatic 188–199
Polyserositis 83
Popcorn calcification 163
Pores of Cohn 28
Postoperative chest 200–203
Poststenotic pneumonia with necrosis 45

PPD, *see* purified protein derivative
– test 64
Primary tuberculous complex 49, 50
– calcified 50
Prostate carcinoma, lymphangitis carcinomatosis 160
Proteinuria 85
Pseudomonas aeruginosa 30, 108
Ptosis 145
Pulmonary artery(-ies) 2, 3, 17–19
– angiogram 20
– in CT 23
– dilated 5, 108, 120, 254–258
– – sarcoidosis stage IV 70
– in MRI 24
– occlusion in upper lobe 181
– prominent 5
Pulmonary calcifications 62
Pulmonary contusion 196, 197
Pulmonary edema 168, 173–176
– batwing type 174, 175
– heart failure 173
– high altitude 176
– interstitial 168, 169, 173–175
– – radiographic signs 168
– reexpansion 223
Pulmonary embolism 180–185
– radiographic signs 180
– streptokinase 184
– transcatheter fibrinolytic therapy 184
– ventilation-perfusion scanning 180
Pulmonary fibrosis, asbestosis 122
– collagen vascular diseases 83
– idiopathic 103
– progressive massive 112, 118
– reactive 122
– sarcoidosis, stage III 69
Pulmonary hemorrhage, Wegener granulomatosis 85
Pulmonary herniation 230
Pulmonary hypertension 258
– emphysema 92
– sarcoidosis stage IV 70
Pulmonary infact 180, 182, 183
Pulmonary leiomyosarcoma, pneumonectomy 210
Pulmonary markings, abnormal, emphysema 94
Pulmonary nodule(-s), aspergilloma 72
– benign tumor 163
– multiple 46
– peripheral lung cancer 126, 128
– postirradiation 87
– solitary, tuberculoma 56, 57
– Wegener granulomatosis 85
Pulmonary perfusion, wedge-shaped defect 180, 181
Pulmonary sequestration 210–213
– connection to esophagus 210
– extralobar 210, 212
– intralobar 210, 211, 213
Pulmonary tuberculosis 49–61
– classification 49
– oleothorax 231
– thoracoplasty 231
Pulmonary vascular congestion 168–179
– chronic 177
– mitral stenosis 177

Pulmonary vascular flow, cephalization 39, 169–171, 177, 254
Pulmonary veins 17
Pulmonary vessels 3, 17–20
– central, dilatated 168, 177
– decrease in number 60
– dilated 177
– – emphysema 92
– displacement, tuberculosis 60
– radiation damage 86
Purified protein derivative (PPD) test 54, 55
Pus formation, lung abscess 45
Pyelonephritis 194

R

Radiation fibrosis 86–88
– paramediastinal 88
Radiation pneumonitis 86–88
Ranke complex 49
Reflux esophagitis 83
Relaxation atelectasis 226
Renal cell carcinoma, pulmonary metastasis 158
– rib metastases 277
Renal failure 174
Respiratory failure, acute 188
Retrocardiac space, encroachment 254
– narrowing 178, 179
Retrosternal space, encroachment 254
Rheumatic fever 252, 254
– with carditis 254
Rheumatoid arthritis, chronic hydropneumothorax 228
Rheumatoid nodules 84, 85
Rib, bifid 9
– cervical 9
– enchondroma 276
– osteolytic destruction 146, 277
Rib cage configurations 4, 5
– athletic individual 4
– osteoporotic patient 4
– overweight individual 4
Rib destruction, Pancoast tumor 145, 146
Rib fractures, multiple, hemopneumothorax 191
– – pneumomediastinum 191
– – segmental 190
– – traumatic pneumatocele 196
– – pneumothorax 188, 189
Rib resection 276
Right ventricular hypertrophy 256
Ring shadows, bronchogenic cysts 209, 210
Rounded atelectasis 225
– comet-tail 225
Rye classification, Hodgkin lymphoma 149

S

Sarcoidosis 64–70
– stage I 64, 65
– stage II 67–68
– stage III 69
– stage IV 70
Scapula, lateral border 2, 8
– medial border 2, 6
– spine of 8
Scar formation, tuberculosis 60, 61
Schede thoracoplasty 232

Schwannoma 244
Scimitar syndrome 215
Scleroderma 83
Sclerosis, of clavicle 275
Scoliosis 274
– deformed thorax 274
– due to neurofibromatosis 276
– rib cage configuration 5
– thoracogenic 60
Secondary lobules, inflammation 36
Segmental bronchus 19
Segmental consolidation, Wegener granulomatosis 85
Segmental pneumonia 30
Sepsis 192
– staphylococcal, ARDS 194
– tuberculosa Landouzy 49
Septal defects 256, 257
Septic embolization 45, 46
Septic shock, ARDS 195
Shaggy heart 122
Shock lung 192
– posttraumatic 192
Shoulder region 8
Shoulder/arm pain, Pancoast tumor 145, 146
Silicosis 112, 113, 120, 121
– course of disease 120, 121
– eggshell calcifications 113
– multiple calcifications 42
Simon's apical foci 49
Sinus venosus, ASD 256
Skinfold 7
Small cell carcinoma 139, 140
– adrenal metastases 139
– chemotherapy 139
Spinal canal, tumor invasion 145
Spine of scapula 8
Splenic flexure 2
Spontaneous pneumothorax 89, 226, 227
– cervical emphysema 280
– subcutaneous emphysema 280
Sporothrix schenckii 70
Sporotrichosis 74
Squamous cell carcinoma 126, 133–136
– bronchogenic 142
– central 142, 143, 144
– lymph node involvement 133
– peripheral 129
– postobstructive pneumonia 135
Sternoclavicular joint 8
Sternocleidomastoid muscle 2, 4, 7
Sternum, body of 9
Stokes collar 147
Stomach bubble 9, 10
Stomach carcinoma, lymphangitis carcinomatosis 160
Streptokinase, pulmonary embolism 184
Stridor 242
Stripe, azygoesophageal 12, 13, 29, 165
– paraspinal 12
Subclavian artery(-ies), in CT 23
– in MRI 24
Subclavian puncture 199
Subclavian veins, collateral circulation 148
– in CT 23

– in MRI 24, 25
– occlusion 147
Subcutaneous emphysema, pneumomediastinum 191
– posttraumatic 189, 191
– spontaneous pneumothorax 280
Subcutaneous pouch, infected, pacemaker battery 279
Subpleural edema 172
Superior sulcus tumor 145
Surfactant factor, discoid atelectasis 186
Swyer-James syndrome 103
– hyperlucent lung 103
Sympathetic trunk, tumor invasion 145

T

T-cell lymphoma 154
Tension pneumothorax 188, 223, 226
Tetralogy of Fallot 258–261
Thoracic aorta 246–251
– descending 2
– dilatation 246
– elongation 246
Thoracic spine, lower 8
– upper 8
Thoracic veins, internal 147
Thoracoplasty 231
Thorax, deformed, scoliosis 274
– overview 2, 3
Thymic hyperplasia 240, 241
Thymic involution 240
Thymoma 240, 241
Thymus, replacement by fat 240
Thyroid gland, calcified nodular adenoma 238
– cold nodule 239
– enlarged 238
– suppressed 239
Trachea 3, 18, 19
– narrowing, caused by goiter 238
Tracheal stenosis, after tracheostomy 200
Tracheobronchial cartilages, calcification 62
Tracheostomy 200
Tracheostomy tube 198
Tram tracks sign, bronchiectases 104
Transcatheter fibronolytic therapy, pulmonary embolism 184
Transverse colon, retrosternal location 270
Trauma 187–203
Traumatic pneumatocele 196
Traumatic pneumothorax 188–190
– check-valve mechanism 188
Tuberculin (PPD) test 54, 55
Tuberculoma 58, 59
– granulomatous form 56, 57
– solitary pulmonary nodule 56, 57
Tuberculosis 49–61
– bronchogenic spread 58
– cavitary 49
– cavitation 58, 59
– fibrous postprimary 60, 61
– hematogemous dissemination 49
– laryngeal 58
– miliary 49, 51–53

– multiple calcifications 42
– pleural peel 230
– postprimary 39, 49, 102
– primary 49
– scar formation 60
Tuberculous cavity 59,
– draining bronchus 59
Tuberculous granuloma, calcified 57
Tuberculous pleurisy 49, 50
Tuberculous pneumonia 54, 55, 58
– progressive 55
Tumor volume, doubling time 127, 128

U

Upper lobe, cavitary tuberculous pneumonia 50
– occlusion of pulmonary artery 181
– oligemia 180
– pneumonia 31–35
– solitary pulmonary nodule 56, 57
Upper lobe bronchus 3
– in CT 23
Upper lobe vessels 17, 19
– distended 39
Uveitis 64
Uveoparotid fever of Heerfordt 64

V

Vanishing lung 100
Vanishing tumor 220
Varicella pneumonia 42, 43
Vascular malformations, of lung 214–216
Vasculitis, collagen vascular diseases 83
– Wegener granulomatosis 85
Vena cava, in CT 23
– inferior 18, 93, 99, 203
– in MRI 24
– superior, left jugular line 199
– – obstruction 147, 148
– – – by bronchogenic carcinoma 147
Venous confluence 19
Venous return, impaired 147
Venous valves 198
Ventricular septal defect (VSD) 256, 258
Ventilation-perfusion mismatch, emphysema 92
Ventilation-perfusion scan, pulmonary embolism 180
Ventricular aneurysm 253
– calcified 253
Vertebral bodies, destruction, Pancoast tumor 145
Vineyard sprayer's lung disease 124

W

Waterlily sign 81
Weber-Rendu-Osler disease 214
Wegener granulomatosis 85
– pulmonary hemorrhage 85
– pulmonary nodules 85
– segmental consolidation 85
– vasculitis 85
Westermark sign 180